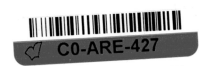

Drug Therapy in Pregnancy

Third Edition

Drug Therapy in Pregnancy
Third Edition

Editors

Jerome Yankowitz, M.D.

Associate Professor
Director, Division of Maternal-Fetal Medicine
and Fetal Diagnosis and Therapy Unit
Department of Obstetrics and Gynecology
The University of Iowa Hospital and Clinics
Iowa City, Iowa

Jennifer R. Niebyl, M.D.

Professor and Chair
Department of Obstetrics and Gynecology
The University of Iowa Hospital and Clinics
Iowa City, Iowa

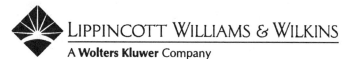

LIPPINCOTT WILLIAMS & WILKINS
A **Wolters Kluwer** Company
Philadelphia • Baltimore • New York • London
Buenos Aires • Hong Kong • Sydney • Tokyo

Acquisitions Editor: Lisa McAllister
Developmental Editor: Raymond E. Reter
Production Editor: Jeff Somers
Manufacturing Manager: Benjamin Rivera
Cover Designer: Patricia Gast
Compositor: The PRD Group
Printer: Maple Press

© **2001 by LIPPINCOTT WILLIAMS & WILKINS**
530 Walnut Street
Philadelphia, PA 19106 USA
LWW.com

Previous edition published by Lea and Febiger as "Drug Use in Pregnancy, Second Edition."

Printed in the USA

Library of Congress Cataloging-in-Publication Data
Drug therapy in pregnancy / editors, Jerome Yankowitz, Jennifer Niebyl.—3rd ed.
　　p. ; cm.
　　Rev. ed. of: Drug use in pregnancy / [edited by] Jennifer R. Niebyl. 2nd ed. 1988.
　　Includes bibliographical references and index.
　　ISBN 0-683-30708-8 (alk. paper)
　　　1. Obstetrical pharmacology.　2. Fetus—Effect of drugs on.　I. Yankowitz, Jerome.
　　II. Niebyl, Jennifer R.　III. Drug use in pregnancy.
　　　[DNLM: 1. Drug Therapy—methods—Pregnancy.　2. Fetus—drug effects.
　　3. Pharmaceutical Preparations—administration & dosage—Pregnancy.　4. Substance-Related
　　Disorders—Pregnancy. WQ 200 D79375 2001]
RG528 .D78　2001
618.2′061—dc21　　　　　　　　　　　　　　　　　　　　00-052016

Care has been taken to confirm the accuracy of the information presented and to describe generally accepted practices. However, the editors, authors, and publisher are not responsible for errors or omissions or for any consequences from application of the information in this book and make no warranty, expressed or implied, with respect to the currency, completeness, or accuracy of the contents of the publication. Application of this information in a particular situation remains the professional responsibility of the practitioner.

The editors, authors, and publisher have exerted every effort to ensure that drug selection and dosage set forth in this text are in accordance with current recommendations and practice at the time of publication. However, in view of ongoing research, changes in government regulations, and the constant flow of information relating to drug therapy and drug reactions, the reader is urged to check the package insert for each drug for any change in indications and dosage and for added warnings and precautions. This is particularly important when the recommended agent is a new or infrequently employed drug.

Some drugs and medical devices presented in this publication have Food and Drug Administration (FDA) clearance for limited use in restricted research settings. It is the responsibility of the health care provider to ascertain the FDA status of each drug or device planned for use in their clinical practice.

10　9　8　7　6　5　4　3　2　1

This book is dedicated to our spouses, Diana Kawai Yankowitz and Allan Poots; and to our children, Hana Brit Yankowitz and Peter Robinson Niebyl.

Contents

Contributing Authors

Alexander D. Allaire, M.D., M.S.P.H. *Staff Physician, Department of Obstetrics and Gynecology, National Capitol Uniformed Services, National Naval Medical Center, Bethesda, Maryland*

Robert H. Ball, M.D. *Departments of Obstetrics and Gynecology, University of Utah Health Sciences Center, 50 N. Medical Drive Salt Lake City, Utah*

George Bergus, M.D. *Department of Family Medicine, University of Iowa Hospital Center, Iowa City, Iowa*

Gail Best, M.D. *Fellow, Maternal/Fetal Medicine, Department of Obstetrics and Gynecology, University of Rochester, Strong Memorial Hospital, Rochester, New York*

John W. Ely, M.D., M.S.P.H. *Associate Professor, Department of Family Medicine, University of Iowa, Iowa City, Iowa*

Martin Fielder, M.D. *University of North Carolina at Chapel Hill, Chapel Hill, North Carolina*

Melissa H. Fries, M.D., F.A.C.O.G. *Program Director, OB/GYN Residency, 81 MSGS/SGCG, Keesler Medical Center, Keesler Air Force Base, Mississippi*

Alfredo F. Gei, M.D. *Department of Obstetrics and Gynecology, The University of Texas Medical Branch at Galveston, Galveston, Texas*

James D. Goldberg, M.D. *Director, Reproductive Genetics Unit, Department of Obstetrics, Gynecology and Reproductive Sciences, University of California, San Francisco, San Francisco, California*

Jeffrey A. Kuller, M.D. *Associate Professor, Department of Obstetrics and Gynecology, University of North Carolina at Chapel Hill, Chapel Hill, North Carolina*

Clayton E. Littell, R.Ph, B.C.P.S. *Assistant Professor, School Adjunct of Pharmacy, Washington State University Sacred Heart Medical Center, Spokane, Washington*

Michael J. McMahon, M.D., M.P.H. *Assistant Professor, Department of Obstetrics and Gynecology, University of North Carolina School of Medicine, Chapel Hill, North Carolina*

Jennifer R. Niebyl, M.D. *Professor and Chair, Department of Obstetrics and Gynecology, The University of Iowa Hospital and Clinics, Iowa City, Iowa*

Mary E. Norton, M.D. *Assistant Professor, Department of Obstetrics, Gynecology and Reproductive Services, University of California, San Francisco, San Francisco, California*

Errol R. Norwitz, M.D., Ph.D. *Department of Obstetrics and Gynecology, Brigham and Women's Hospital, Harvard Medical School, Boston, Massachusetts*

Gayle L. Olson, M.D. *Assistant Professor, Department of Obstetrics and Gynecology, The University of Texas Medical Branch at Galveston, Galveston, Texas*

Stephen D. Ratcliffe, M.D., M.S.P.H.   *Division Chief and Program Director of Family Practice, Department of Family and Preventive Medicine, University of Utah, Salt Lake City, Utah*

William F. Rayburn, M.D.   *Professor and Chair, Department of Obstetrics & Gynecology, The University of New Mexico Health Sciences Center, Albuquerque, New Mexico*

John T. Repke, M.D.   *Department of Obstetrics and Gynecology, Brigham and Women's Hospital, Harvard Medical School, Boston, Massachusetts*

Asha Rijhsinghani, M.D.   *Associate Professor, Department of Obstetrics and Gynecology, University of Iowa Hospitals and Clinics, Iowa City, Iowa*

Julian N. Robinson, M.D., Ph.D.   *Department of Obstetrics and Gynecology, Brigham and Women's Hospital, Harvard Medical School, Boston, Massachusetts*

George R. Saade, M.D.   *Professor, Department of Obstetrics and Gynecology, The University of Texas Medical Branch at Galveston, Galveston, Texas*

Ellen Louise Sakornbut, M.D.   *Acting Chair, Department of Family Medicine, University of Tennessee–Memphis, Memphis, Tennessee*

Lori L. Schoonover, Pharm.D, B.C.P.S.   *Scientific Manager, U.S. Medical and Regulatory Affairs, Aventis Pharmaceuticals, Spokane, Washington*

Mark S. Shahin, M.D.   *Fellow, Division of Gynecologic Oncology, Department of Obstetrics and Gynecology, University of Iowa Hospitals and Clinics, Iowa City, Iowa*

Stephen D. Silberstein, M.D.   *Professor of Neurology, Department of Medicine, Thomas Jefferson University, Philadelphia, Pennsylvania*

Joel I. Sorosky, M.D.   *Professor, Department of Obstetrics and Gynecology, University of Iowa Hospitals and Clinics, Iowa City, Iowa*

Laura A. Tavernier, M.D., M.Ed.   *Assistant Professor, Department of Family Medicine, University of Tennessee–Memphis, Covington, Tennessee*

John M. Thorp, Jr., M.D.   *Associate Professor, Department of Obstetrics and Gynecology, University of North Carolina School of Medicine, Chapel Hill, North Carolina*

James R. Woods, Jr., M.D.   *Professor and Associate Chair, Department of Obstetrics and Gynecology, University of Rochester, Strong Memorial Hospital, Rochester, New York*

Michele Wylen, M.D.   *Assistant Professor, Department of Obstetrics and Gynecology, Georgetown University, Washington, D.C.*

Jerome Yankowitz, M.D.   *Associate Professor, Director, Division of Maternal Fetal Medicine and Fetal Diagnosis and Therapy, Department of Obstetrics & Gynecology, University of Iowa Hospitals and Clinics, Iowa City, Iowa*

Preface

The first edition of this book was published as part of a series edited by Dr. Frederick P. Zuspan, Current Concepts in Obstetrics and Gynecology, published by Lea & Febiger. The second edition was published in 1988, just before Dr. Jennifer Niebyl left Johns Hopkins Hospital to be Head of the Department of Obstetrics and Gynecology at The University of Iowa. Dr. Jerome Yankowitz, Director of the Division of Maternal-Fetal Medicine at the University of Iowa Hospitals and Clinics, joins in editing this third edition.

This book covers the use of therapeutic medications by topic. In contrast to other resources in which one looks up individual drug names, this book describes medical and pharmacological management of disease processes. In this edition we have added several new chapters and markedly revised others. The general principles chapter has been completely rewritten to include the most recent developments in FDA classification. Also, chapters have been added in pharmacokinetics, urinary tract infections, psychotropic drugs, radiologic imaging procedures, poisoning, alternative and complimentary health care, and antiviral drugs. In addition, the panel of authors has been expanded to foster interest by primary care providers as well as sub-specialists. The authors now include not only perinatologists but also family physicians and a pharmacologist. We hope that this book will serve as a useful reference for anyone who provides medical care for the pregnant or breast-feeding woman.

Jerome Yankowitz, MD
Jennifer R. Niebyl, MD

Drug Therapy in Pregnancy

Third Edition

1

Use of Medications in Pregnancy: General Principles, Teratology, and Current Developments

Jerome Yankowitz

Division of Maternal-Fetal Medicine and Fetal Diagnosis and Therapy, Department of Obstetrics and Gynecology, University of Iowa Hospitals and Clinics, Iowa City, Iowa

Pharmacologic treatment in pregnancy is a broad topic and requires an in-depth discussion of a broad array of illnesses, conditions, and patient habits. The first principle of treating a pregnant woman with a disease is to ask what would be the appropriate treatment in the nonpregnant state? The answer to this almost always guides proper management of the pregnant or postpartum woman. Usually, there are several choices for pharmacologic management and for this reason the second principle is to evaluate the relative safety of these choices to the patient and the fetus. This requires a knowledge of teratogenicity and fetal effects. A corollary to these two principles is that the pregnant woman should not expose herself to or be prescribed unnecessary treatments. Each chapter in this book provides specific information about each principle relative to specific conditions or groups of agents. A general background of teratology and a discussion of two recent developments in drug therapy during pregnancy, which are the explosion of personal computer use and the Internet follow, and the potential overhaul of the pregnancy-labeling system for drugs and biologics by the US Food and Drug Administration (FDA).

TERATOLOGY

Derived from the Greek *teras* meaning "monster," teratology is the study of abnormal development or the production of defects in the fetus (1). Birth defects can be due to deformation, disruption, dysplasia, or malformation (2). Although traditionally teratogens were defined as agents that produce a structural defect in an embryo or fetus that was developing normally before exposure to the agent, the definition has been expanded to include agents that cause any deviation from normal morphology or function (1). The latter includes growth restriction and developmental or behavioral abnormalities (3). Scant information was available about teratogenesis before 1950, when most defects were believed to be genetic in origin (3,4).

In the United States, birth defects affect 2%–3% of neonates (2) but account for approximately 20% of infant mortality (1). Exogenous causes of birth defects, including radiation, infections, maternal metabolic disorders, and drugs or environmental and chemical, account for almost 10% of all birth defects and therefore affect only 0.2% to 0.3% of all births. However, it is often necessary to treat a variety of problems during pregnancy, including colds, nausea, urinary tract infections, hypertension, diabetes, epilepsy, and others (5); thus, it is paramount that physicians understand the principles of teratology and be aware of which medications are safe to use.

Criteria to prove that an agent is a human teratogen are:

• Proven exposure at a critical time in prenatal development

- Consistent findings by two or more epidemiologic studies of high quality
- Careful delineation of clinical cases
- Rare environmental exposure associated with a rare defect

Although not absolutely required, proof of teratogenicity ideally includes:

- Teratogenicity in experimental animals
- An association that is biologically plausible
- Experimental proof that the agent acts in an unaltered state (6)

Other concepts related to teratology include specificity, timing, dose, maternal physiology, embryology, and genetics. Specificity indicates that a substance may be teratogenic in some species but not others. For example, thalidomide produces phocomelia in primates but not rodents, and cortisone is a teratogen in rodents but not in humans. It is for this reason that this book contains almost no data from animal studies—such data are too often not applicable to humans. Timing is also critical. When administered between 35 and 37 days, thalidomide produces ear malformations, but between 41 and 44 days, it produces amelia or phocomelia. Dose is also important. In most cases, administration of a low dose will result in no effect, whereas malformations occur at intermediate doses and death at higher doses. Death may cause organ-specific teratogenic action to go unnoticed. The route of administration, possibly secondary to absorption, is also important. Small doses over several days may have an effect different than that of the same total dose given at once. Sequential dosing as opposed to a bolus may induce an enzyme to metabolize the substance, which potentially causes less damage. Constant exposure may destroy cells that would have catabolized the drug if administered in periodic doses. Maternal physiology altered by the pregnant state can affect absorption, distribution, metabolism, and excretion. Placental transfer must also be considered. For example, coumarin derivatives easily cross the placenta and have teratogenic potential, in contrast with the heparins, which are highly charged and do not cross the placenta. As noted for thalidomide, timing of exposure relative to embryologic events is important. Teratogen exposure in the first 2 to 3 weeks after conception is generally thought to have no effect or result in spontaneous loss (all-or-nothing phenomenon). The period of susceptibility to teratogenic agents is during the period of organogenesis, which occurs primarily at 3 to 8 weeks postconception (35 to 70 days after the last menstrual period) or to 10 weeks from the last menstrual period. After this period, embryonic development is characterized primarily by increasing organ size (10 to 12 weeks); thus, the principal effect of exposure will be growth restriction and/or effects on the nervous system and gonadal tissue. These systems continue to develop throughout pregnancy. During organogenesis, each organ system will have different critical periods of sensitivity. A teratogen can act by causing cell death, altering tissue growth (hyperplasia, hypoplasia, or asynchronous growth), or interfering with cellular differentiation or other basic morphogenic processes.

The genotype of the mother and fetus can affect individual susceptibility to an agent. For example, fetuses with low levels of the enzyme epoxide hydrolase are more likely to manifest the fetal hydantoin syndrome than those with normal levels of epoxide hydrolase (7). Combinations of agents may produce different degrees of malformation and/or growth restriction than if given individually. Fetuses whose mothers are on combination antiepileptic agents are at the highest risk for malformations including neural tube defects and facial dysmorphic features.

The FDA introduced a drug classification system in 1979 (8,9), the purpose of which was to discourage nonessential use of medication during pregnancy. Unfortunately, maternal anxiety related to medication use can lead to unnecessary pregnancy terminations. Several characteristics of the FDA drug classification process contribute to public perception of the dangers of medication use during pregnancy. Although only 20 to 30 commonly used drugs are known teratogens, 7% of the more than 1,000 medications listed in the *Physicians' Desk Reference* (PDR) are classified as category X (9,10). Category X indicates that studies in animals or humans or investigational or postmarketing reports have shown fetal risk that clearly outweighs any possible benefit to the patient. The definitions of the

TABLE 1.1. *U.S. Food and Drug Administration drug-risk categories*

Category A	Controlled studies in women fail to demonstrate a risk to the fetus in the first trimester (and there is no evidence of a risk in later trimesters), and the possibility of fetal harm appears remote.
Category B	Either animal reproduction studies have not demonstrated fetal risk but no controlled studies in pregnant women have been reported or animal reproduction studies have shown an adverse effect (other than a decrease in fertility) that was not confirmed in controlled studies in women in the first trimester (and there is no evidence of risk in later trimesters).
Category C	Either studies in animals have revealed adverse effects on the fetus (teratogenic, embryocidal, or other) but no controlled studies in women have been reported or studies in women and animals are not available. Drugs should be given only if the potential benefit justifies the potential risk to the fetus.
Category D	Positive evidence of human fetal risk exists, but the benefits from use in pregnant women may be acceptable despite the risk (e.g., if the drug is needed for a life-threatening condition or for a serious disease for which safer drugs cannot be used or are ineffective).
Category X	Studies in animals or human beings have demonstrated fetal abnormalities, evidence exists of fetal risk based on human experience, or both, and the risk in pregnant women clearly outweighs any possible benefit. The drug is contraindicated in women who are or may become pregnant.

categories are given in Table 1.1. All new medications are classified as category C, leading to an elevated impression of the danger of the medication. The percentages of medications in each category are shown in Table 1.2. The Teratology Society suggests abandoning the FDA classification (9). When counseling patients or responding to queries from physicians, we recommend avoiding the PDR and instead using specific descriptions in teratogen databases to provide accurate information.

Proposed Changes in the Pregnancy-labeling System for Drugs and Biologics by the FDA

In 1994, the Teratology Society Public Affairs Committee recommended that the FDA use-in-pregnancy ratings be deleted from drug labeling and be replaced by narrative statements that summarize and interpret available data regarding hazards of developmental toxicity and provide

TABLE 1.2. *Percentage of drugs in each U.S. Food and Drug Administration risk category as listed in the Physicians' Desk Reference*

Category	Percentage
A: Controlled studies show no risk	0.7
B: No evidence of risk in humans	19
C: Risk cannot be ruled out	66
D: Positive evidence of risk	7
X: Contraindicated in pregnancy	7

estimates of teratogenic risk (9). In 1997, the FDA announced a public meeting to discuss labeling (http://www.fda.gov, search site for "pregnancy" and "labeling"). This public hearing was held in September 1997. There was consensus that the category labeling currently in use is relied on but is probably oversimplified and confusing, does not address the range of clinical situations and the range of effects, and should be replaced with narrative labeling. A concept paper was presented on May 20, 1999 that outlined a model for labeling and included suggested sections titled, "clinical management statement," "summary risk assessment," and "discussion of data"(http://www.fda.gov) for both pregnancy and lactation sections.

It is expected that the FDA will release a series of three drafts starting in the Fall 2000 (FDA, personal communication, 2000) that will outline different aspects of the proposed new labeling format. After a period of public comment and input, this new format will probably be put into use. I agree with this change and have counseled patients without use of the specific categories rather supplying them with a narrative.

Although Sweden also uses a classification system with categories from A to D that was implemented in 1978, their system seems to have resulted in wider physician acceptance (11). This would appear to be owing to differences in the categories in that the FDA system requires an unrealistically high quality of data. The authors compare the distribution of drugs within each category, which differs in the Swedish and FDA systems.

COMPUTER AND INTERNET USE

Several databases are available for personal computer use. The University of Iowa utilizes RE-PROTEXT, REPROTOX, TERIS, and Shepard's Catalog of teratogenic agents (12). These and other databases can be purchased and installed in personal computers (http://www.reprotox.org/, http://depts.washington.edu/terisweb/).

More important in terms of the potential for widespread access by both health care providers and patients are on-line Internet sources. A synopsis of *Drugs in Pregnancy and Lactation* is available on-line (13,14). Other sites include FDA classification and lactation information among a vast array of other data (http://www.rxlist.com/). Links to general teratology services and organizations are also available (15).

Professional organizations also offer drug information including the American Academy of Pediatrics web site, which contains the entire document concerning "The Transfer of Drugs and Other Chemicals Into Human Milk" (16). For the layperson, any drug name and pregnancy can be entered into a search engine such as Dogpile (http://www.dogpile.com) and thousands of sites with information become available. General sites concerning breast-feeding that contain drug information are available (www.breastfeeding.com, www.babyfriendly.org.uk). This will require greater knowledge on the part of health care providers who must understand not only the potential interactions of many drugs during pregnancy and lactation, but who must be savvy in their ability to also use books and on-line resources to gather appropriate information for an individual patient.

SUMMARY

Health care workers should be knowledgeable about the basic principles of teratology. Emphasis should be placed on counseling pregnant or lactating patients based on results of studies or case series and not merely a category designation. This same philosophy is leading to changes in the current FDA classification system. Rapid expansion of computer- or Internet-based information allows health care providers and patients greater access to drug information.

REFERENCES

1. Sever LE, Mortensen ME. Teratology and the epidemiology of birth defects: occupational and environmental perspectives. In: Gabbe SG, Niebyl JR, Simpson JL, eds. *Obstetrics: normal and problem pregnancies,* 3rd ed. New York: Churchill-Livingstone, 1996.
2. Aase JM. *Diagnostic dysmorphology.* New York: Plenum, 1990.
3. Hanson JW. Human teratology. In: Rimoin DL, Connor JM, Pyeritz RE, eds. *Principles and practice of medical genetics,* 3rd ed. New York: Churchill-Livingstone, 1996.
4. Jones KL. Effects of therapeutic, diagnostic, and environmental agents. In: Creasy RK, Resnik R, eds. *Maternal-fetal medicine: principles and practice,* 3rd ed. Philadelphia: WB Saunders, 1994.
5. McMahon MJ, Katz VL. Clinical teratology. In: Kuller JA, Chescheir NC, Cefalo RC, eds. *Prenatal diagnosis and reproductive genetics.* Baltimore: Mosby-Year Book, 1996.
6. Shepard TH. "Proof" of human tertogenicity. *Teratology* 1994;50:97–98.
7. Buehler BA, Delimont D, van Waes M, et al. Prenatal prediction of risk of the fetal hydantoin syndrome. *N Engl J Med* 1990;322:1567–1572.
8. Briggs GG, Freeman RK, Yaffe SJ. *Drugs in pregnancy and lactation,* 4th ed. Baltimore: Williams & Wilkins, 1994.
9. Teratology Society Public Affairs Committee. FDA Classification of drugs for teratogenic risk. *Teratology* 1994;49:446–447.
10. Friedman JM. Report of the Teratology Society Public Affairs Committee Symposium on FDA Classification of Drugs. *Teratology* 1993;48:5–6.
11. Sannerstedt R, Lundborg P, Danielsson BR, et al. Drugs during pregnancy: an issue of risk classification and information to prescribers. *Drug Saf* 1996;14:69–77.
12. Computer Teratology and Reproductive Risk Information Database. MICROMEDEX Inc. 1974–2000 MICROMEDEX(R) Healthcare Series Vol. 105 9/2000.
13. Briggs GG, Freeman RK, Yaffe SJ. *Drugs in pregnancy and lactation,* 5th ed. Baltimore: Williams & Wilkins, 1998.
14. http://prl.humc.edu/obgyn/PUBLIC/TEARATOG/riska-c.HTM
15. http://orpheus.ucsd.edu/otis/links.htm, Organization of teratology information services.
16. American Academy of Pediatrics. The transfer of drugs and other chemicals into human milk. *Pediatrics* 1994;93:137–150. http://www.aap.org/policy/00026.html

2

Pharmacokinetics of Drugs During Pregnancy and Lactation

Lori L. Schoonover* and Clayton E. Littell[†]

*U.S. Medical and Regulatory Affairs, Aventis Pharmaceuticals, Spokane, Washington
[†] School of Pharmacy, Washington State University, Sacred Heart Medical Center, Spokane, Washington

Appropriate dosing of medications during pregnancy can be difficult because there are few pharmacokinetic studies in this population. Recommendations for dose adjustment are readily available for pediatric patients or for those with renal failure, but rarely are recommendations for the adjustment of dosing in pregnancy published. Physiologic changes occur throughout pregnancy that can cause a deviation from the expected pharmacokinetic processes in the nonpregnant patient and necessitate dose adjustments (1–4).

As many as 35% of women report taking at least one drug during pregnancy (2). Women with chronic illnesses, who are stabilized on drug therapy and become pregnant, may have to continue treatment throughout pregnancy to prevent morbidity to themselves and their fetus. Fortunately, the majority of medications are safe to use during pregnancy, and few compounds used in clinical practice today are proven human teratogens (2), including new, innovative pharmacologic therapies for the treatment of asthma, epilepsy, psychiatric disorders, and infection (5,6). Nevertheless, the lack of information on dose adjustment in pregnancy leaves the clinician with incomplete data from which to create a safe, effective dosing regimen.

Women have, in general, been excluded from most drug development studies because of ethical, practical, and liability concerns (7). A recent survey analyzing the gender composition of studies published in two major pharmacology journals from 1969 to 1991 found that only approximately 50% included women (8). Yet, in the majority of studies that included both men and women, the results were grouped together, without providing an analysis of gender differences (8). The US Food and Drug Administration, the National Institutes of Health, and other regulatory agencies have changed their policies in an attempt to create more gender-balanced research in drug therapy (7). A significant lag time is expected until this type of information becomes widely available.

Physiologic changes take place during pregnancy that influence the pharmacokinetic parameters of drug absorption, distribution, metabolism, and elimination. A full understanding of each pharmacokinetic characteristic is important so that appropriate drug therapy can be provided during pregnancy. Information on specific drugs that have undergone pharmacokinetic study during pregnancy is helpful; however, for many medications, data are not available and clinicians must individualize care.

PHARMACOKINETICS

Pharmacokinetics describes the absorption, distribution, metabolism, and excretion of a drug and its metabolites in the body (1). These principles, along with the dosage of medication, determine the amount of active drug that will be present at the site of action and the degree of its effect (1). Variability in the pharmacokinetics of a compound can be seen between individuals. Identical doses of a drug can produce large differences in pharmacologic response between individuals and in patient populations, such as those with renal disease, congestive heart failure, or pregnancy (9). Understanding the basic principles of pharmacokinetics and the variability that can exist in the pregnant population is essential to optimize drug therapy, while limiting toxicity to the mother and fetus.

Drug Absorption

Drug absorption into the bloodstream can be achieved through numerous pathways, including the gastrointestinal tract, skin, lungs, and muscles, or the drug can be directly administered by the intravenous route. The bioavailability of a drug defines its rate and extent of absorption. Factors that can affect the ability of a drug to reach the systemic circulation include the drug formulation; simultaneous administration with food or other drugs; chemical composition; metabolism by gut bacteria, mucosa, or the liver (first-pass elimination); gastric emptying time; intestinal motility; and blood flow to the target organ (10).

Gastrointestinal Absorption

Increased progesterone production, occurring maximally in the third trimester of pregnancy, is thought to decrease intestinal motility and contribute to the 30% to 50% increase in gastric emptying time seen during pregnancy (3). As a result, the absorption and onset of drug response may be delayed, as has been shown for acetaminophen use in late pregnancy (11,12). If a quick, reliable drug response is desired, intravenous administration may be the preferred route of delivery, particularly for acute analgesic therapy.

An additional consequence of prolonged gastric emptying and reduced intestinal motility is an increase in drug dissolution time, which could lead to an increase in the absorption of poorly water-soluble drugs, as has been shown with digoxin (13). Conversely, increased exposure to metabolism by gut bacteria or mucosa can result in a decrease in bioavailability for some drugs, like chlorpromazine (14).

Other causes of reduced gastrointestinal drug absorption during pregnancy include the concurrent use of medications, like sucralfate or antacids and nutritional supplements (e.g., calcium, iron, and vitamins) that can bind and inactivate some drugs (4). Nausea and vomiting occur frequently during pregnancy and can affect drug absorption (10).

Lung Absorption

During pregnancy, both cardiac output and respiratory minute volume increase by approximately 50%, which leads to an increase in the alveolar uptake and systemic absorption of drugs given through the lungs (14). Dose requirements for inhalational anesthetic agents, like halothane and isoflurane, decrease in the pregnant population (15). This effect could occur with any inhaled medication.

Transdermal, Subcutaneous, and Intramuscular Absorption

Skin perfusion is significantly increased during pregnancy due to an increase in cardiac output, potentially altering absorption of drugs across the skin. This is likely the major cause of enhanced absorption of lipophilic drugs given transdermally (16). Also, because of an increase in total body water, there is increased extravascular water and skin hydration. By increasing the water content of the skin, an increase in the rate and extent of transdermal absorption of iontophoretically administered, water-soluble drugs might be seen in pregnancy (16). Lidocaine is an example of a moderately water-soluble drug that could be given transdermally during pregnancy for topical anesthesia (6). An increase in transdermal absorption and steady-state concentration of this drug could occur; however, the effects would more than likely be diminished by the observed increase in volume of distribution and rate of elimination (9). This topic remains theoretical as no concrete data currently exist.

In general, the intramuscular absorption of drugs is more rapid and complete than after subcutaneous administration because of greater blood flow (1). In view of the recognized changes in hemodynamics during pregnancy, drugs given intramuscularly may result in enhanced systemic absorption and a faster onset of action. An exception in late pregnancy is that blood flow to the lower extremities is reduced; therefore, the absorption of intramuscular injections at this site may be decreased (14).

Drug Distribution

The next step after drug absorption is the transfer or distribution of drugs from plasma into extravascular fluids and tissues. The volume of distribution (Vd) of a drug is defined as the volume it would occupy if the concentration throughout the body were equal to that in plasma (4). The extent to which a drug distributes is a function of its lipid solubility, tissue affinity, and plasma protein-binding characteristics (1). Drugs with significant lipid solubility and/or tissue affinity tend to have Vds that are large (e.g., bupropion) (3). The opposite usually holds true for drugs with low lipid solubility and high plasma protein-binding (e.g., omeprazole) (3). It is currently accepted that a drug is considered to be in its pharmacologically active form when it is "free" and not bound to proteins in the plasma (1). Variations in body weight, total body water, plasma volume, plasma protein concentration, and protein-binding affinity can significantly change the concentration of drug available at the site of action and thus its effect (1).

The Vd of drugs is often increased during pregnancy because the plasma volume is expanded by 50% (10). Mean total body water is also increased by 8 L, 60% of which belongs to the fetus, amniotic fluid, and placenta (17). Drugs that distribute predominantly to water and have a low Vd (e.g., cephalosporins) will exhibit the greatest reduction in drug plasma concentration (4). Lipophilic drugs (e.g., amiodarone) are already extensively distributed throughout the body and tend to be affected minimally by this change (16). In the application of pharmacokinetics, an increased Vd of a drug leads to an increased half-life unless there is an off-setting increase in clearance by metabolism or excretion. The relationship of these kinetic parameters is described with the following equation: half-life = (volume of distribution × 0.693)/clearance (3).

Body fat increases by 3 to 4 kg during pregnancy and may act as a reservoir for lipophilic drugs (4). Drugs with lipophilic properties (e.g., ondansetron or fentanyl) may need to be initially dosed on kilograms of total body weight to achieve therapeutic concentrations at the site of action. The extra fat stores that develop in pregnancy are mobilized during labor and delivery, as evidenced by an increase in serum lipid levels observed during this time (18). Long-term use of a lipophilic drug can lead to accumulation and prolonged effects even after the drug has been discontinued.

Protein Binding

By the third trimester of pregnancy, plasma albumin concentrations are reduced by approximately 1 g/dL because of the dilutional effect caused by the increased plasma volume (18). In addition, plasma concentrations of free fatty acids and steroid hormones, which compete against drugs for albumin binding sites, are increased late in pregnancy (19). The net result of these interactions may be an increased unbound or free fraction of drug available to cause pharmacologic effects. Drugs that are highly protein bound to albumin, such as most anticonvulsants and serotonin reuptake inhibitors, may be displaced and lead to an increased effect. Conversely, some studies have shown that unbound drugs are more susceptible to accelerated clearance by the kidney and liver, actually leading to lower drug levels and effects (20). Table 2.1 lists drugs that are significantly bound to albumin (5).

In comparison to albumin, concentrations and binding characteristics of α_1-acid glycoprotein, which bind most basic drugs (e.g., opioid analgesics, tricyclic antidepressants, and beta blockers), are not significantly altered during pregnancy (21).

Fetal-Maternal Distribution

The placenta, amniotic fluid, and fetus (i.e., the products of conception) comprise a complex organ to which drugs can distribute, undergo metabolism, and return to the maternal circulation or accumulate in fetal tissues. The

TABLE 2.1. *Drugs used in pregnancy with significant protein binding to albumin*

Amiodarone (Cordarone)
Bupropion (Zyban/Wellbutrin)
Buspirone (BusPar)
Cetirizine (Zyrtec)
Cisapride (Propulsid)
Doxepin (Sinequan)
Fluoxetine (Prozac)
Fluvoxamine (Luvox)
Gemfibrozil (Lopid)
Haloperidol (Haldol)
Hydralazine (Apresoline)
Indinavir (Crixivan)
Lansoprazole (Prevacid)
Loratadine (Claritin)
Mirtazapine (Remeron)
Nefazodone (Serzone)
Nifedipine (Procardia)
Olanzapine (Zyprexa)
Omeprazole (Prilosec)
Ondansetron (Zofran)
Paroxetine (Paxil)
Phenytoin (Dilantin)
Propafenone (Rythmol)
Risperidone (Risperdal)
Ritonavir (Norvir)
Sertraline (Zoloft)
Tiagabine (Gabitril)
Trazodone (Desyrel)
Valproic Acid (Depakote)
Venlafaxine (Effexor)
Zafirlukast (Accolate)
Zileuton (Zyflo)
Zolpidem (Ambien)

Drugs listed here are >75% bound to albumin. Dose adjustment is not necessarily recommended (5).

fetoplacental unit increases body water by 4 to 5 L and will act as a compartment for any drug that has the ability to cross the placenta (14). Characteristics of drugs that allow penetration to the placenta include high lipid solubility, low molecular size, low protein binding, and low ionization (1). Transplacental transfer of drugs increases during the third trimester because of increased maternal and placental blood flow, decreased placental thickness, and a resultant increase in surface area of the placenta. Because of a more acidic fetal circulation, "ion trapping" of basic drugs (e.g., meperidine or propranolol) may produce drug concentrations in the fetus that exceed those in the maternal circulation (2). *In vitro* and *in vivo* pharmacokinetic models for placental transfer have been created in an attempt to understand better drug penetration and handling by the fetoplacental unit (20). A true grasp of this complex concept has yet to be reached, however, for most drugs that are used long enough to achieve fetal-maternal steady state, fetal blood concentrations tend to be 50% to 100% of maternal blood concentrations (22).

Fetal Protein Binding

Fundamentally, drugs cannot cross the placenta when bound to proteins. Although once they penetrate this barrier, they are free to bind to the proteins that exist in fetal plasma (4). Fetal plasma proteins have been shown to bind several drugs (e.g., diazepam and propranolol), some with higher affinity than that bound in maternal plasma (23). Whereas maternal plasma albumin concentrations gradually decrease throughout pregnancy, fetal albumin concentrations progressively increase to approximately 20% greater than the corresponding maternal concentration (24). It has been shown that plasma protein binding alters the total concentration of drugs between the maternal and fetal plasma; however, the free concentrations of drugs do not differ as a result of this effect (22). Importantly, drug exposure to the fetus depends on the free concentration of drug (1).

Unlike albumin, there is a significant decrease in fetal α_1-acid glycoprotein concentration. Changes in the amount of unbound basic drugs like propranolol, meperidine, and amitriptyline could occur (21). To minimize toxicity to the fetus, discontinuation of drugs such as propranolol a few days before delivery is recommended so that levels in the newborn can decline (25). Meperidine, however, is usually only administered on a short-term basis during labor and delivery. No dose adjustment is recommended, but close observation for neonatal toxicity (i.e., respiratory depression) is the standard of care (24).

Drug Elimination

Metabolism

The metabolism of drugs primarily occurs in the liver. Lipophilic drugs must be converted in the liver to a more water-soluble form to be renally eliminated. Drugs that are hydrophilic are eliminated primarily by the kidney. The clearance of medications by the liver depends not only on liver enzyme activity but also on liver blood flow, and the plasma concentration of the unbound drug (1). High extraction drugs (e.g., lidocaine, meperidine, and metoprolol) are mainly dependent on liver blood flow for their metabolic clearance and usually undergo a significant first-pass effect (24). Low extraction drugs (e.g., phenytoin, theophylline, and fluoxetine) depend primarily on liver enzyme activity for their systemic clearance (1). There are several drug-metabolizing enzymes present in the liver that increase drug hydrophilicity. The majority of drugs undergoing biotransformation are either oxidized, reduced, hydrolyzed, or conjugated (i.e., phase I or II reactions); however, the most clinically important metabolic pathway is oxidation involving the P-450 enzyme system (3). It was demonstrated that a multitude of endogenous and exogenous substances can affect the ability of this enzyme system to metabolize drugs including nicotine, ethanol, estrogen, and progesterone (4). A detailed evaluation of the mechanism of the P-450 enzyme system and factors affecting its function is beyond the scope of this chapter but was recently reviewed elsewhere (26).

Despite an increase in cardiac output and plasma volume, liver blood flow has been shown to remain normal during pregnancy, which means that the elimination rate of high extraction drugs (e.g., lidocaine) is relatively unchanged (27).

Hepatic enzyme activity has been found to be altered during pregnancy leading to changes in the metabolism of drugs (28). Progressive fluctuations in estrogen and progesterone concentrations throughout pregnancy are presumed to be responsible for this modification (29). Estrogen may competitively inhibit enzyme activity leading to drug accumulation (4). High levels of progesterone may inhibit some enzymes of the P-450 system (e.g., CYP1A2) leading to decreased hepatic elimination of drugs like theophylline, caffeine, and zileuton (10,29). Conversely, the activity of other P-450 enzymes (e.g., CYP3A4 and CYP2C9) may be increased by progesterone, leading to an increase in hepatic elimination of drugs like phenytoin or sertraline (29). Table 2.2 lists drugs that are significantly metabolized by the P-450 enzyme system (5,10,20,21).

TABLE 2.2. *Drugs used in pregnancy that undergo significant liver metabolism*

Amiodarone (Cordarone)
Amitriptyline (Elavil)
Carbamazepine (Tegretol)[a]
Carisoprodol (Soma)
Cisapride (Propulsid)
Clarithromycin (Biaxin)
Clomipramine (Anafranil)
Clozapine (Clozaril)
Desipramine (Norpramin)
Erythromycin (Ery-Tab)
Fexofenadine (Allegra)
Fentanyl (Sublimaze)
Fluoxetine (Prozac)
Fluvoxamine (Luvox)
Haloperidol (Haldol)
Hydrocodone (in Lortab)
Imipramine (Tofranil)[a]
Indinavir (Crixivan)
Lansoprazole (Prevacid)
Loratadine (Claritin)
Maprotiline (Ludiomil)
Metoprolol (Lopressor)[a]
Nefazodone (Serzone)
Nifedipine (Procardia/Adalat)
Nortriptyline (Pamelor)[a]
Olanzapine (Zyprexa)[b]
Omeprazole (Prilosec)
Oxycodone (in Percocet)
Paroxetine (Paxil)
Perphenazine (Trilafon)
Phenytoin (Dilantin)[a]
Propafenone (Rhythmol)
Propranolol (Inderal)
Risperidone (Risperdal)
Ritonavir (Norvir)
Saquinavir (Invirase)
Sertraline (Zoloft)
Theophylline (Theo-Dur)[b]
Thioridazine (Mellaril)
Tramadol (Ultram)
Trazodone (Desyrel)
Venlafaxine (Effexor)
Verapamil (Calan)
Zileuton (Zyflo)[b]
Zolpidem (Ambien)

Drugs listed here are metabolized by the P-450 isozyme system. Dose adjustment is not necessarily recommended for all patients (5,10).
[a]Small studies have demonstrated increased drug clearance.
[b]Metabolized by the P-450 CYP1A2 isozyme.

Placental and Fetal Metabolism

The placenta not only acts as a physical barrier to drugs but has a complement of cytochrome P-450 system enzymes with the ability to metabolize drugs (27). It contains approximately half the level of enzymes as adult liver (4). The placenta also contains other enzymes, such as catechol-O-methyl transferase and monoamine oxidase, which are thought to impede the ability of endogenous compounds to cross the placenta and enter the fetal circulation (4). The effect that all these enzymes have on fetomaternal pharmacokinetics is poorly understood but probably plays a minor role in the biotransformation of drugs compared with the role of the adult liver (30).

All enzymatic processes including phase I and II metabolism have been shown to exist in the fetal liver as early as 7 to 8 weeks postconception (31). The degree of metabolizing activity of these enzymes, as well as their ability to be induced, is low relative to adult liver enzymes (4). Overall, the fetus relies heavily on the maternal system for the clearance of drugs (31). Yet, fetal metabolism could produce water-soluble metabolites that possess pharmacologic activity and are unable to readily diffuse back into the maternal circulation (10). This can lead to drug accumulation in the fetus and potential toxicity. Studies on the use of meperidine in pregnancy showed that the half-life of its neurotoxic metabolite normeperidine is prolonged in the neonate and may contribute to toxicity (32).

Renal Clearance

The kidney is the most important organ for elimination of drugs and their metabolites. Renal excretion of drugs involves three processes: glomerular filtration, active tubular secretion, and passive reabsorption (1). Water-soluble drugs tend to be eliminated by filtration. The rate of filtration of a drug depends on the volume of fluid that is filtered in the glomerulus and the unbound concentration of drug in plasma, because protein bound drugs are not filtered. Lipid-soluble drugs are not readily eliminated by the kidney and are generally reabsorbed. Protein-bound drugs may be eliminated by active tubular secretion. The clearance of drugs excreted unchanged is directly proportional to creatinine clearance, allowing the prediction of drug elimination by the kidney (1). Overall, the clearance of drugs by the kidney is influenced by blood flow, protein binding, and the number of functioning nephrons.

Renal blood flow increases by 80% during early pregnancy but returns to normal during the third trimester (33). The glomerular filtration rate increases as high as 50% throughout pregnancy (33). Creatinine clearance, which closely reflects the glomerular filtration rate, increases to a maximum at 34 weeks (4). The result of these changes may lead to an increase in clearance of renally excreted drugs, such as β-lactam antibiotics, aminoglycosides, digoxin, and lithium. Table 2.3 lists drugs that are significantly renally eliminated (5,34,35).

TABLE 2.3. *Drugs used in pregnancy with significant renal clearance*

Acyclovir (Zovirax)
Amoxicillin (generic)
Ampicillin (generic)[a]
Atenolol (Tenormin)
Bupropion (Zyban/Wellbutrin)[a]
Cefazolin (Kefzol)[a]
Cefixime (Suprax)
Cefotaxime (Claforan)
Cefprozil (Cefzil)
Ceftazidime (Fortaz)
Ceftibuten (Cedax)
Cefuroxime (Zinacef/Ceftin)
Cephalexin (Keflex)
Cetirizine (Zyrtec)
Digoxin (Lanoxin)[a]
Famciclovir (Famvir)
Fluconazole (Diflucan)
Gabapentin (Neurontin)
Gentamicin (generic)[b]
Levofloxacin (Levaquin)
LMWt Heparin (Lovenox)
Lithium (Lithobid)[a]
Loracarbef (Lorabid)
Nitrofurantoin (Macrodantin)
Penicillin (Pen-Vee K)
Procainamide (Procanbid)[c]
Pseudoephedrine (Sudafed)
Ranitidine (Zantac)
Sotalol (Betapace)[c]
Tobramycin (generic)[b]
Topiramate (Topamax)
Trimethoprim/sulfamethoxazole (Bactrim/Septra)[b]
Valacyclovir (Valtrex)

Drugs listed here are cleared predominantly by the kidney. Dose adjustment is not necessarily recommended (5,20,34,35).
[a]Small studies have shown increased clearance in pregnancy.
[b]Small studies have shown no change in clearance in pregnancy.
[c]Metabolites of clinical significance cleared by kidney.
LMWt, low molecular weight.

TABLE 2.4. *Potential changes of pharmacokinetic parameters of drugs in pregnancy*

Absorption	↑/↓
Onset of action	↓
Duration of action	↑/↓
Volume of distribution	↑
Protein binding	↓
Hepatic metabolism	↑
Renal excretion	↑

↑, increased; ↓, decreased.
From Schoonover LL, Littell CE. How pregnancy affects pharmacokinetics. *The Female Patient* 1998; 16:13–24, with permission.

SUMMARY

Pregnancy causes a multitude of physiologic alterations that lead to differences in the way medications are pharmacokinetically handled in the body. These alterations lead to changes in drug absorption, volume of distribution, protein binding, and clearance (Table 2.4). Most of these changes have been identified; however, their clinical significance still remains to be determined, especially with new therapies. If the basic concepts of these changes are realized, along with data on the disposition of drugs that have been studied and show variance in the pregnant population, one might be able to cautiously extrapolate this information to other medications with similar disposition characteristics to individualize more prudently drug therapy during pregnancy.

Specific Medications

Physiologic changes that occur during pregnancy are variable over the 9 months. In general, the most pronounced pharmacokinetic changes are during the third trimester. Table 2.5 lists the medications that would most likely have clinically important pharmacokinetic changes occur during pregnancy (9). It is important for clinicians to evaluate the clinical effects of these medications as reasons for making dose alterations.

Antibiotics

Antimicrobials are among the most commonly used medications during pregnancy and delivery. Data are available on several specific antimicrobial agents. The primary effect of pregnancy

TABLE 2.5. *Medications potentially requiring dosage adjustment during pregnancy*

Drug	Serum conc.	PB alteration	Vd	Cl	$t_{1/2}$	Ref.
Antibiotics						
Aminoglycosides	↓	N	↑			34
Ampicillin	↓	N	↑	↑	↓	34
Cefazolin	↓	N	↑	↑	↓	34
Antiepileptics						
Carbamazepine		N		↑	↓	28, 45
Phenobarbital		N		↑	↓	28, 45
Phenytoin	↓	Y	↑	↑	↓	28, 45
Primidone		N		↑		28, 45
Valproic acid	↓	Y	↑	↑	↓	3, 45
Antihypertensives						
Metoprolol	↓	N		↑		3
Sotalol	↓	N		↑	↓	51
Psychiatric therapy						
Lithium	↓	N		↑	↓	3
Tricyclic antidepressants	↓					62
Miscellaneous						
Theophylline	↑	N			↑	46

conc., concentration; PB, protein binding; Vd, volume of distribution; Cl, Clearance; $t_{1/2}$, half-life; Ref., reference; N, no; Y, yes; ↑, increased; ↓, decreased.
Reprinted by permission of the publisher from Schoonover LL, Littell CE. How Pregnancy Affects Pharmacokinetics. The Female Patient, vol 23, pp 22, copyright 1998, by Quadrant Healthcom, Inc.

on the penicillins and cephalosporins is an increase in renal clearance, although the increased volume of distribution also causes a decrease in serum concentrations (3). The profound increase in glomerular filtration rate is likely the primary reason for the accelerated clearance of these compounds. Ampicillin is estimated to produce serum concentrations that are approximately 50% of those seen in nonpregnant women (34). Penicillin, piperacillin, cefazolin, and imipenem concentrations are similarly affected (34–37). Ceftriaxone serum concentrations during the third trimester have been shown to be similar to those in nonpregnant control subjects (38). Ceftriaxone uses both renal and hepatic pathways for elimination, which may explain some of the differences with this antibiotic relative to the majority of other drugs in this category (38).

Gentamicin, tobramycin, and amikacin serum concentrations are reduced during pregnancy, possibly because of the increased volume of distribution (34). Standard recommendations are to monitor serum drug concentrations when these medications are used for more than 48 hours. Pregnant women may require higher aminoglycoside doses to achieve therapeutic serum levels. Therapeutic serum concentrations for selected medications used during pregnancy are provided in Table 2.6 (39). The concept of extended interval dosing of aminoglycosides has recently been proposed (40). This approach to therapy has not been studied in pregnant women but is effective for postpartum therapy.

Vancomycin pharmacokinetics was reported in one patient who was treated for chorioam-nionitis at 26 weeks' gestation (41). There was an increase in the volume of distribution and the total plasma clearance for this patient, whereas the half-life of the drug was unchanged. Serum vancomycin concentrations should be monitored during therapy and maintained within the acceptable therapeutic range (Table 2.6).

The wide interpatient variation of serum erythromycin concentrations have made studies of this compound inconclusive. No data are available regarding the newer generation macrolides azithromycin and clarithromycin in this patient population. These drugs primarily reside intracellularly and therefore serum concentrations are very low (42). The serum concentrations of trimethoprim, sulfamethoxazole, and clindamycin are not significantly affected in pregnancy (34). Information on pharmacokinetic alterations with metronidazole during pregnancy has not been published.

Anticonvulsants

Women with epilepsy are typically continued on anticonvulsant therapy during pregnancy. Although some believe that phenobarbital and carbamazepine may have lower teratogenic potential compared with phenytoin (43,44), the most effective agent for the individual patient should be used. The pharmacokinetics of phenytoin are complex, regardless of the patient population being treated. When phenytoin is used during pregnancy, it has been shown to have an increased clearance, resulting in lower serum concentrations and potentially less effective seizure control. This change is greatest in the second and

TABLE 2.6. *Selected therapeutic serum drug concentrations*

Drug name	Therapeutic concentration
Carbamazepine	4–12 μg/mL
Digoxin	0.8–2 ng/mL
Gentamicin[a]	Peak, 4–8 μg/mL; trough, <2 μg/mL
Lithium	0.6–0.8 mEq/L
Phenytoin	10–20 μg/mL
Free phenytoin	1–2 μg/mL
Theophylline	5–20 μg/mL
Valproic acid	50–100 μg/mL
Vancomycin	peak, <40–50 μg/mL; trough, 5–10 μg/mL

[a]Values for tobramycin are the same. Values obtained from ref. 39.

third trimesters. Altered phenytoin absorption during pregnancy may also contribute to the reduced levels (45). Additionally, plasma protein binding of phenytoin is diminished secondary to the decline in albumin concentration during pregnancy (45). Phenytoin displays great interpatient pharmacokinetic variability. This is particularly problematic because the levels at which toxicity develops are very close to the levels needed to prevent seizures. Monitoring serum concentrations can be useful. Obtaining a free phenytoin level may be therapeutically helpful in determining appropriate dosing needs (Table 2.6).

Carbamazepine clearance is accelerated in pregnancy, potentially resulting in lower serum levels or greater fluctuation in levels (45). Other data suggest that the active epoxide metabolite of carbamazepine may be increased during pregnancy (10). Studies that considered the increase in body weight during pregnancy showed no significant difference in carbamazepine clearance; however, there was considerable variation among the small number of patients studied (45). Because of this variability, serum concentrations can be monitored (Table 2.6).

Valproic acid serum concentrations commonly decline during pregnancy, most notably in the third trimester. Without dose alterations, plasma concentrations reportedly declined from 100 to 150 μg/mL in the first trimester to 30 to 50 μg/mL in the third trimester (45). An increased volume of distribution and hepatic clearance of valproic acid explain these reductions in serum concentrations. There may also be decreased gastric absorption of the drug (45). If valproic acid is used, maternal serum α-fetoprotein and targeted ultrasound should be offered to the patient because of the concern over neural tube defects in the fetus.

Asthma Therapy

Antiinflammatory agents are now considered primary therapy for asthma. Most patients can be controlled with inhaled steroids and beta-agonists; however, some patients with severe asthma may require theophylline. Theophylline serum concentrations can be elevated during pregnancy. Unfortunately, theophylline has a narrow therapeutic index and toxicity can occur at levels close to the high end of the therapeutic range. Carter et al. (46) published a study of eight patients who received theophylline during pregnancy. Serum drug concentrations were obtained on three separate occasions during gestation and once postpartum. Theophylline clearance was statistically significantly reduced during pregnancy. Three of these patients had theophylline concentrations exceeding 20 μg/mL. A reduction in dose and close monitoring of serum concentrations are recommended in patients who must continue taking theophylline during pregnancy.

Also, because of the potential for increased lung absorption during pregnancy, one may see increased toxicity from inhaled agents used in asthma treatment. If an increase in systemic absorption occurs while using beta-agonist inhalation treatment (i.e., albuterol) in a pregnant asthmatic patient, tachycardia may occur, requiring a dose reduction (17).

Cardiovascular Agents

Patients with chronic hypertension typically require continued therapy during gestation. Diastolic blood pressure greater than 100 mm Hg should be treated during pregnancy (47).

Beta blockers are the most extensively studied class of medications. Serum concentrations of propranolol, labetalol, and atenolol are not clinically significantly different in pregnant women (48–50). However, lowered serum concentrations during pregnancy have been demonstrated with metoprolol. Increased hepatic clearance is speculated as the reason for the reduction in serum levels (48). A cross-over study of six women given sotalol found reduced concentrations of this compound during gestation (51). Angotensin-converting enzyme inhibitors have serious effects on the fetal kidneys and should not be used after the first trimester (see Chapter 9).

The pharmacokinetics of digoxin during pregnancy are poorly understood. The determination of any changes in pharmacokinetics is made more difficult because endogenous compounds, similar in structure to digoxin, are produced by the fetus and placenta. These digoxin-like substances interact with the radioimmunoassay used to determine digoxin concentrations (48). In addition, there is poor correlation between digoxin serum concentrations and therapeutic efficacy or toxicity. Patients requiring therapy with digoxin during gestation should be closely observed for responses to therapy and signs of toxicity.

Teratogenesis from the use of coumadin makes heparin the drug of choice for treatment and prevention of thromboembolic disorders during pregnancy (43). One study of six women at 24 to 30 weeks' gestation and six nonpregnant controls reported significant reductions in heparin levels and little change in activated partial thromboplastin time (aPTT) in the pregnant subjects. Patients were given a single dose of heparin 143 U/kg (10,000 U for a 70-kg patient). Peak plasma heparin concentrations were 0.11 U/mL in the pregnant subjects and 0.23 U/mL in the nonpregnant individuals. The aPTT did not change from baseline for the pregnant subjects but reached a mean of 50 seconds in the control subjects (52). The use of aPTT to monitor the therapeutic response to heparin may be altered owing to physiologic changes induced by pregnancy. Monitoring heparin levels directly has been suggested as an alternative, although not all clinical laboratories are equipped to do this testing. Heparin levels of 0.05 to 0.2 U/mL obtained at the middle of the dosing interval have been suggested to be therapeutic (52–54). The pharmacokinetics of dalteparin, a low molecular weight heparin, has been reported for patients in the third trimester of pregnancy. The study lacked a control population. When compared with previously published data in nonpregnant individuals, reduced activity of dalteparin, as measured by anti-factor Xa activity, was reported (55). Decreased absorption of subcutaneously administered drugs late in pregnancy could have contributed to this effect.

Human Immunodeficiency Virus Therapies

It has been shown that zidovudine treatment in pregnant women infected with the human immunodeficiency virus (HIV) reduces the rate of transmission to the fetus (56). It is now recognized that combination therapy for the treatment of acquired immunodeficiency syndrome (AIDS) is necessary to adequately control the virus (57). Generally, zidovudine is used for prevention of mother-to-fetus transmission of the virus in women with CD4 cell counts greater than 500 cells/mm^3 and low viral loads. In the pregnant woman with a CD4 cell count less than 500 cells/mm^3, usual combination therapy for AIDS should be employed (57). There are conflicting data regarding zidovudine pharmacokinetics. It was reported to have unchanged pharmacokinetics during pregnancy, whereas other investigators demonstrated more rapid clearance rates and a reduced area under the concentration-time curve (58–60). Lamivudine (3TC) has been reported to produce pharmacokinetic parameters during pregnancy that are similar to those that occur in nonpregnant patients (61). Human data regarding pharmacokinetics of the other antiretroviral agents administered during the gestational period have not been reported. HIV-1 RNA levels should be monitored and therapy adjusted to achieve the lowest possible viral load.

Psychiatric Therapies

It may be necessary to continue therapy for clinical depression during pregnancy. Although the teratogenic potential of these agents must be taken into account, if the decision to employ medical therapy for depression is made, appropriate dosing should be used. Data are limited to one uncontrolled study that based the study outcomes on control of only the most notable depressive symptom. Eight women with severe recurrent major depression treated with tricyclic antidepressants (six treated with nortriptyline, one with clomipramine, and one with imipramine) were studied. The mean increase in dose required to control symptoms in these patients was 1.6 times the initial dose. Steady-state serum concentrations in the women showed that, despite an increase in dose, individual serum concentrations were lower (62). This small uncontrolled observation suggests that patients should be closely monitored for reduced efficacy of antidepressant therapy.

The clearance of lithium is also increased during pregnancy as a result of the considerable increase in renal clearance. In patients with severe bipolar disorder, maintenance of lithium therapy during pregnancy may be needed despite the possible association with congenital heart disease (2). An increased dose of lithium will likely be required during pregnancy. Serum levels should be obtained to guide dosing changes (Table 2.6). Renal clearance rapidly returns to prepregnancy levels after parturition; therefore, it is recommended that the lithium dose be reduced to the prepregnancy dose at the start of labor (3).

DRUG THERAPY DURING LACTATION

There is a vast array of conditions that affect the concentrations of medications in breast milk. The maternal pharmacokinetics, as reviewed, affects the serum concentration of the medication. Blood flow to the breast, pH of the plasma and breast milk, mammary tissue composition, breast-milk composition, and the rate of breast-milk production are all physiologic variables that affect the amount of drugs delivered to the infant through breast milk. There are also several characteristics of the medication itself that play an important role. These include lipid solubility, molecular weight, degree of ionization in the plasma and breast milk, and the extent to which the drug is protein bound (63). The chemical characteristics of drugs that are most likely to pass into breast milk are lipid solubility, low protein binding, and being a weak base (10). Most drugs enter breast milk by passive diffusion; therefore, as the concentration in the breast milk increases and the plasma concentration declines, movement of the drug from the breast milk back into the plasma could occur (63).

The milk-to-plasma ratio for a drug is often used to describe the potential exposure of the infant to medications in the breast milk (10,63). Several issues must be considered when interpreting this number. Many reports come from a single drug measurement. Time from drug administration to sampling, dose, and length of lactation is information that is often not provided. Additionally, the infant's ability to metabolize and eliminate the drug must also factor into the equation. The potential adverse effects and the expected overall length of exposure are also

important considerations in determining whether a woman should breast-feed her infant while taking medications (10,63).

The American Academy of Pediatrics lists the following medications as contraindicated during breast-feeding: bromocriptine, cyclophosphamide, cyclosporin, doxorubicin, ergotamine, lithium, methotrexate, and radioactive isotopes (10,64). This list of medications only serves as a guide. It is necessary to weigh the benefits of treatment of the mother with the potential risks to the fetus from exposure to the drug relative to the importance of breast-feeding.

Antibiotics

Most antibiotics are excreted into breast milk in low concentrations. Development of an allergic reaction, altering the bowel flora so as to induce diarrhea or candidiasis, or interference with culture results, if the child requires such tests, are theoretical concerns that are probably of less importance than the benefits of breast-feeding (63,65). Special consideration may be needed for some agents. It is generally considered reasonable to continue breast-feeding while taking sulfonamides; however, in premature infants with hyperbilirubinemia or glucose-6-phosphate deficiency, it should be avoided (63,65). Diarrhea was reported in a breast-fed infant whose mother was taking metronidazole (65). Treatment of trichomoniasis requires only single dose therapy, so in that instance it is recommended that the mother discontinue breast-feeding for 12 to 24 hours to allow clearance of the drug (64). Chloramphenicol, even in low concentrations in breast milk, should be avoided because of the potential for idiosyncratic bone marrow suppression (64).

Anticonvulsants

Because of low concentrations found in breast milk, phenytoin, carbamazepine, and valproic acid are considered compatible with breast-feeding (10,63). Phenobarbital clearance is reduced in young infants; therefore, the potential for accumulation exists. For mothers requiring therapy with phenobarbital or the related compound primidone, infants should be monitored for symptoms of sedation and phenobarbital serum concentrations (10). Ethosuximide similarly accumulates (10).

Asthma Therapies

Only a small amount (1% of maternal serum concentrations) of theophylline appears in breast milk (63). It is unlikely to be problematic; however, if signs of irritability, hyperactivity, or excessive wakefulness occur in the infant of a woman taking theophylline who is breast-feeding, theophylline may be the culprit (63). No data exist, but it is unlikely that the serum concentrations of the inhaled products used in asthma, such as inhaled steroids or beta-agonists, would achieve sufficiently high serum levels as to contribute to breast-milk composition.

Cardiovascular Agents

For the treatment of hypertension, beta blockers, captopril, enalapril, and calcium channel blockers are considered compatible with breast-feeding (63,64). Atenolol, acebutolol, nadolol, and sotalol are weak bases or have low protein binding relative to the other beta blockers, therefore breast-milk concentrations are higher (10,48). Verapamil achieves lower breast-milk levels compared with nifedipine (63).

Digoxin is highly protein bound and has low milk-to-plasma ratios of 0.6 to 0.9. It is considered compatible with breast-feeding (63,64). The diuretics chlorothiazide, furosemide, and spironolactone are excreted in only small amounts in breast milk, so infant exposure is minimal (63). Diuretics may decrease breast milk production, which should be considered and discussed if they are to be prescribed for the nursing mother.

Amiodarone and its major metabolite desethylamiodarone accumulate in breast milk. There is the potential to induce hyperthyroidism or hypothyroidism in the nursing infant owing to the iodine moieties incorporated in the molecular structure of the drug (66).

Heparin has a large molecular weight and coumadin is highly protein bound, so neither of these anticoagulants passes into breast milk to any great degree (63). During gestation, coumadin is contraindicated, and heparin therapy is used. After parturition, the nursing mother could be switched over to coumadin without major concerns for the infant.

HIV Therapies

The risk of vertical transmission of HIV virus from breast-feeding precludes this practice for HIV-positive women (56). Therefore, the amount of these drugs present in the breast milk is inconsequential.

Psychiatric Therapies

Treatment of depression may be necessary postpartum. The tricyclic antidepressants nortriptyline, amitriptyline, and desipramine have been shown not to accumulate in breast milk (67). Comparable maternal and infant serum concentration of the N-desmethyldoxepin metabolite of doxepin have been reported (67–69).

Fluoxetine and norfluoxetine are excreted into breast milk. It is estimated that the infant receives approximately 11% of the maternal dose of the medication (70). The prolonged elimination half-life of fluoxetine and its metabolite means that interruption of breast-feeding would be of little benefit. Sertraline and desmethylsertraline are also detectable in breast milk. Four of 11 infants studied had detectable serum sertraline concentrations, whereas nine of 11 were found to have desmethylsertraline present (71).

The American Academy of Pediatrics classifies amitriptyline, desipramine, doxepin, fluoxetine, imipramine, trazodone, and fluvoxamine as drugs whose effect on nursing infants is unknown but may be of concern (64). Other authors suggested that in nursing mothers amitriptyline, nortriptyline, desipramine, clomipramine, and sertraline are the agents of choice for the treatment of depression in this setting (67).

For the treatment of mood disorders, valproic acid and carbamazepine are considered compatible with nursing, whereas lithium is contraindicated (64). Low concentrations of haloperidol, chlorpromazine, and the benzodiazpines lorazepam and diazepam have been found in breast milk (63). These drugs are classified as having unknown effects on the nursing infant but may be of concern (64).

CONCLUSION

The β-lactam antibiotics, aminoglycosides, lithium, and most anticonvulsants, in general, produce lower serum concentrations in women who are pregnant. Other compounds, such as theophylline, may have decreased drug clearance resulting in increased serum concentrations during the gestational period.

Many medications are excreted into breast milk; however, concentrations are generally low and infant exposure minimal. A small number of medications are contraindicated in women planning to breast-feed (64). The benefits of breast-feeding are numerous. In most instances, the mother who wishes to breast-feed can do so, after the clinician considers the specific medications involved, identifies alternatives that may produce lower breast-milk concentrations, evaluates the infant's ability to eliminate the medications, and discusses with the parent a plan for monitoring the infant if needed.

Because of the issues related to studying pregnant women, there are few concrete data on dosing guidelines or pharmacokinetic changes for most medications. This leaves the clinician with monitoring the patient's clinical response to make decisions regarding dose adjustments. General knowledge of the changes in pharmacokinetic parameters seen during pregnancy and specific information on some of the medications that are most affected can help the clinician make more informed decisions and better anticipate patient response.

REFERENCES

1. Gibaldi M. *Biopharmaceutics and clinical pharmacokinetics,* 4th ed. Philadelphia: Lea & Febiger, 1990.
2. Murray L, Seger D. Drug therapy during pregnancy and lactation. *Emerg Med Clin North Am* 1994;12:129–149.
3. Mucklow JC. The fate of drugs in pregnancy. *Clin Obstet Gynecol* 1986;13:161–175.
4. Reynolds F, Knott C. Pharmacokinetics in pregnancy and placental drug transfer. *Oxf Rev Reprod Biol* 1989;11:389–449.
5. Briggs GG, Freeman RK, Yaffe SJ. *Drugs in pregnancy and lactation. A reference guide to fetal and neonatal risk,* 5th ed. Baltimore: Williams & Wilkins, 1999.
6. Koren G, Pastuszak A, Ito S. Drugs in Pregnancy. *N Eng J Med* 1998;338:1128–1137.
7. Berg MJ. Status of research on gender differences. *J Am Pharm Assoc (Wash)* 1997;NS37:43–56.
8. Schumucker DL, Vessell ES. Under-representation of women in clinical drug trials. *Clin Pharmacol Ther* 1993;54:11–15.
9. Schoonover LL, Littell CE. How pregnancy affects pharmacokinetics. *Female Patient* 1998;23:13–24.
10. Loebstein R, Lalkin A, Koren G. Pharmacokinetic changes during pregnancy and their clinical relevance. *Clin Pharmacokinet* 1997;33:328–343.
11. Simpson KH, Stakes AF, Miller M. Pregnancy delays paracetamol absorption and gastric emptying in patients undergoing surgery. *Br J Anaesth* 1988;60:24.
12. Nimmo WS, Wilson J, Prescott LF. Naracotic analgesics and delayed gastric emptying during labour. *Lancet* 1975;1:890–893.
13. Luxford AM, Kellaway GS. Pharmacokinetics of digoxin in pregnancy. *Eur J Clin Pharmacol* 1983;25:117–121.
14. Jeffries WS, Bochner F. The effect of pregnancy on drug pharmacokinetics. *Med J Aust* 1988;149:675–677.
15. Palahniuk RJ, Shnider SM, Eger EL. Pregnancy decreases the requirement for inhaled anesthetic agents. *Anesthesiology* 1974;41:82–3.
16. Mattison DR. Transdermal drug absorption during pregnancy. *Clin Obstet Gynecol* 1990;33:718–727.
17. Krauer B, Krauer F, Hytten FE. Pregnancy and its effect on drug handling: the influence of physiological changes in pregnancy. In: Lind T, Singer A, eds. *Current reviews in obstetrics and gynaecology.* Edinburgh: Churchill-Livingstone, 1984:19–50.
18. Hytten FE, Chamberlain GV, eds. *Clinical physiology in obstetrics.* Oxford: Blackwell Scientific Publications, 1980:163–233.
19. Dean M, Stock B, Patterson RJ, et al. Serum protein binding of drugs during and after pregnancy in humans. *Clin Pharmacol Ther* 1980;28:253–260.
20. Bourget P, Roulot C, Fernandez H. Models for placental transfer studies of drugs. *Clin Pharmacokinet* 1995;28:161–180.
21. Wood M, Wood AJJ. Changes in plasma drug binding and alpha-1 acid glycoprotein in mother and newborn infant. *Clin Pharmacol Ther* 1981;29:522–526.
22. Hill MD, Abramson FP. The significance of plasma protein binding on the fetal maternal distribution of drugs at steady-state. *Clin Pharmacokinet* 1988;14:156–170.
23. Krauer B, Nau H, Dayer P, et al. Serum protein binding of diazepam and propranolol in the feto-maternal unit from early to late pregnancy. *Br J Gynaecol* 1986;93:322–328.
24. Wood AJJ. Drug disposition and pharmacokinetics. In: Wood M, Wood AJJ, eds. *Drugs and anesthesia. Pharmacology for anesthesiologists,* 2nd ed. Baltimore: Williams & Wilkins, 1990:3–41.
25. Rayburn WF, Lavin JP. Drug prescribing for chronic disorders during pregnancy: an overview. *Am J Obstet Gynecol* 1986;155:565–569.

26. Slaughter RL, Edwards DJ. Recent advances: the cytochrome P450 enzymes. *Ann Pharmacother* 1995; 6:619–624.

27. Juchau MR. Drug biotransformation in the placenta. *Pharmacol Ther* 1980;8:501–524.

28. Bologa M, Tang B, Klein J, et al. Pregnancy induced changes in drug metabolism in epileptic women. *J Pharmacol Exp Ther* 1991;257:735–740.

29. Harris RZ, Benet LZ, Schwartz JB. Gender effects in pharmacokinetics and pharmacodynamics. *Drugs* 1995;50:222–239.

30. Juchau MR. The role of the placenta in developmental toxicology. In: Snell K, ed. *Developmental toxicology*. London: Croom Helm, 1982:189–209.

31. Juchau MR, Chao ST, Omiecinski CJ. Drug metabolism by the human fetus. In: Gibaldi M, Prescott L, eds. *Handbook of clinical pharmacokinetics*. New York: Adis, 1983:58–78.

32. Santos AC, Pederson H, Finster M. Obstetric anesthesia. In: Barash P, Cullen B, Stoelting R, eds. *Clinical anesthesia*. Philadelphia: Lippincott–Raven, 1997:1061–1090.

33. Dunlop W. Serial Changes in renal haemodynamics during normal human pregnancy. *Br J Obstet Gynaecol* 1981;88:1–9.

34. Philipson A. Pharmacokinetics of antibiotics in pregnancy and labour. *Clin Pharmacokinet* 1979;4:297–306.

35. Heikkila A, Erkkola R. The need for adjustment of dosage regimen for penicillin V during pregnancy. *Obstet Gynecol* 1993;81:919–921.

36. Heikkila A, Erkkola R. Pharmacokinetics of piperacillin during pregnancy. *J Antimicrob Chemother* 1991;28:419–423.

37. Heikkila A, Renkonen OV, Erkkola R. Pharmacokinetics and transplacental passage of imipenem during pregnancy. *Antimicrob Agents Chemother* 1992;36:2652–2655.

38. Bourget D, Fernandez H, Quinquis V, et al., Pharmacokinetics and protein binding of ceftriaxone during pregnancy. *Antimicrob Agents Chemother* 1993;37:54–59.

39. Winter ME. *Basic clinical pharmacokinetics,* 3rd ed. Vancouver, WA: Applied Therapeutics, 1994.

40. Bates RD, Nahata MC. Once-daily administration of aminoglycosides. *Ann Pharmacother* 1994;28:757–766.

41. Bourget P, Fernandez H, Delouis C, et al. Transplacental passage of vancomycin during the second trimester of pregnancy. *Obstet Gynecol* 1991;78:908.

42. Lode H. The pharmacokinetics of azithromycin and their clinical significance. *Eur J Clin Microbiol Infect Dis* 1991;10:807–812.

43. McCombs J. Therapeutic considerations in pregnancy and lactation. In: DiPiro JT, Talbert RL, Yee GC, et al., eds. *Pharmacotherapy, a pathophysiologic approach,* 3rd ed. Stamford, CT: Appleton & Lange, 1997:1565–1583.

44. Brodie MJ. Management of epilepsy during pregnancy and lactation. *Lancet* 1990;336:426–427.

45. Nau H, Kuhnz W, Egger HJ, et al. Anticonvulsants during pregnancy and lactation: transplacental, maternal, and neonatal pharmacokinetics. *Clin Pharmacokinet* 1982;7:508–543.

46. Carter BL, Driscoll CE, Smith GD. Theophylline clearance during pregnancy. *Obstet Gynecol* 1986;68:555–559.

47. Neerhof MG. Pregnancy in the chronically hypertensive patient. *Clin Perinat* 1997;24:391–406.

48. Mitani GM, Steinberg I, Lien EJ, et al. The pharmacokinetics of antiarrhythmic agents in pregnancy and lactation. *Clin Pharmacokinet* 1987;12:253–291.

49. Thorley KJ, McAinsh J, Cruickshank JM. Atenolol in the treatment of pregnancy-induced hypertension. *Br J Clin Pharmacol* 1981;12:725–730.

50. Rubin PC, Buttners L, Kelman AW, et al. Labetolol disposition and concentration-effect relationships during pregnancy. *Br J Clin Pharmacol* 1983;15:465–470.

51. O'Hare MF, Leahey W, Murnaghan GA, et al. Pharmacokinetics of sotalol during pregnancy. *Eur J Clin Pharmacol* 1983;24:521–524.

52. Brancazio LR, Roperti KA, Stierer R, et al. Pharmacokinetics and pharmacodynamics of subcutaneous heparin during the early third trimester of pregnancy. *Am J Obstet Gynecol* 1995;173:1240–1245.

53. Dahlman TC, Hellgren MSE, Blombäck M. Thrombosis prophylaxis in pregnancy with use of subcutaneous heparin adjusted by monitoring heparin concentration in plasma. *Am J Obstet Gynecol* 1989;161:420–425.

54. Bremme K, Lind H, Blombäck M. The effect of prohylactic heparin treatment on enhanced thrombin generation in pregnancy. *Obstet Gynecol* 1993;81:78–83.

55. Blombäck M, Bremme K, Hellgren M, et al. A pharmacokinetic study of dalteparin (Fragmin®) during late pregnancy. *Blood Coagul Fibrinolysis* 1998;9:343–350.

56. Connor EM, Sperling RS, Gelber R, et al. Reduction of maternal-infant transmission of human immunodeficiency virus type 1 with zidovudine treatment. *N Engl J Med* 1994;331:1173–1180.

57. Minkoff H, Augenbraun M. Antiretroviral therapy for pregnant women. *Am J Obstet Gynecol* 1997;176:478–489.

58. O'Sullivan MJ, Boyer PJJ, Scott GB, et al. The pharmacokinetics and safety of zidovudine in the third trimester of pregnancy for women infected with human immunodeficiency virus and their infants: phase I acquired immunodeficiency syndrome clinical trials group study (protocol 082). *Am J Obstet Gynecol* 1993;168:1510–1516.

59. Sperling RS, Roboz J, Dische R, et al. Zidovudine pharmacokinetics during pregnancy. *Am J Perinatol* 1992;9:247–249.

60. Watts DH, Brown ZA, Tartaglione T, et al. Pharmacokinetic disposition of zidovudine during pregnancy. *J Infect Dis* 1991;163:226–232.

61. Johnson MA, Goodwin C, Yuen GJ, et al. The pharmacokinetics of 3TC administered to HIV-1 infected women (pre-partum, during labor, and post-partum) and their offspring. Proceedings from the XI International Conference on AIDS, Vancouver, Canada, July 1996, volume 1:249–250(abst Tu.C. 445).

62. Wisner KL, Perel JM, Wheeler SB. Tricyclic dose requirements across pregnancy. *Am J Psychiatry* 1993; 150;1541–1542.

63. Dillon AE, Wagner CL, Wiest D, et al. Drug therapy in the nursing mother. *Obstet Gynecol Clin North Am* 1997;24:675–696.

64. Committee on Drugs, American Academy of Pediatrics. The transfer of drugs and other chemicals in to human milk. *Pediatrics* 1994;93:137–150.

65. Niebyl JR. Use of antibiotics for ear, nose, and throat disorders in pregnancy and lactation. *Am J Otolaryngol* 1992;13:187–192.

66. Plomp TA, Vulsma T, deVijlder JJM. Use of amiodarone during pregnancy. *Eur J Obstet Gynecol Reprod Biol* 1992;43:201–207.
67. Wisner KL, Perel JM, Findling RL. Antidepressant treatment during breast-feeding. *Am J Psychiatry* 1996;153:1132–1137.
68. Matheson I, Pande H, Alertsen AR. Respiratory depression caused by N-desmethyldoxepin in breast milk [Letter]. *Lancet* 1985;2:1124.

69. Kemp J, Ilett KF, Booth J, et al. Excretion of doxepin and N-desmethyldoxepin in human milk. *Br J Clin Pharmacol* 1985;20:497–499.
70. Taddio A, Ito S, Koren G. Excretion of fluoxetine and its metabolite, norfluoxetine in human breast milk. *J Clin Pharmacol* 1996;36:42–47.
71. Stowe ZN, Owens MJ, Landry JC, et al. Sertraline and desmethylsertraline in human breast milk and nursing infants. *Am J Psychiatry* 1997;154:1255–1260.

3

Antibiotics and Other Antimicrobial Agents in Pregnancy and During Lactation

Jennifer R. Niebyl

Department of Obstetrics and Gynecology, University of Iowa Hospitals and Clinics, Iowa City, Iowa

Antibiotics are widely used during pregnancy. Because of the potential for maternal and fetal side effects, they should be used only when the indication is clear and the risk:benefit ratio justifies their use. Pregnant patients should be warned that they are particularly susceptible to yeast infections resulting from antibiotic use and may need therapy later with antifungal agents should such symptoms occur.

PENICILLINS

The penicillins have a wide margin of safety and lack toxicity for both the pregnant woman and the fetus (1). Penicillin is the antibiotic of choice in the treatment of numerous serious bacterial infections, including syphilis. Ampicillin and amoxicillin are the most frequently used drugs in the treatment of respiratory and urinary tract infections during pregnancy. Adverse effects, however, may include nausea, epigastric distress, diarrhea, and candidal vaginitis.

Before therapy, it is important to ascertain that the patient is not allergic to penicillin. The severity of reactions ranges from a mild rash to anaphylaxis. One patient had a stillborn infant attributed to an anaphylactic reaction to penicillin (2), and anaphylaxis after ampicillin administration during labor has been described (3). There is no evidence that penicillin or its derivatives are teratogenic. In the Collaborative Perinatal Project, 3,546 mothers took penicillin derivatives in the first trimester of pregnancy, with no increased risk of anomalies (1).

Of 86 women exposed to dicloxacillin in the first trimester, there was no increase in birth defects (4).

Pharmacology

Several studies revealed that the serum levels of the penicillins are lower and their renal clearance is higher throughout pregnancy compared with the nonpregnant state (5–7). The increase in maternal renal function, because of an increase in both renal blood flow and glomerular filtration rate, results in a higher renal excretion of drugs. The expansion of the maternal intravascular volume during the late stages of pregnancy is another factor that affects antibiotic therapy. If the same dose of penicillin or ampicillin is given to both nonpregnant and pregnant women, lower serum levels are attained during pregnancy because of the distribution of the drug in a larger intravascular volume.

The transplacental passage of penicillin is by simple diffusion. The free-circulating portion of the antibiotic crosses the placenta, resulting in a lower maternal serum level of the unbound portion of the drug. Maternal administration of penicillins with high protein binding (e.g., oxacillin, cloxacillin, dicloxacillin, and nafcillin) results in lower fetal tissue and amniotic fluid levels than the administration of poorly bound penicillins (e.g., penicillin G, ampicillin, and methicillin) (8,9). The antibiotic is ultimately excreted in the fetal urine and thus into the amniotic fluid. The delay in appearance of different types of penicillins in the amniotic fluid depends primarily on the rate of transplacental diffusion, the amount of protein binding in fetal serum, and the adequacy of fetal enzymatic and renal function. A time delay may occur before effective levels of the antibiotic appear in the amniotic fluid.

At term, maternal serum and amniotic fluid concentrations of penicillin G are equal at 60 to 90 minutes after intravenous administration (10), representing rapid passage into the fetal circulation and amniotic fluid. Continuous intravenous infusions caused equal concentrations of penicillin G at 20 hours in maternal serum, cord serum, and amniotic fluid (10). Ampicillin rapidly crosses the placenta, and fetal serum levels can be detected within 30 minutes and equilibrate in an hour.

Amoxicillin is similar to ampicillin in its spectrum of activity but is stable in the presence of gastric acid and may be given without regard to meals. It has been used effectively as a 3-g single dose to treat bacteriuria in pregnancy (11).

Methicillin crosses rapidly into the fetal circulation and amniotic fluid. After a 500-mg intravenous dose over 10 to 15 minutes, equilibration occurred within 1 hour in fetal tissues (12).

Carbenicillin crosses the placenta and distributes to fetal tissues. After a 4-g intramuscular dose, mean peak concentrations in cord and maternal serum occurred at 2 hours and were similar (13). Ticarcillin rapidly crosses the placenta into the fetal circulation and amniotic fluid (14). Dicloxacillin and oxacillin cross the placenta only in low concentrations because of the high degree of maternal protein binding (12,15).

Most penicillins are primarily excreted unchanged in the urine, with only small amounts being inactivated in the liver. This is of significance in patients with impaired renal function, which requires reduction in dose.

Breast-feeding

Penicillin G is excreted into breast milk in low concentrations (16). Although no adverse effects are clearly attributable to penicillin in breast milk, three problems theoretically might be seen in the nursing infant: modification of bowel flora (possible diarrhea, candidiasis), allergic response, and interference with the interpretation of culture results.

The benefits of continued breast-feeding usually outweigh these potential risks. When these drugs are used to treat mastitis or other infections in nursing mothers, nursing should be allowed to continue. Ampicillin and amoxicillin are excreted into breast milk in low concentrations (17,18).

Oxacillin, dicloxacillin, and ticarcillin are highly protein bound and are excreted into breast milk in only very small amounts. After a 1-g intravenous dose of ticarcillin was given to five patients, only trace amounts of the drug were measured at intervals up to 6 hours (14).

CEPHALOSPORINS

The use of cephalosporins in obstetrics has been extensive. They are used as prophylactic agents in cesarean section and in the treatment of septic abortion, pyelonephritis, and amnionitis, but they have not been well studied in the first trimester.

In a study of 5,000 Michigan Medicaid recipients, there was a suggestion of possible teratogenicity (25% increase in birth defects) with cefaclor, cephalexin, and cephradine, but not other cephalosporins (19). Because other antibiotics that have been used extensively (e.g., penicillin, ampicillin, amoxicillin, and erythromycin) have not been associated with an increased risk of congenital defects, they should be first-line therapy when such treatment is needed in the first trimester.

Pharmacology

Maternal serum levels attained with these drugs during pregnancy are lower than those in nonpregnant patients receiving equivalent doses because of a shorter half-life in pregnancy and an increased volume of distribution. This is true not only for well-established cephalosporin drugs [e.g., cephalothin (20), cephalexin, and cefazolin], but also for the newer cephalosporins [e.g., cefoxitin, cephradine, and cefuroxime (21,22)]. Renal elimination is increased in pregnancy (23).

These drugs readily cross the placenta to the fetal bloodstream and ultimately the amniotic fluid (24). Transplacental transfer of these drugs is fairly rapid, and adequate bactericidal concentrations are attained in both fetal soft tissues and the amniotic fluid (20–22,25–27). Repeated high bolus doses of cephalosporins have been shown to result in higher levels in fetal serum and amniotic fluid than continuous intravenous infusions of the same amount of drug (28).

The average fetal cord blood level achieved ranges from 10% to 40% of the maternal serum levels, depending on the timing and the particular drug used. Studies reporting cord levels only a few hours after a drug dose may not reveal the full picture. For example, when ceftizoxime was administered in a 2-g intravenous dose, the mean fetal:maternal ratio was 0.28. However, after reaching steady state after three doses of 2 g every 8 hours, ceftizoxime was concentrated on the fetal side of the placenta, achieving a fetal serum level two times that in the maternal serum and, in the amniotic fluid, a level four times that of the maternal serum (29).

Breast-feeding

The cephalosporins are excreted into breast milk in sufficiently low concentrations that the infant receives an insignificant dose. Although the same theoretical concerns exist as with penicillins, the advantages of continued breast-feeding during treatment usually outweigh these risks.

SULFONAMIDES

The sulfonamides are often used for treatment of urinary tract infections in pregnancy. Among 1,455 human infants exposed to sulfonamides during the first trimester, no teratogenic effects were noted (1).

The administration of sulfonamides should be avoided in glucose-6-phosphate dehydrogenase–deficient women. A dose-related toxic reaction may occur in these individuals, resulting in red cell hemolysis.

Sulfonamides cause no known damage to the fetus *in utero* because the fetus can clear free bilirubin through the placenta. These drugs might theoretically have deleterious effects if present in the blood of the neonate after birth, however. The sulfonamides compete with bilirubin for binding sites on albumin, thus raising the levels of free bilirubin in the serum and increasing the risk of hyperbilirubinemia or kernicterus in the neonate (30,31). For that reason, it is recommended that an alternate antibiotic be used in the third trimester, if possible. However, kernicterus in the neonate after *in utero* exposure has not been reported.

Pharmacology

The sulfonamides are easily absorbed orally and readily cross the placenta, achieving fetal plasma levels 50% to 90% of those attained in the maternal plasma (32). Ylikorkala and colleagues (33) studied the pharmacokinetics of trimethoprim-sulfamethoxazole in 10 pregnant women in the first trimester and found the maternal serum levels of the drug to be comparable with nonpregnant individuals. The elimination half-life of this combination drug was shorter, however, in the pregnant women, and trimethoprim was cleared faster from the maternal serum than sulfamethoxazole (33).

Use with Trimethoprim

Trimethoprim is often given with sulfa in treatment of urinary tract infections. Two trials including 131 women failed to show any increased risk of birth defects after first-trimester exposure (34,35). However, in 2,296 Michigan Medicaid recipients first-trimester trimethoprim exposure was associated with a slightly increased risk of birth defects, particularly cardiovascular (36), and in a retrospective study, the odds ratio was 2.3 (37).

Sulfasalazine

Sulfasalazine is used for treatment of ulcerative colitis and Crohn's disease because of its relatively poor oral absorption. However, it does cross the placenta to the fetal circulation, with fetal concentrations approximately the same as maternal concentrations, although both are low. Neither kernicterus nor severe neonatal jaundice has been reported after maternal use of sulfasalazine, even when the drug was given up to the time of delivery (38,39).

Breast-feeding

Sulfonamides are excreted into breast milk in low concentrations. The milk:plasma ratio is approximately 0.5 (40). The amount of sulfonamide ingested by an infant would be sufficiently low not to have any toxicity (less than 1% of the maternal dose), and so breast-feeding is usually continued during administration of these drugs. When sulfasalazine was taken by breast-feeding mothers, the drug was undetectable in all milk samples. However, during the first 5 days of life or with premature infants when hyperbilirubinemia may be a problem, sulfa drugs are best avoided (41).

NITROFURANTOIN

Nitrofurantoin is an antimicrobial agent used in the treatment of acute uncomplicated lower urinary tract infections as well as for long-term suppression in patients with chronic bacteriuria. Nitrofurantoin is capable of inducing hemolytic anemia in patients deficient in glucose-6-phosphate dehydrogenase (42).

No reports linking the use of nitrofurantoin with congenital defects were found. In the Collaborative Perinatal Project (1), 590 infants were exposed, 83 in the first trimester, with no significantly increased risk of anomalies or other adverse effects. Other studies suggested no fetal toxicity from nitrofurantoin exposure (43,44).

Pharmacology

Nitrofurantoin absorption from the gastrointestinal tract varies with the form administered. The macrocrystalline form is absorbed more slowly than the crystalline and is associated with less gastrointestinal intolerance. Because of rapid elimination, the serum half-life is 20 to 60 minutes. Therapeutic serum levels are not achieved; therefore, this drug is not indicated when there is a possibility of bacteremia such as with pyelonephritis. Approximately one third of an oral dose appears in the active form in the urine.

Breast-feeding

Nitrofurantoin is excreted into breast milk in very low concentrations. The drug could not be detected in 20 samples from mothers receiving 100 mg four times a day (45,46).

TETRACYCLINES

The tetracyclines readily cross the placenta and are firmly bound by chelating to calcium in developing bone and tooth structures (47). This produces brown discoloration of the teeth, hypoplasia of the enamel, inhibition of bone growth (48), and other skeletal abnormalities. The yellowish brown staining of the teeth usually occurs in the second or third trimesters of pregnancy after 24 weeks, whereas bone incorporation can occur earlier. Depression of skeletal growth was particularly common among premature infants treated with tetracycline. A 40% inhibition of fibular growth in the second trimester was demonstrated in patients who subsequently underwent termination of pregnancy, but the effect was reversible when the drug was stopped. Alternate antibiotics are currently recommended during pregnancy.

Hepatotoxicity has been reported in pregnant women treated with large doses of intravenous tetracyclines. This has been presumed to be an overdose effect and has not been reported with brief courses of therapy at lower doses. Tetracycline-induced hepatotoxicity differs from acute fatty liver of pregnancy in that it is not unique to pregnant women and reversal of the disease does not occur with pregnancy termination.

First-trimester exposure to tetracycline was not found to have any teratogenic risk in 341 women in the Collaborative Perinatal Project (1), in 174 women in another study (4), or in 63 women treated with doxycycline (49).

Breast-feeding

Tetracycline is excreted into breast milk in low concentrations. Tetracycline was not detectable in the serum of breast-feeding infants, and delayed bone growth from tetracycline has not been reported after the drug was taken by breast-feeding mothers. This may be owing to the high binding of the drug to calcium and protein, limiting absorption from the milk.

AMINOGLYCOSIDES

Aminoglycosides are commonly used with penicillin or clindamycin in the treatment of postpartum endometritis, septic abortion, or endometritis. They should be given during pregnancy only when serious gram-negative infections are suspected. Gentamicin is preferred over tobramycin and amikacin, as it has been more extensively studied.

Streptomycin and kanamycin have been associated with congenital deafness in the offspring of mothers who took these drugs during pregnancy. Ototoxicity was reported with doses as low as 1 g streptomycin biweekly for 8 weeks during the first trimester, and it is recommended to limit doses to a total of 20 g during the last half of pregnancy (50). Eighth cranial nerve damage has been reported after *in utero* exposure to kanamycin. Of 391 mothers who had received 50 mg/kg for prolonged periods during pregnancy, nine children were found to have hearing loss (2.3%) (51). Ototoxicity may be increased with simultaneous use of ethacrynic acid (52).

Nephrotoxicity may be increased when the drug is given in combination with cephalosporins, and this should be avoided. Neuromuscular blockade may be potentiated by the combined use of these drugs and curariform drugs; therefore, the dose should be reduced appropriately. Potentiation of magnesium sulfate–induced neuromuscular weakness has also been reported in a neonate exposed to magnesium sulfate and gentamicin (53).

No known teratogenic effect is associated with the use of these drugs in the first trimester other than ototoxicity. In 135 infants exposed to streptomycin in the Collaborative Perinatal Project (1), no teratogenic effects were observed. In a group of 1,619 newborns whose mothers were treated for tuberculosis during pregnancy with multiple drugs, including streptomycin, the incidence of congenital defects was the same as that of the healthy control group (54).

Pharmacology

The aminoglycosides are poorly absorbed after oral administration and are rapidly excreted by the normal kidney. Because the rate of clearance is related to the glomerular filtration rate, the dose must be reduced in the presence of abnormal renal function.

The serum aminoglycoside levels are usually lower in pregnant than in nonpregnant patients receiving equivalent doses because of more rapid elimination. Thus, it is important to monitor levels to prevent subtherapeutic dosing (55,56). Wide interpatient variation in gentamicin levels has been observed in obstetric patients, varying with the volume of distribution of the drug (56). The concentrations in fetal blood are lower than those in maternal blood at full term (57). After 40- to 80-mg intramuscular doses given to patients in labor, peak cord serum levels averaging 30% to 40% of maternal levels were obtained at 1 to 2 hours (56,57). At term, cord serum levels of amikacin are one half to one third of maternal serum levels, and measurable amniotic fluid levels appear at approximately 5 hours postinjection (58).

One dose per day is recommended for gentamicin, as it increases efficacy (59) and decreases toxicity and cost (60). It has been studied in chorioamnionitis and endometritis and shown to be safe and effective (61).

Breast-feeding

Limited information is available about excretion of gentamicin into breast milk. Other aminoglycosides (e.g., amikacin, kanamycin, streptomycin, and tobramycin) are known to be excreted in low levels into breast milk (62). Because oral absorption of these drugs by the infant is poor, ototoxicity or other side effects would not be expected.

ERYTHROMYCIN

Erythromycin is the alternate drug of choice to penicillin for many diseases in pregnancy and is used for primary treatment for mycoplasma and chlamydia.

Erythromycin estolate has been associated with subclinical reversible hepatotoxicity during pregnancy (63). Thus, other forms that are thought to be relatively nontoxic are usually recommended.

No teratogenic risk of erythromycin has been reported. In 79 patients in the Collaborative Perinatal Project (1) and 260 in another study (49), no increased risk of birth defects was noted.

Pharmacology

Erythromycin and its salts are not consistently absorbed from the gastrointestinal tract of pregnant women, and transplacental passage is unpredictable. Both maternal and fetal serum levels achieved after the administration of the drug in pregnancy are low and vary considerably (64,65). For treatment of syphilis in pregnancy, desensitization and treatment with penicillin are still the treatment of choice, as many erythromycin treatment failures have occurred (66). Fetal tissue levels increase after multiple doses (65). Fetal plasma concentrations are 5% to 20% of those in maternal plasma. The usual oral dose is 250 to 500 mg every 6 hours, but the higher dose may not be well tolerated in pregnant women who are susceptible to nausea and gastrointestinal symptoms.

Breast-feeding

Erythromycin is excreted into breast milk in small amounts, and no reports of adverse effects of infants exposed to erythromycin in breast milk have been noted.

CLINDAMYCIN

Clindamycin should be used in pregnancy only when anaerobic infections are suspected that are not sensitive to other antibiotics. Most authorities would agree that this drug should not be used for prophylaxis before cesarean section, reserving its use for therapeutic indications.

If diarrhea develops during the administration of this drug, the patient should be evaluated for the possibility of pseudomembranous colitis, which has been reported in as many as 10% of patients.

Of 647 infants exposed to clindamycin in the first trimester, no increased risk of birth defects was noted (67).

Pharmacology

Clindamycin crosses the placenta, achieving maximum cord serum levels of approximately 50% of the maternal serum (65). It is 90% bound to serum protein, and fetal tissue levels increase after multiple dosing (65). Maternal serum levels after dosing at various stages of pregnancy are similar to those of nonpregnant patients (55).

Clindamycin is nearly completely absorbed after oral administration, and a small percentage is absorbed after topical application. Most of the drug is metabolized in the liver to products excreted in the urine and bile, and only 10% of the drug is excreted unchanged in the urine.

Breast-feeding

Clindamycin is excreted into breast milk in low levels, and nursing is usually continued during administration of this drug. Two bloody stools were observed in one nursing infant whose mother was receiving clindamycin and gentamicin (68), and this symptom cleared when the breast-feeding was stopped. Except for this one case, no other adverse effects in nursing infants have been reported.

QUINOLONES

The quinolones (e.g., ciprofloxacin and norfloxacin) have a high affinity for bone tissue and cartilage and may cause arthropathies in children. However, no malformations or musculoskeletal problems were noted in 38 infants exposed *in utero* in the first trimester (69). The manufacturer recommends against use in pregnancy and in children.

METRONIDAZOLE

Metronidazole possesses trichomonacidal and amebicidal activity as well as effectiveness against certain bacteria, especially anaerobes.

Controversy regarding the use of metronidazole during pregnancy was initiated when the drug was shown to be positive in the Ames test, which correlates with carcinogenicity in animals. However, doses used were much higher than the doses used clinically, and carcinogenicity in humans has not been confirmed (70). Because some have advised against the use of this drug in pregnancy (71), it should only be used for clear-cut indications.

Studies have failed to show any increase in the incidence of congenital defects among the newborns of mothers treated with metronidazole during early or late gestation. In a study of 1,387 prescriptions filled, no risk of birth defects could be determined (72), and a metaanalysis confirmed no teratogenic risk (73).

Metronidazole remains the most effective drug for trichomoniasis. Because of the past controversy surrounding this drug, some would defer therapy until after the first trimester, whereas other specialists believe that such prohibition is unwarranted. Treatment with metronidazole and erythromycin resulted in reduced rates of premature delivery in women with bacterial vaginosis and a previous preterm delivery in one study (74), but this has not been confirmed in the general obstetric population (75).

Pharmacology

Metronidazole crosses the placenta to the fetus throughout gestation with a cord:maternal plasma ratio at term of approximately 1.0 (76).

Breast-feeding

Metronidazole is excreted into breast milk in small amounts. One infant had diarrhea while the mother was receiving metronidazole; otherwise, no adverse effects in metronidazole exposed nursing infants have been reported. The American Academy of Pediatrics recommends interrupting breast-feeding after a single 2-g oral dose for 12 to 24 hours to allow clearance of the drug (41).

ACYCLOVIR

The Acyclovir Registry has recorded 601 exposures during pregnancy, including 425 in the first trimester, with no increased risk of abnormalities in the infants (77).

Maternal systemic acyclovir has also been used near term to prevent recurrent genital herpes, with no adverse effects on the infants (78,79). The Centers for Disease Control and Prevention recommend that pregnant women with disseminated infection, e.g., herpetic encephalitis or hepatitis or varicella pneumonia, be treated with acyclovir (80).

LINDANE

Lindane (Quell) has been administered to pregnant women for the treatment of scabies and lice. Treatment should be such that only a minimal amount of the drug is absorbed percutaneously, as high doses applied in this way have produced convulsions.

Toxicity in humans after topical use of 1% lindane has been observed almost exclusively after overexposure to the agent. However, approximately 10% of the dose is recovered in the urine after application to the skin. Because this drug is a potent neurotoxin, its use during pregnancy should be limited. The manufacturer recommends no more than two treatments during pregnancy. Although no specific reproductive damage attributable to lindane has been reported, pregnant women should be advised to wear gloves when shampooing their children's hair, as absorption could easily occur across the skin of the hands of the mother. Alternate drugs are usually recommended, specifically pyrethrins with piperonyl butoxide (RID) or permethrin (NIX).

Pharmacology

Lindane is absorbed through the skin after local application, and more is absorbed in patients with excoriated skin.

Breast-feeding

No reports describing the use of lindane in lactating women have been noted. However, the amount of lindane ingested in breast milk would be less than the amount absorbed from direct topical application to the infant.

TABLE 3.1. *Teratogenic effects of antibiotics*

Drug	First trimester teratogen	Perinatal effects
Penicillins	No	No
Cephalosporins	? Some	No
Sulfonamides	No	Compete with bilirubin for albumin binding sites, increased risk of jaundice
Sulfasalazin	No	No
Trimethoprim	?	No
Nitrofurantoin	No	No
Tetracyclines	No	Tooth discoloration, decreased bone growth
Aminoglycosides	No	Ototoxicity (deafness)

PYRETHRINS WITH PIPERONYL BUTOXIDE (RID)

Pyrethrins with piperonyl butoxide constitute a combination product used topically for the treatment of lice. This product is considered the drug of choice for lice in pregnancy, as topical absorption is poor, so potential toxicity should be less than that with lindane.

PERMETHRIN

Permethrin is an effective therapy for treatment of lice and scabies, but it has not been studied in human pregnancy. Topical application is unlikely to have an adverse effect (81).

ANTITUBERCULOSIS DRUGS

There is no evidence of any teratogenic effect of isoniazid, paraaminosalicylic acid, rifampin, or ethambutol. The American Thoracic Society states that therapy with isoniazid for a positive purified protein derivative test with a negative chest radiograph should be delayed until after delivery because of a small risk of maternal liver toxicity (82).

ANTIFUNGAL AGENTS

Nystatin, miconazole, and clotrimazole are commonly used topically during pregnancy for monilial infections. Nystatin is poorly absorbed from intact skin and mucous membranes; consequently, topical use would not be expected to be associated with teratogenesis. In the Collaborative Perinatal Project (1), however, of 142 exposures, there were 14 malformations, which was a statistically increased risk. This was attributed to adjunctive use with other drugs. Another study of 176 infants has not confirmed any risk with use in pregnancy (49).

Clotrimazole has not been implicated as a teratogen (83). Only small amounts are absorbed from the skin and vaginal mucosa (84), and 0.15% of the dose was recovered in the urine after it had been applied to inflamed skin.

Miconazole is also absorbed in small amounts from the vagina. Use in the first trimester of pregnancy was not shown to be associated with congenital malformations in the Michigan Medicaid data (7,266 exposures) (85). In one study, however, a slightly increased risk of first-trimester abortion was noted after use of this drug, although many associations were examined. These findings were considered not to be definitive evidence of risk (86).

First-trimester exposure to fluconazole as one 150-mg dose did not increase congenital anomalies or pregnancy loss in 226 exposures (87).

Breast-feeding

Because nystatin is poorly absorbed orally, it is unlikely to be found in serum and breast milk.

No data are available with miconazole or clotrimazole in breast milk, but because only small amounts are absorbed vaginally, this would not be expected to be a problem.

TABLE 3.2. *Antibiotics compatible with breast feeding*

Penicillins
Cephalosporins
Trimethoprim
Nitrofurantoin
Tetracyclines
Aminoglycosides

TABLE 3.3. *Antimicrobials whose effects on nursing infants are unknown but may be of concern*

Metronidazole (Flagyl)
Sulfonamides

Infant exposure to ketoconazole in human milk was 0.4% of the therapeutic dose, unlikely to cause adverse effects (88).

CONCLUSIONS

Most antibiotics are safe to use during pregnancy, but because there is potential for fetal effects that are still unrecognized, they should be used only when clearly indicated. A summary of drug effects in pregnancy is presented in Table 3.1, and effects in breast-feeding mothers in Tables 3.2 and 3.3.

REFERENCES

1. Heinonen PO, Slone D, Shapiro S. *Birth defects and drugs in pregnancy*. Littleton, MA: Publishing Sciences Group, 1977.
2. Kosim H. Intrauterine fetal death as a result of anaphylactic reaction to penicillin in a pregnant woman. *Dapim Refuiim* 1959;18:136.
3. Heim K, Alge A, Marth C. Anaphylactic reaction to ampicillin and severe complication in the fetus. *Lancet* 1991;337:859.
4. Aselton P, Jick H, Milunsky A, et al. First-trimester drug use and congenital disorders. *Obstet Gynecol* 1985;65:451.
5. Philipson A. Pharmacokinetics of antibiotics in pregnancy and labour. *Clin Pharmacokinet* 1979;4:297.
6. Heikkila AM, Erkkola RU. The need for adjustment of dosage regimen of penicillin V during pregnancy. *Obstet Gynecol* 1993;81:919.
7. Philipson A. Pharmacokinetics of ampicillin during pregnancy. *J Infect Dis* 1977;136:370.
8. Kunin CM. Clinical pharmacology of the new penicillins. I. The importance of serum protein binding in determining antimicrobial activity and concentration in serum. *Clin Pharmacol Ther* 1966;7:166.
9. Macaulay MA, Berg SA, Charles D. Placental transfer of dicloxacillin at term. *Am J Obstet Gynecol* 1968;102:1162.
10. Woltz J, Zintel H. The transmission of penicillin to amniotic fluid and fetal blood in the human. *Am J Obstet Gynecol* 1945;50:338.
11. Masterson RG, Evans DC, Strike PW. Single-dose amoxicillin in the treatment of bacteriuria in pregnancy and the puerperium: a controlled clinical trial. *Br J Obstet Gynaecol* 1985;92:498.
12. Depp R, Kind A, Kirby W, et al. Transplacental passage of methicillin and dicloxacillin into the fetus and amniotic fluid. *Am J Obstet Gynecol* 1970;107:1054.
13. Elek E, Ivan E, Arr M. Passage of penicillins from mother to foetus in humans. *Int J Clin Pharmacol Ther Toxicol* 1972;6:223.
14. Cho N, Nakayama T, Vehara K, et al. Laboratory and clinical evaluation of ticarcillin in the field of obstetrics and gynecology. *Chemotherapy* 1977;25:2911.
15. Prigot A, Froix C, Rubin E. Absorption, diffusion, and excretion of new penicillin, oxacillin. *Antimicrob Agents Chemother* 1962;402.
16. Greene H, Burkhart B, Hobby G. Excretion of penicillin in human milk following parturition. *Am J Obstet Gynecol* 1946;51:732.
17. Wilson J, Brown R, Cherek D, et al. Drug excretion in human breast milk: principles, pharmacokinetics and projected consequences. *Clin Pharmacol Ther* 1980;5:1.
18. Kafetzis D, Siafas C, Georgakopoulos P, et al. Passage of cephalosporins and amoxicillin into the breast milk. *Acta Paediatr Scand* 1981;70:285.
19. Briggs GG, Freeman RK, Yaffe SJ. *Drugs in pregnancy and lactation,* 5th ed. Baltimore: Williams & Wilkins, 1998:151.
20. Morrow S, Palmisano P, Cassady G. The placental transfer of cephalothin. *J Pediatr* 1968;73:262.
21. Dubois M, Delapierre D, Demonty J, et al. Transplacental and mammary transfer of cephoxitin. 11th International Congress of Chemotherapy and 19th Interscience Conference on Antimicrobial Agents and Chemotherapy. Boston, 1979.
22. Philipson A, Stiernsted TG. Pharmacokinetics of cephradine in pregnancy. 11th International Congress of Chemotherapy and 19th Interscience Conference on Antimicrobial Agents and Chemotherapy. Boston, 1979.
23. Nathorst-Boos J, Philipson A, Hedman A, et al. Renal elimination of ceftazidime during pregnancy. *Am J Obstet Gynecol* 1995;172:163.
24. Sheng KT, Huang NN, Promadhattavedi V. Serum concentrations of cephalothin in infants and children and placental transmission of the antibiotic. *Antimicrob Agents Chemother* 1964:200.
25. Dubois M, Delapierre D, Demonty J, et al. Transplacental and mammary transfer of cephoxitin. 11th International Congress of Chemotherapy and 19th Interscience Conference on Antimicrobial Agents and Chemotherapy. Boston, 1979.
26. Craft I, Mullinger BM, Kennedy MRK. Placental transfer of cefuroxine. 11th International Congress of Chemotherapy and 19th Interscience Conference on Antimicrobial Agents and Chemotherapy. Boston, 1979.
27. Macaulay MA, Charles D. Placental transfer of cephalothin. *Am J Obstet Gynecol* 1968;100:940.
28. Hirsch HA, Herbst S, Lang R, et al. Transfer of a new cephalosporin antibiotic to the foetus and the amniotic fluid during a continuous infusion (steady state) and single repeated intravenous injections to the mother. *Arkh Gynakol* 1974;16:1.
29. Fortunato SJ, Bawdon RE, Welt SI, et al. Steady-state cord and amniotic fluid ceftizoxime levels continuously surpass maternal levels. *Am J Obstet Gynecol* 1988;159:570.
30. Harris RC, Lucey JF, MacLean JR. Kernicterus in premature infants associated with low concentration of bilirubin in the plasma. *Pediatrics* 1950;23:878.
31. Nyhan WL. Toxicity of drugs in the neonatal period. *J Pediatr* 1961;59:1.
32. Monif GFG. *Infectious diseases in obstetrics and gynecology*. New York: Harper & Row, 1974:26.

33. Ylikorkala O, Sjostedt E, Jarvinen PA, et al. Trimethoprim-sulfonamide combination administered orally and intravaginally in the first trimester of pregnancy: its absorption into serum and transfer to amniotic fluid. *Acta Obstet Gynecol Scand* 1973; 52:229.

34. Colley DP, Kay J, Gibson GT. A study of the use in pregnancy of co-trimoxazole and sulfamethizole. *Aust J Pharm* 1982;63:570.

35. Bailey RR. Single-dose antibacterial treatment for bacteriuria in pregnancy. *Drugs* 1984;27:183.

36. Briggs GG, Freeman RK, Yaffe SJ. *Drugs in pregnancy and lactation,* 5th ed. Baltimore: Williams & Wilkins, 1998:1061.

37. Czeizel A. A case-control analysis of the teratogenic effects of co-trimoxazole. *Reprod Toxicol* 1990;4: 305.

38. Jarnerot G, Into-Malmberg MB, Esbjorner E. Placental transfer of sulphasalazine and sulphapyridine and some of its metabolites. *Scand J Gastroenterol* 1981;16: 693.

39. Modadam M. Sulfasalazine IBD, pregnancy [Reply]. *Gastroenterology* 1981;81:194.

40. Foster FP. Sulfanilamide excretion in breast milk: report of a case. *Proc Staff Meet Mayo Clin* 1939;14:153.

41. Committee on Drugs. American Academy of Pediatrics. The transfer of drugs and other chemicals into human milk. *Pediatrics* 1994;93:137.

42. Briggs GG, Freeman RK, Yaffe SJ. *Drugs in pregnancy and lactation,* 5th ed. Baltimore: Williams & Wilkins, 1998:772.

43. Hailey FJ, Fort H, Wiiliams JR, et al. Foetal safety of nitrofurantoin, macrocrystals therapy during pregnancy: a retrospective analysis. *J Int Med Res* 1983;11: 364.

44. Lenke RR, VanDorsten JP, Schifrin BS. Pyelonephritis in pregnancy: a prospective randomized trial to prevent recurrent disease evaluating suppressive therapy with nitrofurantoin and close surveillance. *Am J Obstet Gynecol* 1983;146:953.

45. Hosbach RE, Foster RB. Absence of nitrofurantoin from human milk. *JAMA* 1967;202:1057.

46. Varsano I, Fischl J, Shochet SB. The excretion of orally ingested nitrofurantoin in human milk. *J Pediatr* 1973;82:886.

47. Kline AH, Blattner RT, Lunin M. Transplacental effects of tetracycline on teeth. *JAMA* 1964;118:178.

48. Cohlan SQ, Bevelander G, Tiamsic T. Growth inhibition of prematures receiving tetracycline. *Am J Dis Child* 1963;105:453.

49. Czeizel AE, Rockenbauer M. Teratogenic study of doxycycline. *Obstet Gynecol* 1997;89:524.

50. Robinson GC, Cambon KG. Hearing loss in infants of tuberculous mothers treated with streptomycin during pregnancy. *N Engl J Med* 1964;271:949.

51. Nishimura H, Tanimura T. *Clinical aspects of the teratogenicity of drugs.* Amsterdam: Excerpta Medica, 1976:131.

52. Jones HC. Intrauterine ototoxicity: a case report and review of literature. *J Natl Med Assoc* 1973;65:201.

53. L'Hommedieu CS, Nicholas D, Armes DA, et al. Potentiation of magnesium sulfate-induced neuromuscular weakness by gentamicin, tobramycin, and amikacin. *J Pediatr* 1983;102:629.

54. Marynowski A, Sianozecka E. Comparison of the incidence of congenital malformations in neonates from healthy mothers and from patients treated because of tuberculosis. *Ginekol Pol* 1972;43:713.

55. Weinstein AJ, Gibbs RS, Gallagher M. Placental transfer of clindamycin and gentamicin in term pregnancy. *Am J Obstet Gynecol* 1976;124:688.

56. Zaske DE, Cipolle RJ, Strate RG, et al. Rapid gentamicin elimination in obstetric patients. *Obstet Gynecol* 1980;56:559.

57. Yoshioka H, Monma T, Matsuda S. Placental transfer of gentamicin. *J Pediatr* 1972;80:121.

58. Matsuda C, Mori C, Maruno M, et al. A study of amikacin in the obstetrics field. *Jpn J Antibiot* 1974;27:633.

59. Nicolau DP, Freeman CD, Belliveau PP, et al. Aminoglycoside program administered to 2,184 adult patients. *Antimicrob Agents Chemother* 1995;39:650.

60. Munckhof WJ, Grayson ML, Turnidge JD. A meta-analysis of studies on the safety and efficacy of aminoglycosides given either once daily or as divided doses. *J Antimicrob Chemother* 1996;37:645.

61. Mitra AG, Whitten K, Laurent SL, et al. A randomized, prospective study comparing once-daily gentamicin versus thrice-daily gentamicin in the treatment of puerperal infection. *Am J Obstet Gynecol* 1997;177: 786.

62. Wilson JT. Milk/plasma ratios and contraindicated drugs. In: Wilson JT, ed. *Drugs in breast milk.* Balgowlah, Australia: ADIS Press, 1981:79.

63. McCormack WM, George H, Donner A, et al. Hepatotoxicity of erythromycin estolate during pregnancy. *Antimicrob Agents Chemother* 1977;12:630.

64. Philipson A, Sabath LD, Charles D. Erythromycin and clindamycin absorption and elimination in pregnant women. *Clin Pharmacol Ther* 1976;19:68.

65. Philipson A, Sabath LD, Charles D. Transplacental passage of erythromycin and clindamycin. *N Engl J Med* 1973;288:1219.

66. South MA, Short DH, Knox JM. Failure of erythromycin estolate therapy in in utero syphilis. *JAMA* 1964; 190:70.

67. Briggs GG, Freeman RK, Yaffe SJ. *Drugs and pregnancy and lactation,* 5th ed. Baltimore: Williams & Wilkins, 1998:223.

68. Mann CF. Clindamycin and breast-feeding. *Pediatrics* 1980;66:1030.

69. Berkovitch M, Pastuszak A, Gazarian M, et al. Safety of the new quinolones in pregnancy. *Obstet Gynecol* 1994;84:535.

70. Beard CM, Noller KL, O'Fallon WM, et al. Lack of evidence for cancer due to use of metronidazole. *N Engl J Med* 1979;301:519.

71. Finegold SM. Metronidazole. *Ann Intern Med* 1980; 93:585.

72. Piper JM, Mitchel EF, Ray WA. Prenatal use of metronidazole and birth defects: no association. *Obstet Gynecol* 1993;82:348.

73. Burtin P, Taddio A, Ariburnu O, et al: Safety of metronidazole in pregnancy: a meta-analysis. *Am J Obstet Gynecol* 1995;172:525.

74. Hauth JC, Goldenberg RL, Andrews WW, et al. Reduced incidence of preterm delivery with metronidazole and erythromycin in women with bacterial vaginosis. *N Engl J Med* 1995;333:1732.

75. Carey JC, Klebanoff MA, Hauth JC, et al. Metronidazole to prevent preterm delivery in pregnant women with asymptomatic bacterial vaginosis. *N Engl J Med* 2000;342:534.

76. Karhunen M. Placental transfer of metronidazole and tinidazole in early human pregnancy after a single infusion. *Br J Clin Pharmacol* 1984;18:254.

77. Centers for Disease Control. Pregnancy outcomes following systemic prenatal acyclovir exposure—June 1, 1984–June 30, 1993. *MMWR Morb Mortal Wkly Rep* 1992;42:806.

78. Scott LL, Sanchez PJ, Jackson GL, et al. Acyclovir suppression to prevent cesarean delivery after first-episode genital herpes. *Obstet Gynecol* 1996:87:69.

79. Stray-Pedersen B. Acyclovir in late pregnancy to prevent neonatal herpes simplex. *Lancet* 1990;336:756.

80. Andrews EB, Yankaskas BC, Cordero JF, et al. Acyclovir in pregnancy registry: six years' experience. *Obstet Gynecol* 1992;79:7.

81. Brandenburg K, Deinhard AS, DiNapoli J, et al. 1% permethrin cream rinse vs. 1% lindane shampoo in treating pediculosis capitis. *Am J Dis Child* 1986;140: 894.

82. American Thoracic Society. Treatment of tuberculosis and tuberculosis infection in adults and children. *Am J Respir Crit Care Med* 1994;149:1359–1374.

83. Briggs GG, Freeman RK, Yaffe SJ. *Drugs in pregnancy and lactation,* 5th ed. Baltimore: Williams & Wilkins, 1998:235.

84. Tan CG, Good CS, Milne WR, et al. A comparative trial of six day therapy with clotrimazole and nystatin in pregnant patients with vaginal candidiasis. *Postgrad Med* 1974;50:102.

85. Briggs GG, Freeman RK, Yaffe SJ. *Drugs in pregnancy and lactation,* 5th ed. Baltimore: Williams & Wilkins, 1998:728.

86. Rosa FW, Baum C, Shaw M. Pregnancy outcomes after first-trimester vaginitis drug therapy. *Obstet Gynecol* 1987;69:751.

87. Mastroiacovo P, Mazzone T, Rotto LD, et al. Prospective assessment of pregnancy outcomes after first-trimester exposure to fluconazole. *Am J Obstet Gynecol* 1996;175:1645.

88. Moretti ME, Ito S, Koren G. Disposition of maternal ketoconazole in breast milk. *Am J Obstet Gynecol* 1995;173:1625.

4

Treatment of Upper Respiratory Complaints in Pregnancy

John W. Ely

Department of Family Medicine, University of Iowa, Iowa City, Iowa

INTRODUCTION

Background

The common cold is the most frequent acute illness affecting humans (1–3). Most colds are self-diagnosed and self-treated (4,5), but because they are so common, physicians are often consulted. Patients frequently request antibiotics for severe episodes or for suspected sinusitis. Although colds are often regarded as minor problems, they can challenge physicians both diagnostically and therapeutically; diagnostically because the common cold is mimicked by other illnesses for which specific treatments are indicated; therapeutically because there is conflicting evidence on the efficacy of symptomatic treatment (6). Over-the-counter cold preparations are among the most common medications in household medicine cabinets (4,5) and among the most commonly used during pregnancy (7). Colds affect women more than men (8,9), and during pregnancy, they can be aggravated by estrogen-mediated nasal congestion (10).

Traditionally, physicians have reassured women that cold viruses are not teratogenic. However, concern has been raised by a Finnish study in which 393 mothers of anencephalic children and their time-area matched controls were asked about first-trimester illnesses. Among mothers of anencephalic children, 70 reported a first-trimester cold compared with only 17 controls (adjusted odds ratio, 4.5; 95% confidence interval, 2.2 to 9.1) (11). This association could not be explained by medications used to treat the colds, and there was no association with other infectious diseases. Second-trimester colds were not associated with anencephaly. Of course, recall bias can affect any retrospective study.

Clinical Presentation

Although cold viruses can result in asymptomatic infections, 70% to 90% of transmitted infections result in complaints of fatigue, malaise, rhinorrhea, nasal congestion, cough, and sore throat (12). Usually there is no fever or only a low-grade fever. The incubation period is 24 to 72 hours (12). Colds are communicable for 2 to 3 days after the onset of symptoms, which usually peak around the third day and resolve within 1–2 weeks, although the cough may last longer (8,12).

Epidemiology

In temperate climates, colds peak in the fall and again in the spring. Rhinoviruses are the most common cause (30% to 40% of all colds), followed by coronaviruses, respiratory syncytial virus, adenovirus, parainfluenza virus, influenza virus, and others (8). Known risk factors include emotional stress (13) and smoking (14), but colds are not caused by getting cold or damp.

The major means of transmission is from the donor's nose to the donor's hand, and from there to the recipient's hand, and from there to the recipient's nose or eye (8,15). Fomites can also transmit colds because rhinoviruses remain infectious for at least 3 hours after drying on hard surfaces (8). The transmission rate among household contacts is 38%, but hand washing can help to prevent colds (12). Pregnancy can exacerbate cold symptoms and predispose to sinus infection because of sinus ostia occlusion and decreased ciliary activity (10,16).

DIAGNOSIS

The common cold can progress to bacterial sinusitis, and the two diseases can be difficult to distinguish because the clinical findings overlap (17). The distinction is important because sinusitis is treated with antibiotics, whereas the common cold is treated symptomatically. A sense of facial pressure and sinus tenderness do not reliably predict sinusitis (17,18). Even computed tomography scans may be misleading because patients with colds often have radiographic findings that are indistinguishable from bacterial sinusitis (19).

Williams et al. (17,18) identified five clinical findings that predict sinusitis in patients with acute upper respiratory complaints: maxillary toothache, purulent nasal secretions on physical examination, poor response to decongestants, abnormal transillumination of the maxillary sinuses, and history of colored nasal discharge. In their study, a patient with all five findings had a 92% chance of having plain-film evidence of sinusitis, whereas a patient with none of the findings had only a 9% chance. However, most patients fell between these extremes and had intermediate probabilities. Thus, physicians are left with few practical tools to distinguish between colds and sinusitis. Treatment decisions often depend on the tension between patient wishes and physician beliefs about the overuse of antibiotics (20).

Patients with allergic rhinitis complain of rhinorrhea and nasal congestion, but they tend to have more chronic complaints. They usually have other manifestations of atopic disease such as sneezing, itching, and watery eyes, and these symptoms may have seasonal exacerbations. Vasomotor rhinitis is a poorly understood entity that is thought to result from abnormal autonomic responsiveness. It is characterized by chronic nasal congestion that can be aggravated by temperature changes and strong odors (21). Nonallergic rhinitis with eosinophilia (NARES) mimics allergic rhinitis but is not immunoglobulin-E mediated. NARES is often accompanied by asthma and nasal polyps, and patients tend to be intolerant of aspirin (22).

Pregnant women commonly develop a physiologic nasal congestion, sometimes called "rhinitis of pregnancy" (23,24). High levels of estrogen inhibit acetylcholinesterase activity, which stimulates additional acetylcholine production (10,25). The resulting edema of the nasal mucosa causes symptomatic congestion in 20% of pregnant women. Colds and allergic rhinitis can be exacerbated by this underlying congestion, which commonly begins late in the first trimester or early in the second. The symptoms worsen in the third trimester but usually resolve by the third week postpartum (23).

Patients with sore throats should be evaluated to distinguish between viral and streptococcal infection. A common strategy is to make the distinction based on clinical findings if they are obvious and to obtain an antigen test if they are not (26). Patients with mildly scratchy throats accompanied by rhinorrhea or cough and an unremarkable examination require only symptomatic treatment without laboratory evaluation. Patients with severe sore throat and fever accompanied by purulent pharyngitis and tender cervical lymph nodes can be given antibiotics without further testing. When the clinical findings are equivocal, a rapid streptococcal antigen test can help. These tests have high specificity (95%) but low sensitivity (as low as 60%). Therefore, many physicians treat with antibiotics if the antigen test is positive and obtain a routine throat culture if it is negative (26,27).

TREATMENT

Common Cold

Although there is no cure for the common cold, a variety of medications has provided symptomatic relief in randomized clinical trials (6). The most popular medications include antihistamines, decongestants, and cough remedies.

In 1997, a list of the 100 most commonly prescribed drugs in the United States included three antihistamines [loratadine (Claritin), cetirizine (Zyrtec), and fexofenadine (Allegra)] (28). Antihistamines fall into two groups: sedating (e.g., chlorpheniramine, diphenhydramine, pyrilamine, triprolidine) and nonsedating (e.g., astemizole, loratadine, cetirizine, fexofenadine). When taking sedating antihistamines, patients should not drive or operate dangerous equipment. The nonsedating antihistamine astemizole (Hismanal) can lead to life-threatening arrhythmias in patients with impaired hepatic metabolism, either from liver disease or concomitant administration of certain drugs (e.g., erythromycin, clarithromycin, ketoconazole, itraconazole). Arrhythmias have not been associated with the other nonsedating antihistamines (e.g., loratadine, cetirizine, fexofenadine) (29,30).

In cold sufferers, the beneficial effects of antihistamines probably result from their atropine-like drying action rather than their antihistamine action (31). Clinical trials in patients with colds demonstrated symptom relief with the use of some antihistamines [e.g., chlorpheniramine (Chlor-Trimeton), clemastine (Tavist)] but not others [e.g., diphenhydramine (Benadryl), triprolidine (Actifed)] (6,8).

Commonly used oral decongestants include phenylephrine (Codimal), pseudoephedrine (Sudafed), and phenylpropanolamine (Entex) (In November 2000, the FDA asked that products containing phenylpropanolamine no longer be marketed because of a possible association with hemorrhagic stroke). These drugs cause vasoconstriction of the nasal mucosa and a reduction in rhinorrhea. Side effects include elevated heart rate and diastolic blood pressure, palpitations, fatigue, and dizziness (6). Pseudoephedrine and phenylpropanolamine relieved cold symptoms in clinical trials (6,32). Many oral preparations combine a decongestant with an antihistamine, and such combinations can also relieve cold symptoms (6,33).

The most common topical decongestants are phenylephrine (Neo-Synephrine), which is short acting, and oxymetazoline (Afrin), which is long acting. Neither should be used for more than 3 days because of their tendency to cause rebound congestion (rhinitis medicamentosa). Oral decongestants do not cause rebound nasal congestion (34).

Colds are often accompanied by coughs, which can interfere with sleep. Cough medicines fall into three categories: antitussives, expectorants, and mucolytics. Expectorants (e.g., guaifenesin, ipecac, terpin hydrate, iodine products) and mucolytics (e.g., acetylcysteine) have little benefit in reducing cough or sputum production (6,35). Codeine and dextromethorphan are the most commonly used antitussives and both are effective (36). Benzonatate (Tessalon) is related to tetracaine and, when taken orally, inhibits coughing by anesthetizing the stretch receptors in the bronchioles and pleura (34). Over-the-counter cough drops often contain menthol, which can provide a local counterirritant effect.

Zinc has shortened the duration of cold symptoms in some studies but not in others (37–40). Intranasal ipratropium was found to decrease nasal secretions in one study (41). Naproxen treatment did not alter virus shedding in subjects with experimental rhinovirus colds, but it reduced headache, malaise, myalgia, and cough (42). Chicken soup was found to increase nasal mucous velocity and decrease airflow resistance in 15 healthy volunteers (43). Other purported treatments and preventive agents without firm evidence of benefit include inhaled steam, vitamin C, and interferon (8,31,44). Various herbs have been used but with little evidence of efficacy (45).

Bacterial Sinusitis

Bacterial sinusitis can present with either acute or chronic symptoms. In either case, antibiotics are prescribed along with measures to reduce nasal congestion. Acute sinusitis is usually caused by *Streptococcus pneumoniae, Haemophilus influenzae,* or *Moraxella catarrhalis* (46). Antibiotics of choice that are relevant in pregnancy include amoxicillin/clavulanate, cefuroxime axetil, clarithromycin, and cefprozil (27). Chronic sinusitis, which is often associated with anaerobic bacteria, should be managed in consultation with an otolaryngologist.

Allergic Rhinitis

Allergic rhinitis is best treated by avoiding the offending allergen. This strategy is more practical for perennial rhinitis (e.g., pets, dust, molds) than for seasonal rhinitis (e.g., pollens). When avoidance is not possible, treatment includes nonsedating antihistamines and topical steroids. The nonsedating antihistamines are as effective as the sedating antihistamines and have fewer anticholinergic effects such as dry mouth and constipation. Topical nasal steroids, which do not cause adrenal suppression at recommended doses, are considered first-line therapy for allergic rhinitis (47). Azelastine (Astelin) is an antihistamine nose spray that is effective in relieving allergic rhinitis symptoms, but oral antihistamines and nasal steroids are preferred (48). If medications are ineffective, allergy immunotherapy can be considered, but immunotherapy is costly and inconvenient, and most patients can be managed without it.

Other Causes of Nasal Congestion

The physiologic nasal congestion that occurs during pregnancy is sometimes severe enough to warrant treatment with an antihistamine-decongestant combination (Tables 4.1 and 4.2). Topical steroids have also been used for this condition (10). Topical decongestants should not be used because rhinitis of pregnancy is a chronic condition, and chronic use of topical decongestants can lead to rhinitis medicamentosa.

Vasomotor rhinitis is often refractory to treatment, but antihistamines and decongestants have been used. Patients are advised to avoid strong odors when possible, and they should be warned about the dangers of prolonged use of decongestant sprays. Treatment of NARES involves avoidance of aspirin (22) and chronic therapy with topical steroids using the lowest effective dose.

Sore Throat

Many patients with sore throat require only confirmation that they do not have streptococcal pharyngitis. Patients who request symptomatic relief can be treated with throat lozenges, saline gargles, and oral analgesics. For streptococcal pharyngitis, the antibiotic of choice is penicillin G (e.g., Pen VK 500 mg twice daily for 10 days). Patients should be advised to complete the full 10-day antibiotic course to prevent rheumatic fever. Penicillin-allergic patients can be treated with a macrolide (e.g., erythromycin, azithromycin) or a second-generation cephalosporin (27).

DRUG SAFETY DURING PREGNANCY

Antihistamines

Sedating Antihistamines

Most sedating antihistamines are safe during pregnancy (Table 4.3). In the Collaborative Perinatal Project, only brompheniramine (Bromfed) was associated with malformations (49). Among 65 women exposed to brompheniramine during the first trimester, there were 10 malformed infants (relative risk, 2.34; $p < 0.05$) (49). Analysis of these data showed that the defects were mild with markedly varying rates at the participating institutions. The increased relative risk is therefore probably not of clinical significance. Other antihistamines in this study were not associated with an increased malformation rate. These included chlorpheniramine, diphenhydramine, trimethobenzamide, methapyrilene, thonzylamine, pyrilamine, tripelennamine, phenyltoloxamine, and buclizine.

In the Boston Collaborative Drug Surveillance Program, only five (3%) of 172 brompheniramine-exposed women delivered malformed infants, which was not more than expected (50). A meta-analysis found no evidence to implicate brompheniramine as a teratogen (51). In the Boston Collaborative Program, none of the sedating antihistamines was associated with malformations nor were two combination products: triprolidine with pseudoephedrine (Actifed) and phenylpropanolamine with chlorpheniramine (Ornade). In a cohort of 1,502 San Diego women, antihistamines were not associated with congenital malformations (52). This study included 269 women exposed to chlorpheniramine (Chor-Trimeton). Azatadine (Trinalin) was not found to be teratogenic among 127 Michigan Medicaid recipients (53).

In a study of 3,026 premature infants weighing less than 1,750 g, retrolental fibroplasia was more common among infants exposed to

TABLE 4.1. *Over-the-counter combination cold and cough preparations*

Trade name	Antihistamine	Decongestant	Cough remedy	Analgesic
Actifed Cold & Allergy	TR	PS	—	—
Actifed Allergy Daytime	—	PS	—	—
Actifed Nighttime	DI	PS	—	—
Actifed Cold & Sinus	TR	PS	—	AC
Actifed Sinus Daytime	—	PS	—	AC
Actifed Sinus Nighttime	DI	PS	—	AC
Advil Cold & Sinus	—	PS	—	IB
Alka-Seltzer Plus Cold & Cough	CH	PP	DM	AS
Alka-Seltzer Plus Night-Time Cold	DO	PP	DM	AS
Alka-Seltzer Plus Cold	CH	PP	—	AS
Alka-Seltzer Plus Cold & Sinus	—	PP	—	AS
Alka-Seltzer Plus Cold & Flu	CH	PP	DM	AC
Allerest Maximum Strength	CH	PS	—	—
Allerest No Drowsiness	—	PS	—	AC
Benylin Adult Formula Cough Suppressant	—	—	DM	—
Benylin Cough Suppressant Expectorant	—	—	GU, DM	—
Benylin Multi-Symptom	—	PS	GU, DM	—
Comtrex Cold & Flu Reliever	CH	PS	DM	AC
Comtrex Cold & Flu Reliever	CH	PP	DM	AC
Comtrex Cold & Flu Reliever Liquid[a]	CH	PS	DM	AC
Comtrex Deep Chest Cold & Congestion Relief	—	PP	GU, DM	AC
Comtrex Non-Drowsy	—	PS	DM	AC
Contac Day Cold & Flu	—	PS	DM	AC
Contac Night Cold & Flu	DI	PS	—	AC
Contac 12 Hour	CH	PP	—	—
Contac Severe Cold & Flu	CH	PP	DM	AC
Contac Severe Cold & Flu Non-Drowsy	—	PS	DM	AC
Coricidin HBP Cold & Flu	CH	—	—	AC
Coricidin HBP Cough & Cold	CH	—	DM	—
Coricidin HBP Nighttime Cold & Cough	DI	—	—	AC
Coricidin D Decongestant	CH	PP	—	AC
Dimetapp Allergy	BR	—	—	—
Dimetapp Allergy Sinus	BR	PP	—	AC
Dimetapp Cold & Cough	BR	PP	DM	—
Dimetapp Elixir	BR	PP	—	—
Dimetapp DM Elixir	BR	PP	DM	—
Dimetapp Extentabs	BR	PP	—	—
Dimetapp	BR	PP	—	—
Dristan Sinus	—	PS	—	IB
Dristan Cold	CH	PH	—	AC
Drixoral Cold & Allergy	BR[b]	PS	—	—
Drixoral Nasal Decongestant	—	PS	—	—
Drixoral Cold & Flu	BR[b]	PS	—	AC
Drixoral Allergy/Sinus	BR[b]	PS	—	AC
Novahistine Elixir	CH	PH	—	—
Novahistine DMX	—	PS	GU, DM	—
Robitussin	—	—	GU	—
Robitussin Cold & Cough	—	PS	GU, DM	—
Robitussin Cold, Cough & Flu	—	PS	GU, DM	AC
Robitussin Severe Congestion	—	PS	GU	—
Robitussin-CF	—	PP	GU, DM	—
Robitussin-DM			GU, DM	
Robitussin-PE	—	PS	GU	—
Robitussin Cough Suppressant	—	—	DM	—
Robitussin Cough & Cold	—	PS	DM	—
Robitussin Night-Time Cold	DO	PS	DM	AC

Continued

TABLE 4.1. Continued

Trade name	Antihistamine	Decongestant	Cough remedy	Analgesic
Sinarest	CH	PS	—	AC
Sine-Off Sinus	CH	PS	—	AC
Sine-Off No Drowsiness		PS	—	AC
Sine-Off Night Time Formula Sinus, Cold & Flu	DI	PS	—	AC
Sinutab Non-Drying	—	PS	GU	—
Sinutab Sinus Allergy	CH	PS	—	AC
Sinutab Sinus	—	PS	—	AC
Sudafed	—	PS	—	—
Sudafed Cold & Allergy	CH	PS	—	—
Sudafed Cold & Cough	—	PS	GU, DM	AC
Sudafed Cold & Sinus	—	PS	—	AC
Sudafed Non-Drying Sinus	—	PS	GU	—
Sudafed, Severe Cold	—	PS	DM	AC
Sudafed Sinus	—	PS	—	AC
Tavist-1	CL	—	—	—
Tavist-D	CL	PP	—	—
Tavist Sinus	—	PS	—	AC
Thera Flu, Flu and Cold	CH	PS	—	AC
Thera Flu, Flu, Cold & Cough	CH	PS	DM	AC
Thera Flu Flu and Cold for Sore Throat	CH	PS	—	AC
Thera Flu Nighttime	CH	PS	DM	AC
Thera Flu Non-Drowsy	—	PS	DM	AC
Thera Flu Non-Drowsy Sinus	—	PS	—	AC
Triaminic AM Cough & Decongestant	—	PS	DM	—
Triaminic AM Decongestant	—	PS	—	—
Triaminic Expectorant	—	PP	GU	—
Triaminic Nighttime Cough and Cold	CH	PS	DM	—
Triaminic Sore Throat	—	PS	DM	AC
Triaminic	CH	PP	—	—
Triaminicol Cold & Cough	CH	PP	DM	—
Triaminic-DM	—	PP	DM	—
Triaminicin	CH	PP	—	AC
Tylenol Cold No Drowsiness	—	PS	DM	AC
Tylenol Cold Multi-Symptom	CH	PS	DM	AC
Tylenol Cold Severe Congestion Multisymptom	—	PS	GU, DM	AC
Tylenol Cough Multi-Symptom	—	—	DM	AC
Tylenol Cough Multi-Symptom with Decongestant	—	PS	DM	AC
Tylenol Flu No Drowsiness	—	PS	DM	AC
Tylenol Flu Nighttime	DI	PS	—	AC
Tylenol Severe Allergy	DI	—	—	AC
Tylenol Allergy Sinus Nighttime	DI	PS	—	AC
Tylenol Allergy Sinus	CH	PS	—	AC
Tylenol Sinus	—	PS	—	AC
Vicks 44 Cough[a]	—	—	DM	—
Vicks 44D Cough & Head Congestion[a]	—	PS	DM	—
Vicks 44E Cough & Chest Congestion[a]	—	—	GU, DM	—
Vicks 44M Cough, Cold & Flu[a]	CH	PS	DM	AC
Vicks Dayquil	—	PS	DM	AC
Vicks Dayquil Sinus	IB	PS	—	—
Vicks Nyquil Adult Nighttime Cold/Flu	DO	PS	DM	AC
Vicks Nyquil[a]	DO	PS	DM	AC

[a]Contains alcohol.
[b]Dexbrompheniramine.

Antihistamines: CH, chlorpheniramine; CL, clemastine; DI, diphenhydramine; DO, doxylamine. Decongestants: PH, phenylephrine; PP, phenylpropanolamine; PS, pseudoephedrine; TR, triprolidine. Analgesics: AC, acetaminophen; AS, aspirin; IB, ibuprofen. Cough preparations: DM, dextromethorphan; GU, guaifenesin.

(In November 2000, the FDA asked that products containing phenylpropanolamine no longer be marketed because of a possible association with hemorrhagic stroke.)

TABLE 4.2. *Prescription combination cold and cough preparations*

Trade name	Antihistamine	Decongestant	Cough remedy
Actifed with codeine	TR	PS	CO
Claritin-D 12 hour	LO	PS	—
Claritin-D 24-Hour	LO	PS	—
Codimal DH	PY	PH	HY
Codimal DM	PY	PH	DM
Codimal-L.A.	CH	PS	—
Codimal PH	PY	PH	CO
Deconamine	CH	PS	—
Deconamine SR	CH	PS	—
Entex	—	PP	GU
Entex LA	—	PP	GU
Histussin D	—	PS	HY
Histussin HC	CH	—	HY
Humibid DM	—	—	DM, GU
Naldecon	CH	PP	—
Ornade Spansules	CH	PP	—
Phenergan with Dextromethorphan	PR	—	DM
Phenergan VC	PR	—	—
Phenergan VC with codeine	PR	—	CO
Robitussin A-C	—	—	GU, CO
Robitussin-DAC	—	PS	GU, CO
Rondec Syrup	CA	PS	—
Rondec-DM Syrup	CA	PS	DM
Rynatan	CH, PY	—	—
Tessalon Pearles	—	—	BE

Antihistamines: CA, carbinoxamine; CH, chlorpheniramine; LO, loratadine; PR, promethazine; PY, pyrilamine; TR, triprolidine. Cough preparations: BE, benzonatate; CO, codeine; DM, dextromethorphan; GU, guaifenesin; HY, hydrocodone. Decongestants: PH, phenylephrine; PP, phenylpropanolamine; PS, pseudoephedrine.

(In November 2000, the FDA asked that products containing phenylpropanolamine no longer be marketed because of a possible association with hemorrhagic stroke.)

TABLE 4.3. *Antihistamines*

Generic name	Trade name	Comment
Azatadine	Optimine	—
Astemizole	Hismanal	Nonsedating, dangerous drug interactions[a]
Brompheniramine	Dimetane	Associated with malformations in CPP, infant irritability with breast-feeding
Carbinoxamine	Rondec	—
Cetirizine	Zyrtec	Nonsedating
Chlorpheniramine	Chor-Trimeton	—
Clemastine	Tavist	Infant irritability with breast-feeding
Diphenhydramine	Benadryl	Antiprurutic, very sedating
Doxylamine	Unisom	Antinauseant
Fexofenadine	Allegra	Nonsedating
Hydroxyzine	Atarax, Vistaril	Antiprurutic, very sedating
Loratadine	Claritin	Nonsedating
Meclizine	Antivert	Used for vertigo
Promethazine	Phenergan	—
Pyrilamine	Codimal	—
Triprolidine	Actifed	—

[a]Contraindicated with cisapride, erythromycin, itraconazole, ketoconazole, and others
CPP, Collaborative Perinatal Project (49).

antihistamines within 2 weeks of premature delivery (54). Nineteen of 86 (22%) exposed to antihistamines developed retrolental fibroplasia compared with 324 of 2,940 (11%) unexposed infants (rate ratio, 2.0; 95% confidence interval, 1.3 to 3.1). These findings persisted after controlling for many potential confounders. The specific antihistamines involved were not reported.

Nonsedating Antihistamines

Limited safety information is available for the newer nonsedating antihistamines (Table 4.3). In a cohort study, 114 astemizole (Hismanal)-exposed women were matched with 114 women exposed to nonteratogens (e.g., dental x-rays, acetaminophen) (55). There were two major malformations in the astemizole group and two in the control group. In a study of 39 women exposed to cetirizine (Zyrtec), there was no increase in malformations compared with a control group (56). Animal studies with cetirizine have also been reassuring (57). There are no controlled human studies for loratadine (Claritin) or fexofenadine (Allegra), but these drugs were not teratogenic in animals (manufacturers' data).

Antihistamines with Nonrespiratory Indications

Several antihistamines have primary indications not directly related to upper respiratory complaints. Hydroxyzine (Atarax, Vistaril) is used for pruritus, meclizine (Antivert) for dizziness, diphenhydramine (Benadryl) for sleep and pruritus, and one of the most studied drugs in pregnancy, doxylamine (a component of Bendectin), was used in the past for nausea and vomiting of pregnancy. Promethazine (Phenergan), a phenothiazine antihistamine, is a component of cough remedies and is also used as an anti-nauseant. There were nine malformations among 114 promethazine exposures (relative risk, 1.17; not significant) in the Collaborative Perinatal Project (49). A metaanalysis of antihistamines used mostly for nonrespiratory complaints found a protective effect against malformations (odds ratio, 0.76; 95% confidence interval, 0.60 to 0.94) (58). This apparent benefit may have resulted from the association between maternal nausea and good fetal outcomes rather than from a direct effect of antihistamines.

Oral Decongestants

The most common oral decongestants, which are all sympathomimetic agents, include pseudoephedrine (Sudafed), phenylephrine (Codimal), and phenylpropanolamine (Entex) (Table 4.4) (In November 2000, the FDA asked that products containing phenylpropanolamine no longer be marketed because of a possible association with hemorrhagic stroke). In the Collaborative Perinatal Project, the relative risk of malformations for all sympathomimetics was 1.19 ($p < 0.05$) (49). There were 102 (8%) malformations among 1,249 infants exposed to phenylephrine, but the standardized relative risk (1.23) did not reach statistical significance. In this study, there was one malformation among 39 women exposed to pseudoephedrine (Sudafed) with a nonsignificant relative risk of 0.35. Among 726 women exposed to phenylpropanolamine, there were 71 (10%) malformed infants with a significant relative risk (1.4, $p < 0.01$) (49). Sympathomimetics not associated with malformations in this study included ephedrine and naphazoline.

In the Boston Collaborative Program, 421 women were exposed to pseudoephedrine and only seven (1.7%) infants had congenital disorders

TABLE 4.4. *Decongestants*

Generic name	Trade name	Comments
Oxymetazoline	Afrin	Avoid topical use for more than 3 days
Phenylephrine	Neo-Synephrine	Avoid topical use for more than 3 days
Phenylpropanolamine	Entex	—
Pseudoephedrine	Sudafed	—
Xylometazoline	Otrivin	Avoid topical use for more than 3 days

(50). In this study, only one infant of 129 (0.8%) exposed to phenylephrine had a malformation. There were two (2.4%) malformations among 82 women who took a combination product (Ornade) containing phenylpropanolamine and chlorpheniramine. Among Michigan Medicaid recipients, 940 newborns were exposed to pseudoephedrine during the first trimester, and 37 (3.9%) had major malformations (40 expected) (53).

In a case-control study, gastroschisis was associated with first trimester use of pseudoephedrine (relative risk, 3.2; 95% confidence limits, 1.3 to 7.7) (59). This association was considered plausible because gastroschisis is thought to be related to disruption of the omphalomesenteric artery (53,60). However, when other conditions thought to be related to vascular malformations were studied, no association was found (53,59).

Topical Preparations

Topical Nasal Decongestants

Two common topical nasal decongestants, oxymetazoline (Afrin) and phenylephrine (Neo-Synephrine), are considered safe during pregnancy. If used for more than 3 to 4 days, however, both can lead to rhinitis medicamentosa. In the Boston Collaborative Program, there were only two (1.3%) malformations among 155 first-trimester exposures to oxymetazoline (50). Xylometazoline (Otrivin), another topical decongestant, was associated with five congenital disorders in 207 exposures (2.4%), but this rate was not greater than expected (50).

Baxi et al. (60) reported a nonreactive nonstress test in a woman at 41 weeks gestation who overused oxymetazoline (Dristan Nasal Spray; six uses in 16 hours). A spontaneous contraction stress test showed late decelerations that continued after amniotomy. After the drug was metabolized (6 hours later), the fetal heart rate pattern became normal (60). In a subsequent study, there were no significant effects on maternal or fetal circulation in 12 healthy gravidas after a single dose of oxymetazoline (61).

Phenylephrine was associated with eye and ear malformations in the Collaborative Perinatal Project, but it was not clear which exposures were topical and which systemic (49). Because of this association, oxymetazoline (Afrin) is considered the topical decongestant of choice during pregnancy (62).

Topical Nasal Steroids

The commonly used topical nasal steroids include beclomethasone, (Vancenase, Beconase), budesonide (Rhinocort), dexamethasone (Decadron), flunisolide (Nasalide), fluticasone (Flonase), and triamcinolone (Nasacort). They are relatively new preparations, and neither the Collaborative Perinatal Program nor the Boston Collaborative Drug Surveillance Program collected information about them. Inhaled topical steroids when used for the treatment of asthma in pregnancy are not associated with malformations (52). In a study of inhaled beclomethasone (used for asthma), there was one cardiac malformation among 45 pregnancies (63). However, the mother of the affected infant had diabetes and took many other medications. Among 229,101 Michigan Medicaid recipients, there were 16 (4.1%) major birth defects among 395 newborns exposed to beclomethasone (16 expected) (53). Oral dexamethasone is not considered a teratogen (53). Human experience with inhaled steroids is reassuring, and it seems reasonable to generalize these findings to nasal steroids.

Cough and Sore Throat Remedies

Codeine and dextromethorphan are commonly used cough suppressants, and neither is associated with fetal malformation (Table 4.5). In the Collaborative Perinatal Program, 948 women

TABLE 4.5. *Cough remedies*

Generic name	Trade name	Comments
Benzonatate	Tessalon Perles	—
Codeine	—	—
Dextromethorphan	Benylin DM	—
Hydrocodone	Hycodan	—
Guaifenesin	Robitussin	Expectorant
Terpin hydrate	—	Expectorant

took cough medications, and there were 71 malformed children (7.5%; relative risk, 1.10; not significant). Three hundred women took dextromethorphan, and there were 24 malformed children (8%; relative risk, 1.24; not significant). Codeine was taken by 563 women, and there were 48 malformations (9%; relative risk, 1.27; not significant).

In a study comparing 1,427 malformed infants and 3,001 controls, narcotic use in the first trimester was associated with inguinal hernias, cardiac defects, cleft lip and palate, and dislocated hip (64). In a Finnish study, narcotic use during the first trimester was associated with oral clefts (65,66). Among 229,101 Michigan Medicaid recipients, there were 7,640 first-trimester exposures to codeine and 375 (4.9%) major birth defects (325 expected) (53). Other factors such as the mother's illness and concurrent drug use were not controlled in this analysis (53). In the Boston Collaborative Program, there was one malformation among 59 infants exposed to dextromethorphan, which is considered the cough suppressant of choice during pregnancy (67,68). Benzonatate (Tessalon) is occasionally used as a cough suppressant, but there are insufficient data to recommend its use in pregnancy (34).

Guaifenesin (glyceryl guaiacolate) and terpin hydrate are expectorants with little efficacy, but they are included in many cough preparations. Among 197 women who took guaifenesin in the Collaborative Perinatal Project, there were 14 (7%) children with malformations (adjusted relative risk, 1.03) (49). In the Boston Collaborative Program, there were five (2%) malformed infants among 241 exposed to guaifenesin in the first trimester (50). There were 10 (7%) malformations among the 146 women who took elixir of terpin hydrate (relative risk, 1.47; not significant) in the Collaborative Perinatal Project (49). In the Boston Collaborative Program, there was one malformation among 144 infants (1%) exposed to terpin hydrate with codeine (50). Among 1,338 Michigan Medicaid recipients exposed to expectorants during the first trimester, there were 63 major birth defects (57 expected) (53). Saturated solution of potassium iodide, which is rarely used as an expectorant, should be avoided during pregnancy because it can cause fetal goiters.

Some cough syrups contain alcohol, which should generally be avoided during pregnancy (Table 4.1). Chasnoff et al. (69) reported a case of fetal alcohol syndrome in an infant whose mother drank as many as seven bottles daily of an over-the-counter cough suppressant (Ambenyl-D Decongestant Cough Formula) throughout the pregnancy (69).

Little is known about the safety of throat lozenges and cough drops during pregnancy. In the Boston Collaborative Program, there were nine (3.1%) congenital disorders among 292 infants exposed to cetylpyridinium chloride (Cepacol lozenges) during the first trimester (relative risk, 2.0; 95% confidence interval, 1.0 to 3.8) (50). There are no published data on the safety of menthol, another common ingredient in throat lozenges.

Antibiotics

Most antibiotics are considered safe during pregnancy. Trimethoprim/sulfamethoxazole is often used for sinusitis, but it should not be used during the first trimester because trimethoprim is a folate antagonist and may be teratogenic (70). Also, the sulfa component may lead to neonatal hyperbilirubinemia if given near delivery (71). The penicillins and cephalosporins, such as amoxicillin/clavulanate, cefuroxime axetil, and cefprozil, are considered safe during pregnancy (70). Clavulanate is a β-lactamase inhibitor that is combined with amoxicillin to form amoxicillin clavulanate (Augmentin). There were 24 (4.3%) major malformations (24 expected) among 556 newborns exposed to clavulanic acid in a large series of Michigan Medicaid patients (53). There were three (2.1%) major malformations (six expected) among 143 newborns exposed to cefuroxime during the first trimester (53). There are no human data on cefprozil, but no increased rates of malformations have been found in animal studies (70).

Clarithromycin was introduced in 1991, and there is little published information about its use in pregnancy. In a series of 34 exposures to clarithromycin during the first and early second trimesters, there were eight abortions (four spontaneous, four voluntary), 20 normal newborns, and one with a 0.5-cm brown mark on the temple (72). Pregnancy outcome was pending for the remaining five exposures. These outcomes were not considered unusual (53,72). Because of a paucity of data, clarithromycin should not be used as a first-line agent in pregnancy.

Other Treatments and Alternative Medicine

Ipratropium, an anticholinergic compound related to atropine, is used for severe asthma and has also been used to treat nasal congestion (41). Among 37 Michigan Medicaid recipients who took ipratropium for asthma, there was one malformation (a renal obstruction) (53).

High doses of vitamin C (more than 400 mg per day) were associated with a "conditioned scurvy" among two infants in a 1965 report (73). In a later case report, an anencephalic fetus was delivered by a woman who took high doses of vitamin C and other vitamins (74). However, doses as high as 2,000 mg per day were not associated with malformations in a third study (75).

In one study, zinc levels in cord blood were higher among infants with neural tube defects than among controls (76). When used as a dietary supplement, zinc has been found to increase the birth weights and head circumferences of infants born to zinc-deficient mothers (77) but not unselected healthy gravidas (78).

Naproxen, a nonsteroidal antiinflammatory agent, can lessen the symptoms of a cold (42), but drugs in this class should be avoided. In the third trimester, they can cause premature closure of the ductus arteriosus (79,80) and decreased urine production in the second and third trimesters. These drugs should not be used in women trying to conceive because they may block blastocyst implantation (81).

There are insufficient data to affirm the safety of interferon alpha and interferon beta during pregnancy. In any case, their use to prevent colds is controversial, and they are best avoided on that basis (82). There are insufficient safety data for herbal treatments of respiratory complaints, but herbal medications during pregnancy may have significant adverse effects (83,84).

BREAST-FEEDING

Most cold remedies are safe to use while breast-feeding. Antihistamine use during lactation was reviewed by Lione and Scialli (85) in 1996. Other than occasional case reports of infant irritability (with clemastine and brompheniramine), no consistent adverse effects were noted. Because of their anticholinergic properties, antihistamines could theoretically lead to decreased milk production, but this has not been reported.

Adverse effects from decongestants during breast-feeding have not been reported. Pseudoephedrine is concentrated in breast milk, but the American Academy of Pediatrics considers it compatible with breast feeding (86). There are no published data on the safety of dextromethorphan or guaifenesin during breast-feeding. The American Academy of Pediatrics considers codeine safe during lactation (86). The penicillins and cephalosporins are also safe to use during lactation (86). No breast-feeding data are available for clavulanate or clarithromycin.

SUMMARY

During pregnancy, upper respiratory tract complaints should be treated with a minimal number of drugs chosen based on the patient's specific signs and symptoms. Polypharmacy should be avoided. If rhinorrhea and nasal congestion from a cold require treatment, pseudoephedrine (Sudafed) 30 to 60 mg four times a day is a reasonable choice. A combination product containing chlorpheniramine and pseudoephedrine could also be used (Tables 4.1 and 4.2). For cough relief, a product containing dextromethorphan but not alcohol, such as Robitussin DM (10 mL every 4 hours as needed), would be a good choice. For allergic rhinitis, one or two inhalations in each nostril once a day of a nasal steroid such as beclomethasone (Beconase AQ, Vancenase AQ) could be given. If this is not effective, an oral nonsedating antihistamine, such as cetirizine (Zyrtec) 5 to 10 mg once daily could be added. For more information concerning the recent findings connecting phenylpropanolamine and the risk of hemorrhagic stroke, see work published in 2000 by Kernan and Viscoli et al. (87).

REFERENCES

1. Monto AS, Ullman BM. Acute respiratory illness in an American community: the Tecumseh study. *JAMA* 1974;227:164–169.
2. Dingle JH, Badger GF, Jordan WS, eds. *Illness in the home: a study of 25,000 illnesses in a group of Cleveland families.* Cleveland: Press of Western Reserve University, 1964.
3. National Center for Health Statistics. *Vital and health statistics: ambulatory care visits to physician offices, hospital outpatient departments, and emergency departments: United States, 1995, series 13.* Hyattsville, MD: U.S. Department of Health and Human Services, 1997.
4. Knapp DA, Knapp DE. Decision-making and self-medication. *Am J Hosp Pharm* 1972;29:1004–1012.
5. Levin LS, Idler EL. Self-care in health. *Annu Rev Public Health* 1983;4:181–201.
6. Smith MBH, Feldman W. Over-the-counter cold medications: a critical review of clinical trials between 1950 and 1991. *JAMA* 1991;269:2258–2263.
7. Hill RM, Craig JP, Chaney MD, et al. Utilization of over-the-counter drugs during pregnancy. *Clin Obstet Gynecol* 1977;20:381–394.
8. Lorber B. The common cold. *J Gen Intern Med* 1996;11:229–236.
9. Monto AS, Bryan ER, Ohmit S. Rhinovirus infections in Tecumseh, Michigan: frequency of illness and number of serotypes. *J Infect Dis* 1987;156:43–49.
10. Lekas MD. Rhinitis during pregnancy and rhinitis medicamentosa. *Otolaryngol Head Neck Surg* 1992;107:845–849.
11. Kurppa K, Holmberg PC, Kuosma E, et al. Anencephaly and maternal common cold. *Teratology* 1991;44:51–55.
12. Gwaltney JM Jr. The common cold. In: Mandell GL, Bennett JE, Dolin R, eds. *Principles and practice of infectious diseases,* 4th ed. New York: Churchill-Livingstone, 1995:561–566.
13. Cohen S, Tyrrell DAJ, Smith AP. Psychological stress and susceptibility to the common cold. *N Engl J Med* 1991;325:606–612.
14. Cohen S, Tyrrell DA, Russell MA, et al. Smoking, alcohol consumption, and susceptibility to the common cold. *Am J Public Health* 1993;83:1277–1283.
15. Gwaltney JM Jr. Hand-to-hand transmission of rhinovirus colds. *Ann Intern Med* 1978;88:463–467.
16. Lewis JH. Surgery of the ear, nose and throat in pregnancy. In: Barber HRK, Graber EA, eds. *Surgical diseases in pregnancy.* Philadelphia: WB Saunders, 1974:248–253.
17. Williams JW, Simel DL. Does this patient have sinusitis? Diagnosing acute sinusitis by history and physical examination. *JAMA* 1993;270:1242–1246.
18. Williams JW Jr, Simel DL, Roberts L, et al. Clinical evaluation for sinusitis. Making the diagnosis by history and physical examination. *Ann Intern Med* 1992;117:705–710.
19. Gwaltney JM, Phillips CD, Miller RD, et al. Computed tomographic study of the common cold. *N Engl J Med* 1994;330:25–30.
20. Gonzales R, Steiner JF, Sande MA. Antibiotic prescribing for adults with colds, upper respiratory tract infections, and bronchitis by ambulatory care physicians. *JAMA* 1997;278:901–904.
21. Knight A. The differential diagnosis of rhinorrhea. *J Allergy Clin Immunol* 1995;95[5 Pt 2 Suppl]:1080–1083.
22. Moneret-Vautrin DA, Hsieh V, Wayoff M, et al. Nonallergic rhinitis with eosinophilia syndrome a precursor of the triad: nasal polyposis, intrinsic asthma, and intolerance to aspirin. *Ann Allergy* 1990;64:513–518.
23. Crawford LV, Cohen RM. Therapy for allergic rhinitis. *Compr Ther* 1985;11:60–69.
24. Mabry RL. The management of nasal obstruction during pregnancy. *Ear Nose Throat J* 1983;62:28–33.
25. Marbry RL. Rhinitis of pregnancy. *South Med J* 1986;79:965–971.
26. Komaroff AL. Sore throat in adult patients. In: Panzer RJ, Black ER, Griner PF, eds. *Diagnostic strategies for common medical problems.* Philadelphia: American College of Physicians, 1991:186–195.
27. Gilbert DN, Moellering RC Jr, Sande MA. *The Sanford guide to antimicrobial therapy,* 28th ed. Vienna, VA: Antimicrobial Therapy, Inc., 1998.
28. Anonymous. Top 200 drugs of 1997. *Pharm Times* 1998;April:31–49.
29. Rizack MA. *The Medical Letter handbook of adverse drug interactions.* New Rochelle, NY: The Medical Letter Inc., 1998.
30. Hardman JG, Limbird LE, Molinoff PB, Ruddon RW, Gilman AG, eds. *Goodman & Gilman's The pharmacological basis of therapeutics,* 9th ed. New York: McGraw-Hill, 1996.
31. Lowenstein SR, Parrino TA. Management of the common cold. *Adv Intern Med* 1987;32:207–234.
32. Bye CE, Cooper J, Empey DW, et al. Effects of pseudoephedrine and triprolidine, alone and in combination, on symptoms of the common cold. *BMJ* 1980;281:189–190.
33. Curley FJ, Irwin RS, Pratter MR, et al. Cough and the common cold. *Am Rev Respir Dis* 1988;238:305–311.
34. Hornby PJ, Abrahams TP. Pulmonary pharmacology. *Clin Obstet Gynecol* 1996;39:17–35.
35. Brucker MC. Management of common minor discomforts in pregnancy. Part I. Managing upper respiratory infections in pregnancy. *J Nurse Midwifery* 1987;32:349–356.
36. Parvez L, Vaidya M, Sakhardande A, et al. Evaluation of antitussive agents in man. *Pulm Pharmacol* 1996;9:299–308.
37. Mossad SB, Macknin ML, Medendorp SV, et al. Zinc gluconate lozenges for treating the common cold: a randomized, double-blind, placebo-controlled study. *Ann Intern Med* 1996;125:81–88.
38. Macknin ML, Piedmonte M, Calendine C, et al. Zinc gluconate lozenges for treating the common cold in children. *JAMA* 1998;279:1962–1967.
39. Gadomski A. A cure for the common cold? Zinc again. *JAMA* 1998;279:1999–2000.
40. Jackson JL, Peterson C, Lesho E. A meta-analysis of zinc salts lozenges and the common cold. *Arch Intern Med* 1997;10:2373–2376.

41. Borum P, Olsen L, Winther B, et al. Ipratropium nasal spray: a new treatment for rhinorrhea in the common cold. *Am Rev Respir Dis* 1981;123:418–420.

42. Sperber SJ, Hendley JO, Hayden FG, et al. Effects of naproxen on experimental rhinovirus colds: a randomized, double-blind, controlled trial. *Ann Intern Med* 1992;117:37–41.

43. Saketkhoo K, Januszkiewicz A, Sackner M. Effects of drinking hot water, cold water, and chicken soup on nasal mucus velocity and nasal airflow resistance. *Chest* 1978;74:408–410.

44. Hemila H. Does vitamin C alleviate the symptoms of the common cold? A review of current evidence. *Scand J Nutr* 1994;67:1–6.

45. Tyler VE. *Herbs of choice. The therapeutic use of phytomedicinals.* New York: Pharmaceutical Products Press, 1994.

46. Gwaltney JM. Acute community-acquired sinusitis. *Clin Infect Dis* 1996;23:1209–1235.

47. Mabry RL. Topical pharmacotherapy for allergic rhinitis. *South Med J* 1992;85:149–154.

48. Anonymous. Azelastine nasal spray for allergic rhinitis. *Med Lett* 1997;39:45–47.

49. Heinonen OP, Slone D, Shapiro S. *Birth defects and drugs in pregnancy.* Littleton, MA: Publishing Sciences Group, Inc., 1977.

50. Aselton P, Jick H, Milunsky A, et al. First trimester drug use and congenital disorders. *Obstet Gynecol* 1985;65:451–455.

51. Seto A, Einarson T, Koren G. Evaluation of brompheniramine safety in pregnancy. *Reprod Toxicol* 1993;7:393–395.

52. Schatz M, Zeiger RS, Harden K, et al. The safety of asthma and allergy medications during pregnancy. *J Allergy Clin Immunol* 1997;100:301–306.

53. Briggs GG, Freeman RK, Yaffee SJ. *Drugs in pregnancy and lactation*, 5th ed. Baltimore: Williams & Wilkins, 1998.

54. Zierler S, Purohit D. Prenatal antihistamine exposure and retrolental fibroplasia. *Am J Epidemiol* 1986;123:192–196.

55. Pastuszak A, Schick B, D'Alimonte D, et al. The safety of astemizole in pregnancy. *J Allergy Clin Immunol* 1996;98:748–750.

56. Einarson A, Bailey B, Jung G, et al. Prospective controlled study of hydroxyzine and cetirizine in pregnancy. *Ann Allergy Asthma Immunol* 1997;78:183–186.

57. Kamijima M, Sakai Y, Kinoshita K, et al. Reproductive and developmental toxicity studies of cetirizine in rats and rabbits. *Clin Rep* 1994;28:1877–1903.

58. Seto A, Einarson T, Koren G. Pregnancy outcome following first trimester exposure to antihistamines: meta-analysis. *Am J Perinatol* 1997;14:119–124.

59. Werler MM, Mitchell AA, Shapiro S. First trimester maternal medication use in relation to gastroschisis. *Teratology* 1992;45:361–367.

60. Baxi LV, Gindoff PR, Pregenzer GJ, et al. Fetal heart rate changes following maternal administration of a nasal decongestant. *Am J Obstet Gynecol* 1985;153:799–800.

61. Rayburn WF, Anderson JC, Smith CV, et al. Uterine and fetal Doppler flow changes from a single dose of a long-acting intranasal decongestant. *Obstet Gynecol* 1990;76:180–182.

62. Schatz M, Zeiger RS. Diagnosis and management of rhinitis during pregnancy. *Allergy Proc* 1988;9:545–554.

63. Greenberger PA, Patterson R. Beclomethasone dipropionate for severe asthma during pregnancy. *Ann Intern Med* 1983;98:478–480.

64. Bracken MB, Holford TR. Exposure to prescribed drugs in pregnancy and association with congenital malformations. *Obstet Gynecol* 1981;58:336–344.

65. Saxen I. Epidemiology of cleft lip and palate: an attempt to rule out chance correlations. *Br J Prev Soc Med* 1975;29:103–110.

66. Saxen I. Associations between oral clefts and drugs taken during pregnancy. *Int J Epidemiol* 1975;4:37–44.

67. Rayburn WF. OTC drugs and pregnancy. *Perinatol Neonatol* 1984;8:21–27.

68. Report of the Working Group on Asthma and Pregnancy. Executive summary: management of asthma during pregnancy. *J Allergy Clin Immunol* 1994;93:139–162.

69. Chasnoff IJ, Diggs G, Schnoll SH. Fetal alcohol effects and maternal cough syrup abuse. *Am J Dis Child* 1981;135:968.

70. Anonymous. Antimicrobial therapy for obstetric patients. *ACOG Educ Bull* 1998;245:1–10.

71. Landers DV, Green JR, Sweet RL. Antibiotic use during pregnancy and the postpartum period. *Clin Obstet Gynecol* 1983;26:391–406.

72. Schick B, Hom M, Librizzi R, et al. Pregnancy outcome following exposure to clarithromycin. Abstracts of the Ninth International Conference of the Organization of Teratology Information Services, May 2–4, 1996, Salt Lake City, Utah. *Reprod Toxicol* 1996;10:162(abst).

73. Cochrane WA. Overnutrition in prenatal and neonatal life: a problem? *Can Med Assoc J* 1965;93:893–899.

74. Averback P. Anencephaly associated with megavitamin therapy. *Can Med Assoc J* 1976;114:995.

75. Ingalls TH, Draper R, Teel HM. Vitamin C in human pregnancy and lactation. II. Studies during lactation. *Am J Dis Child* 1938;56:1011–1019.

76. Zimmerman AW. Hyperzincemia in anencephaly and spina bifida: a clue to the pathogenesis of neural tube defects? *Neurology* 1984;34:443–450.

77. Goldenberg RL, Tamura T, Neggers Y, et al. The effect of zinc supplementation on pregnancy outcome. *JAMA* 1995;274:463–468.

78. Jonsson B, Hauge B, Larsen MF, et al. Zinc supplementation during pregnancy: a double blind randomised controlled trial. *Acta Obstet Gynecol Scand* 1996;75:725–729.

79. Rudolph AM. The effects of nonsteroidal antiinflammatory compounds on fetal circulation and pulmonary function. *Obstet Gynecol* 1981;58[Suppl]:63S–67S.

80. Levin DL. Effects of inhibition of prostaglandin synthesis on fetal development, oxygenation, and the fetal circulation. *Semin Perinatol* 1980;4:35–44.

81. Dawood MY. Nonsteroidal antiinflammatory drugs and reproduction. *Am J Obstet Gynecol* 1993;169:1255–1265.

82. Sperber SJ, Sorrentino JV, Riker DK, et al. Ineffectiveness of recombinant interferon-beta serine nasal drops for prophylaxis of natural colds. *J Infect Dis* 1989;160:700–705.

83. Jones TK, Lawson BM. Profound neonatal congestive heart failure caused by maternal consumption of blue cohosh herbal medication. *J Pediatr* 1998;132:550–552.

84. Mabina MH, Pitsoe SB, Moodley J. The effect of traditional herbal medicines on pregnancy outcome. The King Edward VIII Hospital experience. *South Afr Med J* 1997;87:1008–1010.

85. Lione A, Scialli AR. The developmental toxicity of the H1 histamine antagonists. *Reprod Toxicol* 1996;10:247–255.

86. Anonymous. American Academy of Pediatrics Committee on Drugs: the transfer of drugs and other chemicals into human milk. *Pediatrics* 1994;93:137–150.

87. Kernan WN, Viscoli CM, Brass LM, et al. Phenylpropanolamine and the risk of hemorrhagic stroke. *N Engl J Med* 2000;343:1826–1832.

5

Therapy of Asthma During Pregnancy

Ellen Louise Sakornbut and Laura A. Tavernier

Department of Family Medicine, University of Tennessee—Memphis, Memphis, Tennessee

INTRODUCTION

The most common chronic respiratory condition occurring in women during the reproductive years is asthma. Asthma, despite a better understanding of its pathogenesis and improved treatment regimens, continues to increase in prevalence, morbidity, and mortality in the United States and other industrialized nations. Asthma affects 4% to 10% of the population in the United States and constitutes approximately 1% of total health care expenditures. Approximately half the cost is attributed to emergency care, much of which could be avoided if appropriate management were provided in a longitudinal fashion (1,2).

Asthma affects 4% to 6% of all pregnancies, and status asthmaticus complicates approximately 0.2% of all pregnancies in the United States (3). Early studies on asthma in pregnancy documented statistically significant increases in preterm birth low birth weight and increased neonatal morbidity in pregnant patients with asthma compared with healthy pregnant patients. More recently, Schatz et al. (4) conducted a prospective case-controlled study in which pregnant patients with actively managed asthma were compared with healthy control obstetric patients. There were no statistically significant differences in preeclampsia, preterm birth, low birth weight, intrauterine growth restriction, congenital malformation, or perinatal mortality between the two groups. The conclusion from this study is that overall perinatal prognosis for women with well-controlled asthma during pregnancy is similar to that of their healthy counterparts. This same study did find a higher rate of pregnant asthmatics with chronic hypertension.

Inadequate treatment of asthma during pregnancy, primarily attributed to unsubstantiated fear of fetal effects of medication, is a major problem in the management of asthma in pregnancy (5). Issues addressed in this chapter include pertinent pathophysiology of asthma and how it may affect pregnancy, pregnancy outcomes, use of medication during pregnancy and lactation, non-pharmacologic measures, and treatment of acute exacerbations of asthma in the antepartum and intrapartum setting.

PHYSIOLOGIC PULMONARY CHANGES IN PREGNANCY

Pulmonary physiologic changes resulting in increased ventilation secondary to deeper inspiration are presumed to help meet increased basal oxygen consumption and metabolic rates (21% and 14%, respectively). This effective increase in ventilation, but not respiratory rate, results in alveolar hyperventilation with a resting carbon dioxide tension of 28 to 35 mm Hg. Chronic respiratory alkalosis during pregnancy is partially compensated (pH 7.45) by renal excretion of bicarbonate ($HCO_3 \sim 20$ mEq/L).

In the second trimester, distention of the abdominal cavity by the enlarging uterus causes a mechanical displacement of the diaphragm, reducing the functional residual capacity by approximately 18%. The resulting changes in lung volumes include decreases in expiratory reserve volume and residual volume. Vital capacity may increase by 100 to 200 mL and inspiratory capacity may increase by 300 mL at term (6).

PATHOPHYSIOLOGY OF ASTHMA

Asthma, once viewed as an intermittent disease process related to bronchospastic events, is now understood to be a chronic disease process involving both airway inflammation and bronchial hyperreactivity. This manifests itself clinically by varying degrees of airway obstruction. Asthma as an obstructive pulmonary disease process is associated with a decrease in expiratory airflow and a resultant increase in functional residual capacity. This increase in functional residual capacity leads to an increased work of breathing, with recruitment of accessory muscles of respiration, in an attempt to overcome the ventilation–perfusion mismatch and associated hypoxemia. Ultimately these accessory muscles become fatigued, leading to hypercapnia and increased pulmonary vascular resistance. Without treatment, severe obstruction-impaired ventilation and carbon dioxide retention result.

Asthma as an inflammatory disease involves eosinophils, neutrophils, TH2 lymphocytes, mast cells, and antigen-presenting cells. The inflammatory response is mediated by a number of humoral factors, including cytokines and leukotrienes (7). These produce mucous secretion, mucosal edema, bronchial edema, and bronchoconstriction.

New specific therapies available for the treatment of asthma target the conversion to or binding of leukotrienes A_4, B_4, C_4, D_4, and E_4. The production of leukotrienes from free arachidonic acid requires activation of the enzyme 5-lipoxygenase (5-LO) by binding to a membrane-associated 5-LO–activating protein (FLAP). One approach to the treatment of asthma is to inhibit FLAP (FLAP inhibitors are not currently approved for use in the United States). After activation, 5-LO may be inhibited by zileuton (a 5-LO inhibitor). Uninhibited 5-LO will convert arachidonic acid into leukotriene A_4. This, in turn, is converted by an epoxide hydrolase to leukotriene B_4. Leukotriene B_4 is a potent chemotactic factor for neutrophils but

does not affect smooth muscle in the airways. Alternately, leukotriene A_4 may be converted by LTC_4 synthase to leukotriene C_4, which itself is biologically active, but is rapidly converted to leukotriene D_4 and thence to leukotriene E_4 (8). Leukotrienes C_4, D_4, and E_4 are collectively referred to as cysteinyl leukotrienes; these were originally referred to as the slow-reacting substances of anaphylaxis (9). They initiate biological activity by binding to a common leukotriene receptor known as the cysteinyl-LT-1 (Cys-LT1) receptor. Zafirlukast and montelukast are Cys-LT1 receptor antagonists.

Further investigations at this time involve the role of adhesion molecules and the movement of inflammatory cells from the vascular space into the airways, the role of immunoglobulin E in initiation of the immediate asthmatic response, and the role of thromboxane A_2, neurokinins, interleukins, and other chemotactic factors.

Pathophysiology of Asthma in Pregnancy

Because of differences in fetal hemoglobin-dissociation properties (normal fetal pO_2 is approximately 33 mm Hg), decreases in maternal (and consequently) fetal pO_2 rapidly result in fetal hemoglobin oxygen desaturation and fetal hypoxemia. These decreases become most rapid and profound at maternal pO_2 less than 60 mm Hg and oxygen saturations less than 90%.

In addition, the interpretation of arterial blood gas data should be altered in the pregnant patient. Normally, asthmatic patients presenting with an acute attack will manifest initial hypocapnia. This is followed, as the attack progresses, with a decrease in pO_2 and normalization of the pCO_2. However, because the normal pCO_2 of patients in the second and third trimesters of pregnancy is in the low 30s, a pCO_2 of 40 mm Hg should be interpreted as hypercarbia, demonstrating a more serious progression of the attack and impending respiratory failure (6).

NATURAL HISTORY OF ASTHMA IN PREGNANCY

The overall course of asthma during pregnancy worsens in approximately 20% to 35% of women, remains stable in 40% to 50%, and improves in 20% to 30% (10–12). In a prospective, control-matched group of approximately 200 asthmatic women, 40% of women were successfully managed on the same medication regimen as before pregnancy, 18% needed less medication, and 42% required more medication (13). Acute exacerbations occur with increasing frequency during weeks 24 to 32 of gestation. Studies have shown as many as 46% of patients required hospitalization for asthma (14,15).

Before the advent of aggressive modern asthma treatment, patients with uncontrolled asthma were more likely to experience a poorer outcome than that of the general population. Large, population-based cohort studies from the early 1990's showed an increased odds ratio (OR) for preterm birth [OR, 1.36; 95% confidence interval (CI), 1.18 to 1.55], low birth weight (OR, 1.32; 95% CI, 1.10 to 1.58), preeclampsia (OR, 2.18; 95% CI, 1.68 to 2.83), cesarean delivery (OR, 1.62; 95% CI, 1.46 to 1.80) (16), and neonatal hyperbilirubinemia in infants of women taking steroids (OR, 1.9; 95% CI, 1.1 to 3.4) (17). A smaller case-controlled study from a tertiary center demonstrated an increase in respiratory and urinary tract infections in asthmatic women compared with nonasthmatic women during pregnancy ($p < 0.001$), but no association with pregnancy-induced hypertension or low birth weight (18). Interpretation of these studies is complex given the changes in asthma treatment over the past decade and the difference in study methodology. However, well-controlled asthmatic patients in more recent studies do not show these outcomes except an increase in incidence of chronic hypertension in asthmatic women (12).

Asthma has been classified according to the frequency and severity of symptoms and findings: mild asthma is classified as patients experiencing symptoms less than three times per week and nocturnal symptoms less than two times per month, forced expiratory volume in 1 second (FEV_1) or peak expiratory flow rate (PEFR) <80% of norm for the patient. Moderate asthma is classified as more than three episodes of symptoms per week with exacerbations that affect sleep or activity and FEV_1 or PEFR of 60% to 80%. Severe asthma is defined as daily symptoms, limiting activity, with frequent nocturnal symptoms and frequent exacerbations, and pulmonary functions less than 60% of the norm (3).

LIFESTYLE ISSUES AND THEIR ROLE IN ASTHMA TREATMENT DURING PREGNANCY

Patients who are receiving desensitization immunotherapy and experiencing no adverse reactions and who appear to be receiving benefit may continue to receive desensitization during pregnancy. It should not be initiated as a new treatment because of possible unpredictable reactions (19).

All patients with asthma should receive influenza vaccination on a yearly basis except in cases of allergy to eggs and thimerosal (the preservative). The Centers for Disease Control and Prevention recommend routine vaccination against influenza in all women who will be in the second or third trimester of pregnancy during the influenza season, with avoidance of vaccination during the first trimester (20).

Environmental issues that may need attention by the pregnancy care provider include patient avoidance of specific allergens, such as animal dander, pollen, house dust mites, and cockroach allergen. Avoidance of smoking and passive smoke inhalation is strongly encouraged for all asthmatic patients and for all pregnant patients. In the pregnant asthmatic, patient education must include realistic discussion about the possibility of acute exacerbations within the pregnancy resulting in a poor outcome.

The safety of nicotine gum and nicotine patches for smoking cessation has not been established in pregnancy. Nicotine has been demonstrated to decrease mean beat intervals, short-term variability, and accelerations of the fetal heart rate (21–23). Methodology and results vary in Doppler studies of maternal and fetal blood flow with administration of nicotine in various forms. Some studies in animals and humans appear to indicate increased uterine artery resistance and decreased fetal cerebral blood flow (23–25), whereas other studies of acute effects of nicotine gum and nicotine patches do not show short-term negative effects (26–28). In addition, the use of a 21-mg transdermal nicotine patch has been shown to result in maternal blood nicotine concentrations and fetal cerebral resistance indices similar to those from hourly smoking (23). Nicotine gum appears to deliver less nicotine than smoking (26). Because nicotine use has been implicated in long-term effects on the developing brain (29), it is not clear that any form of nicotine replacement therapy is without risk in pregnancy. Nonetheless, compared with the direct effects of tobacco in provoking bronchial mucosal irritation in the pregnant asthmatic, the use of short-term nicotine replacement may be considered in the lowest doses possible to facilitate smoking cessation.

Buproprion, although classified as US Food and Drug Administration Pregnancy Category B, has not been studied in pregnancy (30). It may be useful in smoking cessation in the nonpregnant patient. Its risks in pregnancy would be similar to the risks from antidepressant use, which have not been well studied.

ASTHMA MEDICATIONS IN PREGNANCY AND LACTATION

Table 5.1 provides an overview of medication classes in pregnancy. The following specific information on medications and strategies for use of medications are discussed with reference to severity of asthma. It should be emphasized that the overall emphasis in pharmacotherapy is to use sufficient types and amounts of medication to achieve as few symptoms as is reasonably possible with avoidance of acute exacerbations and potential complications. Rather than avoiding medication to prevent ill effects to the fetus, the asthmatic patient and her physician should be aware of the potential for normalization of perinatal outcomes with active and appropriate drug use.

Beta-sympathomimetic Agents

Short-acting beta-sympathomimetic agents that have been used to treat asthma include terbutaline, albuterol, metaproterenol, and pirbuterol. The duration of action of bitolterol mesylate is intermediate, whereas salmeterol is a long-acting agent. For purposes of discussion, short- and long-acting beta-sympathomimetic medications are discussed separately because their role in asthma treatment is somewhat different.

Short-acting Beta-sympathomimetics

Indications

First-line treatment for acute exacerbations of asthma includes short-acting inhaled beta-sympathomimetic agents. The principal agent used for this indication in the United States currently is albuterol (also referred to as salbutamol), which has previously been used in systemic

TABLE 5.1. *Summary of medications for asthma in pregnancy and lactation*

Medication class	Indication	Comments
Beta agonists	Acute treatment, chronic for long-acting, exercise-induced	May be only medication used in patients with mild, intermittent symptoms
Theophylline/aminophylline	Acute and chronic treatment	Not first line, toxicity concerns
Cromolyn	Chronic	Not as effective as steroids
Inhaled corticosteroids	Chronic	First-line therapy as antiinflammatory
Nedocromil	Chronic	Efficacy similar to that of cromolyn
Leukotriene receptor antagonists	Chronic	Zafirlukast contraindicated in lactation, for severe asthma refractory to traditional prescriptions
Systemic corticosteroids	Acute and chronic	Multiple systemic effects
Anticholinergic medications	Controversial, adjuvant acute therapy	Indicated for alpha-1 antitrypsin deficiency
5-Lipoxygenase inhibitor	Chronic	For severe asthma refractory to traditional prescriptions

formulations as a tocolytic agent. Intermittent positive-pressure breathing administration carries no advantage over simple nebulizer treatments administered in sterile saline unless atelectasis is present. Patients using inhaled short-acting beta-sympathomimetics for ambulatory treatment frequently benefit from the use of a spacer device because of the difficulty encountered by many in using metered-dose inhalers properly.

Overall Precautions

Beta-sympathomimetic medications have all been associated with tachycardia, transient hyperglycemia and subsequent increased release of insulin, hypokalemia, and feelings of jitteriness, anxiety, and insomnia. Demargination of white blood cells is manifested as a leukocytosis. Cardiac arrhythmias may occur, including ectopic ventricular beats and tachyarrhythmias. Metaproterenol and isoproterenol are less beta$_2$ selective than terbutaline, albuterol, and pirbuterol and, thus, have greater potential for cardiovascular effects.

Dosage of Medication

Dosage of medication information is shown in Table 5.2. For further discussion of treatment in the acute exacerbation of asthma, see the section

on acute asthma exacerbations in pregnancy later in this chapter.

Possible Effects on Pregnancy

Terbutaline: Administered intravenously, it can preserve or increase uteroplacental blood flow compromised by uterine contractions. Serious side effects that are observed with continuous infusion include pulmonary edema, myocardial ischemia, cardiac arrhythmias, cerebral vasospasm, hypotension, hyperglycemia, increased serum lactate levels, and decreased measured hemoglobin concentration (31,32). Maternal hyperglycemia can increase serum insulin and result in neonatal hypoglycemia if administered close to or at the time of delivery. Only rare reports of serious maternal and fetal toxicity have occurred since the inception of its use approximately 25 years ago (33).

Albuterol: Adverse reactions in humans include maternal and fetal tachycardia, decrease in maternal blood pressure with both systolic and diastolic dropping more than 30 mm Hg (34). Other more serious but rarely reported adverse effects include acute congestive heart failure, pulmonary edema, and death. These effects have been seen with systemic albuterol. However, a study of maternal and fetal circulation with inhaled albuterol demonstrated no significant changes (35). Transient maternal

TABLE 5.2. *Beta-sympathomimetic medications for asthma*

Medication	Dosage	Comments
Albuterol inhalers: Proventil, Ventolin (0.5% solution for inhalation)	2 puffs every 4–6 h p.r.n. or 2.5 mg or 0.5 mL in 3 mL NS every 4–6 h[a]	Short acting
Bitolterol mesylate (Tornalate MDI)	2 puffs every 4–6 h p.r.n.	Intermediate acting
Pirbuterol (Maxair)	2 puffs every 4–6 h p.r.n.	Short acting
Terbutaline (Brethaire)	2 puffs every 4–6 h p.r.n.	Short acting
Metaproterenol inhaler	2–3 puffs every 3–4 h p.r.n. orally 20 mg every 6–8 h,	Short acting, less beta$_2$-selective
5% solution for inhalation	0.01 mL/kg (maximum of 0.3 mL) every 4 h diluted in normal saline to 2.5 cc	
tablets	20 mg every 8 h	
syrup	10 cc t.i.d or q.i.d	
Salmeterol (Serevent)	2 puffs every 12 h	Long acting

[a]More frequent or continuous albuterol via nebulizer may be considered in a monitored patient for severe exacerbations while initiating systemic corticosteroid therapy.

hyperglycemia with increased serum insulin as well as neonatal hypoglycemia may occur with albuterol as with all beta-sympathomimetics; these effects are more likely to occur in diabetics (36). Fetal arrhythmias have been documented with high doses of inhaled albuterol, including atrial flutter with 2:1 conduction. This resolved spontaneously (37).

Metaproterenol: Like all beta-sympathomimetics, metaproterenol may be associated with maternal and fetal tachycardia, maternal hypotension, and maternal hyperglycemia with subsequent neonatal hypoglycemia (38).

Pirbuterol: Pirbuterol is more $beta_2$ selective than older medications in the same class. Again all beta-sympathomimetics may be associated with maternal and, to a lesser degree, fetal tachycardia, maternal hypotension, maternal hyperglycemia, and fetal hypoglycemia.

Teratogenicity

A Michigan Medicaid study of more than 200,000 births with more than 1,000 first-trimester exposures to albuterol and smaller numbers of exposures to metaproterenol, terbutaline, and isoproterenol failed to demonstrate any significant teratogenic risk in humans (39). Nonhuman reproductive studies with pirbuterol reveal no mutagenesis at as much as 6,250 times the maximum recommended human dose (product information, Maxair Autohaler, 3M Pharmaceuticals, St. Paul, MN, 1996). No association with human congenital anomalies has been reported since its introduction in 1988.

Alterations in Metabolism

There are no alterations known in pregnancy for any of the beta-sympathomimetic drugs.

Use During Lactation

Terbutaline has been studied in lactation, with newborns receiving approximately 0.7% of the maternal ingested dose (40). No short-term deleterious effects have been found, and this drug is considered safe in lactation. Although no direct information is available about other short-acting beta-sympathomimetics, their use in lactation is probably safe.

Long-acting Beta-sympathomimetics

Indications

Although short-term sympathomimetics are indicated as rescue medications in acute asthmatic attacks, long-acting beta-sympathomimetics may be viewed as chronic or maintenance medications. Clearly salmeterol belongs in this class, with bitolterol being somewhat intermediate in its duration of action. These medications are useful for nighttime administration, with prevention of night symptoms prominent in some asthmatics. These drugs are generally indicated in patients with moderate asthma requiring regular $beta_2$-agonist therapy in conjunction with anti-inflammatory agents (41).

Overall Precautions

Salmeterol does not appear to be associated with significant cardiovascular effects (42).

Dosage

Table 5.2 provides dosage information for long-acting beta-sympathomimetics.

Possible Effects on Pregnancy

Salmeterol xinafoate: The duration of action is approximately 12 hours. The mechanism of action is the same as that of all beta-sympathomimetics but is more $beta_2$ selective than older short-acting agents (43). Few data on human pregnancy are available on this relatively new, long-acting, more $beta_2$-selective sympathomimetic agent.

Bitolterol: Bitolterol is a relatively long-acting beta-agonist with a duration of action of approximately 6 to 7 hours.

Teratogenicity

Nonhuman reproductive studies of salmeterol indicated no significant effects on fetal development at up to 12 times the recommended clinical dose (Serevent Inhaler, GlaxoWellcome,

Research Triangle Park, NC, 1998). Bitolterol has not been associated with congenital anomalies since its introduction in 1985. Nonhuman studies have shown no mutagenesis. Like other beta-agonist studies indicating dose-dependent increases in the incidence of cleft palate in nonhuman subjects, these results have not proven applicable to human populations at recommended doses.

Alterations in Metabolism with Pregnancy

There are no alterations in metabolism.

Use in Lactation

Few data are available, but these drugs are probably acceptable with breast-feeding because they are in the same class as terbutaline, which is considered safe.

Theophylline

Indications

Theophylline has waned as a first-line drug in the treatment of asthma. Its use should be restricted to patients who have failed to be well-controlled with inhaled corticosteroids and inhaled beta-agonists (moderate to severe asthma). Intravenous aminophylline given with inhaled beta-agonists has not been shown to decrease hospital length of stay or shorten response time in pregnant women hospitalized with acute asthma compared with pregnant women treated with systemic steroids and inhaled beta-agonists (44). The role of its intravenous equivalent, aminophylline, appears limited for most patients requiring acute treatment. Theophylline as long-term therapy has the advantage of oral administration with twice a day dosing in most sustained-release preparations and relatively low cost.

Overall Precautions

Theophylline has a narrow therapeutic range, usually measured as 8 to 12 μ/mL (in some literature 10 to 15 μg/mL), with toxicity being encountered more frequently when levels exceed 20 μ/mL. Even before a toxic level is reached, some patients will experience unpleasant or harmful side effects, such as jitteriness, nausea and vomiting, and palpitations. Theophylline has been implicated in a significant number of drug–drug interactions, including elevation of blood levels with concomitant use of common medications such as erythromycin (product information, Theodur, Key Pharmaceuticals, Kenilworth, NJ, 1997).

Dosage of Medication

Oral theophylline dosage varies widely from 400 to 1,600 mg per day to achieve a serum level of 8 to 12 μ/mL. Parenteral dosing of aminophylline is usually accomplished with a loading dose of 6 mg/kg of ideal body weight (IBW) and subsequent infusion rates of 0.5 mg/kg per hour, with adjustment depending on hepatic and cardiac factors and follow-up levels.

Possible Negative Effects on Pregnancy

Theophylline is a smooth muscle relaxant of the bronchial musculature and stimulates increased contractility of diaphragmatic musculature. It has been found to increase fetal breathing movements, so interpretation of the biophysical profile should take this into account (45). Theophylline has mild uterine relaxant or tocolytic properties (46), but it has not been demonstrated to inhibit term labor.

Teratogenicity

Theophylline has not been implicated in specific patterns of fetal malformations in the Collaborative Perinatal Project (47), although there was a slight increase over expected rate of birth defects in the Michigan Medicaid study (39).

Alterations in Clearance or Metabolism

Theophylline is approximately 40% bound to serum proteins, especially albumin. The reduction in plasma protein binding during the third trimester of pregnancy increases the active drug available. Thus, pregnant women may manifest toxicity at lower levels than in the nonpregnant state (48). Its metabolism is primarily through the hepatic route. However, a case control study of more than 200 women treated with slow-release theophylline failed to demonstrate adverse outcomes associated with its use (49). Maternal theophylline use has resulted in severely toxic levels in premature infants (50). Hepatocellular disease and passive congestion of the liver may alter (decrease) theophylline metabolism.

Lactation

Use of theophylline during lactation is not contraindicated but may cause signs of irritability or mild toxicity in a breast-feeding infant. Serum and breast milk concentrations of theophylline are approximately equal. A breast-feeding infant may receive as much as 10 to 20 mg of theophylline in a day, which would be unlikely to cause serious injury (30). Greater concern should probably be directed toward the breast-feeding premature infant in whom reduced protein binding may potentiate toxicity.

Antiinflammatory Agents

Cromolyn Sodium

Indications

Cromolyn sodium is used in atopic patients as long-term therapy. It has no use in the acute attack. Cromolyn is a mast-cell stabilizer that prevents them from releasing histamine. Cromolyn is also effective in some patients with exercise-induced asthma. This medication is not as effective an antiinflammatory agent as inhaled corticosteroids.

Overall Precautions

There are no known serious effects.

Dosage

Cromolyn is administered by inhaler in two to four puffs four times daily or orally (200 mg) four times daily.

Possible Negative Effects in Pregnancy

There are no known serious effects. Although minute amounts are absorbed systemically, it is not known whether it crosses the placenta.

Teratogenicity

This mast-cell stabilizer has been used for more than 25 years without reported association with congenital defects (39).

Alteration in Metabolism with Pregnancy

There are no alterations.

Use in Lactation

There are no obvious risks to the newborn, and its use is appropriate for lactation.

5-LO Inhibitors

Indications

Zileuton is the currently available 5-LO inhibitor in the United States. Its use appears to be for moderate to severe asthma to decrease the need for beta-agonist rescue medication, possibly in conjunction with inhaled corticosteroids. There is one experimental model that used a 5-LO inhibitor to treat amniotic fluid embolism (51).

Overall Precautions

This medication is contraindicated in patients with liver disease or transaminase elevations greater than or equal to three times the upper limit of normal. Liver function monitoring is recommended for all patients at the time of initiation of therapy and monthly thereafter for the first 3 months.

Dosage

Zilevton is administered orally, 600 mg four times daily.

Possible Negative Effects in Pregnancy

Very little information is available.

Teratogenicity

Because this agent is so new and human data are so few, its use should be limited in pregnancy to situations in which more traditional and well-proven medications have failed.

Alteration in Metabolism with Pregnancy

There are no data available.

Use in Lactation

Data are not available, and therefore these drugs should be avoided.

Leukotriene Receptor Antagonists, Zafirlukast and Montelukast

Indications

Leukotriene receptor antagonists are selective competitive antagonists of the leukotriene D_4 and E_4 components of the slow-reacting substance of anaphylaxis. They inhibit bronchoconstriction and have been shown to be effective against various antigen and histamine challenges. Their use is restricted to the chronic treatment of asthma. They have no role in acute treatment of bronchospasm. Their efficacy is similar to inhaled steroids (52). When used in steroid-treated and steroid-dependent asthmatics, they have been shown to be effective in decreasing the patient's need for corticosteroids (53).

Overall Precautions

Zafirlukast is metabolized by the liver with 90% excretion in feces and 10% renal excretion. Its bioavailability is decreased by administration with food. A rare side effect is elevation of liver enzymes with nausea, fatigue, lethargy, jaundice, and flu-like symptoms (product information, Accolate, Zeneca Pharmaceuticals, Wilmington, DE). An additional rare condition associated with zafirlukast presents as an eosinophilic vasculitis consistent with Churg-Strauss syndrome, generally seen in patients who are being treated with or tapering systemic corticosteroid therapy (54). Drug interactions include increased serum half-life of both zafirlukast and warfarin when used concomitantly and increased serum levels of zafirlukast in combination with aspirin (product information). Theophylline toxicity has been reported in combination with this drug (product information). Montelukast is metabolized in the liver. No dosage adjustment is needed in patients with mild to moderate hepatic insufficiency or renal insufficiency, and there are no significant interactions with digoxin, warfarin, theophylline, prednisone, or oral contraceptives. Its metabolism may be increased by potent cytochrome P-450 inducers, such as phenobarbital. The side-effect profile is very low.

Dosage of Medication

The recommended dosage of Zafirlukast is 20 mg twice a day orally taken at least 1 hour before or 2 hours after meals. The recommended dosage of montelukast is 10 mg orally at bedtime.

Possible Negative Effects on Pregnancy

Metabolic information regarding zafirlukast and montelukast during pregnancy is unavailable. Because little information is available about use in human pregnancy, it should only be utilized in complicated cases in which patients require systemic steroids or in patients in whom the risks are clearly outweighed by potential benefits.

Teratogenicity

No human data are available.

Use During Lactation

Zafirlukast is excreted into human breast milk at levels approximately one fifth of serum levels. Because of concerns about tumorigenicity, zafirlukast should not be used during lactation. Montelukast is excreted into breast milk in rats, but no human studies exist to document its excretion into human breast milk. There are no studies on the safety of montelukast in children younger than 6 years of age. Because of a lack of information, montelukast should probably not be used in lactation.

Nedocromil

Indications

Nedocromil sodium is an inhaled antiinflammatory agent of the pyranoquinoline class that is primarily useful in patients with mild to moderate, atopic asthma. It prevents bronchoconstriction in response to various antigens, exercise, and cold. It has no systemic effects when taken in prescribed doses and has no role in the treatment of acute bronchospasm. It should be used as maintenance therapy as an alternative to agents such as cromolyn.

Overall Precautions

There are no regularly occurring adverse events associated with nedocromil. The side-effect profile is low. Used as prescribed, it has no known systemic activity and has low bioavailability. It is excreted into the urine. It may be used in conjunction with other inhaled asthma medications such as corticosteroids and cromolyn sodium without adverse effect or interference with other medications. There are no known drug–drug interactions.

Dosage

The dosage is two inhalations four times daily.

Teratogenicity

No human data are available.

Possible Negative Effects on Pregnancy

There are no known negative effects, and the potential for adverse effects appears low because its mechanism of action is local and not systemic. However, unless a patient has been on nedocromil with good response before pregnancy, the efficacy and safety of inhaled corticosteroids are better documented at this time in pregnancy.

Use During Lactation

It is not known whether nedocromil is excreted into human milk. Safety in children younger than 6 years of age has not been established. Because nedocromil has low bioavailability when taken via inhalation, there may be little opportunity for absorption by the infant. Nonetheless, inhaled cromolyn has been utilized more extensively in children and may be a safer alternative in a breastfeeding mother.

Inhaled Corticosteroids

Indications

Inhaled corticosteroids have become first-line therapy in all asthmatic patients except those with very sporadic, mild symptoms and patients with exercise-induced asthma only (i.e., mild to moderate, persistent asthma and severe asthma). Even in patients needing intermittent or long-term use of systemic steroids, inhaled corticosteroid therapy is helpful in reducing the dose of systemic steroids and, thus, the risk or severity of steroid-related side effects.

Mechanism of Action

The mechanisms of action are suppression of inflammation and decrease in bronchial hyperresponsiveness.

Overall Precautions

Inhaled corticosteroids have been demonstrated to slow linear growth in children and adolescents, possibly with little effect on final adult height (55). Decreased bone density, cataract formation, dermal thinning, and glaucoma have all been reported, generally in patients using higher than standard doses. The risk of oral candidiasis can be reduced by using a spacer device and by rinsing the mouth after use.

TABLE 5.3. Inhaled corticosteroids

Medication	Strength/type	Dosage range
Beclomethasone dipropionate (Beclovent, Vanceril)	MDI 42 μg/puff	4–8 puffs b.i.d.
Vanceril DS	MDI 84 μg/puff	2–4 puffs b.i.d.
Budesonide (Pulmicort Turbuhaler)	Dry powder inhaler 200 or 400 μg/inhalation	400 μg b.i.d. or 1–2 inhalations b.i.d.
Flunisolide (AeroBid)	MDI 250 μg/puff	2–4 puffs b.i.d.
Fluticasone propionate (Flovent)	MDI 44, 110, and 220 μg/puff	2–4 puffs b.i.d. (44 μg)
Flovent Rotadisk	Dry powder inhaler 50, 100, and 250 μg/inhalation	1 inhalation b.i.d. (100 μg)
Triamcinolone acetonide (Azmacort)	MDI 100 μg/puff	2 puffs t.i.d. or q.i.d. or 4 puffs b.i.d.

Possible Negative Effects on Pregnancy

Circadian rhythms of cortisol, corticotropin (ACTH), 17β-estradiol, and estriol levels and fetal heart rate circadian and ultradian patterns are modified by administration of triamcinolone acetonide to healthy pregnant women (56). Several studies demonstrated an increase in preeclampsia among asthmatic women treated with oral corticosteroids (17). Inhaled corticosteroids that have been studied in pregnancy include beclomethasone and triamcinolone acetonide. No studies of newer, potent corticosteroids such as fluticasone, budesonide, and flunisolide have been published. Antenatal beclomethasone therapy has been associated with transient decreases in neonatal glucocorticoids, but with no effects on mineralocorticoids (57).

Teratogenicity

A large population-based, case-control study of teratogenicity in humans failed to show any association between oral and topical corticosteroid use and congenital abnormalities, including women treated during the second and third trimesters of pregnancy (58). In addition, the Michigan Medicaid study did not find evidence of teratogenicity with inhaled corticosteroids (39). Ongoing studies using inhaled corticosteroids should further delineate safety concerns about these medications (59).

Dosage of Medication

Inhaled corticosteroids fall into several groups based on the potency of the medication and the delivery system. In general, dry-powder inhalations require fewer inhalations on a twice daily dosing schedule, whereas some inhalers, such as triamcinolone, require multiple inhalations per day. Table 5.3 lists dosages.

Alterations in Clearance or Metabolism

There are no known alterations during pregnancy.

Systemic Corticosteroids

Indications

The indications are the same as in nonpregnant patients. Patients with acute exacerbations who do not readily clear with beta-agonist nebulizer treatments are candidates for systemic therapy, usually with a rapid taper over 10 days after stabilization. Patients requiring long-term steroid therapy because of failure to control symptoms despite inhaled corticosteroids, beta-agonist medication, and appropriate treatment of underlying conditions, such as environmental modifications described previously in this chapter, are candidates for oral steroid treatment. Doses will vary but should be kept to the lowest dose that produces control of symptoms and adequate airway function, utilizing alternate-day therapy if tolerated, because of the decreased effect on the hypothalamic-pituitary-adrenal axis.

Overall Precautions

Both short- and long-term systemic corticosteroid use has been associated with glucose intolerance and overt hyperglycemia, hypertension, demineralization of bone, immunosuppression, and multiple other metabolic effects. In addition, corticosteroids may be accompanied by neuropsychiatric symptoms, which include euphoria, agitation, steroid psychosis, nightmares, and mood disorders. As an additional precaution, it should be remembered that patients who have been on long-term systemic steroids should be provided with stress doses of corticosteroids for events such as trauma, surgery, acute illness, or labor and delivery, generally in the range of 100 mg of hydrocortisone every 8 hours intravenously or its equivalent.

Possible Negative Effects on Pregnancy

Steroid-induced hyperglycemia and bone demineralization are of particular concern in pregnancy.

Dosage of Medication

The dosage is the same as in the nonpregnant state. Acute exacerbations may be treated with methylprednisolone 1 mg/kg intravenously every 6 hours for severe exacerbations or oral burst therapy using 40 to 60 mg orally as an initial dose, with a moderately rapid taper as the patient stabilizes.

Alterations in Clearance or Metabolism with Pregnancy

There are no alterations in clearance or metabolism.

Role in Overall Treatment of Asthma

Its use is confined to significant acute exacerbations that are unrelieved by beta-agonist inhalations and long-term treatment of the severe asthmatic unresponsive to combinations of beta-agonists, inhaled corticosteroids, and other anti-inflammatory medications such as cromolyn and nedocromil. In nonpregnant patients, leukotriene receptor antagonists and 5-LO inhibitors should be tried before long-term oral steroid use. In the pregnant patient, theophylline should be added before consideration of maintenance or long-term oral steroids.

Teratogenicity

As stated previously, there is no evidence of teratogenicity for oral or inhaled steroids.

OVERALL TREATMENT PLANS FOR ASTHMA IN PREGNANCY

Patients should be carefully questioned about previous episodes of asthma and/or wheezing. Many patients will give a history of childhood asthma that has since remitted. It is common for these patients to experience reexacerbation of their condition as they grow older, in association with upper respiratory infections, allergens, or tobacco exposure. Asthma severity should be assessed. Patients who experience only infrequent exacerbations, do not require regular or frequent medication, and have no history of hospitalization for asthma can be considered as mild, intermittent and may be observed with occasional use of beta-sympathomimetic inhalant medication as needed. They should receive influenza vaccination.

Even if a patient does not take medication on a regular basis, a history of exacerbations that were severe enough to warrant emergency department visits or hospitalizations raises the likelihood of exacerbation during pregnancy. These patients should be considered for prophylactic treatment with inhaled steroids because these have been shown to decrease the incidence of acute attacks of asthma in pregnancy (60). All patients with moderate to severe asthma should be on inhaled corticosteroids.

Exercise-induced asthma may be treated with albuterol inhalation 30 minutes before exercise or cromolyn as long-term therapy.

If a patient has regular, daily, or almost daily symptoms requiring the use of a rescue beta-agonist therapy, she should be started on an inhaled steroid with the hope that use of rescue medication will be reduced. In patients with moderate or severe asthma, control of nighttime symptoms may improve with long-acting beta-sympathomimetics, such as bitolterol or salmeterol. Other medications that may be considered in the severe asthmatic include cromolyn sodium or nedocromil in combination with inhaled corticosteroids and beta-agonists or the addition of theophylline.

Patients with moderate to severe asthma should be taught the use of daily PEFR monitoring and instructed on a protocol for self-management of symptoms and when to call her physician. Hand-held peak flow meters are easy to use and relatively inexpensive. The patient should establish her personal best and utilize this as a means of self-monitoring (3).

Patients on repeated use of systemic steroids should be treated as much as possible with a combination of inhaled steroids and beta-sympathomimetic inhalant medications, with the use of nedocromil or cromolyn as demonstrated to be effective by use of daily PEFR monitoring. If systemic steroids are necessary for long-term therapy despite the above measures, they should be used at the lowest dose effective to prevent acute exacerbation.

Newer agents, such as the leukotriene receptor antagonists or 5-LO inhibitors, usually should not be used in most pregnant women with asthma because little information is available regarding these medications in human pregnancy. If a patient with severe asthma has been treated successfully before pregnancy with antileukotrienes and experienced improvement, this may justify use during pregnancy. Relative risks and benefits of systemic corticosteroids versus those of newer agents must then be weighed.

Other exacerbating conditions, such as allergic rhinitis and sinusitis, should be treated using topical agents on a preferential basis. Nasal corticosteroids, antihistamines, and nasal cromolyn are considered safe in pregnancy (61). Other antihistamines (hydroxyzine and cetirizine) have been studied and show no evidence of teratogenicity or poor pregnancy outcome (62).

If the patient develops acute bacterial sinusitis, then she should be vigorously treated with antibiotic coverage for β-lactamase–resistant *Haemophilus influenzae*, *Moraxella catarrhalis*, and *Streptococcus pneumoniae*. Antibiotic therapy should extend for a minimum of 14 days for sinusitis and possibly 21 days. Nasal steroids will decrease overall inflammation and treat underlying allergic rhinitis, if present. Nasal decongestant sprays may be used for as long as 3 days to help in opening up swollen sinus ostia, which can assist in the drainage of the infection. Small doses of pseudoephedrine may also be helpful for decongestant purposes, but its use should be restricted to the amount necessary for symptomatic relief. Expectorants, such as guaifenesin, have not been shown to be effective compared with an increase in oral fluids and humidification.

ACUTE ASTHMA EXACERBATIONS IN PREGNANCY

Treatment of acute exacerbations of asthma in pregnancy are the same as for nonpregnant patients with similar exacerbations. Optimization of traditional bronchodilatory and antiinflammatory therapies with a low threshold for initiation of medications to inhibit immediate- and slow-reacting mediators of inflammation associated with reversible obstructive pulmonary disease. Aggressive treatment of acute exacerbations of this chronic disease preclude previously discussed disparities in morbidity during pregnancy compared with that of a healthy population.

The National Asthma Education Project Working Group on Asthma in Pregnancy recommends a home "rescue" approach to early symptoms (3). If the patient experiences symptoms such as coughing, chest tightness, wheezing, or shortness of breath, she should utilize a short-acting beta-agonist (albuterol) two to four puffs every 20 minutes up to 1 hour. If the patient experiences resolution of symptoms and her PEFR is greater than 70% of her personal best, then she may resume usual activities. If symptoms do not resolve or if fetal activity is decreased, she should seek medical attention.

Oxygen should be liberally prescribed to maintain saturation of 95% or more. Findings suggestive of a serious attack include an initial FEV_1 less than 1.0 L, a PEFR less than 100 L, or oximetry less than 90% on presentation for medical care. These patients should be started on intravenous corticosteroids and frequent or continuous albuterol via nebulizer, and may need intensive care unit admission and/or intubation. The use of intravenous aminophylline or subcutaneous terbutaline should be individualized.

MANAGEMENT OF ASTHMA COMPLICATIONS IN PREGNANCY

Sinus infections have already been addressed in this chapter as they relate to the asthmatic pregnant woman. Patients with an acute exacerbation of asthma during the influenza season accompanied by profuse myalgias and upper respiratory symptoms may be suspected of antecedent influenza. Given the excess mortality and morbidity attributed to the condition of pregnancy during certain influenza epidemics, it is prudent to keep a high index of suspicion for complicated cases, including women with viral pneumonitis and superimposed bacterial pneumonia. An ill-appearing patient with asthma and apparent influenza or other viral infection (such as *Varicella*) should be evaluated with a chest radiograph, shielding the abdomen. Laboratory evaluation of the acutely ill patient must be tempered with caution when interpreting leukocytosis and a leftward shift in patients who have received either beta-sympathomimetic medication or corticosteroids with demargination of white blood cells.

Patients with either atypical scattered infiltrates or areas of lobar or subsegmental consolidation should be hospitalized and followed closely with initiation of antiviral or antibiotic therapy as indicated. Classic secondary pneumonias after viral infection include group A streptococci and *Staphylococcus aureus*.

Steroid-induced hyperglycemia may be encountered in the asthmatic patient with chronic or acute corticosteroid therapy. Although dietary therapy may be helpful in the chronic situation, the acutely ill asthmatic with hyperglycemia should be managed with protocols similar to those for insulin-dependent diabetics. Steroid taper as the patient stabilizes may permit reduction in insulin dose or its elimination. Inhaled corticosteroids should be started in these patients in the hope that systemic steroid taper will be facilitated. Inhaled steroids should have no effect on serum glucose levels given in standard dosing schedules.

MANAGEMENT OF ASTHMA IN LABOR

The usual asthma medications that controlled the patient through pregnancy should be continued during labor. As many as 10% of asthmatic women have been reported to experience acute intrapartum exacerbations (62). A high clinical suspicion for exacerbations during delivery should be maintained, and immediate aggressive treatment instituted as indicated. Some authors recommend consideration of PEFRs at the time of admission and every 12 hours thereafter as an objective means to determine the need for additional intrapartum asthma therapy (63). Appropriate analgesia and adequate hydration can decrease the risk of bronchospasm during labor.

Oxytocin and E-series prostaglandins may be safely used in labor management. Magnesium sulfate or terbutaline, depending on patient circumstances, may be used for tocolysis for asthmatics in preterm labor. Magnesium sulfate is also a bronchodilator. Indomethacin should be avoided, as it may induce bronchospasm in the aspirin-sensitive patient. Data regarding the use of calcium channel blockers in pregnant asthmatics are not available. Patients who have been on systemic corticosteroid therapy within the past year should receive "stress doses" of 100 mg hydrocortisone every 8 hours (or its equivalent) throughout labor and for 24 hours postpartum (3).

Pain relief may be accomplished with fentanyl [other narcotics, including Demerol (meperidine), nalbuphine, and butorphanol, are associated with histamine release] or epidural anesthesia, as it decreases oxygen consumption and minute volume during labor (64). Minimal risk of bronchospasm may be accomplished during cesarean section by use of regional anesthesia or general anesthesia with ketamine induction (65).

Asthmatic patients are at increased risk of postpartum hemorrhage; this is believed to be secondary to hemostatic alterations related to altered arachidonic acid metabolism, deficient platelet aggregation, and increased levels of endogenous circulating heparin. F-series prostaglandins (66) and methylergonovine may trigger bronchospasm and should be avoided in asthmatics. Given these pharmacologic limitations, the physician may wish to type and cross match the asthmatic patient with other risk factors for hemorrhage as a precaution before delivery.

POSTPARTUM AND LACTATION CONCERNS

The overall course of asthma tends to resume its prepregnancy level of severity within 3 months postpartum. Lactation concerns have been addressed previously, but almost all asthma medications appear to be compatible with breast-feeding with the exception of antileukotrienes and 5-LO inhibitors. The importance of breast-feeding for newborn and maternal well-being can be safely emphasized in the majority of patients.

SUMMARY

Standard treatment of asthma, as recommended by the National Asthma Education Program, is, for the most part, applicable in pregnancy. Outcomes of pregnancy appear to be improved and similar to those of the general population if asthma is actively managed. Newer forms of treatment, such as leukotriene receptor antagonists and 5-LO inhibitors, are not recommended in the majority of patients at this time because of the availability of older agents with known safety profiles and proven efficacy.

REFERENCES

1. Weiss KB, Gergen PJ, Hodgon TA. An economic evaluation of asthma in the United States. *N Engl J Med* 1992;326:862–866.
2. Weiss KB. National Asthma Education and Prevention Program Task Force report on the cost effectiveness, quality of care, and financing of asthma care. *Am J Resp Crit Care Med* 1996;154(Suppl):S81–130.
3. National Asthma Education Program. *Management of Asthma During Pregnancy. Report of the Working Group on Asthma and Pregnancy,* 1993. Publication no. NIH 93-3279.
4. Schatz M, Zeiger RS, Harden K, et al. The safety of asthma and allergy medications during pregnancy. *J Allergy Clin Immunol* 1997;100:301–306.
5. McDonald CF, Burdon GW. Asthma in pregnancy and lactation. A position paper for the Thoracic Society of Australia and New Zealand. *Med J Aust* 1996;165:485–488.
6. De Swiet M. The respiratory system. In: Hyten F, Chamberlain G, eds. *Clinical physiology in obstetrics,* 2nd ed. London: Blackwell Scientific Publications, 1991:83–100.
7. Louis R, Shute J, Biagi S, et al. Cell infiltration, ICAM-1 expression, and eosinophil chemotactic activity in asthmatic sputum. A*m J Resp Crit Care Med* 1997;155:466–472.
8. Dahlen S-E, Hedqvist P, Hammarstrom S, et al. Leukotrienes are potent constrictors of human bronchi. *Nature* 1980;288:484–486.
9. Kellaway CH, Trethewie RE. The liberation of slow reacting smooth muscle stimulating substance of anaphylaxis. *Q J Ext Physiol* 1940;30:121–145.
10. Sims C, Chamberlain G, De Swiet M. Lung function test in bronchial asthma before, during, and after pregnancy. *Br J Obstet Gynecol* 1976;83:434–437.
11. Burdon JGW, Goss G. Asthma and pregnancy. *Aust N Z J Med* 1994;24:3–4.
12. Schatz M, Harden K, Forsythe A, et al. The course of asthma in pregnancy, post-partum, and with successive pregnancies: a prospective analysis. *J Allergy Clin Immunol* 1988;81:509–517.
13. Stenius-Aarniala B, Piirila P, Teramo K. Asthma and pregnancy: a prospective study of 198 pregnancies. *Thorax* 1988;43:12–18.
14. Mabie WC, Barton JR, Wasserstrum N, et al. Clinical observations on asthma in pregnancy. *J Matern Fetal Med* 1992;1:45–50.
15. Perlow JH, Montgomery D, Morgan MA, et al. Severity of asthma and perinatal outcome. *Am J Obstet Gynecol* 1992;167:963–967.
16. Demissie K, Breckenridge MB, Rhoads GG. Infant and maternal outcomes of pregnancies in asthmatic women. *Am J Resp Crit Care Med* 1998;158:1091–1095.
17. Alexander S, Dodds L, Armson BA. Perinatal outcomes in women with asthma during pregnancy. *Obstet Gynecol* 1998;92:435–440.
18. Minerbi-Codish I, Fraser D, Avnun L, et al. Influence of asthma in pregnancy on labor and the newborn. *Respiration* 1998;65:130–135.
19. Shaikh WA. A retrospective study on the safety of immunotherapy in pregnancy. *Clin Exp Allergy* 1993;23:857–860.
20. Prevention and control of influenza: recommendations of the Advisory Committee on Immunization Practices. *MMWR Morb Mortal Wkly Rep* 1999;48:1–28.
21. Sindberg Eriksen P, Gennser G, Lindvall R, et al. Acute effects of maternal smoking on fetal heart beat intervals. *Acta Obstet Gynecol Scand* 1984;63:385–390.
22. Goodman JD, Visser FG, Dawes GS. Effects of maternal cigarette smoking on fetal trunk movements, fetal breathing movements, and fetal heart rate. *Br J Obstet Gynecol* 1984;91:657–661.
23. Oncken CA, Hardardottir H, Hatsukami DK, et al. Effects of transdermal nicotine or smoking on nicotine concentrations and maternal-fetal hemodynamics. *Obstet Gynecol* 1997;90:569–574.
24. Bruner JP, Forouzan I. Smoking and buccally administered nicotine. Acute effect on uterine and umbilical

artery Doppler flow velocity waveforms. *J Reprod Med* 1991;36:435–440.

25. Arbeille P, Fignon A, Bose M, et al. [Changes in the utero-placental and fetal cerebral circulations induced by nicotine in the ovine fetus]. *J Gynecol Obstet Biol Reprod (Paris)* 1994;23:51–56.

26. Oncken CA, Hatsukami DK, Lupo VR, et al. Effects of short-term use of nicotine gum in pregnant smokers. *Clin Pharmacol Ther* 1996;59:654–661.

27. Lindblad A, Marsal K. Influence of nicotine chewing gum on fetal blood flow. *J Perinat Med* 1987;15:13–19.

28. Wright LN, Thorp JM Jr, Kuller JA, et al. Transdermal nicotine replacement in pregnancy: maternal pharmacokinetics and fetal effects. *Am J Obstet Gynecol* 1997;176:1090–1094.

29. Slotkin TA. Fetal nicotine exposure or cocaine exposure: which one is worse? *J Pharmacol Exp Ther* 1998;285:931–945.

30. Briggs GG, Freeman RK, Yaffe SJ. *Drugs in pregnancy and lactation,* 5th ed. Baltimore: Williams & Wilkins, 1998.

31. Haller Dl. The use of terbutaline for premature labor. *Drug Intell Clin Pharm* 1980;14:757–764.

32. Katz M, Robertson PA, Creasy RK. Cardiovascular complications associated with terbutaline treatment for premature labor. *Am J Obstet Gynecol* 1981;139:605–608.

33. Ingemarsson I, Bengtsson B. A five year experience with terbutaline for preterm labor: low rate of severe side effects. *Obstet Gynecol* 1985;66:176–180.

34. Hastwell GB, Halloway CP, Taylor TLO. A study of 208 patients in premature labor treated with orally-administered salbutamol. *Med J Aust* 1978;1:465–469.

35. Rayburn WF, Atkinson BD, Gilbert K, et al. Short-term effects of inhaled albuterol on maternal and fetal circulations. *Am J Obstet Gynecol* 1994;171:770–773.

36. Wagner J, Fredholm B, Lunelle NO, et al. Metabolic and circulatory effects of intravenous and oral salbutamol in late pregnancy in diabetic and non-diabetic women. *Acta Obstet Gynecol Scand Suppl* 1982;108:41–46.

37. Baker ER, Flanagan MF. Fetal atrial flutter associated with maternal beta-sympathomimetic drug exposure. *Obstet Gynecol* 1997;89:861.

38. Zilianti M, Aller J. Action of orciprenaline on uterine contractility during labor, maternal cardiovascular system, fetal heart rate, and acid-base balance. *Am J Obstet Gynecol* 1971;109:1073–1079.

39. Rosa F. Databases in the assessment of the effect of drugs during pregnancy. *J Allergy Clin Immunol* 1999;103:S360–S361.

40. Committee on Drugs, American Academy of Pediatrics. The transfer of drugs and other chemicals into human milk. *Pediatrics* 1994;93:137–150.

41. Kelly HW. Asthma pharmacotherapy: current practices and outlook. *Pharmacotherapy* 1997;17:13S–21S.

42. Tranfa CME, Pelaia G, Grembiale RD, et al. Short-term cardiovascular effects of salmeterol. *Chest* 1998;113:1272–1276.

43. Manchee GR, Barrow A, Kulkarni S, et al. Disposition of salmeterol xinafoate in laboratory animals and humans. *Drug Metab Dispos* 1993;21:1022–1028.

44. Wendel PJ, Ramin SM, Barnett-Hamm C, et al. Asthma treatment in pregnancy: a randomized controlled study. *Am J Obstet Gynecol* 1996;175:150–154.

45. Ishikawa M, Yoneyama Y, Power GG, et al. Maternal theophylline administration and breathing movements in late-gestation human fetuses. *Obstet Gynecol* 1996;88:973–978.

46. Lipshitz J. Uterine and cardiovascular effects of aminophylline. *Am J Obstet Gynecol* 1978;131:716–718.

47. Heinonen OP, Slone D, Shapiro S. *Birth defects and drugs in pregnancy.* Littleton, MA: Publishing Sciences Group, 1977:367, 370.

48. Nagahama H, Nagano K, Yamanaka I, et al. [Severe theophylline toxicity in a pregnant asthmatic patient]. *Masui* 1993;42:1076–1080.

49. Stenius-Aarniala B, Riikonen S, Teramo K. Slow-release theophylline in pregnant asthmatics. *Chest* 1995;107:642–647.

50. Strauss AA, Modanlou HD, Komatsu G. Theophylline toxicity in a preterm infant: selected clinical aspects. *Pediatr Pharmacol* 1985;5:209–212.

51. Azegami M, Mori N. Amniotic fluid embolism and leukotrienes. *Am J Obstet Gynecol* 1986;155:1119–1124.

52. Smith LJ. A risk-benefit assessment of antileukotrienes in asthma. *Drug Saf* 1998;19:205–218.

53. Calhoun WJ. Summary of clinical trials with zafirlukast. *Am J Respir Crit Care Med* 1998;157:S238–S248.

54. Holloway J, Ferriss J, Groff J, et al. Churg-Strauss syndrome associated with zafirlukast. *J Am Osteopath Assoc* 1998;98:275–278.

55. Sorkness CA. Establishing a therapeutic index for the inhaled corticosteroids: Part II. *J Allergy Clin Immunol* 1998;102:S52–S64.

56. Arduini D, Rizzo G, Parlati E, et al. Modifications of ultradian and circadian rhythms of fetal heart rate after fetal-maternal adrenal gland suppression: a double blind study. *Prenat Diagn* 19866:409–417.

57. Dorr HG, Versmold HT, Sippell WG, et al. Antenatal betamethasone therapy: effects on maternal, fetal, and neonatal mineralocorticoids, glucocorticoids, and progestins. *J Pediatr* 1986;108:990–993.

58. Ceizel AE, Rockenhauer M. Population-based case-control study of teratogenic potential of corticosteroids. *Teratology* 1997;56:335–340.

59. Dombrowski M, Thom E, McNellis D. Maternal-fetal medicine units studies of inhaled corticosteroids during pregnancy. *J Allergy Clin Immunol* 1999;103:S356–S359.

60. Stenius-Aarniala BS, Hedman J, Teramo KA. Acute asthma during pregnancy. *Thorax* 1996;51:411–414.

61. Mazzotta P, Loebstein R, Koren G. Treating allergic rhinitis in pregnancy. Safety considerations. *Drug Saf* 1999;20:361–375.

62. Mabie WC, Barton JR, Wasserstrum N, et al. Clinical observation on asthma in pregnancy. *J Matern Fetal Med* 1992;1:45–50.

63. Dombrowski MP. Pharmacologic therapy of asthma in pregnancy. *Obstet Gynecol Clin North Am* 1997;24:559–575.

64. Hagerdahl M, Jarvinen M, Kava T, et al. Minute ventilation and oxygen consumption during labor with epidural anesthesia. *Anesthesiology* 1983;59:425–427.

65. Hirschman CA, Downes H, Farbood A, et al. Ketamine block of bronchospasm in experimental canine asthma. *Br J Anaesth* 1979;51:8:713–718.

66. Hankins GDV, Berryman GK, Scott RT, et al. Maternal arterial desaturation with 15-methyl prostaglandin F2-alpha for uterine atony. *Obstet Gynecol* 1988;72:367.

6

Urinary Tract Infections in Pregnancy

George Bergus

Department of Family Medicine, University of Iowa Hospital Center, Iowa City, Iowa

INTRODUCTION

Urinary tract infection (UTI) is a frequent complication of pregnancy. This infection can be divided into three categories: asymptomatic bacteriuria (ASB), cystitis, and pyelonephritis. Of the three, ASB is the most common and is of concern because of the risk of progression to pyelonephritis and possible relationship to preterm birth and low birth weight children.

Background: UTI in Nonpregnant Women

Females of all ages are at a much higher risk for UTI than males except during the neonatal period. During the third and fourth decades of life, this gender difference is at its maximum with women at 40 to 50 times greater risk. Young adult women have the highest incidence of UTI of any group and average one infection every other year (1).

The usual route of infection is one in which bacteria ascend from the perineum, pass through the urethra, and invade the bladder. Glycolipid adherence factors enhance the ability of some strains of *Escherichia coli* to bind to urinary epithelium, but these strains cause most UTIs (2–4). Infections most often remain within the lower urinary tract but infrequently can ascend through the ureters and invade the upper urinary tract to cause pyelonephritis. Infections within the urinary tract are rarely from a blood-borne source.

Some individuals are at higher risk for developing UTI. Ten percent to 20% of women have epithelium to which uropathogenic *E. coli* adhere more easily and as a result are more prone to UTI (5–7). Having a history of at least two UTIs is a marker of having this type of epithelium and is a strong predictor of subsequent infections. Other well-defined physiologic risk factors for UTI include conditions that increase the risk of bladder contamination with perineal organisms. Sexual activity is one such condition and increases the risk of UTI in women with a dose–response relationship (1). Another physiologic risk factor is urine stasis in the bladder as this enhances bacterial growth. Infrequent voiding or incomplete bladder emptying are two common causes of stasis.

UTI IN PREGNANCY

Epidemiology

Significant bacteriuria is defined as the presence of more than 10^5 colony-forming units per milliliter of a single organism in a midstream, clean-catch urine specimen, whether or not symptoms are present. ASB is defined as the presence of significant bacteriuria with the absence of urinary symptoms.

The prevalence of bacteriuria during pregnancy is similar to that of age-matched, sexually active, nonpregnant women. Based on the prevalence of ASB in nonpregnant women, one would predict that 4% to 7% of women will be bacteriuric during pregnancy, a percentage that has been confirmed by various studies. Prevalence is doubled in groups of lower socioeconomic class, with sickle cell trait, or with diabetes. Women with a history of UTI are at higher risk of developing bacteriuria during pregnancy.

Bacteriuria is associated with significant morbidity to the mother and fetus; thus, it is important to identify it early and eradicate it for the duration of gestation (8). Although the frequency of ASB does not appear to be related to pregnancy, the morbidity associated with this condition is. In a nonpregnant cohort, ASB is little more than a curiosity because it is not related to symptomatic infection or illness (8a). In pregnancy, however, ASB can frequently progress to pyelonephritis (9).

Anatomic/Physiologic Changes of the Urinary Tract Associated with Pregnancy

During pregnancy, the urinary tract undergoes several distinct changes that increase the risk of urinary tract infection. Urine production increases because of increased blood volume associated with pregnancy and increased glomerular filtration rate. Urine also provides a better culture medium for bacteria during pregnancy because of gestational glucosuria and higher levels of amino acids. The ureters dilate under hormonal influence and the enlarged uterus can cause a functional obstruction of the ureters, particularly on the right side. Additionally, the bladder of a pregnant woman can tolerate double the normal filling volume before triggering the sensation of the need to void. These combined effects result in urinary stasis and a favorable bacterial growth environment, predisposing pregnant women to ascending urinary infections and pyelonephritis.

Microbiology

The pathogens cultured during pregnancy are much the same as those found in nonpregnant women. Most UTIs are caused by bacteria that normally inhabit the colon. Nearly 80% to 90% of community-acquired UTIs are caused by *E. coli* (10,11). Other gram-negative organisms, including *Proteus* species, *Klebsiella pneumoniae*, and *Pseudomonas aeruginosa*, cause infections but are much less common with the exception of hospitalized patients, immunocompromised patients, or patients who have undergone recent urinary tract catheterization or instrumentation. Gram-positive organisms including *Staphylococcus saprophyticus*, *Staphylococcus aureus*, group B streptococci, and *Enterococcus faecium* are uropathogens but are less common causes of UTI. Anaerobic bacteria and fastidious organisms predominate in the gut but almost never cause UTI in nonpregnant women. However, during pregnancy, these organisms can be cultured from 10% to 15% of women. *Gardnerella vaginalis* is one of the most common isolates followed by lactobacilli, microaerophilic streptococci, and *Ureaplasma urealyticum*. It is unclear whether these organisms cause disease in pregnant women (12,13).

Complications of UTIs

Although pyelonephritis is a rare outcome of uncomplicated UTI among nonpregnant women, the incidence during pregnancy is 1% to 4%. Among pregnant women, 20% to 40% of those with bacteriuria will develop pyelonephritis compared with less than 2% of those with an initial negative urine culture (14). Also, in contrast to healthy nonpregnant women, pregnant women are likely to have persistent bacteriuria until treated, with most untreated patients remaining culture positive for the duration of gestation.

The risk of pyelonephritis from ASB can be reduced by detecting ASB and eradicating the bacteriuria. Only 6.5 women with ASB need to be treated to prevent one case of pyelonephritis (15). Some, but not all, data suggest that ASB, independent of its progression to pyelonephritis, places a mother at higher risk of preterm birth and low birth weight infant, although the mechanism of this relationship is unknown (16).

Because of the risks associated with ASB and the fact that it is asymptomatic by definition, both the U.S. Preventive Task Force and the American College of Obstetricians and Gynecologists recommend that physicians actively screen for this condition. Additionally, although a history of UTI places pregnant women at higher risk for ASB, this history alone cannot be used to identify the subgroup of women who are at markedly higher risk of having ASB. Thus, laboratory evaluation of urine samples is central to screening. ACOG recommends screening all women for asymptomatic bacteriuria during the first prenatal visit. If screening is by urine dipstick, ACOG recommends confirming the presence of bacteriuria by culture (17). The U.S. Preventive Services Taskforce recommends that all women be screened at 12 to 16 weeks gestation with urine culture (18). Using the urinalysis alone for screening will miss 25 to 50% of women with asymptomatic bacteriuria (19). Epidemiological data suggest that urine culture at the 16th gestational week produces the greatest number of bacteriuria-free gestational weeks (20). The U.S. Preventive Services Task Force recommends that all pregnant women be screened at 12 to 16 weeks gestation with urine culture (21). Using the urinalysis alone for screening will miss 25% to 50% of women with ASB (22). Epidemiologic data suggest that urine culture at the 16th gestational week produces the greatest number of bacteriuria-free gestational weeks (14).

Symptoms

Cystitis is suggested by complaints of dysuria, hematuria, urinary frequency, urgency, or suprapubic discomfort. Elements of the history that localize the infection to the upper urinary tract include the presence of fever, chills, abdominal pain, flank pain, or vomiting (Table 6.1). These systemic symptoms are suggestive of an upper tract infection, but clinical localization within the upper or lower urinary tract is difficult. More than 30% of women with symptoms suggestive of lower tract infection can have renal involvement, and in some studies as many as one third of patients with lower tract infections had fever and flank pain. Most of the research on differentiating upper tract and lower tract infections has been undertaken in nonpregnant women, but those data that are available suggest that these findings also apply to pregnant women.

TABLE 6.1. *Clinical factors useful in localizing urinary tract infections to the upper urinary tract*

	Sensitivity (%)	Specificity (%)
Flank pain	48	67
Fever	44	80
Chills and rigors	32	87
Nausea and vomiting	24	84

Data from ref. 57.

Detection of UTI in Pregnancy

Dipstick Urinalysis

Physicians generally use the urinalysis to diagnose UTI in nonpregnant women. The urinalysis includes a dry reagent test strip (the dipstick) and microscopy of a centrifuged urine sample. The dipstick, which detects blood, nitrite, and leukocyte esterase (LE) in the urine, is simple to perform and takes less than 5 minutes from sample collection to test result. The dipstick is not a sensitive means of detecting ASB because of the lack of inflammation associated with this type of infection.

The LE test detects the presence of an esterase found in white blood cells (WBCs) and has a reported sensitivity for detecting symptomatic infection in the range of 70% to 90% (23,24). The LE is less sensitive in patients with only mild symptoms and more sensitive in patients with severe symptoms (25). It is likely that there is a relationship between the severity of symptoms and leukocyte counts in the urine as both are related to urinary tract inflammation. False positives can occur because of contamination by vaginal leukocytes and leukocytes from chlamydial urethritis as well as by a high urine pH, high levels of urine glucose, or from tetracycline, cephalexin, gentamicin, imipenem, or clavulanate in the urine (26).

Dietary nitrates are excreted into the urine and converted by gram-negative bacteria to nitrites. This conversion usually requires that the urine and gram-negative organisms have several hours of contact; therefore, the first voided specimen in the morning is most likely to be positive for nitrites in a patient with UTI. This test has a sensitivity of only 20% to 45% (22,23,27,28). Gram-positive and *Pseudomonas* species will not be detected with this test as these bacteria do not convert nitrates to nitrites. The specificity of this test is more than 95%; therefore, when the nitrite test is positive, it is highly likely that UTI is present. Using LE and nitrate in combination so that the dipstick is considered positive if either is positive is a better predictor of symptomatic UTI than is either of the two tests individually (29). Combining these two tests has little impact on the sensitivity of the dipstick for detecting ASB.

Tincello and Richmond (28) reported their experience based on 960 women in the first trimester of pregnancy. Although they used a liberal definition of a positive test (any positive nitrite or LE or more than a trace of blood or protein), the dipstick detected only one third of all the infected urine samples. A second study with more than 1,000 women similarly found a low sensitivity (50%) for a dipstick that assessed nitrites and LE (22).

Microscopy

Direct microscopy of the urinary sediment is used to look for white cells (pyuria), red cells (hematuria), bacteria (bacteriuria), and white cell casts. The sediment is prepared by centrifuging a test tube of freshly voided urine, decanting the urine, and then resuspending the sediment with the urine that adheres to the sides of the test tube. The microscopy results are influenced by how long the urine is allowed to sit after collection, the duration and speed of centrifugation, the technique used to decant the urine and resuspend the sediment, and finally the technique of the individual performing the microscopy. Although the number of leukocytes per high-power field (HPF or 400× magnification) in the resuspended urine sediment is commonly used to diagnose UTI, there is not agreement about how many leukocytes define the presence of infection. Some authors suggested that as few as two WBCs per HPF can be used to identify infected urine, whereas other authors suggested that 15 WBCs is a more appropriate cutoff point (30,31). Additionally, pyuria is not a sensitive test for detecting ASB. The sensitivity of 10 or more leukocytes per HPF is reported to be less than 30% (22,32).

The presence of bacteria under an oil-immersion magnification (400×) is also suggestive of UTI. Finding at least one bacterium under these conditions has a sensitivity and specificity of approximately 90%. Increasing the definition of bacteriuria to at least two bacteria per HPF improves specificity (95%) but is associated with a lower sensitivity (83%) (22). Similar test characteristics were reported for the presence of bacteria in the urine of nonpregnant individuals (33).

White cell casts can also be found in the urine sediment and are identified by their tube-like, granular appearance. Their presence suggests inflammation within the kidney such that WBCs are collecting within the renal tubules. Infection is the primary cause of these casts, although interstitial nephritis can also produce them.

Urine Culture

The urine culture remains the test of choice for detection of ASB despite its significant cost. The culture is simple and reliable. Although more expensive than a urine dipstick, the culture is a sensitive means of detecting ASB and provides antibiotic sensitivities to help with clinical decision making. A typical culture does not provide any information for 48 hours, but this does not represent a major problem for ASB because the culture is being used as a means of screening.

The ideal specimen for culture is clean-catch midstream urine properly collected with minimal vaginal contamination. When the urine produces a colony count of more than 10^5 of the same organism, there is an 80% chance that the patient has a significant bacteriuria. When two consecutive cultures grow out the same organism, the probability of a true bacteriuria increases to more than 95%. There are more specific methods of obtaining urine for culture. Suprapubic aspiration is safe in pregnancy, but this invasive procedure is not clinically used to obtain a sample for a screening test. Bladder catheterization carries a risk of introduction of infection and therefore is not used as a screening test.

Cost-effectiveness analysis (34,35) suggests that screening for ASB using culture can be cost-effective because of the marked decrease in costs for hospitalizations arising from women developing pyelonephritis. Although the analysis reported screening with a urine dipstick saves more money than screening with culture, screening with urine culture prevented about twice as many cases of pyelonephritis. Because of the cost of urine culture, efforts have been made to find a quick, inexpensive, and reliable screening test to predict which patients need the standard urine culture. At this time, such a test is not readily available.

Therapy

After bacteriuria has been identified, the goal is to eradicate it for the duration of the pregnancy.

Patients with a negative initial culture require no further screening for infection unless they develop urinary symptoms later. Women with positive cultures must be promptly treated with the appropriate antibiotics.

The health care professional is faced with two decisions after deciding that antibiotic therapy is indicated: the specific drug and the duration of therapy. There is wide agreement about drug type but less agreement about duration of therapy. In pregnancy, antibiotics should be selected using specific knowledge of the potential risks and the potential benefits.

There are several excellent references that can be used to guide physicians in antibiotic selection during pregnancy and lactation (36–38). Easily accessible references about drug use in pregnancy and lactation can be found on the Internet (http://www.perinatology.com/exposures/druglist.htm and http://www.rxlist.com).

Virtually all antibiotics cross the placenta, and many antibiotics appear in breast milk when taken by lactating women. However, not all antibiotics are associated with adverse effects in the fetus or the breast-feeding woman. Selection should be carefully made and risks of therapy should always be weighed against the benefits.

Drugs That Can Be Used as First-line Therapy in Pregnancy

Amoxicillin and Ampicillin

Amoxicillin and ampicillin rapidly cross the placenta and enter the fetal circulation. These antibiotics have been widely used without evidence of toxicity.

Amoxicillin and ampicillin are excreted in human milk in very small amounts but cause few adverse effects. In general, amoxicillin and ampicillin appear to be safe to administer to a breast-feeding woman.

Amoxicillin and Clavulanate Potassium

Both agents rapidly cross the placenta. There are, however, no adequate and well-controlled studies in pregnant women, and so this drug should be used during pregnancy only if clearly needed. Clinical trials using amoxicillin and clavulanate

potassium have not found any significant fetal or maternal toxicity (39).

Amoxicillin is excreted into the milk but appears to pose little danger to breast-feeding infants. It is unknown whether clavulanate potassium passes into breast milk. This drug appears to be safe to use with breast-feeding women.

Cephalosporins

Cephalosporins have been widely used in treating pregnant women. They are effective, and to date there have not been reports of adverse effects to the fetus. They appear to be safe during gestation; however, no adequate and well-controlled studies have been performed in pregnant women.

Cephalosporins are excreted into human milk in low concentration but appear to have little adverse impact on infants. They can be considered safe for use in breast-feeding women.

Erythromycin and Azithromycin

These drugs pass at low levels across the placenta. Erythromycin has been widely used in pregnancy and appears to be safe. Studies have found that azithromycin is better tolerated during pregnancy than is erythromycin owing to a lower incidence of gastrointestinal side effects (40).

Erythromycin is excreted into breast milk but is safe when administered to a breast-feeding woman. Azithromycin is excreted into human milk and appears to accumulate in breast milk owing to its lipid solubility. Azithromycin is approved for use in children 6 months and older, but studies on this drug's use in breast-feeding are not available.

Nitrofurantoin

There are no data linking this drug with congenital malformations. Nitrofurantoin poses a risk of hemolytic anemia in infants with G6PD deficiency. Otherwise, there are no reports of hemolysis in infants from this drug. Thus, in general, nitrofurantoin is regarded as safe for use during pregnancy.

Nitrofurantoin has been detected in breast milk in trace amounts. This drug appears to be safe when taken by breast-feeding mothers as long as their infants do not have a G6PD deficiency.

Antibiotics That Can Be Used as Second-line Therapy in Pregnancy

Aminoglycosides

Aminoglycosides rapidly cross the placenta. They appear to pose no risks specifically associated with pregnancy but should not be used as first-line therapy because of their potential nephrotoxicity and ototoxicity. Ototoxicity from gentamicin has not been documented from fetal exposure, but there are reports of irreversible bilateral congenital deafness in children whose mothers received streptomycin during pregnancy. Serious side effects to the mother, fetus, or newborn have not been reported in the treatment of pregnant women with other aminoglycosides.

Aminoglycosides pass into breast milk at low levels, but they have poor oral absorption. These drugs appear to be safe when administered to breast-feeding women.

Trimethoprim

Trimethoprim (TMP) is a potential teratogen, and, if possible, its use should be avoided during the first trimester. TMP crosses the placenta and results in a fetal drug level 70% to 90% of maternal levels. Although there are no large, well-controlled studies on the use of TMP in pregnant women, a retrospective study found no increase in congenital abnormalities (41).

TMP is excreted into human milk at very low levels. The risk to breast-feeding infants appears to be negligible.

Trimethoprim/Sulfamethoxazole

Trimethoprim/sulfamethoxazole (TMP/SMX) has been widely used in pregnancy but because of the concern of the antifolate effect of trimethoprim and the neonatal hyperbilirubinemia that can occur if sulfonamides are used late in pregnancy, TMP/SMX is recommended only in the second trimester. Although there are no large, well-controlled studies on the use of TMP/SMX

in pregnant women, Brumfitt and Pursell (42), in a retrospective study, reported no increase in the incidence of congenital abnormalities.

Low concentrations of SMX pass into breast milk. There are rare reports of adverse effects with breast-feeding infants. Breast-feeding appears to be safe as long as exposure is avoided with premature infants, medically ill infants, infants with hyperbilirubinemia, or infants with glucose-6-phosphate dehydrogenase (G6PD) deficiency.

Route and Duration of Therapy

There have been many recommendations about the duration of therapy of UTIs ranging from 1 to 10 days, depending on whether the patient has upper or lower tract disease and whether she is pregnant (17). Three days of antibiotic treatment appear to be optimal in many cases of ASB or cystitis. Three-day therapy results in a cure rate close to that achieved with 7 to 10 days of treatment but with many fewer antibiotic complications (43). Single-dose therapy has been advocated but has a lower cure rate than does multiple-day therapy. TMP/SMX is the most cost-effective antibiotic because of its low cost, high cure rate, and only moderate level of side effects (44).

Therapy of ASB and Cystitis

Discussion of treatment of these conditions is combined here because antibiotic therapy is similar for both. Although there is debate about the duration of therapy, there is agreement about the class of antibiotics that is effective. Studies have shown that TMP/SMX, the cephalosporins, and nitrofurantoin are safe and effective. Increasingly, amoxicillin is not a good empiric choice because 20% to 30% of the gram-negative organisms that cause UTI are resistant (Table 6.2).

Single-dose oral therapy has been advocated to help with patient compliance and reduce adverse effects of therapy. Most of the studies comparing single- with multiple-dose therapy have not found significant differences. However, the studies have been small and the lack of difference could arise from lack of statistical power.

TABLE 6.2. *Standard therapy for asymptomatic bacteriuria and cystitis*

Antibiotic	Dose (mg)	Frequency	Duration
Amoxicillin	500	t.i.d.	3–5 days
Cephalexin	500	q.i.d.	3–5 days
TMP/SMX[a]	DS	b.i.d.	3–5 days
Nitrofurantoin	100	q.i.d.	3–5 days

[a]TMP/SMX is not recommended early in the first trimester or within 2 weeks of delivery.

TMP/SMX, trimethoprim-sulfamethoxazole; DS, double strength.

TABLE 6.3. *Standard initial therapy for pyelonephritis*

Antibiotic	Dosage
Ampicillin	2 g every 6 h
Gentamicin[a]	2 mg/kg load then 1.7 mg/kg every 8 h
Cefazolin	1 g every 6 h
Gentamicin[a]	2 mg/kg load then 1.7 mg/kg every 8 h
Piperacillin	4 g every 8 h
Ceftriaxone	1 g every 24 h
Cefotaxime	1 g every 6 h

[a]Dose of gentamicin to be adjusted for renal function and levels need to be monitored.

Therapy should be modified based on culture result and clinical course.

The question of antibiotic duration is the subject of a recent Cochrane review based on seven individual trials (45). Although the authors could not demonstrate a difference in the effectiveness between single-dose therapy and therapies of 4 to 7 days, they also caution that there was significant heterogeneity of the trials. As a result, the authors reported that the effectiveness of single-dose therapy has not been confirmed. At this time, it appears reasonable to treat women with ASB or cystitis for 3 to 5 days. Of greater importance than duration of therapy is the follow-up that is required because these women are at high risk of a recurrence of infection and the morbidity that is associated with UTI during pregnancy.

Pyelonephritis

Traditionally, all pregnant women with pyelonephritis have been hospitalized for parenteral therapy, intravenous hydration, and close observation. Initial choice of antibiotic should be ampicillin and gentamicin or a cephalosporin given parenterally (Table 6.3). Fifteen percent of these patients will have bacteremia, so blood cultures should be obtained before starting parenteral antibiotics (46,47). Intravenous antibiotics need to be continued until the patient has been afebrile for 24 hours and then can be switched to an oral agent for a total of 10 to 14 days. Women with pyelonephritis commonly have coexisting dehydration owing to the fever and vomiting associated with the infection. Thus, vigorous intravenous fluid rehydration with normal saline is indicated to improve perfusion of vital organs including the uterus.

The typical clinical course of pyelonephritis during pregnancy can be summarized based on drug efficacy trials (48). Despite the presence of septicemia, few women will develop septic shock. Fever typically lasts into the second hospital day and the average length of hospitalization is 4 days. Within 24 hours of starting antibiotics, approximately half of all patients will be afebrile, and within 48 hours, 85% of women will no longer have fever. Transient renal dysfunction occurs in one fourth of women with pyelonephritis, but this dysfunction is temporary and resolves quickly (49). When patients do not improve after 72 hours of parenteral therapy, imaging is indicated to identify a perinephric abscess, an intrarenal abscess, unrecognized anatomic abnormality, or ureteral obstruction. Sonography can be used to identify these complications. Abscess or obstruction is an indication for urologic consultation. Complicated infections should be treated for at least 21 days.

Although hospital-based care remains the usual standard, this practice has been challenged by research on outpatient therapy of pyelonephritis. Nonhospital-based care has clearly been shown to be safe and effective in carefully selected nonpregnant women as long as the patients are medically stable and can maintain hydration by oral fluids. Using oral antibiotics at home, these women do as well as if they are admitted to the hospital and treated with parenteral antibiotics (50). There are several studies that suggest that outpatient therapy of pregnant women can also be as safe but more cost-effective than hospitalization. Angel et al. (47), in 1990, published a report on 90 women randomized to inpatient therapy using oral cephalexin or parenteral cephalothin therapy. All women received initial hydration with normal saline. Cure rates were almost identical and more than 90% in both groups. More recently, Sanchez-Ramos et al. (51) compared once-a-day ceftriaxone to multiple doses of cefazolin. This study of 178 patients found no difference between the groups in relation to treatment failure, length of febrile morbidity, or duration of hospitalization. The authors of this study suggested that their findings raise the possibility of outpatient management of pyelonephritis with systemic antibiotics administered by a visiting nurse. Millar et al. (52), in the same year, reported such a study based on 120 women. All women were initially evaluated in the emergency department where their ability to tolerate oral hydration was confirmed. Patients admitted to the hospital were treated with intravenous cefazolin, whereas those sent home were treated with intramuscular ceftriaxone. Clinical outcomes were similar in both groups except for the need to broaden antimicrobial coverage of more of the hospitalized women because of worsening clinical picture or a prolonged febrile course while on cefazolin alone. This study suggests that in properly selected patients, outpatient therapy may be safe and effective.

FOLLOW-UP AFTER THERAPY FOR UTI DURING PREGNANCY

Repeat cultures should be obtained 7 days after treatment to confirm eradication of bacteriuria. Persistent infections after a 3- to 5-day course of oral antibiotics will occur in 20% of women. A second course of antibiotics, using a different agent and based on *in vitro* sensitivities should be prescribed for 7 to 10 days.

Because one third of women with a first episode of UTI during pregnancy will develop a relapse or recurrence, all these women should be cultured monthly until delivery (53). The risk of recurrence is not associated with the duration of treatment. If repeat cultures revert to being positive, antibiotic sensitivities should be reassessed

TABLE 6.4. *Antibiotic prophylaxis for recurrent urinary tract infections during pregnancy*

Antibiotic	Dosage
Nitrofurantoin	100 mg/day
Cephalexin	250 mg/day
TMP/SMX	One single-strength tablet/day

TMP/SMX, trimethoprim-sulfamethoxazole.

and bacteriuria treated with a different drug. Approximately 50% of women who develop a second infection will develop another infection after successful treatment (54). Suppressive antibiotic therapy for the duration of pregnancy is indicated for patients who experience more than one relapse of bacteriuria.

Because eradication of bacteriuria has a substantial impact on improving obstetric and neonatal outcome, physicians have been encouraged to be more liberal in their use of prophylaxis (55). Recommended regimens are shown in Table 6.4. An alternative to everyday use of prophylaxis is the use of a single postcoital dose of 250 mg cephalexin or 50 mg nitrofurantoin (56). Postcoital treatment is effective and exposes the pregnant woman to significantly smaller amounts of antibiotics than does daily dosing.

SUMMARY

Although pregnancy is not associated with a higher rate of bacteriuria, women with ASB are at a high risk of developing pyelonephritis. Detection and antibiotic treatment significantly reduce prenatal morbidity associated with bacteriuria. The standard urine culture, performed once near the sixteenth week of pregnancy, is currently the optimal screening test.

Every pregnant woman with ASB should be treated with a 3- to 5-day course of antibiotics. An extended second course of antibiotic therapy should be used if the initial course of antibiotics does not result in a sterile urine. Follow-up cultures must be done after all courses of therapy to ensure eradication of infection. Pyelonephritis requires rapid initiation of parenteral antibiotic therapy and rehydration. Cephalosporins or ampicillin and gentamicin are safe and effective during pregnancy.

REFERENCES

1. Hooton TM, Scholes D, Hughes JP, et al. A prospective study of risk factors for symptomatic urinary tract infection in young women. *N Engl J Med* 1996;335: 468–474.
2. Svanborg C, Godaly G. Bacterial virulence in urinary tract infection. *Infect Dis Clin North Am* 1997;11:513–529.
3. Measley RE Jr, Levison ME. Host defense mechanisms in the pathogenesis of urinary tract infection. *Med Clin North Am* 1991;75:275–286.
4. Johnson JR. Virulence factors in *Escherichia coli* urinary tract infection. *Clin Microbiol Rev* 1991;4:80–128.
5. Schaeffer AJ, Jones JM, Dunn JK. Association of *in vitro* Escherichia coli adherence to vaginal and buccal epithelial cells with susceptibility of women to recurrent urinary-tract infections. *N Engl J Med* 1981;304:1062–1066.
6. Stapleton A. Host factors in susceptibility to urinary tract infections. *Adv Exp Med Biol* 1999;462:351–358.
7. Sobel JD. Pathogenesis of urinary tract infection. Role of host defenses. *Infect Dis Clin North Am* 1997;11:531–549.
8. Smaill F. Antibiotic vs no treatment for asymptomatic bacteriuria in pregnancy (Cochrane review). In: *The Cochrane Library*, issue 4. Oxford: Update Software, 1998.
8a. Hooton TM, Scholes D, Stapleton AE, et al. A prospective study of asymptomatic bacteriuria in sexually active young women. *N Engl J Med* 2000;343(14):992–997.
9. Norden CW, Kass EH. Bacteriuria of pregnancy–a critical appraisal. *Annu Rev Med* 1968;19:431–470.
10. Wilkie ME, Almond MK, Marsh FP. Diagnosis and management of urinary tract infection in adults. *BMJ* 1992;305:1137–1041.
11. Lucas MJ, Cunningham FG. Urinary infection in pregnancy. *Clin Obstet Gynecol* 1993;36:855–868.
12. Hay PE, Lamont RF, Taylor-Robinson D, et al. Abnormal bacterial colonisation of the genital tract and subsequent preterm delivery and late miscarriage. *BMJ* 1994;308:295–298.
13. Patterson TF, Andriole VT. Detection, significance, and therapy of bacteriuria in pregnancy. *Infect Dis Clin North Am* 1997;11:593–608.
14. Stenqvist K, Dahlen-Nilsson I, Lidin-Janson G, et al. Bacteriuria in pregnancy. *Am J Epidemiol* 1989;129:372–379.
15. Smaill F. Antibiotic vs no treatment for asymptomatic bacteriuria. In: Enkin MW, Keirse MJNC, Renfrew MJ, et al., eds. *Pregnancy and childbirth module of the Cochrane database of systematic reviews.* London: BMJ Publishing Group, 1995.
16. Romero R, Oyarzun E, Mazor M, Sirtori M, Hobbins JC, Bracken M. Meta-analysis of the relationship between asymptomatic bacteriuria and preterm delivery/low birth weight. *Obstet Gynecol* 1989;73(4):576–582.
17. The American Academy of Obstetricians and Gynecologists (ACOG). Antimicrobial therapy for obstetric patients. *ACOG Educational Bulletin* 1998;245.
18. *Guide to Clinical Preventive Services, 2nd ed.* Baltimore, MD: Williams & Wilkins, 1996:347–359.
19. Bachman JW, Heise RH, Naessens JM, Timmerman MG. A study of various tests to detect asymptomatic urinary tract infections in an obstetric population. *JAMA* 1993;270(16):1971–1974.
20. Stenqvist K, Dahlen-Nilsson I, Lidin-Janson G, et al. Bacteriuria in pregnancy. Frequency and risk of acquisition. *Am J Epidemiol* 1989;129(2):372–379.
21. U.S. Preventive Task Force. *Guide to clinical preventive services,* 2nd ed. Baltimore: Williams & Wilkins, 1996:347–359.
22. Bachman JW, Heise RH, Naessens JM, et al. A study of various tests to detect asymptomatic urinary tract infections in an obstetric population. *JAMA* 1993;3270:1971–1974.
23. Pfaller MA, Koontz FP. Laboratory evaluation of leukocyte esterase and nitrite tests for the detection of bacteriuria. *J Clin Microbiol* 1985;21:840–842.
24. Blum RN, Wright RA. Detection of pyuria and bacteriuria in symptomatic ambulatory women. *Gen Intern Med* 1992;7:140–144.
25. Lachs MS, Nachamkin I, Edelstein PH, et al. Spectrum bias in the evaluation of diagnostic tests: lessons from the rapid dipstick test for urinary tract infection. *Ann Intern Med* 1992;117:135–140.
26. Beer JH, Vogt A, Neftel K, et al. False positive results for leucocytes in urine dipstick test with common antibiotics. *BMJ* 1996;313:25.
27. Roy JB, Wilkerson RG. Fallibility of Griess (nitrite) test. *Urology* 1984;23:270–271.
28. Tincello DG, Richmond DH. Evaluation of reagent strips in detecting asymptomatic bacteriuria in early pregnancy: prospective case series. *BMJ* 1998;316:435–437.
29. Hurlbut TA, Littenberg B. The diagnostic accuracy of rapid dipstick tests to predict urinary tract infection. *Am J Clin Pathol* 1991;96:582–588.
30. Alwall N. Pyuria: deposit in high-power microscopic field- WBC/hpf-versus WBC/mm3 in counting chamber. *Acta Med Scand* 1973;194:537–540.
31. Wigton RS, Hoellerich VL, Ornato JP, et al. Use of clinical findings in the diagnosis of urinary tract infection in women. *Arch Intern Med* 1985;145:2222–2227.
32. Soisson AP, Watson WJ, Benson WL, et al. Value of a screening urinalysis in pregnancy. *J Reprod Med* 1985;30:588–90.
33. Jenkins RD, Fenn JP, Matsen JM. Review of urine microscopy for bacteriuria. *JAMA* 1986;255:3397–3403.
34. Campbell-Brown M, McFadyen IR, Seal DV, et al. Is screening for bacteriuria in pregnancy worthwhile? *BMJ* 1987;294:1579–1582.
35. Rouse DJ, Andrews WW, Goldenberg RL, et al. Screening and treatment of asymptomatic bacteriuria of pregnancy to prevent pyelonephritis: a cost-effectiveness and cost-benefit analysis. *Obstet Gynecol* 1995;86:119–123.
36. Briggs GB, Freeman RK, Yaffe SJ. *Drugs in pregnancy and lactation: a reference guide to fetal and neonatal risk,* 5th ed. Baltimore: Williams & Wilkins, 1998.
37. Lawrence RA. *Breastfeeding: a guide for the medical profession,* 4th ed. St. Louis: Mosby, 1994.
38. Committee on Drugs. The transfer of drugs and other chemicals into human milk. *Pediatrics* 1994;93:137–150.
39. Pedler SJ, Bint AJ. Comparative study of amoxicillin-clavulanic acid and cephalexin in the treatment of bacteriuria during pregnancy. *Antimicrob Agents Chemother* 1985;27:508–510.
40. Wehbeh HA, Ruggeirio RM, Shahem S, et al. Single-dose azithromycin for chlamydia in pregnant women. *J Reprod Med* 1998;43:509–514.
41. Czeizel A. A case-control analysis of the teratogenic effects of co-trimoxazole. *Reprod Toxicol* 1990;4:305–313.

42. Brumfitt W, Pursell R. Trimethoprim-sulfamethoxazole in the treatment of bacteriuria in women. *J Infect Dis* 1973;128[Suppl]:657–665.

43. Duff P. Urinary tract infections. *Prim Care Update Ob/Gyn* 1994;1:12.

44. Hooton TM, Winter C, Tiu F, et al. Randomized comparative trial and cost analysis of 3-day antimicrobial regimens for treatment of acute cystitis in women. *JAMA* 1995;273:41–45.

45. Villar J, Lydon-Rochelle MT, Gülmezoglu AM. Duration of treatment for asymptomatic bacteriuria during pregnancy (Cochrane review). In: *The Cochrane Library*, issue 4. Oxford: Update Software, 1998.

46. Johnson JR, Lyons MF, Pearce W, et al. Therapy for women hospitalized with acute pyelonephritis: a randomized trial of ampicillin versus trimethoprim-sulfamethoxazole for 14 days. *J Infect Dis* 1991;163:325–330.

47. Angel JL, O'Brien WF, Finan MA, et al. Acute pyelonephritis in pregnancy: a prospective study of oral versus intravenous antibiotic therapy. *Obstet Gynecol* 1990;76:28–32.

48. Sanchez-Ramos L, McAlpine KJ, Adair CD, et al. Pyelonephritis in pregnancy: once-a-day ceftriaxone versus multiple doses of cefazolin. A randomized, double-blind trial. *Am J Obstet Gynecol* 1995;172:129–133.

49. Whalley PJ, Cunningham FG, Martin FG. Transient renal dysfunction associated with acute pyelonephritis of pregnancy. *Obstet Gynecol* 1975;46:174–177.

50. Pinson AG, Philbrick JT, Lindbeck GH, et al. Oral antibiotic therapy for acute pyelonephritis: a methodologic review of the literature. *J Gen Intern Med* 1992;7:544–553.

51. Sanchez-Ramos L, McAlpine KJ, Adair CD, et al. Pyelonephritis in pregnancy: once-a-day ceftriaxone versus multiple doses of cefazolin. A randomized, double-blind trial. *Am J Obstet Gynecol* 1995;172:129–133.

52. Millar LK, Wing DA, Paul RH, et al. Outpatient treatment of pyelonephritis in pregnancy: a randomized controlled trial. *Obstet Gynecol* 1995;86:560–564.

53. Leveno KJ, Harris RE, Gilstrap LC, et al. Bladder versus renal bacteriuria during pregnancy: recurrence after treatment. *Am J Obstet Gynecol* 1981;139:403–406.

54. Whalley PJ, Cunningham FG. Short-term versus continuous antimicrobial therapy for asymptomatic bacteriuria in pregnancy. *Obstet Gynecol* 1977;49:262–265.

55. Stapleton A, Stamm WE. Prevention of urinary tract infection. *Infect Dis Clin North Am* 1997;11:719–733.

56. Pfau A, Sacks TG. Effective prophylaxis for recurrent urinary tract infections during pregnancy. *Clin Infect Dis* 1992;14:810–814.

57. Sanford JP. Urinary tract symptoms and infections. *Annu Rev Med* 1975;26:485–497.

7

Caffeine

James D. Goldberg

Department of Obstetrics, Gynecology and Reproductive Sciences, University of California, San Francisco, San Francisco, California

Caffeine is present in a variety of edibles including coffee, tea, soft drinks, cocoa, chocolate, and several over-the-counter drugs. As a result, caffeine is widely used in pregnancy, the most common source being coffee. It has been estimated that 70% to 80% of pregnant women use caffeine daily (1,2). Caffeine is rapidly absorbed from the digestive tract and has been detected in essentially all body fluids. Caffeine is metabolized more slowly during pregnancy, and thus blood levels may be higher than in the nonpregnant state (3). There is some evidence that pregnant women may decrease their coffee intake during pregnancy, possibly related to the nausea of early pregnancy (4).

Caffeine (1,3,7-trimethylxanthine) is an alkaloid present in several different plants. Caffeine is a dioxypurine and is related to uric acid and the purine DNA bases adenine and guanine. Because of this, there has been concern regarding possible teratogenic effects of caffeine. Based on a number of animal studies that showed teratogenic effects after exposure to large amounts of caffeine (generally the equivalent of approximately 25 cups of coffee per day), the US Food and Drug Administration (FDA) in 1980 cautioned pregnant women to limit their intake of coffee (5). After a review of subsequent literature, the FDA in 1986 issued a statement that they had "significantly less concern" regarding caffeine and stated that "there is insufficient evidence to conclude that caffeine adversely affects reproductive function in humans" (6).

Studies of the effects of caffeine in pregnancy have been confounded by differences in study populations and study design, outcome ascertainment, determination of amount and timing of caffeine exposure, and lack of adjustment for confounding factors. This chapter reviews the reported effects of caffeine in the areas of congenital malformations, low birth weight, delayed fertility, and spontaneous abortion. Review of the literature focuses on those papers published since the 1986 FDA statement.

SOURCES OF CAFFEINE

Caffeine has been identified in more than 60 plant species. Almost all the caffeine available in the United States is imported, mainly in the form of coffee, tea, cocoa, kola nuts, and caffeine itself. One of the major difficulties in studying the effects of caffeine has been the wide variation in caffeine content of various products. Table 7.1 presents average values of caffeine content as reported in the literature (7). However, there may be wide variations in these standard values. For example, one investigator reported the caffeine content of a "cup" (25 to 330 mL) of drip coffee varied from 37 to 148 mg of caffeine (8).

Caffeine is also present in many prescription and over-the-counter medications (Table 7.2). This should be kept in mind for the patient trying to limit caffeine intake.

CONGENITAL MALFORMATIONS

Despite the evidence that caffeine causes chromosomal breakage *in vitro,* there is no evidence that this occurs *in vivo* (9). In addition, several studies showed no association with caffeine intake and congenital malformations. A

TABLE 7.1. *Standard values for caffeine content*

Coffee	
Ground roasted	85 mg/5 oz (150 mL)
Instant	60 mg/5 oz (150 mL)
Decaffeinated	3 mg/5 oz (150 mL)
Tea	
Leaf or bag	30 mg/5 oz (150 mL)
Instant	20 mg/5 oz (150 mL)
Cola	18 mg/6 oz (180 mL)
Cocoa, hot chocolate	4 mg/5 oz (150 mL)
Chocolate milk	4 mg/6 oz (180 mL)
Chocolate candy	1.5–6.0 mg/oz
	(5–20 mg/100 g)

Note: Modified from ref. 7.

study from Finland using national malformation registry data looked at more than 700 malformations including those of the central nervous system, cleft lip/palate, skeletal malformations, and congenital heart defects (10). They found no association with coffee consumption. Two large United States studies also found no relationship between coffee intake and congenital malformations (11,12). A Canadian study of 80,319 pregnancies found no increase in malformations related to coffee intake (13). Thus, despite strong evidence of teratogenicity in animals, there is no evidence to suggest such an effect in humans.

LOW BIRTH WEIGHT

The effect of caffeine on the incidence of low birth weight and intrauterine growth retardation is controversial. Recent articles showed both an effect on birth weight (1,14,15) and no association (16–18). One of the only prospective studies showed no effect on fetal growth with less than 300 mg per day of caffeine consumption (17). This study has been criticized, however, because it included few women who consumed more than 300 mg per day of caffeine.

Another prospective study looked at the association of caffeine intake by measuring blood caffeine and cotinine (to assess for effects of smoking) levels on stored plasma (19). This was done to avoid the potential reporting bias regarding caffeine intake inherent in almost all other studies. The authors reported that birth weight was unrelated to blood caffeine concentration overall after adjusting for cotinine concentration.

SPONTANEOUS ABORTION

Two prospective studies suggested an increased pregnancy loss rate associated with caffeine intake in pregnancy. Srisuphan and Bracken (20), in a population of 3,135 women, reported a

TABLE 7.2. *Caffeine content of medications (from 1975–1999 Micromedex Inc., Vol. 101, expires Sept. 1999)*

Drug	Caffeine content (mg)
BC Cold-Sinus Powder	33.3
Darvon Compound-65 Pulvules	32.4
Esgic-Plus	40.0
Excedrin Aspirin Free Caplets	65.0
Excedrin Extra Strength Tablets and Excedrin Migraine Tablets	65.0
Fioricet tablets, Fioricet codeine capsules, Fiorinal capsules, Fiorinal with Codeine capsules	40.0
Goody's Extra Strength Headache Powder	32.5
Goody's Extra Strength Pain Relief	16.25
Hycomine Compound Tablets	30.0
Maximum Strength Midol Menstrual Formula	60.0
NoDoz Maximum Strength Caplets	200.0
Norgesic Forte tablets	30.0
Vanquish Caplets	33.3
Vivarin	200.0
Wigraine tablets	100.0

Note: Dozens of other multiingredient preparations are available in the United States and Europe per Martindale: The Complete Drug Reference Copyright 1982–1999, The Royal Pharmaceutical Society of Great Britain.

relative risk of 2.0 ($p = 0.07$) for pregnancy loss in women who consumed 151 mg or more per day of caffeine. This study has been criticized because of its low background spontaneous loss rate (2.2%). In addition, the losses examined were only late first trimester or second trimester losses. The other prospective study, by Dlugosz et al. (21), which involved 2,849 women, also had a low background loss rate of 4.5%. In addition, the median time of interview was 12 weeks after the last menstrual period, somewhat late. This study showed a relative risk of 2.6 [95% confidence interval (CI), 1.3 to 5.3] of loss in women who consumed 300 mg or more per day of caffeine.

A large, case-control study published by Infante-Rivard et al. (22) reported a relative risk of loss of 1.9 (95% CI, 1.2 to 1.9) in women who consumed more than 321 mg per day of caffeine before pregnancy and a relative loss of 2.6 (95% CI, 1.4 to 5.0) in women who consumed more than 321 mg per day during pregnancy. This study has been criticized on the grounds that residual confounding factors might have been present (23). For example, among the group of less than 16 weeks of gestation, a total of 60% of controls reduced their intake compared with 50% of cases. In addition, the mean age at interview was 2 weeks earlier for cases compared with controls.

The largest prospective study to date was reported by Fenster et al. (24). In this prospective study of 5,144 women, the odds ratio (OR) for fetal losses in women who consumed more than 300 mg per day of caffeine was 1.3 (95% CI, 0.8 to 2.1). This was after adjustment for maternal age, pregnancy history, cigarette and alcohol consumption, employment, race, gestational age at interview, and marital and socioeconomic status. Mills et al. (25), in a prospective cohort study, evaluated 431 women beginning early after conception and calculated caffeine exposure at 5,6,8,10, and 12 weeks after the last menstrual period. They found no evidence that caffeine consumption of less than 300 mg per day was associated with fetal loss. Kline et al. (26) reported on prepregnancy and early pregnancy use of caffeine in women who had chromosomally normal fetal losses. They found no association with caffeine intake.

FERTILITY

An initial study by Wilcox et al. (27) reported that women with high caffeine intake had a longer interval to conceive compared with women with low intakes. These data were confirmed in three other American studies (28–30). These studies showed a relative risk of approximately 2 in women who consumed more than four cups of coffee in their ability to become pregnant (generally within a 12-month period). A prospective Danish study of 10,886 mothers revealed no association with difficulty in conceiving and caffeine consumption after controlling for maternal age, gravidity, education, and alcohol consumption (31). In addition, data from the Ontario Farm Family Health Study showed no difference in fecundity in women who consumed more than 100 mg per day of caffeine (32). In contrast, fecundity was reduced in a retrospective study of 1,430 women (33). Of those who consumed more than 300 mg per day of caffeine and were nonsmokers, the fecundity ratio was 0.74 (95% CI, 0.59 to 0.92). A large retrospective European Multicenter Study showed a slightly increased OR for delayed fertility (OR, 1.45; 95% CI, 1.03 to 2.04) in women who drank more than 500 mg per day of caffeine (34). Thus, there is no clear answer regarding the effects of caffeine consumption on fertility. Most studies, however, report little or no effect on intakes of less than 300 mg per day.

BREAST-FEEDING

After maternal consumption, caffeine rapidly passes into breast milk but at much lower concentrations than in maternal serum. Moderate caffeine consumption has not been shown to have any adverse effect on the nursing infant (35,36). The maternal serum half-life of caffeine postpartum is approximately 5 hours. Newborns have a much longer half-life of approximately 80 hours (37).

SUMMARY

Based on available data, it would appear safe for the woman attempting to conceive or who is already pregnant to ingest three caffeinated beverages or as much as 300 mg of caffeine per day. Information concerning the safety of intake above this amount is sparse or confounded by other factors. For the woman with fertility problems, multiple miscarriages, or pregnancy complications such as preterm labor or fetal arrhythmia, limitation of caffeine intake to 300 mg is a prudent option.

REFERENCES

1. Caan BJ, Goldhaber MK. Caffeinated beverages and low birthweight: a case-control study. *Am J Public Health* 1989;79:1299–300.
2. Dlugosz L, Bracken MB. Reproductive effects of caffeine: a review and theoretical analysis. *Epidemiol Rev* 1992;14:83–100.
3. Knutti R, Rothweiler H, Schalter C. The effect of pregnancy on the pharmacokinetics of caffeine. *Arch Toxicol* 1982;5[Suppl]:187–192.
4. Hook EB. Dietary cravings and aversions during pregnancy. *Am J Clin Nutr* 1978;31:1355–1362.
5. US Food and Drug Administration, Statement by Jere E. Goyan, Commissioner of Food & Drugs. HHS News (No. P80-36). Washington: US Department of Health and Human Services, Sept. 5, 1980.
6. FDA Consumer, US Food and Drug Administration. Washington, December 1987–January 1988.
7. Barone JJ, Roberts HR. Caffeine consumption. *Food Chem Toxicol* 1996;34:119–129.
8. Stavric B, Klassen R, Watkinson B, et al. Variability in caffeine consumption from coffee and tea: possible significance for epidemiological studies. *Food Chem Toxicol* 1988;26:111–118.
9. Al-Hachim GM. Teratogenicity of caffeine: a review. *Eur J Obstet Gynecol Reprod Biol* 1989;31:237–247.
10. Kurpa K, Holmberg PC, Kuosma E, et al. Coffee consumption during pregnancy and selected congenital malformations: a nationwide case-control study. *Am J Public Health* 1983;73:1397–1399.
11. Rosenberg L, Mitchell AA, Shapiro S, et al. Selected birth defects in relation to caffeine-containing beverages. *JAMA* 1982;247:1429–1432.
12. Linn S, Schoenbaum SC, Monson RR, et al. No association between coffee consumption and adverse outcomes of pregnancy. *N Engl J Med* 1982;306:141–145.
13. McDonald AD, Armstrong BG, Sloan M. Cigarette, alcohol and coffee consumption and congenital defects. *Am J Public Health* 1992;82:91–93.
14. Fortier I, Marcoux S, Beaulac-Baillargeon L. Relation of caffeine intake during pregnancy to intrauterine growth retardation and preterm birth. *Am J Epidemiol* 1993;137:931–940.
15. Martin TR, Bracken MD. The association between low birth weight and caffeine consumption during pregnancy. *Am J Epidemiol* 1987;126:813–821.
16. Santos IS, Victora CG, Huttly S, et al. Caffeine intake and low birth weight: a population-based case-control study. *Am J Epidemiol* 1998;147:620–627.

17. Shu XO, Hatch MC, Mills J, et al. Maternal smoking, alcohol drinking, caffeine consumption, and fetal growth: results from a prospective study. *Epidemiology* 1995;6:115–120.
18. Larroque B, Kaminski M, Lelong N, et al. Effects on birth weight of alcohol and caffeine consumption during pregnancy. *Am J Epidemiol* 1993;137:941–950.
19. Cook DG, Peacock JL, Feyerabend C, et al. Relation of caffeine intake and blood caffeine concentrations during pregnancy to fetal growth: prospective population based study. *BMJ* 1996;313:1358–1362.
20. Srisuphan W, Bracken M. Caffeine consumption during pregnancy and association with late spontaneous abortion. *Am J Obstet Gynecol* 1986;154:14–20.
21. Dlugosz L, Belanger K, Hellenbrand K, et al. Maternal caffeine consumption and spontaneous abortion: a prospective cohort study. *Epidemiology* 1996;7:250–255.
22. Infante-Rivard C, Fernandez A, Gauthier R, et al. Fetal loss associated with caffeine intake before and during pregnancy. *JAMA* 1993;270:2940–2943.
23. Kline J, Levin B, Kinney A, et al. Fetal loss and caffeine intake [Letter]. *JAMA* 1994;272:27–28.
24. Fenster L, Hubbard AE, Swan SH, et al. Caffeinated beverages, decaffeinated coffee, and spontaneous abortion. *Epidemiology* 1997;8:515–523.
25. Mills JL, Holmes LB, Aarons JH, et al. Moderate caffeine use and the risk of spontaneous abortion and intrauterine growth retardation. *JAMA* 1993;269:593–597.
26. Kline J, Levin B, Silverman J, et al. Caffeine and spontaneous abortion of known karyotype. *Epidemiology* 1991;2:409–417.
27. Wilcox A, Weinberg C, Baird D. Caffeinated beverages and decreased fertility. *Lancet* 1988;2:1453–1456.
28. Christianson RE, Oechsli FW, van der Berg BJ. Caffeinated beverages and decreased fertility. *Lancet* 1989;1:378.
29. Williams MA, Monson RR, Goldman MB, et al. Coffee and delayed conception. *Lancet* 1990;1:1603.
30. Hatch EE, Bracken MB. Association of delayed conception with caffeine consumption. *Am J Epidemiol* 1993;138:1082–1092.
31. Olsen J. Cigarette smoking, tea and coffee drinking and subfecundity. *Am J Epidemiol* 1991;133:734–739.
32. Curtis KM, Savitz DA, Arbuckle TE. Effects of cigarette smoking, caffeine consumption, and alcohol intake on fecundability. *Am J Epidemiol* 1997;146:32–41.
33. Stanton CK, Gray RH. Effects of caffeine consumption on delayed conception. *Am J Epidemiol* 1995;142:1322–1329.
34. Bolumar F, Olsen J, Rebagliato M, et al. Caffeine intake and delayed conception: a European multicenter study on infertility and subfecundity. *Am J Epidemiol* 1997;145:324–334.
35. Berlin CM, Denson HM, Daniel CH, et al. Disposition of dietary caffeine in milk, saliva, and plasma of lactating women. *Pediatrics* 1984;73:59–63.
36. Tyrala EE, Dodson WE. Caffeine secretion in breast milk. *Arch Dis Child* 1979;54:787–800.
37. Nolen GA. *The developmental toxicology of caffeine.* New York: Plenum, 1988.

8

Drug Therapy for the Treatment of Gastrointestinal Disorders in Pregnancy and Lactation

Michael J. McMahon

Department of Obstetrics and Gynecology, University of North Carolina School of Medicine, Chapel Hill, North Carolina

Gastrointestinal disorders, such as nausea, vomiting, hyperemesis gravidarum, gastroesophageal reflux, peptic ulcer disease, intrahepatic cholestasis of pregnancy, and inflammatory bowel disease, are common in pregnancy and can be especially challenging to manage. At the same time, the clinician must remember other conditions, such as appendicitis, gastroenteritis, cholecystitis, pancreatitis, hepatitis, and carcinoma of the gastrointestinal tract, that can occur during pregnancy but may be overlooked as a result of the normal physiologic changes. Whether the disorder is a pregnancy-related problem (nausea, vomiting, hyperemesis gravidarum), a medical complication of pregnancy (peptic ulcer disease, intrahepatic cholestasis of pregnancy), or a preexisting condition (peptic ulcer disease, inflammatory bowel disease), the goal of drug therapy is to limit fetal risk and at the same time improve maternal outcome.

Unfortunately, the ability to establish the risk or safety of specific drugs is limited because of lack of evidence-based data. For patients and physicians alike, this lack of information and an ever-increasing plethora of misinformation available via lay publications and the Internet make medical management and counseling even more difficult (1,2). Ultimately, one must choose between the risk of fetal exposure, the potential for teratogenesis or neonatal toxicity, and the possibility of harm to the mother and fetus if the gastrointestinal disorder is left untreated. Women need to be informed and encouraged to continue medications when indicated and discouraged from taking medications that can be detrimental to the fetus or adversely affect the expectant mother.

SPECIFIC GASTROINTESTINAL DISORDERS

Nausea, Vomiting, and Hyperemesis Gravidarum in Pregnancy

Few randomized controlled trials have been published regarding the management of nausea, vomiting, and hyperemesis gravidarum. Most studies have evaluated nausea and vomiting together and have been retrospective. Recall bias or partial memory and bias in the way women recall their pregnancy-related problems are a potential methodologic flaw in retrospective studies that needs to be taken into consideration. Nausea, for example, is a more subjective symptom that varies from patient to patient, whereas vomiting is more objective and not as likely to be forgotten. In addition, there is no agreed-on definition for hyperemesis gravidarum. This makes comparisons from one study to another difficult and extrapolation of findings more likely.

Nausea and vomiting or "morning sickness" occurs in as many as approximately 90% of all pregnancies. Although the etiology is unknown and is most likely multifactorial, symptoms are generally seen during the first 16 weeks of pregnancy. The symptoms are usually mild but can become debilitating. Vomiting occurs significantly more in primigravidas, those who are young, less educated, nonsmokers, and overweight, and in mothers of twin gestations (3). Early pregnancy vomiting is associated with a lower risk of miscarriage, stillbirth, and preterm delivery (3). Women are more likely to vomit in a future pregnancy if their first pregnancy was associated with significant emesis (3). Hyperemesis gravidarum is the extreme form of nausea and vomiting in pregnancy and is poorly defined. Generally hyperemesis gravidarum occurs when intractable vomiting leads to fluid and electrolyte abnormalities or there is at least a 5% to 10% weight loss compared with the prepregnancy weight. Hospitalization or aggressive outpatient management is required.

Nonpharmacologic Treatment of Nausea, Vomiting, and Hyperemesis Gravidarum in Pregnancy

Nondrug therapy, including alteration in diet, should always be tried before the initiation of antiemetics. Acupressure, ginger, and pyridoxine (vitamin B_6) have been evaluated in clinical trials.

Acupressure reduced nausea, vomiting, and hyperemesis gravidarum in several studies. In a randomized, double-blind, crossover, placebo-controlled trial by De Aloysio and Penacchioni (4), acupressure at the Neiguan point (or pericardium 6-PC 6, which is located on the anterior surface of the forearm, 2 inches proximal to the wrist crease, between the tendons of the flexor carpi radialis and palmaris longus muscles) significantly reduced morning sickness complaints. Bilateral pressure compared with unilateral pressure did not give any added benefit. In a randomized study by Belluomini et al. (5), the use of acupressure at the Neiguan point was effective in reducing symptoms of nausea but not the frequency of vomiting in pregnancy. It is probably impossible to perform a real double-blind trial comparing acupressure with no intervention. Despite the limitations of these studies, the use of acupressure in improving the symptoms of nausea and vomiting in pregnancy may be of benefit and should not be discouraged.

Ginger has been used in the treatment of nausea and vomiting in pregnancy (6,7). In the only study evaluating ginger in the treatment of hyperemesis gravidarum, Fischer-Rasmussen et al. (7) enrolled 27 women in a randomized, double-blind, crossover trial who were admitted for hyperemesis gravidarum. Women received either 250 mg of ginger in a capsule four times per day or a placebo that contained 250 mg of lactose. Both the degree of nausea and the number of bouts of vomiting were significantly reduced in women who received ginger. Of the 27 pregnancies, there was one spontaneous abortion, one elective abortion, and the remaining were born healthy "without evidence of deformities." Despite the reassuring findings of this one study, no conclusions can be made about the potential for teratogenicity and the use of ginger. Of concern, however, is that ginger has been reported to be a potent thromboxane synthetase inhibitor that theoretically could affect testosterone receptor binding and sex steroid differentiation of the fetal brain (8,9). No further experimental or clinical data were available to evaluate this possible association.

Pyridoxine, or vitamin B_6, is inexpensive, readily available, and the most studied agent for the management of nausea and vomiting in pregnancy. It is a water-soluble B-complex vitamin and has been shown to reduce nausea and vomiting in pregnancy. The use of pyridoxine for the management of nausea and vomiting in pregnancy was first reported in 1942 by Willis et al. (10). Women were given intramuscular injections of 10 to 100 mg pyridoxine, with a total dose of as much as 1,500 mg to alleviate nausea and vomiting. Most women experienced relief of their symptoms. Subsequent studies also showed benefit in the use of pyridoxine but were not controlled or double-blinded (11–15). More recent studies also demonstrated that pyridoxine use in pregnancy appears to reduce nausea and vomiting. In a randomized, double-blind, placebo-controlled trial, Sahakian et al. (16) found a significant reduction in severe nausea and vomiting for those pregnant women who took 25 mg pyridoxine orally every 8 hours for 72 hours. No improvement of symptoms was seen for those women with mild to moderate nausea. A second and similar study was also a randomized, double-blind, placebo-controlled trial by Vutya-vanich et al. (17) that found a significant reduction in nausea and nearly a significant reduction in vomiting episodes when pregnant women took 10 mg pyridoxine orally every 8 hours for 5 days.

No substantive evidence exists that associates pyridoxine use with a teratogenic effect despite case reports to the contrary (18). Pyridoxine was a component of Bendectin (along with dicyclomine and doxylamine) that was approved by the US Food and Drug Administration for the treatment of nausea and vomiting in pregnancy. Bendectin was removed from the market after several large legal settlements against the manufacturer claiming the use of the drug caused birth defects. The evidence of an association between pyridoxine use and congenital malformations, however, was unfounded and is also reviewed in the sections related to doxylamine and Bendectin.

Pyridoxine is excreted into breast milk (19–21) in proportion to maternal intake. In well-nourished women, the level of pyridoxine is between 123 and 314 ng/mL (20,21). In women with low nutritional status and who were supplemented with between 0.4 and 40 mg pyridoxine per day, mean milk concentrations were 80 to 158 ng/mL (22). Daily supplements of 0 to 20 mg corresponded to a milk concentration of 93 to 413 ng/mL (21). When pyridoxine is taken in large quantities, such as 600 mg per day, lactation can be inhibited (23). With ingestion of 20 mg pyridoxine per day, there is no effect on lactation (21). The American Academy of Pediatrics has determined that pyridoxine use is compatible with breast-feeding (24), and no adverse effects on the nursing infant have been reported.

Pharmacologic Treatment in the Management of Nausea, Vomiting, and Hyperemesis Gravidarum in Pregnancy

Persistent bouts of nausea and vomiting in pregnancy can become both physically and emotionally exhausting for the expectant mother. For those that fail to respond to nonpharmacologic measures, the use of antiemetics is appropriate. Close follow-up is necessary to monitor for signs of dehydration, ketonuria, and significant weight loss.

The drugs most commonly prescribed for nausea, vomiting, and hyperemesis gravidarum are classified as anticholinergic, antihistaminic, antidopaminergic, and miscellaneous (Table 8.1). Classification of these drugs is of value mostly with respect to the anticipated side effects rather than efficacy.

Anticholinergic(s)

Dicyclomine (Bentyl) is an anticholinergic that was a component of Bendectin used for the treatment of nausea and vomiting in pregnancy but today is mostly prescribed for the management of spastic or irritable colon. Bendectin (dicyclomine, doxylamine, and pyridoxine) was reformulated in 1976 and dicyclomine removed when it was found to add minimal benefit as an antiemetic. Dicyclomine is reviewed for historical perspective as an original component of Bendectin and for the occasional patient who requires its use.

In the Collaborative Perinatal Project, dicyclomine was the most common anticholinergic used by the women studied with more than 1,024 newborns of the 50,282 mother–child pairs studied being exposed in the first trimester (25,26) (see appendix for further information about the Collaborative Perinatal Project). A significant association was found between first-trimester exposure and the likelihood of minor congenital malformations (25,26). In a study published by Aselton et al. (27) in 1985, no increased risk of congenital anomalies in the newborns of approximately 100 women who used this drug early in pregnancy was found. Among 229,101 Michigan Medicaid recipients, 642 newborns had been exposed to dicyclomine during the first trimester. A total of 31 (4.8%) major birth defects was observed; 27 were expected (25). In review of the specific anomalies, only with the finding of polydactyly is there a possible association between dicyclomine use in the first trimester and congenital malformations. The authors were careful to point out that a causal relationship could not be inferred from any of the data to date and that further confirmation by other studies was required. Finally, in a review of commonly used drugs in 1990 (28), the teratogenic risk of dicyclomine was categorized as "none."

TABLE 8.1. *Drugs most commonly used in the management of nausea, vomiting, and hyperemesis gravidarum in pregnancy*

Generic drug name	Trade name	Pharmacologic class of drug	Dosage	Pregnancy use recommendation[a]	Lactation use recommendation[b]
Dicyclomine	Bentyl	Anticholinergic	20 mg p.o. or i.m. q.i.d.	B	D
—	Bendectin	Antihistaminic	—	B	B
Doxylamine	Unisom	Antihistaminic	25 mg p.o. 30 min before bed	A	B
Dimenhydrinate	Dramamine	Antihistaminic	50–100 mg p.o. every 4 h 50 mg i.m. or i.v. every 3–4 h	B	B
Diphenhydramine	Benadryl	Antihistaminic	50 mg p.o. every 6–8 h 20–50 mg i.m. or i.v. every 2–3 h	B	C
Meclizine	Antivert	Antihistaminic	20–50 mg p.o./day	B	C
Hydroxyzine	Vistaril, Atarax	Antihistaminic	25–100 mg p.o. every 6–8 h 25–100 mg i.m. every 4–6 h	C	C
Promethazine	Phenergan	Antihistaminic	12.5 mg p.o., p.r., or i.m. every 4–6 h	B	C
Chlorpromazine	Thorazine	Antidopaminergic	10–25 mg p.o. every 4–6 h 25 mg p.r. every 12 h 25–50 mg i.m. every 3–4 h	C	C
Perphenazine	Trilafon	Antidopaminergic	2–4 mg p.o. every 4–6 h 5 mg i.m. once	C	C
Prochlorperazine	Compazine	Antidopaminergic	5–10 mg p.o. or i.m. 3–4 h 10 mg p.r. 4–6 h	B	C
Droperidol	Inapsine	Antidopaminergic	Individualized with dose adjustments needed (usual dose 1 mg/h)	C	C
Haloperidol	Haldol	Antidopaminergic	1–5 mg p.o. b.i.d. 1–5 mg i.m. every 12 h	C	B
Metoclopramide	Reglan	Antidopaminergic	5–10 mg p.o. q.i.d. 5–20 mg i.m. or i.v. q.i.d.	B	C
Trimethobenzamide hydrochloride	Tigan	Miscellaneous	250 mg p.o. or p.r. every 6–8 h	C	C
Ondansetron	Zofran	Miscellaneous	8 mg p.o. or i.v. every 8 h	B	C
Pyridoxine	Vitamin B$_6$	Vitamin	10–25 mg p.o. t.i.d.	A	A

[a]A, Drug of choice; B, recommended as an alternate drug of choice; C, limited data to support its use and best avoided, if possible; D, contraindicated (not recommended for use).

[b]A, safe to use in usual doses; B, probably safe to use in usual doses, but there are insufficient data to ensure no neonatal effects; C, should be used with caution and best avoided, if possible; D, contraindicated (not recommended for use).

There are no published data regarding the excretion of dicyclomine into breast milk. There is concern about a possible association between neonatal apnea and the use of dicyclomine and women should be counseled against its use if they choose to breast-feed (25).

Antihistaminic(s)

Bendectin was effective for the treatment of nausea and vomiting in pregnancy. During the 1950s and 1960s, Bendectin was the most prescribed drug for the treatment of nausea and vomiting in pregnancy. It was originally a combination of dicyclomine, doxylamine, and pyridoxine hydrochloride. In the 1970s, allegations of an association between the use of Bendectin and congenital malformations led to numerous lawsuits and negative publicity. In 1976, dicyclomine was eliminated from the three-drug combination so that doxylamine-pyridoxine became the proprietary combination. Early reports indicated an increased risk of malformations, including diaphragmatic hernia (29), congenital heart disease (27), and pyloric stenosis (30). Further studies, however, failed to demonstrate any of these specific associations (31–33). In addition, more recent epidemiologic reviews substantiated the findings that the rate of major malformations was similar among the children born to women who used Bendectin during pregnancy compared with the rate from the general population (34,35). The drug was ultimately withdrawn from the American market in 1983. The use of Bendectin in pregnancy is an unfortunate example of a drug taken off the market despite evidence that its use in pregnancy was safe. Currently Bendectin is not available in the United States but is available in Canada under the trade name Diclectin. Although Bendectin is no longer available in the United States, both pyridoxine, as previously reviewed, and doxylamine can be used for the management of nausea and vomiting in pregnancy.

Doxylamine (Unisom) is an antihistamine that is used as a nighttime sleep aid and for the treatment of nausea and vomiting in pregnancy. The usual dose is 25 mg orally, to be taken approximately 30 minutes before bedtime. One-half tablet (12.5 mg) may be taken in the morning and afternoon as needed. The use of doxylamine with or without pyridoxine, as previously reviewed, is safe in pregnancy when used in the first trimester for nausea and vomiting.

Dimenhydrinate (Dramamine) is the chlorotheophylline salt of diphenhydramine that is useful in the treatment of vertigo in addition to nausea and vomiting in pregnancy. It also has antihistamine properties, although its mode of action is unknown. The usual dose is 50 to 100 mg orally every 4 hours or 50 mg intramuscularly or intravenously every 3 to 4 hours. Drowsiness is a significant side effect.

The Collaborative Perinatal Project evaluated first-trimester exposure to dimenhydrinate and the risk of congenital malformation. Of the 50,282 mother-child pairs, 319 women were identified as consuming the drug in the first trimester. Large categories of major and minor malformations were not increased (26). A possible association with individual malformations and the use of dimenhydrinate in the first trimester was noted, however (26). Cardiovascular defects and inguinal hernia were the birth defects observed, but the actual risk for these malformations attributable to dimenhydrinate is unknown.

Diphenhydramine (Benadryl) has antihistamine properties and is used for the treatment of vertigo, motion sickness, and nausea and vomiting in pregnancy. The usual dose is 50 mg orally three to four times per day or 20 to 50 mg intramuscularly or intravenously every 2 to 3 hours. Its duration of action is approximately 4 to 6 hours. Women whose activities require alertness should be counseled about the high incidence of drowsiness and probably discouraged from its use.

In the Collaborative Perinatal Project, 595 of the 50,282 mother-child pairs were identified as having been exposed to diphenhydramine in the first trimester (26). No association between the use of this drug and large categories of major or minor malformations was observed. Several smaller associations with individual malformations were found, but the calculation of actual fetal risk was not able to be determined and follow-up studies are required to determine whether the findings were real. In the Michigan Medicaid surveillance study involving 229,101 pregnancies, there were 1,461 newborns exposed to diphenhydramine in the first trimester (25). A total of 80 (5.5%) major birth defects were identified and 62 were expected. A possible association of exposure to the drug and an increased risk for polydactyly was noted. In summary, there appears to be no increased risk for major or minor malformations with the use of diphenhydramine use in the first trimester. The risk for individual malformations, including polydactyly, might be increased, but further studies are necessary.

Diphenhydramine is excreted into breast milk (36). Diphenhydramine withdrawal has been reported in a newborn whose mother consumed the drug throughout pregnancy (37). Because of the increased sensitivity of newborns to antihistamines, manufacturers have recommended against their use while breast-feeding.

Meclizine (Antivert) is an antihistamine that is used to treat motion sickness and nausea and vomiting in pregnancy. The usual dose is 20 to 50 mg by mouth every day. Side effects include drowsiness, blurred vision, and dry mouth. One advantage of meclizine over other antihistamines is its slower onset and longer duration of action.

There appears to be no relationship between the use of meclizine and the risk of major or minor malformations. The Collaborative Perinatal Project observed no large category major or minor malformations in 1,104 women of 50,282 mother-child pairs who were exposed to meclizine in the first trimester (26). In addition, meclizine was not found to be associated with an increased risk for congenital malformations in several follow-up cohort and case-control studies (38–41).

Hydroxyzine (Vistaril, Atarax) has both antianxiety and antihistamine properties and has been used in the treatment of nausea, vomiting, and anxiety in pregnancy. The usual dosage is 25 to 100 mg orally three to four times per day or 25 to 100 mg intramuscularly every 4 to 6 hours.

In the Collaborative Perinatal Project that monitored 50,282 mother-child pairs, only 50 women were observed to have been exposed to hydroxyzine in the first trimester of pregnancy.

Five children were born with malformations, suggesting a possible teratogenic role for hydroxyzine use in the first trimester. In the Michigan Medicaid surveillance study involving 229,101 completed pregnancies between 1985 and 1992, 828 newborns were found to have been exposed to hydroxyzine in the first trimester (25). Forty-eight major birth defects were observed and 42 were expected (25). A review of the major categories of birth defects revealed that there was an increased risk for oral clefts. No follow-up study to date has confirmed or refuted this finding.

Promethazine (Phenergan), one of the most prescribed drugs for nausea, vomiting, and hyperemesis gravidarum in pregnancy, is unique in the class of phenothiazines in that it has strong antihistaminic activity in addition to central cholinergic blocking activity. The usual dose is 12.5 to 25 mg orally every 4 to 6 hours, 12.5 to 25 mg intramuscularly every 4 to 6 hours, or 12.5 to 25 mg rectally every 4 to 6 hours. Side effects include drowsiness. Extrapyramidal effects are unusual when promethazine is given in these doses.

There appears to be no increased risk for congenital fetal malformations in women who are prescribed promethazine in the first trimester of pregnancy. Wheatley (42) reported no association between promethazine exposure in the first trimester of pregnancy and the risk for fetal malformations. In the Collaborative Perinatal Project 50,282 mother-child pairs were evaluated and 114 found to have been exposed to promethazine in the first trimester of pregnancy (26). No increased risk for large category major or minor malformations was observed. The Michigan Medicaid surveillance study involving 229,101 pregnancies found that 1,197 women were exposed to promethazine in the first trimester of pregnancy and 61 major birth defects were observed (51 expected) and that cardiovascular malformations were slightly increased in those exposed compared with what was expected (25). Two more recent large controlled trials failed to find an association between promethazine use and the frequency of congenital anomalies (27,43).

There is no information about use of the antihistamines in breast-feeding mothers (25).

Antidopaminergic(s)

Chlorpromazine (Thorazine) is a phenothiazine whose antiemetic activity occurs by reducing neural impulses to the vomiting center via antagonism of the dopamine receptors. Chlorpromazine has been used for the treatment of nausea and vomiting throughout pregnancy. Unfortunately, chlorpromazine can cause significant drowsiness and is associated with orthostatic hypotension. The usual dose is 10 to 25 mg orally every 4 to 6 hours or 25 mg rectally every 12 hours. An initial dose of 25 mg is given intramuscularly and blood pressure is monitored closely. If hypotension does not occur, then 25 to 50 mg is given every 3 to 4 hours until symptoms abate. Use in late gestation is contraindicated because of the potential drop in blood pressure that could cause uteroplacental insufficiency and fetal compromise.

There are conflicting data regarding whether the use of phenothiazines, and more specifically chlorpromazine, in pregnancy is associated with an increased risk of birth defects. In the Collaborative Perinatal Project, 50,282 mother-child pairs were followed and 142 found to have been exposed to chlorpromazine in the first trimester. No increase in the risk for malformations was observed (44). The perinatal mortality rate, birth weight, and intelligent quotient scores at 4 years of age were also not affected (44). Farkas and Farkas (45), in a cohort study of 264 pregnant women who received chlorpromazine for the management of hyperemesis gravidarum in the first trimester, also found no increase in the risk for congenital malformations. Conversely, a large prospective French study evaluating the treatment of hyperemesis gravidarum found a statistically significant increase in congenital anomalies in infants exposed to phenothiazines, including chlorpromazine, in the first trimester (43). Malformations in those infants exposed to chlorpromazine in the first trimester included syndactyly and microcephaly, although the authors concluded the microcephaly observed was most likely a result of genetic influences as the mother had previously delivered two children with microcephaly. The incidence of malformations in the chlorpromazine group was 3.5%,

however, which is no higher than is expected in the general population. More recent studies, however, failed to demonstrate a significant teratogenic risk (46) and chlorpromazine appears to be safe for both mother and fetus when used in low doses (47,48).

Phenothiazines, such as chlorpromazine, may induce breast milk production owing to their antagonism of the dopamine receptor. The phenothiazines as a group are also excreted into breast milk (25) with a calculated infant dose of 0.15% of the maternal dose (49). Data regarding excretion of chlorpromazine into breast milk are limited, and the results are somewhat contradictory. Blacker et al. (50) observed no detectable levels of the drug in breast milk after oral administration of 600 mg per day. There were no neonatal problems noted. In contrast, Wiles et al. (51) found levels of chlorpromazine that were higher in breast milk than in maternal plasma. The mothers consumed unknown amounts of chlorpromazine, and one of the neonates became drowsy and lethargic. No other published reports could be found regarding adverse outcomes in breast-fed newborns exposed to chlorpromazine. Although the use of chlorpromazine is not a contraindication to breast-feeding, the American Academy of Pediatrics cautions women to observe the newborn for signs of sedation (24).

Perphenazine (Trilafon) is a phenothiazine that has action at most levels of the central nervous system. The usual dose is 2 to 4 mg orally every 4 to 6 hours or 5 mg intramuscularly. Side effects include blurred vision, extrapyramidal reactions, and drowsiness.

Data on fetal risk and the use of perphenazine in the first trimester are limited but show no increased risk of malformations or other adverse outcomes. In the Collaborative Perinatal Project involving 50,282 mother-child pairs, 63 neonates were exposed to perphenazine in the first trimester (43). No increase in the risk for malformations was observed (26). In addition, perinatal mortality rates, birth weight, and intelligence quotient scores at 4 years of age were unaffected (43). In the Michigan Medicaid surveillance study, 140 newborns exposed to perphenazine in the first trimester were found to have five major birth defects (six were expected)

(25). Of the five observed, four were cardiovascular defects, suggesting a possible association between first-trimester perphenazine use and cardiac malformations. Follow-up studies have not confirmed or refuted this finding.

Perphenazine has the most potent mammotrophic effect of the phenothiazines (52). Perphenazine is also excreted into human milk (49) with a calculated breast milk/plasma ratio of 1.0. No adverse neonatal effects have been reported to date. There appears to be no clear contraindication to the use of perphenazine in the lowest effective dose in lactating women (53,54), but the American Academy of Pediatrics considers the effects of the drug to be unknown and cautions those who require its use (24).

Prochlorperazine (Compazine) is a phenothiazine that blocks dopamine receptors in the medullary chemoreceptor trigger zone. The usual dose is 5 to 10 mg orally every 3 to 4 hours, 5 to 10 mg intramuscularly every 3 to 4 hours, or 10 mg rectally every 4 to 6 hours. Prochlorperazine has significant side effects including drowsiness, dizziness, blurred vision, leukopenia, and extrapyramidal reactions.

The use of prochlorperazine in pregnancy appears to be safe for mother and fetus if used occasionally in low doses. In the Collaborative Perinatal Project, 50,282 mother-child pairs were monitored and 877 found to have been exposed to prochlorperazine in the first trimester (43). No increased risk for malformations, perinatal mortality rate, birth weight, or intelligence quotient scores at 4 years of age were noted. In the Michigan Medicaid surveillance study involving 229,101 pregnancies, 704 newborns were exposed to prochlorperazine in the first trimester without an increase in the risk for fetal malformations (25). Two additional studies also failed to demonstrate any increase in the frequency of congenital birth defects among those infants exposed to prochlorperazine (55,56).

Prochlorperazine, like all phenothiazines, is most likely excreted into breast milk, although no published data could be found confirming this. Breast-feeding is not contraindicated and mothers should observe the nursing infant for signs of sedation.

Droperidol (Inapsine) is a butyrophenone derivative that is related to haloperidol. It is mainly used to reduce nausea associated with surgical and diagnostic procedures by antagonizing the emetic effects of drugs that act on the chemoreceptor trigger zone. The use of droperidol in pregnancy is usually limited to the most severe forms of hyperemesis gravidarum. Droperidol is available only in injectable form and its dosing must be individualized.

There is limited information regarding the use of droperidol and teratogenicity. In a study by Nageotte et al. (57), droperidol was used in combination with diphenhydramine, metoclopramide, and hydroxyzine in 80 women with hyperemesis gravidarum (57). Three of the women delivered neonates with congenital anomalies of which only one could potentially be attributable to a drug effect (hydrocephalus and hypoplasia of the right cerebral hemisphere). The authors concluded the malformation was a result of an *in utero* fetal vascular accident or infection rather than a result of drug exposure.

Haloperidol (Haldol) is a butyrophenone antidopaminergic that is used for the treatment of nausea and vomiting in pregnancy. The antiemetic effect of this drug is through inhibition of stimuli at the chemoreceptor trigger zone. The duration of action is longer than that of droperidol. The usual dose is 1 to 5 mg orally twice per day or 1 to 5 mg intramuscularly every 12 hours. Side effects are similar to other phenothiazines but are rare with small doses and short-term treatment.

Haloperidol has been associated with limb reduction defects in two early reports (58,59). In one of the reports, a high dose of 15 mg per day of haloperidol was taken by the mother (59). Subsequent studies failed to confirm these findings (60–62). Van Waes and Van de Velde (60) evaluated 98 women in the first trimester who were treated for hyperemesis gravidarum and found no adverse effects or fetal abnormalities. In the Michigan Medicaid surveillance study involving 229,101 pregnancies, 56 newborns were exposed to haloperidol in the first trimester (25). Three major birth defects were noted (5.4%) and two were expected. There is no evidence that haloperidol is a teratogen at currently used doses in humans.

Haloperidol is excreted into breast milk with wide variations in the drug concentrations noted (63,64). A milk/plasma ratio of 0.6 to 0.7 was calculated (25) based on the above patients. No adverse effects were found in the nursing infant.

Metoclopramide (Reglan) is an antidopaminergic used to treat nausea and vomiting in pregnancy that also increases the rate of gastric emptying, stimulates motility of the upper gastrointestinal tract, and is recommended for short-term use (usually 4 to 12 weeks). Gastric, biliary, and pancreatic secretions are not increased with the use of metoclopramide. The usual dose is 5 to 10 mg orally, 5 to 20 mg intramuscularly, or 5 to 20 mg intravenously as much as four times per day. Side effects include sedation, diarrhea, and galactorrhea (owing to stimulation of prolactin secretion) with increasing doses.

Although data are limited, there have been no congenital malformations observed after fetal exposure to metoclopramide. In the Michigan Medicaid surveillance study of 229,101 pregnancies, 192 newborns were exposed to metoclopramide in the first trimester without an increased risk for major malformations observed (25).

Metoclopramide is excreted into breast milk (25) with a milk/plasma ratio of 1.8 to 1.9 (65). No adverse effects in the nursing infant have been reported to date. The American Academy of Pediatrics cautions those who require metoclopramide and breast-feed, however, about the possible central nervous system effects the drug can produce in the nursing infant (24). Maternal doses of 45 mg per day or less are probably safe (25) and treatment should be short term.

Miscellaneous

Trimethobenzamide hydrochloride (Tigan) inhibits stimuli at the chemoreceptor trigger zone and alleviates nausea and vomiting. The usual dose is 250 mg orally or 200 mg rectally every 6 to 8 hours. Side effects include Parkinson-like symptoms, blood dyscrasias, and drowsiness.

Limited data are available regarding the risk of malformation and exposure to trimethobenzamide hydrochloride, but no adverse fetal risks have been noted.

Ondansetron hydrochloride (Zofran) is a potent antiemetic. Initially used in the management of chemotherapy-induced nausea and vomiting, ondansetron has been used recently to treat hyperemesis gravidarum (66–68). Dosage has not been standardized, but a regimen of 8 mg intravenously every 8 hours or 8 mg orally every 8 hours is common.

Sullivan et al. (68) conducted one of the few randomized studies specifically looking at therapy for hyperemesis gravidarum. The authors completed a randomized, double-blinded study comparing intravenous ondansetron to intravenous promethazine. They reported no differences in improvement of nausea, weight gain, length of hospital stay, or treatment failure between the women who received ondansetron compared with those who received promethazine. The only difference between the two study groups was that women who received promethazine were more likely to be sedated than those who received ondansetron. The authors did not comment on pregnancy outcomes for either group.

Because of the limited data, no conclusions can be drawn regarding potential fetal effects.

SUMMARY OF MANAGEMENT OF NAUSEA, VOMITING, AND HYPEREMESIS GRAVIDARUM IN PREGNANCY

Pregnant women who desire alternative, non-pharmacologic treatment for the management of nausea, vomiting, and hyperemesis gravidarum have limited options. The use of acupressure over the Neiguan point for the management of nausea and vomiting in early pregnancy should not be discouraged. The use of ginger for the treatment of hyperemesis gravidarum appears promising, but additional studies are needed to evaluate dosage, the potential for teratogenesis, the possible effects of ginger use in the nursing infant, and its role in the management of nausea and vomiting in early pregnancy. Because of these concerns and the theoretical concern about ginger use affecting testosterone receptor binding and sex steroid differentiation of the fetal brain, ginger use cannot be currently recommended for the management of hyperemesis gravidarum. Finally, pyridoxine supplementation in doses of 30 to 75 mg per day may benefit some women with nausea and vomiting and is recommended. No adverse effects on nursing infants have been reported and breast-feeding should not be discouraged. Women who fail to respond to non-pharmacologic treatment for the management of nausea, vomiting, and hyperemesis gravidarum have numerous antiemetics available that are classified according to maternal side effects as anticholinergic, antihistaminic, antidopaminergic, and miscellaneous.

After 48 to 72 hours, if 10 to 25 mg pyridoxine three times per day fails to relieve symptoms, then 25 mg doxylamine twice per day should be added. If the patient fails to respond to this combination, I would recommend 25 mg promethazine orally or rectally every 4 to 6 hours, 25 mg prochlorperazine rectally every 12 hours, 50 to 100 mg dimenhydrinate orally every 4 hours, 50 mg diphenhydramine orally three to four times per day, 20 to 50 mg meclizine orally per day, or 200 mg trimethobenzamide hydrochloride rectally every 6 hours.

There are limited data available to guide the clinician if all these medications fail, and the patient develops significant weight loss or electrolyte abnormalities consistent with hyperemesis gravidarum. An important point is to reevaluate the patient's condition for other medical complications that may be overlooked, such as appendicitis, cholecystitis, or pancreatitis. Hospitalization with replacement of fluids, electrolytes, and calories is usually necessary. A continuous intravenous infusion of promethazine may be helpful. To each liter of fluid, 25 to 50 mg promethazine is added. As much as 6 L per day of fluid replacement may be necessary. The patient should be allowed nothing by mouth. Diet can be slowly advanced once symptoms subside for at least 36 to 48 hours. Intravenous droperidol, intravenous ondansetron, or combinations of the aforementioned drugs are also options. Consultation with a gastroenterologist is also reasonable and should occur early in the hospital admission.

For the few patients who continue to fail medical management, enteral, peripheral, and central nutrition may be necessary.

GASTROESOPHAGEAL REFLUX AND PEPTIC ULCER DISEASE IN PREGNANCY

Gastroesophageal reflux, or heartburn (pyrosis), occurs as a result of regurgitation of stomach contents into the esophagus and is a common complaint in late pregnancy. Upward of 50% to 80% of pregnant women will have symptoms suggestive of gastroesophageal reflux (69,70). Pregnant women will often complain of retrosternal burning as a result of irritation of the esophagus from reflux. Reflux is thought to occur as a result of relaxation of the lower esophageal sphincter (71) in addition to an increase in the abdominothoracic pressure gradient from the enlarging uterus. Initial management should include lifestyle changes such as elevating of the head of the bed at night, loosening tight clothing, eating frequent small meals that are low in fat, avoiding heavy lifting, encouraging smoking cessation, and eliminating foods that exacerbate symptoms. Usually these conservative measures will be of benefit, and the patient can be reassured that the symptoms will resolve shortly after delivery. When conservative measures fail, antacids and various other drugs are available. In addition, clinicians should not hesitate to refer the patient to a gastroenterologist if symptoms become severe and are suggestive of esophagitis that may necessitate endoscopy.

Active peptic ulcer disease is uncommon during pregnancy. The incidence and recurrence risk appear unchanged relative to the nonpregnant population (72). In 1953, Clark (73) evaluated 313 pregnancies in 118 women with known ulcer disease. Remission rates of 90% were achieved during pregnancy. Unfortunately, recurrence occurred within 3 months of delivery in more than one half of the women and in almost every woman by the end of the second year (73). The diagnosis of peptic ulcer disease can usually be made by a history of symptoms of epigastric burning pain, pain that is worse on an empty stomach, pain relieved with antacids or food, and pain that awakens the patient in the early morning. Complications of peptic ulcer disease, including perforation and hemorrhage, have been reported during pregnancy (74,75). Perforation occurs more commonly in the pregnant woman compared with the general population with peptic ulcer disease, whereas hemorrhage is more likely to occur late in pregnancy or in the early postpartum period. As with many medical complications that present during pregnancy, the diagnosis of perforation and hemorrhage as a result of peptic ulcer disease can be delayed as a result of the clinician associating presenting symptoms with the pregnancy and not with the possibility of the potential complication. As soon as the diagnosis of peptic ulcer disease is made, drug therapy can be initiated.

The following drugs are most commonly used for the treatment of gastroesophageal reflux and peptic ulcer disease (Table 8.2).

Antacids

Antacids can be used to treat both gastroesophageal reflux and peptic ulcer disease. Antacids contain aluminum, calcium, and magnesium salts that react with hydrochloric acid in the stomach to form poorly soluble salts that are less acidic. The pH of stomach contents increases to more than 5.0 when adequate doses are consumed. Liquid formulations are considered more effective than tablets. Side effects include diarrhea with the use of magnesium salts and constipation with prolonged use of calcium or aluminum regimens. Antacid use also reduces the bioavailability of cimetidine and ranitidine (76); these drugs should be given at least 1 hour apart. Magnesium hydroxide, calcium carbonate, and aluminum hydroxide preparations are recommended.

There are no well-controlled studies in humans regarding antacids, and it is unlikely that antacids are associated with any significant fetal risk when used judiciously. Adverse neonatal effects, such as hypercalcemia, hypermagnesemia, or hypocalcemia, however, may be associated with long-term use of high-dose antacids.

Histamine$_2$-Receptor Antagonists

Cimetidine (Tagamet) is an H_2-receptor antagonist that inhibits gastric acid secretion and is used

TABLE 8.2. *Drugs most commonly used in the management of gastroesophageal reflux and peptic ulcer disease in pregnancy*

Generic drug name	Trade name	Pharmacologic class of drug	Dosage	Pregnancy use recommendation[a]	Lactation use recommendation[b]
Antacids	—	—	—	A	B
Cimetidine	Tagamet	H$_2$-receptor antagonist	300 mg p.o. a.c. & h.s. 200 mg p.o. a.c. & 400 mg h.s. 400 mg p.o. b.i.d. 500 p.o. h.s.	C	B
Famotidine	Pepcid	H$_2$-receptor antagonist	40 mg p.o. q.h.s. 20 mg p.o. b.i.d.	C	C
Ranitidine	Zantac	H$_2$-receptor antagonist	150 mg p.o. b.i.d. 300 mg p.o. q.h.s.	A	B
Nizatidine	Axid	H$_2$-receptor antagonist	300 mg p.o./day 150 mg p.o. b.i.d.	C	C
Metoclopramide	Reglan	Promotility	10–15 mg p.o. b.i.d. up to q.i.d. to be taken 30 min a.c. & h.s.	C	C
Cisapride	Propulsid	Promotility	10 mg p.o. a.c. & h.s.	C	C
Sucralfate	Carafate	Antisecretory	1 g p.o. q.i.d.	B	A
Omeprazole	Prilosec	Proton pump inhibitor	20 mg p.o. QD	C	C
Lansoprazole	Prevacid	Proton pump inhibitor	15 mg p.o./day	C	C
Misoprostol	Cytotec	Prostaglandin E$_1$ analog	200 mg p.o. q.i.d.	D	D

[a]A, Drug of choice; B, recommended as an alternate drug of choice; C, limited data to support its use and best avoided, if possible; D, contraindicated (not recommended for use).

[b]A, Safe to use in usual doses; B, probably safe to use in usual doses, but there are insufficient data to ensure no neonatal effects; C, should be used with caution and best avoided, if possible; D, contraindicated (not recommended for use).

in the treatment of gastroesophageal reflux and peptic ulcer disease. The usual dose for gastric or duodenal ulcer and reflux esophagitis is 300 mg orally with or immediately after meals and at bedtime for 4 to 6 weeks. Alternative schedules are available and include 200 mg orally with meals and 400 mg orally at bedtime, 400 mg orally twice daily, or 800 mg orally at bedtime. Side effects are rare but include diarrhea, dizziness, and myalgia.

Cimetidine crosses the placenta to the fetus by simple diffusion (77). No congenital malformations have been detected in humans. In the Michigan Medicaid surveillance study involving 229,101 pregnancies, 460 newborns were exposed to cimetidine in the first trimester (25). There was no increase in the frequency of malformations attributable to cimetidine use. The drug, however, has been found to have weak antiandrogenic effects on the male fetus in rats (78,79).

Cimetidine is excreted into breast milk (25). The breast milk/serum ratio is 4.6 to 11.8 (80). The American Academy of Pediatrics recently classified cimetidine as compatible with breast-feeding (24).

Famotidine (Pepcid) is an H_2-receptor antagonist that is used in the treatment of gastroesophageal reflux and peptic ulcer disease. The usual dose to treat ulcers is 40 mg orally at night or 20 mg orally twice daily. For gastroesophageal reflux disease, the dose is 20 mg twice daily for up to 6 weeks. Side effects are similar to those seen with cimetidine and include diarrhea, dizziness, and myalgia.

Limited information is available to draw any conclusions about the relationship between famotidine and teratogenicity.

Famotidine is excreted into breast milk and is more concentrated (25). The breast milk/serum ratio is 0.41 to 1.78 (80). Breast-feeding is not contraindicated.

Ranitidine (Zantac) is an H_2-receptor antagonist that is used for the treatment of gastroesophageal reflux and peptic ulcer disease. The usual dose is 150 mg orally twice daily or 300 mg orally once daily at night for the treatment of active duodenal ulcers or 150 mg orally twice daily for the treatment of gastroesophageal reflux. Side effects are similar to the those of other H_2-receptor antagonists and include diarrhea, dizziness, and myalgia.

There appears to be no increased risk of malformations in newborns exposed to ranitidine in pregnancy, although data are limited. The Michigan Medicaid surveillance study involving 229,101 pregnancies found 516 newborns exposed to the drug in the first trimester (25). No increase in the frequency of malformations was found. No antiandrogenic effects are associated with the use of ranitidine, and its use is recommended over that of cimetidine in pregnancy.

Ranitidine is excreted into breast milk and has a breast milk/serum ratio of 1.9 to 23.8 (80). Breast-feeding is not contraindicated in women requiring ranitidine during lactation.

Nizatidine (Axid) is an H_2-receptor antagonist that is used in the treatment of gastroesophageal reflux and peptic ulcer disease. The usual dose is 300 mg orally once daily or 150 mg orally twice daily for active duodenal ulcers or benign gastric ulcers and 150 mg orally twice daily for gastroesophageal reflux disease. Side effects are similar to those of other H_2-receptor antagonists and include diarrhea, dizziness, and myalgias.

Limited data are available regarding the risk of fetal malformations and the use of nizatidine.

Nizatidine is excreted in breast milk at a significantly reduced amount compared with the other H_2-receptor antagonists (81). The amount excreted is $0.064\% \pm 0.021\%$ of the maternal dose (81). Breast-feeding is not contraindicated, although the effects of nizatidine on the nursing infant are unknown.

Pro-motility Drugs

Metoclopramide (Reglan) has been previously described.

Cisapride (Propulsid) stimulates the gastrointestinal tract and is used in the treatment of gastroesophageal reflux disease. The usual dose is 10 mg orally to be taken 30 minutes before meals and at bedtime.

No information could be found in the literature concerning the use of cisapride for gastroesophageal reflux in pregnancy.

Cisapride is excreted in breast milk (24). The American Academy of Pediatrics does not consider breast-feeding to be contraindicated in those women who nurse and require cisapride (24).

Antisecretory

Sucralfate (Carafate) inhibits pepsin activity and is used in the treatment of peptic ulcer disease. One of the advantages of sucralfate is that it is poorly absorbed, acts locally at the ulcer site with minimal systemic effects, and has few side effects. The usual dose is 1 g orally as much as four times daily.

Limited information is available about the potential teratogenic effects of sucralfate use in pregnancy. In the Michigan Medicaid surveillance study involving 229,101 pregnancies, 183 newborns were exposed to sucralfate in the first trimester (25). No increase in the frequency of congenital malformations was observed (25).

Breast-feeding is not contraindicated in women who require sucralfate. Because the drug has little systemic absorption, excretion into breast milk is unlikely.

Proton Pump Inhibitors

Omeprazole (Prilosec) is a proton pump inhibitor that suppresses gastric acid secretion by inhibiting gastric parietal cells directly. The drug is used to treat both gastroesophageal reflux and peptic ulcer disease. The usual dose is 20 mg orally daily for as long as 8 weeks for acute duodenal ulcers, erosive esophagitis, and poorly responsive gastroesophageal reflux disease. Significant side effects have not been observed with short-term use.

Omeprazole crosses the placenta in small amounts (82). Unfortunately, data are limited with regard to teratogenicity and the use of omeprazole. Successful pregnancy outcomes have been documented with its use (83,84) as have poor pregnancy outcomes. In one report (85), two consecutive pregnancies were terminated as a result of congenital anomalies in a woman who consumed omeprazole for gastroesophageal reflux. The first pregnancy was complicated by anencephaly and the second one by talipes. In addition, the US Food and Drug Administration has received reports of birth defects,

many of which are neural tube defects, with use of omeprazole (25). Until more information is available, omeprazole should probably be avoided in the first trimester of pregnancy and used selectively throughout the remainder of pregnancy in difficult to treat patients.

Lansoprazole (Prevacid) is a proton pump inhibitor that is used in the management of gastroesophageal reflux disease and peptic ulcer disease. Like omeprazole, lansoprazole is a potent inhibitor of acid secretion. The usual dose is 15 mg orally once daily for 4 weeks in the treatment of duodenal ulcers and 15 mg orally once daily for as long as 8 weeks for gastroesophageal reflux. Side effects include headache and diarrhea.

No reports have been published evaluating the use of lansoprazole in human pregnancy. Omeprazole, the other proton pump inhibitor, is known to cross the placenta and is not recommended for use in the first trimester because of possible congenital malformations. Likewise, the use of lansoprazole is not recommended until further information is available concerning teratogenicity.

Prostaglandin(s)

Misoprostol (Cytotec) is a prostaglandin E_1 analog that is used in the treatment of gastric ulcers as a result of the use of nonsteroidal antiinflammatory agents. The usual dose is 200 μg orally four times per day to be taken with food. Misoprostol use is contraindicated in pregnancy for the treatment of ulcer disease as it is a potent uterine stimulant that induces abortion. In addition, the use of misoprostol in the first trimester has been associated with Moebius sequence (86). Gonzalez et al. (86) studied 42 infants in Brazil who were exposed to misoprostol in the first trimester of pregnancy. Seventeen of the infants had equinovarus with cranial nerve defects (Moebius sequence). Ten of the children had equinovarus as part of more extensive arthrogryposis. Deformities were attributed to vascular disruption and theorized to occur as a result of uterine contractions induced by misoprostol use.

Misoprostol use during lactation is not recommended according to the manufacturer, as there is concern for severe drug-induced diarrhea in the nursing infant (87).

SUMMARY OF MANAGEMENT OF GASTROESOPHAGEAL REFLUX AND PEPTIC ULCER DISEASE IN PREGNANCY

Reflux esophagitis and peptic ulcer disease should initially be managed by conservative measures including lifestyle changes such as elevating the head of the bed at night, eating small low-fat meals, encouraging smoking cessation, wearing loose-fitting clothes, and avoiding heavy lifting. Antacids in various combinations such as magnesium hydroxide, aluminum hydroxide, and calcium carbonate would also be recommended. Of the H_2-receptor antagonists, the drug of choice is ranitidine. Ranitidine is recommended over cimetidine in that cimetidine has been associated with weak antiandrogenic effects and the possibility exists for fetal feminization. Cisapride cannot be currently recommended because of the paucity of information regarding its use in pregnancy. In addition, metoclopramide should be used with caution owing to the many untoward side effects and lack of efficacy. Sucralfate is an excellent alternative medication for the treatment of peptic ulcer disease because it acts locally and is poorly absorbed. The use of proton pump inhibitors is not recommended in pregnancy until further data become available regarding fetal risk. The use of misoprostol is contraindicated.

INTRAHEPATIC CHOLESTASIS OF PREGNANCY

Intrahepatic cholestasis of pregnancy is the most common liver disorder in pregnancy and usually presents in the late second or third trimester (87,88). Women experience itching that involves the extremities, trunk, palms, and soles. Typically the pruritus is worse at night, can become severe, will worsen toward term, and then resolves quickly after delivery. Jaundice develops in approximately 20% to 60% of patients and occurs up to 4 weeks after the pruritus begins (87–90). If anorexia, nausea, vomiting, abdominal pain, hepatosplenomegaly, or fever is present, the clinician needs to rule out other medical complications that might be overlooked. Intrahepatic cholestasis of pregnancy is more common

if there is a family history of the disease and in women of Scandinavian, Bolivian, or Chilean descent (91–95). Both maternal and fetal complications may occur. Postpartum hemorrhage is increased in women with intrahepatic cholestasis of pregnancy and thought to be a result of decreased absorption of vitamin K (87,88,90). The risk of prematurity, low birth weight, stillbirth, and fetal distress are increased in women diagnosed with intrahepatic cholestasis of pregnancy (88,90,96–98).

The management of intrahepatic cholestasis of pregnancy includes reducing the severity of the pruritus in addition to close maternal and fetal observation. Unfortunately, most studies completed to date have proven disappointing in significantly reducing the amount or degree of pruritus. Antihistamines have been used with little success. Antacids containing aluminum that bind bile salts are sometimes helpful. Listed below are the drugs most commonly used in the management of intrahepatic cholestasis of pregnancy (Table 8.3).

PHARMACOLOGIC TREATMENT OF INTRAHEPATIC CHOLESTASIS OF PREGNANCY

Cholestyramine (Questran) is a nonabsorbable anion-exchange resin that binds bile acids and is used in the treatment of intrahepatic cholestasis of pregnancy. The drug also binds anionic drugs in addition to fat-soluble vitamins such as vitamin K. The usual dose is 8 to 20 g per day in divided doses and, once started, may take as long as 2 weeks to work. Side effects include constipation and prolongation of the prothrombin time owing to binding of vitamin K. Women who take cholestyramine should also take vitamin K, 10 mg per day, throughout the remainder of pregnancy.

No adverse fetal outcomes have been noted with the use of cholestyramine in pregnancy, although data are limited (25). In the Michigan Medicaid surveillance study of 229,101 pregnancies, 37 newborns were exposed to the drug during pregnancy without any malformations noted (99).

Ursodeoxycholic acid (Actigall) is a naturally occurring hydrophilic bile salt that is used to dissolve gallstones and has been used to treat

TABLE 8.3. *Drugs most commonly used in the management of intrahepatic cholestasis of pregnancy*

Generic drug name	Trade name	Pharmacologic class of drug	Dosage	Pregnancy use recommendation[a]	Lactation use recommendation[b]
—	—	Antihistamines	Various	C	C
Cholestyramine	Questran	Antilipemic	8–20 g/day p.o. in 3–4 divided doses	B	C
			4 g p.o. a.c. & h.s.		
Ursodeoxycholic acid (Ursodiol)	Actigall, URSO	Gallstone-solubilizing agent	300 mg p.o. b.i.d.	C	C
			750–1,000 mg p.o./day		
Phenobarbital	—	Anticonvulsant sedative	90 mg p.o. q.h.s.	C	C
S-Adenosyl-L-methionine (Ademetionine)	—	—	800 mg i.v./day	C	C
Dexamethasone	Decadron, Maxidex	Corticosteroid	6 mg p.o. b.i.d. for 7 days and then taper over the next 3 days	B	C

[a]A, Drug of choice; B, recommended as an alternate drug of choice; C, limited data to support its use and best avoided, if possible; D, contraindicated (not recommended for use).

[b]A, Safe to use in usual doses; B, probably safe to use in usual doses, but there are insufficient data to ensure no neonatal effects; C, should be used with caution and best avoided, if possible; D, contraindicated (not recommended for use).

intrahepatic cholestasis of pregnancy. There is no recommended dosage of ursodeoxycholic acid, but most patients are started on an oral dose of 300 mg twice daily for 20 days. In the few reported series in the literature, doses of 750 to 1,000 mg per day have also been used.

Data are limited with respect to the use of ursodeoxycholic acid and the risk for fetal malformations. To date, there have been no reported adverse fetal effects with the use of the drug (25).

Phenobarbital is an anticonvulsant that has been used in the treatment of intrahepatic cholestasis of pregnancy, especially in those women who fail to respond to cholestyramine. Phenobarbital induces microsomal enzymes, which increase bile salt secretion and bile flow. The recommended dose is 90 mg per day to be taken at bedtime.

There are limited data on the treatment of intrahepatic cholestasis of pregnancy with the use of phenobarbital. Although no fetal complications were noted, the studies showed the therapy was ineffective (100,101) in treating maternal symptoms.

Phenobarbital is excreted into breast milk. The American Academy of Pediatrics recommends that phenobarbital be used with caution in those women contemplating breast-feeding (24) and that the nursing infant be monitored for signs of sedation.

S-adenosyl-L-methionine is an important methyl donor in hepatic transmethylation reactions that has been used to treat intrahepatic cholestasis of pregnancy. Frezza et al. (102) reported in 1985 reversal of intrahepatic cholestasis of pregnancy in women after administration of 800 mg intravenous *S*-adenosyl-L-methionine per day. The study was single blinded and found that both the degree of pruritus and the severity of transaminase abnormalities were reduced.

In a subsequent randomized, double-blind, placebo-controlled study, the observations of Frezza et al. were not confirmed (103).

Few data exist to draw any conclusions about the safety of this drug in pregnancy with respect to fetal teratogenicity.

Dexamethasone (Decadron, Maxidex) is a corticosteroid that is used in the treatment of many medical disorders and has been used in the management of intrahepatic cholestasis of pregnancy.

The usual dose for management is 6 mg orally twice daily for 7 days followed by a taper regimen over the next 3 days. Hirvioja et al. (104) reported improvement of pruritus in addition to liver transaminases in women who received 12 mg dexamethasone per day for 7 days.

SUMMARY OF PHARMACOLOGIC TREATMENT OF INTRAHEPATIC CHOLESTASIS OF PREGNANCY

The pharmacologic treatment available for the management of intrahepatic cholestasis of pregnancy is limited. Initially intrahepatic cholestasis of pregnancy was thought of as a benign process without significant maternal or fetal sequelae. Now this disorder is recognized as contributing to both maternal and fetal morbidity and mortality. Pharmacologic therapy has focused both on decreasing the amount and degree of pruritus and improving transaminase levels. The use of antihistamines has not proven helpful. Antacids containing aluminum bind bile salts and may be helpful. The use of cholestyramine is recommended to treat pruritus. The dosage to begin with varies but should be at least 8 to 20 g per day in three to four divided doses. Vitamin K should be given along with cholestyramine and the patient told that improvement might take several weeks. The use of ursodeoxycholic acid appears promising but more data are needed regarding fetal risk. Phenobarbital and *S*-adenosyl-L-methionine have not proven efficacious. Dexamethasone may be helpful, and consideration should be given to its use if all else fails.

Fortunately, the symptoms of intrahepatic cholestasis of pregnancy are gone soon after delivery and any medications used for treatment stopped. This is especially reassuring to the woman who desires to breast-feed because there are limited data available regarding lactation and the pharmacologic drugs used to treat intrahepatic cholestasis of pregnancy.

INFLAMMATORY BOWEL DISEASE IN PREGNANCY

Ulcerative colitis and Crohn's disease are both forms of inflammatory bowel disease, occur commonly during the reproductive period of a woman's life, and are associated with a variety of complications as a result of the inflammation of the gastrointestinal tract. For the most part, ulcerative colitis and Crohn's disease represent distinct inflammatory disorders of the gastrointestinal tract, although there is some overlap.

Ulcerative colitis is a mucosal disease of the bowel that involves the rectum and moves proximally to involve part of and sometimes the entire colon. There is a genetic predisposition as seen by a 10-fold increased risk for ulcerative colitis in first-degree relatives and an increased risk seen with twins. Patients usually present with diarrhea, often bloody, and minimal abdominal pain. Colonoscopy reveals mucosal granularity and friability with superficial ulceration. Exacerbations and remissions are not uncommon. Complications include toxic megacolon, reactive arthritis, sclerosing cholangitis, uveitis, erythema nodosum, and an increase in the risk of cancer that has been calculated as 1% per year. Treatment of ulcerative colitis includes medical management or proctocolectomy (105,106).

Crohn's disease is an inflammatory bowel disease that involves not only bowel mucosa but also deeper layers with transmural involvement being common. Any region of the gastrointestinal tract can be involved, but the colon and terminal ileum are most common. The rectum is involved only 50% of the time. There is a genetic predisposition for Crohn's disease with an increased risk in identical twins and a 10-fold increased risk in first-degree relatives. Patients usually present with abdominal pain and diarrhea suggestive of an obstructive process. Colonoscopy reveals patchy involvement of the bowel, often described as segmental or "skip" lesions. Exacerbations and remissions are common and surgery is usually required. Complications of Crohn's disease are common and include fistula formation, toxic megacolon, reactive arthritis, and a sixfold increase in the risk of cancer. Treatment of Crohn's disease includes medical management or segmental resection when indicated (105,106).

Overall there is a significant increase in the rate of spontaneous abortion in women diagnosed with active inflammatory bowel disease (107,108), but otherwise pregnancy outcome is unaffected. Pregnancy also does not appear to exacerbate the disease process (107,109,110). If the disease is active at the beginning of pregnancy, then typically the patient is going to have symptoms throughout her pregnancy. The goal of medical management, including the use of drugs, is to gain rapid control of the disease. Frequent prenatal visits and consultation with a gastroenterologist are necessary to ensure an optimal outcome for the mother and baby.

A review of the most commonly used drugs in the management of inflammatory bowel disease is presented in Table 8.4.

PHARMACOLOGIC TREATMENT OF INFLAMMATORY BOWEL DISEASE

Sulfasalazine (Azulfidine) is composed of 5-aminosalicylic acid (5-ASA) and sulfapyridine and is used for the treatment of both ulcerative colitis and Crohn's disease. The usual starting dose is 4 to 6 g orally in divided doses. The maintenance dose is 2 to 4 g orally in divided doses. Sulfasalazine is poorly absorbed in the upper digestive tract but is split in the colon by bacteria into 5-ASA and sulfapyridine. Sulfapyridine is then absorbed by the colon and excreted in the urine. It is the excretion of sulfapyridine that gives urine its orange color with administration of sulfasalazine. In addition, sulfapyridine is responsible for most of the unpleasant side effects that include headache and hypersensitivity reactions. Mesalamine (5-ASA), in contrast, is poorly absorbed by the colon, is excreted by the feces, but is responsible for the antiinflammatory activity. In fact, the antiinflammatory response of mesalamine is equivalent to that of sulfasalazine and is reviewed later. Sulfasalazine may inhibit folic acid absorption and supplementation of 1 mg twice daily should be prescribed.

There appears to be no increased risk for congenital defects after exposure to sulfasalazine (107–110). A few reports of congenital birth defects have been observed after fetal exposure to sulfasalazine (111,112), but the findings have not been confirmed in subsequent studies and could be related to therapy, chance, the disease, or a combination of the above. Sulfonamides can cause jaundice and possible kernicterus when given near term because these drugs displace

TABLE 8.4. *Drugs most commonly used in the management of inflammatory bowel disease in pregnancy*

Generic drug name	Trade name	Pharmacologic class of drug	Dosage	Pregnancy use recommendation[a]	Lactation use recommendation[b]
Sulfasalazine	Azulfidine	Antiinfective	Starting dose: 4–6 g p.o./day in divided doses; Maintenance: 2–4 g p.o./day in divided doses	B	C
Prednisone	Deltasone	Corticosteroid	40–60 p.o./day although dose may be individualized	A	A
Azathioprine	Imuran	Immunosuppressant	—	C	C
6-Mercaptopurine	Purinethol	Antineoplastic	—	C	C
Mesalamine (5-ASA)	Rowasa	Antiinflammatory bowel disease agent	Rectal suspension (4 mg/60 mL); 4 g p.r. q.h.s. retain for 8 h	B	C
	Asacol		Rectal suppository: 500 mg p.r. b.i.d. retain for 1–3 h; 2.4–4.8 g p.o./day active therapy in divided doses; 800 g p.o./day maintenance therapy in divided doses		
	Pentasa		2–4 g p.o./day active therapy in divided doses; 1.5–3 g maintenance therapy in divided doses		
Olsalazine	Dipentum	Antiinflammatory bowel disease agent	Maintenance therapy: 1.5–3 g p.o./day in divided doses	B	C

[a]A, Drug of choice; B, recommended as an alternate drug of choice; C, limited data to support its use and best avoided, if possible; D, contraindicated (not recommended for use).
[b]A, Safe to use in usual doses; B, probably safe to use in usual doses, but there are insufficient data to ensure no neonatal effects; C, should be used with caution and best avoided, if possible; D, contraindicated (not recommended for use).

bilirubin. To date, there has been no report of either of these problems even when sulfasalazine was given until term (113,114).

Sulfasalazine is excreted into breast milk. There is one report of an infant who developed bloody diarrhea who was exclusively breast-fed (115), and the American Academy of Pediatrics cautions women about the potential for serious side effects if they breast-feed and use sulfasalazine (24).

Prednisone (Deltasone) is a corticosteroid used in the treatment of many medical disorders including inflammatory bowel disease. Prednisone has been used extensively in the treatment of inflammatory bowel disease (usually active disease) and is prescribed at doses from 40 to 60 mg orally every day, although the actual dose should be individualized for each patient.

The use of prednisone for the management of inflammatory bowel disease poses little risk to the developing fetus, and there appears to be no increase in the risk for congenital anomalies (107–110).

Minimal amounts of prednisone have been measured in breast milk (116), and no adverse fetal effects have been reported to date. The American Academy of Pediatrics considers breast-feeding safe in those women requiring prednisone (24).

Azathioprine (Imuran) is an immunosuppressant used for long-term treatment of inflammatory bowel disease. Azathioprine use is well tolerated and potential complications include pancreatitis that occurs after a few weeks of therapy and resolves when the drug is stopped, bone marrow suppression, rash, arthralgias, and toxic hepatitis.

Azathioprine has been shown to cause fetal abnormalities in animal studies (117). Hematologic abnormalities resulting from a toxic effect of the azathioprine on the fetus have also been seen (118). Experience with renal transplant patients who became pregnant and required azathioprine, however, led to delivery of normal infants (119). In addition, women being treated with azathioprine who became pregnant delivered normal infants (120). Results of a case-control study by Connell et al. (121) evaluating inflammatory bowel disease and the teratogenic potential of azathioprine were reassuring. Despite the theoretical concerns about teratogenicity, it appears the use of azathioprine is relatively safe and can be used in selected patients.

6-Mercaptopurine (Purinethol) is an antineoplastic used in the treatment of inflammatory bowel disease. Information regarding the use of the drug and potential teratogenic effects is limited. Animal studies have shown a significantly increased risk for fetal abnormalities when exposed to 6-mercaptopurine (117). Similar to azathioprine, women who accidentally became pregnant while on 6-mercaptopurine usually delivered normal newborns (122). No reports of congenital anomalies related to this drug could be found in the literature, although there was little information available regarding the use of 6-mercaptopurine and its use for inflammatory bowel disease in pregnancy.

Mesalamine (Asacol, Penatasa, Rowasa) is an antiinflammatory bowel disease agent used for the treatment of ulcerative colitis that was developed in the 1990s to reduce the side effects of the sulfapyridine component of sulfasalazine (see section on sulfasalazine). Mesalamine has been formulated to maximize its release in the distal ileum and colon and is made both in delayed- and sustained-release forms.

No reported teratogenic effects have been reported to date. Because little of this drug is absorbed systemically and sulfasalazine is safe to use in pregnancy, the use of mesalamine in pregnancy seems reasonable given its fewer side effects.

Small amounts of mesalamine are excreted into breast milk (25). There is a reported case of a nursing infant developing watery diarrhea after mesalamine was begun in a woman who relapsed with ulcerative colitis (123). Because of this possible allergic reaction, the American Academy of Pediatrics recommends caution in those women who desire to breast-feed and use mesalamine.

Olsalazine (Dipentum) is an antiinflammatory bowel disease drug used to treat ulcerative colitis. The drug is poorly absorbed and releases two molecules of aminosalicylic acid after being broken down by bacteria in the colon.

No information is available regarding olsalazine and teratogenicity.

SUMMARY OF PHARMACOLOGIC TREATMENT OF INFLAMMATORY BOWEL DISEASE IN PREGNANCY

Inflammatory bowel disease is not an uncommon medical complication of pregnancy. To ensure optimal maternal-fetal outcome, care must be taken to aggressively follow these patients with frequent visits and observation for evidence of recurrent disease. Fortunately, most women who relapse or present during pregnancy with inflammatory bowel disease can be treated with prednisone, sulfasalazine, or both. Initiating treatment immediately is important. For those women with ulcerative colitis who fail to respond to prednisone or sulfasalazine, I would recommend the use of mesalamine or olsalazine. The use of azathioprine and 6-mercaptopurine should be reserved for exceptional situations in which control of the disease process occurs only with these drugs and the patient has been counseled regarding the risks and benefits of continued therapy. Women who desire to breast-feed can be encouraged to do so if their only medication is prednisone. With all other drugs listed for treatment of inflammatory bowel disease, there is not enough information for or against breast-feeding and individualized counseling seems prudent.

SUMMARY OF GASTROINTESTINAL DISORDERS IN PREGNANCY

Gastrointestinal disorders in pregnancy are not uncommon and can be difficult to medically manage. Ideally, preconceptional evaluation would allow a woman to be informed of the risks and benefits of drug therapy to control the various medical disorders of the gastrointestinal tract that are preexisting. The goal of therapy would be to limit fetal risk while controlling maternal disease. This goal is also the same for medical complications that develop during pregnancy. Unfortunately, many women are misinformed about drug therapy in pregnancy and this can have serious consequences for both the mother and developing fetus. Recommendations have been made for therapy that take into account the potential for fetal risk while attempting to improve maternal outcome. When selected carefully, drug therapy for the management of gastrointestinal disorders of pregnancy can be done safely, with limited fetal risk, and be beneficial for the mother.

REFERENCES

1. Anonymous. Better news on population. *Lancet* 1992; 339:1600.
2. Koren G, Bologa M, Long D, et al. Perception of teratogenic risk by pregnant women exposed to drugs and chemicals during the first trimester. *Am J Obstet Gynecol* 1989;160:1190–1194.
3. Klebanoff MA, Koslowe PA, Kaslow R, et al. Epidemiology of vomiting in early pregnancy. *Obstet Gynecol* 1985;66:612–616.
4. De Aloysio D, Penacchioni P. Morning sickness control in early pregnancy by Neiguan point acupressure. *Obstet Gynecol* 1992;80:852–854.
5. Belluomini J, Litt RC, Lee KA, et al. Acupressure for nausea and vomiting of pregnancy: a randomized, blinded study. *Obstet Gynecol* 1994;84:245–248.
6. Murphy PA. Alternative therapies for nausea and vomiting of pregnancy. *Obstet Gynecol* 1998;91:149–155.
7. Fischer-Rasmussen W, Kjaer SK, Dahl C, et al. Ginger treatment of hyperemesis gravidarum. *Eur J Obstet Gynecol Reprod Biol* 1990;38:19–24.
8. Srivastava KC. Effects of aqueous extracts of onion, garlic and ginger on platelet aggregation and metabolism of arachidonic acid in the blood vascular system: in vitro study. *Prostaglandins Leukot Med* 1984;13:227–235.
9. Backon J. Ginger: inhibition of thromboxane synthetase and stimulation of prostacyclin: relevance for medicine and psychiatry. *Med Hypotheses* 1986;20:271–278.
10. Willis RS, Winn WW, Morris AT, et al. Clinical observations in treatment of nausea and vomiting in pregnancy with vitamins B_1 and B_6. A preliminary report. *Am J Obstet Gynecol* 1942;44:265–271.
11. Weinstein BB, Mitchell GJ, Sustendal GF. Clinical experiences with pyridoxine hydrochloride in treatment of nausea and vomiting of pregnancy. *Am J Obstet Gynecol* 1943;46:283–285.
12. Hart BF, McConnell WT. Vitamin B factors in toxic psychosis of pregnancy and the puerperium. *Am J Obstet Gynecol* 1943;46:283.
13. Varas O. Treatment of nausea and vomiting of pregnancy with vitamin B_6. *Bol Soc Chilena Obstet Ginecol* 1943;8:404 (abstracted in *Am J Obstet Gynecol* 1945;50:347–348).
14. Weinstein BB, Whol Z, Mitchell GJ, et al. Oral administration of pyridoxine hydrochloride in the treatment of nausea and vomiting of pregnancy. *Am J Obstet Gynecol* 1944;47:389–394.
15. Dorsey CW. The use of pyridoxine and suprarenal cortex combined in the treatment of the nausea and vomiting of pregnancy. *Am J Obstet Gynecol* 1949;58:1073–1078.
16. Sahakian V, Rouse D, Sipes S, et al. Vitamin B6 is effective therapy for nausea and vomiting of pregnancy: a randomized, double-blind placebo-controlled study. *Obstet Gynecol* 1991;78:33–36.
17. Vutyavanich T, Wongtrangan S, Ruangsri R. Pyridoxine for nausea and vomiting of pregnancy: a randomized

double-blind placebo-controlled trial. *Am J Obstet Gynecol* 1995;173:881–884.

18. Gardner LI, Welsh-Sloan J, Cady RB. Phocomelia in infant whose mother took large doses of pyridoxine during pregnancy. *Lancet* 1985;1:636.

19. West KD, Kirksey A. Influence of vitamin B_6 intake on the content of the vitamin in human milk. *Am J Clin Nutr* 1976;29:961–969.

20. Thomas MR, Kawamoto J, Sneed SM, et al. The effects of vitamin C, vitamin B_6, vitamin B_{12}, and folic acid supplementation on the breast milk and maternal status of well-nourished women. *Am J Clin Nutr* 1979;32:1679–1685.

21. Styslinger L, Kirksey A. Effects of different levels of vitamin B-6 supplementation on vitamin B-6 concentrations in human milk and vitamin B-6 intakes of breastfed infants. *Am J Clin Nutr* 1985;41:21–31.

22. Deodhar AD, Rajalaskshmi R, Ramakrishnan CV. Studies on human lactation. Part III. Effect of dietary vitamin supplementation and vitamin contents of breast milk. *Acta Pediatr* 1964;53:42–48.

23. Foukas MD. An antilactogenic effect of pyridoxine. *J Obstet Gynaecol Br Commonw* 1973;80:718–720.

24. Committee on Drugs, American Academy of Pediatrics. The transfer of drugs and other chemicals into human milk. *Pediatrics* 1994;93:137–150.

25. Briggs GG, Freeman RK, Yaffe, SJ. *Drugs in pregnancy and lactation,* 5th ed. Baltimore: Williams & Wilkins, 1998.

26. Heinonen OP, Slone D, Shapiro S. *Birth defects and drugs in pregnancy.* Littleton, MA: Publishing Sciences Group, 1977.

27. Aselton P, Jick H, Milunsky A, et al. First-trimester drug use and congenital disorders. *Obstet Gynecol* 1985;65:451–455.

28. Friedman JM, Little BB, Brent RL, et al. Potential human teratogenicity of frequently prescribed drugs. *Obstet Gynecol* 1990;75:594–599.

29. Bracken MB, Berg A. Bendectin (Debendox) and congenital diaphragmatic hernia. *Lancet* 1983;1:586.

30. Eskenazi B, Bracken MB. Bendectin (Debendox) as a risk factor for pyloric stenosis. *Am J Obstet Gynecol* 1982;144:919–924.

31. Mitchell AA, Rosenberg L, Shapiro S, et al. Birth defects related to Bendectin use in pregnancy. I. Oral clefts and cardiac defects. *JAMA* 1981;245:2311–2314.

32. Mitchell AA, Schwingl PJ, Rosenberg L, et al. Birth defects in relation to Bendectin use in pregnancy. II. Pyloric stenosis. *Am J Obstet Gynecol* 1983;147:737–742.

33. Zierler S, Rothman KJ. Congenital heart disease in relation to maternal use of Bendectin and other drugs in early pregnancy. *N Engl J Med* 1985;313:347–352.

34. Einarson TR, Leeder JS, Koren G. A method for meta-analysis of epidemiological studies. *Drug Intell Clin Pharm* 1988;22:813–824.

35. McKeigue PM, Lamm SH, Linn S, et al. Bendectin and birth defects. I. A meta-analysis of the epidemiologic studies. *Teratology* 1994;50:27–37.

36. O'Brien TE. Excretion of drugs in human milk. *Am J Hosp Pharm* 1974;31:844–854.

37. Parkin DE. Probable Benadryl withdrawal manifestations in a newborn infant. *J Pediatr* 1974;85:580.

38. Milkovich L, Van den Berg BJ. An evaluation of the teratogenicity of certain antinauseant drugs. *Am J Obstet Gynecol* 1976;125:244–248.

39. Greenberg G, Inman WHW, Weatherall JAC, et al. Maternal drug histories and congenital anomalies. *BMJ* 1977;2:853.

40. Mellin GW. Drugs in the first trimester of pregnancy and the fetal life of *Homo sapiens. Am J Obstet Gynecol* 1964;90:1169.

41. Nelson MM, Forfar JO. Associations between drugs administered during pregnancy and congenital abnormalities of the fetus. *BMJ* 1971;1:523–527.

42. Wheatley D. Drugs and the embryo. *BMJ* 1964;1:630.

43. Rumeau-Rouquette C, Goujard J, Huel G. Possible teratogenic effects of phenothiazines in human beings. *Teratology* 1976;15:57–64.

44. Slone D, Siskind V, Heinonen OP, et al. Antenatal exposure to the phenothiazines in relation to congenital malformations, perinatal mortality rate, birth weight, and intelligence quotient score. *Am J Obstet Gynecol* 1977;128:486–488.

45. Farkas VG, Farkas G. Teratogenic action of hyperemesis in pregnancy and of medication used to treat it. *Zentralbl Gynakil* 1971;10:325.

46. Kerns LL. Treatment of mental disorders in pregnancy—a review of psychotropic drug risks and benefits. *J Clin Psychopharmacol* 1989;9:78–87.

47. Ayd FJ Jr. Children born of mothers treated with chlorpromazine during pregnancy. *Clin Med* 1964;71:1758–1763.

48. Ananth J. Congenital malformations with psychopharmacologic agents. *Compr Psychiatry* 1975;16:437–445.

49. Oleson OV, Bartel SA, Paulsen JH. Perphenazine in breast milk and serum. *Am J Psychiatry* 1996;147:1378–1379.

50. Blacker KH, Weinstein BJ, Ellman GL. Mother's milk and chlorpromazine. *Am J Psychiatry* 1962;119:178–179.

51. Wiles DH, Orr MW, Kilakowska T. Chlorpromazine levels in plasma and milk of nursing mothers. *Br J Clin Pharmacol* 1978;5:272–273.

52. Ben-David M, Dikstein S, Sulman FG. Production of lactation by non-sedative phenothiazine derivatives. *Proc Soc Exp Biol Med* 1965;118:265–270.

53. Maitra R, Menkes DB. Psychotropic drugs and lactation. *N Z Med J* 1996;109:217–219.

54. Thiels C. Pharmacotherapy of psychiatric disorder in pregnancy and during breastfeeding: a review. *Pharmacopsychiatry* 1987;20:133–146.

55. Jick H, Holmes LB, Hunter JR, et al. First-trimester drug use and congenital defects. *JAMA* 1981;246:343.

56. Milkovich L, van den Berg BJ. An evaluation of the teratogenicity of certain antinauseant drugs. *Am J Obstet Gynecol* 1976;125:244.

57. Nageotte MP, Briggs GG, Towers CV, et al. Droperidol and diphenhydramine in the management of hyperemesis gravidarum. *Am J Obstet Gynecol* 1996;174:1801–1806.

58. Dieulangard P, Coignet J, Vidal JC. Sur un cas d'ectrophocomelie peut-etre d'origine medicamenteuse. *Bull Fed Gynecol Obstet* 1966;18:85–87.

59. Kopelman AE, McCullar FW, Heggeness L. Limb malformations following maternal use of haloperidol. *JAMA* 1975;231:62–64.

60. Van Waes A, Van de Velde E. Safety evaluation of haloperidol in the treatment of hyperemesis gravidarum. *J Clin Pharmacol* 1969;9:224–227.

61. Hanson JW, Oakley GP. Haloperidol and limb deformity. *JAMA* 1975;231:26.

62. Ayd FJ Jr. Haloperidol: fifteen years of clinical experience. *Dis Nerv Syst* 1972;33:459–469.
63. Stewart RB, Karas B, Springer PK. Haloperidol excretion in human milk. *Am J Psychiatry* 1980;137:849–850.
64. Whalley LJ, Blain PG, Prime JK. Haloperidol secreted in breast milk. *BMJ* 1981;282:1746–1747.
65. Kauppila A, Arvela P, Koivisto M, et al. Metoclopramide in breast feeding: transfer into milk and the newborn. *Eur J Clin Pharmacol* 1983;25;819–823.
66. Guikontes E, Spantideas A, Diakakas J. Ondansetron and hyperemesis gravidarum. *Lancet* 1992;340:1223.
67. World MJ. Ondansetron and hyperemesis gravidarum. *Lancet* 1993;341:185.
68. Sullivan CA, Johnson CA, Roach H, et al. A pilot study of intravenous ondansetron for hyperemesis gravidarum. *Am J Obstet Gynecol* 1996;174:1565–1568.
69. Baron TH, Ramirez B, Richter JE. Gastrointestinal motility disorders during pregnancy. *Ann Intern Med* 1993;118:366–375.
70. Olans LB, Wolf JL. Gastroesophageal reflux in pregnancy. *Gastrointest Endosc Clin North Am* 1994;4:699.
71. Van Thiel DH, Gavaler J, Joshi SN, et al. Heartburn of pregnancy. *Gastroenterology* 1997;72:666.
72. Michaletz-Onody PA. Peptic ulcer disease in pregnancy. *Gastroenterol Clin North Am* 1992;21:817–826.
73. Clark DH. Peptic ulcer in women. *BMJ* 1953;2: 1254.
74. Paul M, Tew WL, Holliday RL. Perforated peptic ulcer in pregnancy with survival of mother and child: case report and review of the literature. *Can J Surg* 1976;19: 427.
75. Aston NO, Kalaichandran S, Carr JV. Duodenal ulcer hemorrhage in the puerperium. *Can J Surg* 1991;34:482.
76. Hansten, PD. Drug interactions of ranitidine vs cimetidine. *Drug Interact Newslett* 1983;3:31–34.
77. Schenker S, Dicke J, Johnson RF, et al. Human placental transfer of cimetidine. *J Clin Invest* 1987;80:1428–1434.
78. Finkelstein W, Isselbacher KJ. Cimetidine. *N Engl J Med* 1978;299:992–996.
79. Pinelli F, Trivulzio S, Colombo R, et al. Antiprostatic effect of cimetidine in rats. *Agents Actions* 1987;22:197–201.
80. Feldman M, Burton M. Histamine$_2$-receptor antagonists: standard therapy for acid-peptic diseases. Part I. *N Engl J Med* 1990;323:1672–1680.
81. Obermeyer BD, Bergstrom RF, Callaghan JT, et al. Secretion of nizatidine into human breast milk after single and multiple doses. *Clin Pharmacol Ther* 1990;47:724–730.
82. Ching MS, Morgan DJ, Mihaly GW, et al. Placental transfer of omeprazole in maternal and fetal sheep. *Dev Pharmacol Ther* 1986;9:323–331.
83. Harper MA, McVeigh JE, Thompson W, et al. Successful pregnancy in association with Zollinger-Ellison syndrome. *Am J Obstet Gynecol* 1995;173:863–864.
84. Brunner G, Athmann C, Hollenz MI. Experience with omeprazole in pregnancy. *Gastroenterology* 1991;112: A79(abst).
85. Tsirigotis M, Yazdani N, Craft I. Potential effects of omeprazole in pregnancy. *Hum Reprod* 1995;10:2177–2178.
86. Gonzales CH, Marques-Dias MJ, Kim CA, et al. Congenital abnormalities in Brazilian children associated with misoprostol misuse in first trimester of pregnancy. *Lancet* 1998;351:1624–1627.
87. Reyes H. The spectrum of liver and gastrointestinal disease seen in cholestasis of pregnancy. *Gastroenterol Clin North Am* 1992;21:905–921.
88. Reid R, Ivey KJ, Rencoret RH, et al. Fetal complications of obstetric cholestasis. *BMJ* 1976;1:870–872.
89. Fisk NM, Bye WB, Storey GNB. Maternal features of obstetric cholestasis: 20 years experience at King George V Hospital. *Aust N Z J Obstet Gynaecol* 1988;28:172–176.
90. Johnston WG, Baskett TF. Obstetric cholestasis: a 14 year review. *Am J Obstet Gynecol* 1979;133:299–301.
91. Shaw D, Frolich J, Whitman BA. A prospective study of 18 patients with cholestasis or pregnancy. *Am J Obstet Gynecol* 1982;142:621–625.
92. Laatikainen T, Ikonen E. Serum bile acids in cholestasis of pregnancy. *Obstet Gynecol* 1977;50:313–318.
93. Reyes H, Gonzales MC, Ribalta J. Prevalence of intrahepatic cholestasis of pregnancy in Chile. *Ann Intern Med* 1978;88:487–493.
94. Reyes H, Taboada G, Rabilta J. Prevalence of intrahepatic cholestasis of pregnancy in La Paz, Bolivia. *J Chronic Dis* 1979;32:499–504.
95. Svanborg A, Ohlsson S. Recurrent jaundice of pregnancy. *Am J Med* 1959;27:40–49.
96. Fagan EA. Intrahepatic cholestasis of pregnancy. *BMJ* 1994;309:1243–1244.
97. Alsulyman GM, Ouzounian JG, Ames-Catro M, et al. Intrahepatic cholestasis of pregnancy: perinatal outcome associated with expectant management. *Am J Obstet Gynecol* 1996;175:957–960.
98. Laatikainen T, Tulenheimo A. Maternal serum bile acid levels and fetal distress in cholestasis of pregnancy. *Int J Gynaecol Obstet* 1984;22:91–94.
99. Rosa F. Anti-cholesterol agent pregnancy exposure outcomes. Presented at the 7th International Organization for Teratogen Information Services, Woods Hole, MA, April 1994.
100. Heikkinen J, Maentausta O, Ylostalo P, et al. Serum bile acid levels in intrahepatic cholestasis of pregnancy during treatment with phenobarbital or cholestyramine. *Eur J Obstet Reprod Biol* 1982;14:153–162.
101. Shaw D, Frohlich J, Wittmann BAK, et al. A prospective study of 18 patients with cholestasis of pregnancy. *Am J Obstet Gynecol* 1982;142:621–625.
102. Frezza M, Pozzato G, Chiesa L, et al. Reversal of intrahepatic cholestasis of pregnancy in women after high dose S-adenosyl-L-methionine administration. *Obstet Gynecol Surv* 1985;40:352–353.
103. Ribalta J, Reyes H, Gonzales MC, et al. S-adensoyl-L-methionine in the treatment of patients with intrahepatic cholestasis of pregnancy: a double-blind, placebo controlled study with negative results. *Hepatology* 1991;13:1084–1089.
104. Hirvioja ML, Tuimala R, Vuori J. The treatment of intrahepatic cholestasis of pregnancy by dexamethasone. *Br J Obstet Gynaecol* 1992;99:109–111.
105. Hanauer SB. Inflammatory bowel disease. *Drug Ther* 1996;334:841–848.
106. Podolsky DK. Inflammatory bowel disease (second of two parts). *N Engl J Med* 1991;325:1008–1016.
107. Khosla R, Willoughby CP, Jewell DP. Crohn's disease and pregnancy. *Gut* 1984;25:52–56.

108. Nielson OH, Andreasson B, Bondesen S, et al. Pregnancy in Crohn's disease. *Scand J Gastroenterol* 1984; 19:724–732.

109. Willoughby CP, Truelove SC. Ulcerative colitis in pregnancy. *Gut3* 1980;21:469–474.

110. Neilson OH, Andreasson B, Bondesen S, et al. Pregnancy in ulcerative colitis. *Scand J Gastroenterol* 1983; 18:735–742.

111. Craxi, A, Pagliarello F. Possible embryotoxicity of sulphasalazine. *Arch Intern Med* 1980;140:1674.

112. Newman NM, Correy JF. Possible teratogenicity of sulphasalazine. *Med J Aust* 1983;1:528–529.

113. Jarnerot G, Into-Malmberg MB, Esbjorner E. Placental and mammary transfer of sulphasalazine and sulphapyridine and some of its metabolites. *Scand J Gastroenterol* 1981;16:693–697.

114. Modadam M. Sulphasalazine, IBD, and pregnancy [Reply]. *Gastroenterology* 1981;81:194.

115. Branski D, Kerem E, Gross-Kieselstein E, et al. Bloody diarrhea–a possible complication of sulfasalazine transferred through human breast milk. *J Pediatr Gastroenterol Nutr* 1986;5:316–317.

116. Greenberger PA, Odeh YK, Frederiksen MC, et al. Pharmacokinetics of prednisolone transfer to breast milk. *Clin Pharmacol Ther* 1993;53:324–328.

117. Reimers TJ, Sluss PM. 6-Mercaptopurine treatment of pregnant mice: effect on second and third generation. *Science* 1978;201:65.

118. Cite CJ, Meuwissen HJ, Pickering RJ. Effect on the neonate of prednisone and azathioprine administered to the mother during pregnancy. *J Pediatr* 1974;85:324–328.

119. Davison JM. Pregnancy in renal allograft recipients: problems, prognosis, and practicalities. *Clin Obstet Gynecol* 1994;8:501–525.

120. Alstead EM, Ritchie JK, Lennard-Jones JE, et al. Safety of azathioprine in pregnancy in inflammatory bowel disease. *Gastroenterology* 1990;99:443–446.

121. Connell WR, Kamm MA, Dickson M, et al. Long-term neoplasia risk after azathioprine treatment in inflammatory bowel disease. *Lancet* 1994;343:1249–1252.

122. Korelitz BI. Fertility and pregnancy in inflammatory bowel disease. In: Kirsner JB, Shorter RG, eds, *Inflammatory bowel disease*, 3rd ed. Philadelphia: Lea & Febiger, 1998:319–326.

123. Nelis GF. Diarrhoea due to 5-aminosalicylic acid in breast milk. *Lancet* 1989;1:383.

APPENDIX

Throughout this chapter reference is often made to the Collaborative Perinatal Project. The Collaborative Perinatal Project was a prospective cohort study of 50,282 mother-child pairs that were cared for at 12 hospitals throughout the United States. Extensive data were collected before the birth of each child that included information on drugs taken during pregnancy, maternal illness, and complications of pregnancy. Information was collected and recorded at each prenatal visit and verified by the attending physician or by review of the chart. For drug use, the heaviest exposure category was recorded if use was for at least 8 days in any given month.

An evaluation of congenital malformations was completed after birth. An estimate of the expected number of malformed children exposed to a specific drug was calculated and a standardized relative risk was then obtained that took into account potential confounding factors from all identified risk factors.

Perinatal mortality rates, birth weights, and intelligence quotient scores were also obtained. The intelligence quotient scores were measured at 4 years of age.

For a more complete description of the materials and methods of the Collaborative Perinatal Project, see ref. 26.

9

Antihypertensive Use During Pregnancy

Julian N. Robinson, Errol R. Norwitz, and John T. Repke

*Department of Obstetrics and Gynecology, Brigham and Women's Hospital,
Harvard Medical School, Boston, Massachusetts*

HYPERTENSIVE DISORDERS OF PREGNANCY

Hypertensive disorders of pregnancy are a major cause of maternal morbidity and mortality from cerebrovascular accident, encephalopathy, and/or hemorrhage. Hypertension can also cause significant perinatal morbidity and mortality, directly through uteroplacental insufficiency and abruptio placenta and indirectly owing to prematurity. Hypertension complicates 6% to 8% of pregnancies in the United States and is directly responsible for 15% of all maternal deaths (1). Because there are no universally accepted, highly effective preventive strategies available to clinicians, the management of hypertension in pregnancy and the use of antihypertensive medications in pregnancy are an important skill for practitioners. There are several different clinical scenarios in which antihypertensive medications may be prescribed in pregnancy. These include chronic hypertension, pregnancy-induced hypertension (PIH), preeclampsia (PET), and hypertensive crises.

Chronic or antecedent hypertension tends to follow a benign course and lends itself to pharmacologic treatment. Risk factors for chronic hypertension include family history, prior hypertensive disorder in pregnancy, diabetes, obesity, increased maternal age, and Afro-Caribbean origin (2). It can be difficult to diagnose chronic hypertension in pregnancy if the parturient's prepregnancy blood pressure range is not known. The physiologic lowering of blood pressure in the second trimester may mask the condition. In addition, other hypertensive disorders of pregnancy may present early, thereby mimicking chronic hypertension. Although this condition appears benign, even mild chronic hypertension has been associated with poor perinatal outcome, although this is often owing to the occurrence of superimposed PET (3). Pregnant women with chronic hypertension have an increased risk of developing "superimposed" PET.

PET is defined as new-onset hypertension associated with proteinuria and/or nondependent edema occurring after 20 weeks of gestation. This condition may require emergency treatment with antihypertensive agents and premature delivery. Other features of PET include hyperuricemia, hemoconcentration, and, in severe cases, thrombocytopenia and hepatic dysfunction. In addition to cerebrovascular accidents, encephalopathy, and hemorrhage, particular maternal risks of PET include seizure (eclampsia), pulmonary edema, liver rupture, renal failure, and coagulopathy. Severe PET can often require immediate delivery; however, recent research suggested that cautious expectant management may be appropriate between 28 and 32 weeks (4). There is no benefit to the mother of expectant management of severe PET. If expectant management is instituted, all parties concerned must be aware that significant maternal risk is being incurred in the pursuit of possible gain by the fetus. HELLP syndrome (hemolysis, elevated liver enzymes, and low platelets) is a particularly serious and aggressive hypertensive condition of pregnancy dominated by hematologic and hepatic manifestations. This condition is treated by immediate delivery of the baby along with antihypertensive therapy, and supportive management as required.

PIH, also known as gestational hypertension, is diagnosed as nonproteinuric hypertension in pregnancy after 20 weeks gestation. It is a diagnosis of exclusion, only being firmly reached when diagnoses of chronic hypertension and PET have been ruled out. PIH may follow a course anywhere within the spectrum outlined above for chronic hypertension and PET.

Hypertensive emergency or crisis may require the use of intravenous antihypertensive therapy. Such intervention is often the hallmark of an unstable clinical situation. If multiple doses or continuous infusion of an intravenous agent is required, management is most suitably performed in the intensive care environment. A peripheral arterial line and/or central cardiovascular monitoring in the acute setting may be needed to titrate antihypertensive medication. Echocardiography may be useful to monitor central cardiovascular function.

PRINCIPLES OF ANTIHYPERTENSIVE THERAPY IN PREGNANCY

Antihypertensive therapy in the nonpregnant individual cannot simply be extrapolated to the pregnant woman. Apart from teratogenicity, there are also issues particular to hypertensive disorders of pregnancy that must be considered before prescribing antihypertensive agents. Similarly, the rationale for choosing a particular antihypertensive agent, such as reduced incidence of atherosclerosis, myocardial infarction, cerebrovascular accident, and renal disease with long-term use, does not apply to pregnancy. The two most important issues in pregnancy are efficacy and safety.

The clinician must also be familiar with the many medical conditions that predispose to hypertension in pregnancy, such as collagen vascular disease, renal disease, diabetes mellitus, and antiphospholipid antibody syndrome. Hypertension may therefore be only one manifestation of a complex clinical situation. When there is a medical condition underlying hypertension, the

clinician should be wary of potential drug interactions.

Adding to the complexity of antihypertensive therapy in pregnancy is the dependency of the fetus on the mother's cardiovascular system for adequate placental perfusion. For example, rapid reduction of blood pressure in a pregnant women using a peripheral vasodilator such as hydralazine may have a profound effect on the uteroplacental circulation. The resulting hypotension may be associated with hypoperfusion of the uteroplacental unit. For this reason, there should be close fetal surveillance in all pregnant women undergoing aggressive antihypertensive therapy. Other agents may selectively dilate the uterine vasculature, thereby improving placental perfusion. Similarly, both nifedipine and methyldopa cause selective vasodilation in the maternal cerebral circulation that could counteract vasospasm caused by PET (5). Antihypertensive agents may have other interactions with hypertensive pathological processes. Calcium channel blockers and β-adrenergic blocking agents can inhibit platelet function (6), this could be of importance as platelet function is a feature of PET (7). Nifedipine has been shown to have an anticonvulsant effect that may be of value when treating patients with PET (8).

WHEN TO USE ANTIHYPERTENSIVES IN PREGNANCY

Severe hypertension in pregnancy (defined as sustained systolic pressures of 160 mm Hg or higher or repeated diastolic blood pressures of 110 mm Hg or higher) should be treated to prevent maternal cerebrovascular accident and placental abruption. The benefit of initiating antihypertensive medication for mild or moderate hypertension in pregnancy (defined as repeated systolic pressures of 140 mm Hg or higher or repeated diastolic blood pressures of 90 mm Hg or higher) is less clear. The use of methyldopa or a beta-blocking agent with moderate hypertension substantially reduces the risk of developing severe hypertension (9). However, there is a lesser body of evidence for a decrease in the incidence of intrauterine growth retardation, preterm birth, cesarean section, and perinatal death (9). The advantage of reducing the incidence of severe hypertension, at the cost of the potential iatrogenic side effects in the mother and even harmful effects in the fetus, can be debated. The main advantage would appear to be in terms of fewer office visits and hospital admissions rather than any alteration of pregnancy outcome. Furthermore, the incidence of blood pressures in this range in pregnancy has been reported to be as high as 20% (10). This high incidence would result in significant therapeutic intervention for questionable gain. Until further evidence becomes available, clinicians should limit pharmacologic antihypertensive intervention to severe hypertension of pregnancy.

CLINICAL APPROACH TO ANTIHYPERTENSIVE THERAPY

Severe hypertension may present as gradually rising blood pressures over a period of hours or days or as a hypertensive crisis. A similar management philosophy is adopted in the treatment of each of these presentations, but the choice of drugs is different. In this chapter, we deal with the philosophy of management, analyze the choice of drugs available, and then draw together different protocols for these different clinical presentations.

To optimize control of blood pressure and to limit the side effects of antihypertensive medications, a systematic, stepwise approach to the control of blood pressure is recommended. This management strategy involves increasing the dose of a first-line agent to maximum before adding a second-line drug. On rare occasions, a third agent may be needed. Although this management style has been widely adopted, there are differences of opinion among obstetricians as to which is the best agent for each level of this stepwise approach. The choice of drugs will also differ between the acute and more chronic clinical presentation. Suitable oral therapeutic agents in the less acute setting include methyldopa, beta blockers [labetalol, pindolol, or oxprenolol (the latter is unavailable in the United States)], and calcium channel blockers (nifedipine and

nicardipine). In the more acute setting, intravenous agents may be required, and options include beta blockers (labetalol), hydralazine, nitroglycerin, and sodium nitroprusside. More recently, the use of a selective serotonin$_2$-receptor antagonist (ketanserin) has been recommended (11,12). A survey of obstetricians in the 1980s showed that 70% of practitioners preferred methyldopa as a first-choice agent, 8% favored labetalol, 8% preferred other β-adrenergic blockers, 4% hydralazine, and 4% clonidine hydrochloride. Reserpine, guanethedine, prazosin, and diuretics were used rarely (13). At the time of this report, calcium antagonists were not widely in use. Practice patterns have not changed greatly since the time of this survey. Diuretics are not recommended as a first-line antihypertensive in pregnancy. Although low-dose diuretics can be continued in patients who conceive on them, in general, diuretics should not be started in pregnancy because of the theoretic concern about decreased uteroplacental perfusion (14). However, this dictum was recently challenged by a report recommending the use of a diuretic as an additional therapeutic agent in early severe hypertension in pregnancy (15).

The American College of Obstetricians and Gynecologists currently recommends alpha methyl dopa as first-line therapy in chronic hypertension, with labetalol or atenolol as a second-line agent (1). In the acute situation, hydralazine or labetalol is the first-line drug recommendation.

ANTIHYPERTENSIVE AGENTS

Methyldopa (Table 9.1) has been well studied in pregnancy. Methyldopa is effective but may take as long as 48 hours to exert its antihypertensive effect. It is safe for both mother and fetus. The most common and major side effect of methyldopa, especially at higher doses, is lethargy. However, when used at higher doses, the mother is often hospitalized or on bed rest, thereby lessening the impact of this effect. Use of methyldopa in pregnancy does not affect later growth and development (16). When methyldopa is used, the maximum dose of 2 g per day is often reached before delivery is desired, and

TABLE 9.1. *Methyldopa*

Agent	Alpha methyl dopa
Trade name	Aldomet
Class	Central α-adrenergic inhibitor
Dosage	Starting dose, 250 mg p.o., t.i.d. or q.i.d. Increase to maximum dosage of 2 g/24 h
Preparation	Tablet or oral suspension
Contraindications	Hypersensitivity to methyldopa, history of hepatitis, autonomic dysfunction, patients on monoamine oxidase inhibitors,
Adverse effects	Liver damage, fever, Coombs-positive hemolytic anemia
Common drug interactions	Pseudoephedrine
Breast-feeding	Safe

additional antihypertensive agents have to be added to the therapeutic regimen. However, this should not be viewed as a disadvantage, as its role of delaying the use of, and reducing the necessary dose of, other drugs is in itself beneficial. In its role as a first-line agent, methyldopa is an excellent choice, being both efficacious and safe. We do not advocate the treatment of mild chronic hypertension in pregnancy. However, randomized trials, using methyldopa compared with placebo in this application, have conflicting results. Some studies suggested that it may prolong gestation, reduce perinatal deaths (17), and reduce mid-trimester pregnancy loss (18), whereas others showed no beneficial effect (19,20). In the treatment of PIH, randomized trials reveal methyldopa to be as effective as labetalol (21) and clonidine (22) and to have fewer complications than oxprenolol (23). In the treatment of sudden-onset severe hypertension of pregnancy or in rapidly rising hypertension, methyldopa is found to have too slow an onset of action to be useful by itself. However, concurrent administration of another agent (such as nifedipine) may be useful for the first 48 to 72 hours, until methyldopa is therapeutic.

Adverse Effects of Alpha Methyl Dopa

Although methyldopa is a very safe agent in pregnancy, potentially serious adverse effects can occur. The clinician should be vigilant for Comb's positive hemolytic anemia in patients on this agent. Liver damage is a recognized side effect of methyldopa, and, indeed, severe liver damage has been described with its use in pregnancy (24).

BETA BLOCKERS

Clinical Review of β-Adrenergic Blockers

The introduction of beta blockers (Table 9.2) in the treatment of hypertension inevitably led to

TABLE 9.2. *Beta-blockers*

Agent (most commonly used)	Labetalol
Trade names	Trandate, Normodyne
Class	α-/β-adrenergic blocker
Dosage	100–400 mg p.o. b.i.d.–t.i.d. (maximum dose, 2,400 mg/day), IV bolus 10 mg, if no response, double dose and repeat every 15 min, up to a cumulative maximum dose of 300 mg
Preparation	Tablet or solution
Contraindications	Labetalol hypersensitivity, bradycardia, asthma, heart block, heart failure
Adverse effects	Maternal and fetal bradycardia, hypotension, bronchospasm
Common drug interactions	Clonidine, halothane, oxilofrine
Breast-feeding	Safe

their use in pregnancy. First-generation beta-blocking agents, such as atenolol, had a long half-life and flat dose–response curve that did not lend itself to the potentially labile nature of hypertension in pregnancy. For this reason, shorter acting beta-blocking agents such as labetalol, pindolol, and oxprenolol (the latter is unavailable in the United States) are preferred in pregnancy. Pindolol has mild alpha-blocking actions and labetalol (unlike most of the other beta blockers) has significant alpha-blocking properties. Early reports on the efficacy and safety of beta blockers in pregnancy were encouraging. Rubin et al. (25) reported less proteinuria and fewer hospital admissions when comparing atenolol with a placebo. Hogstedt et al. (26) found no significant difference in pregnancy outcome when studying metoprolol in combination with hydralazine compared with a placebo in the treatment of mild gestational hypertension. Some practitioners now use β-adrenergic blockers as a first-line antihypertensive agent rather than methyldopa. Indeed, pindolol has been associated with better renal function compared with methyldopa (27), and metoprolol has been associated with lower umbilical blood lactate levels compared with methyldopa (28). Review of randomized, placebo-controlled trials using selected beta blockers in the treatment of mild hypertension shows subtle benefits that may help in choosing an optimal agent. Less proteinuria and fewer hospital admissions have been reported with both atenolol and labetalol (25,29). Lower placental weight has been reported when using atenolol compared with pindolol (30). A review of randomized, controlled trials in the setting of severe hypertension in pregnancy favored the use of intravenous labetalol. Although it is reported that there is a large dose range for labetalol compared with hydralazine in this setting (31), it has been reported to give more effective blood pressure control than both dihydralazine (32) and diazoxide (33). It should be noted that these findings are not without dispute, as dihydralazine has been reported to be more effective than labetalol in the treatment of severe hypertension in another randomized trial (34). In all these randomized trials of treatment of severe hypertension in pregnancy, it should be noted that the numbers of subjects are modest.

Adverse Effects of β-Adrenergic Blockers

Initial enthusiasm surrounding the use of β-adrenergic blockers for hypertension in pregnancy was tempered by reports of adverse effects with atenolol and propranolol (35,36). The first reports of adverse effects of propranolol in pregnancy appeared in the late 1970s (35,36). The first of these series reported propranolol to be harmful to the hypoxic fetus (35), and the second reported fetal growth restriction with propranolol use (36). It should be noted that such studies failed to control for smoking. Growth restriction has since been reported with atenolol (37). The potential inhibition of human placental lactogen (38) may be the cause of the significant restriction of fetal growth associated with atenolol (37). Although the effect of fetal growth restriction has also been reported in labetalol (39), this agent continues to be widely used. When these agents were introduced, there was concern that the cardiac effects of these drugs would adversely affect the fetus and newborn; however, this has been proven not to be the case (25,29,40,41). Despite such adverse associations, labetalol and oxprenolol (and to a lesser extent pindolol) continue to be widely used.

There is a recent report of the birth of two infants born with features of severe fetal β-adrenergic blockade (pericardial effusions and myocardial hypertrophy) to mothers who received long-term antihypertensive therapy with labetalol (42). Prolonged fetal beta blockade (hypoglycemia, bradycardia, and hypotension) was also reported in preterm twins after administration of a single intravenous bolus of labetalol to the mother (43). Severe maternal hypotension was also reported with labetalol in pregnancy (44). Practitioners should be aware of these reports but be reassured that, for such a widely used drug, reports of significant adverse effects in pregnancy are rare.

TABLE 9.3. *Calcium channel antagonists*

Agent (most commonly used)	Nifedipine
Trade names	Adalat, Procardia
Class	Calcium channel blocker
Dosage	10–30 mg p.o. t.i.d., slow-release preparation once a day, maximum of 90 mg/day. In acute situations, nifedipine can be given p.o. in a 10-mg dose repeated every 15 min to maximum of 30 mg
Preparation	Capsule, gel capsule, tablet, slow-release tablet
Contraindications	Hypersensitivity to calcium channel blockers, persistent dermatologic reactions, congestive heart failure
Adverse effects	Peripheral edema, headache, dizziness, tachycardia
Common drug interactions	Potentiates cardiac depressive effect of magnesium sulfate
Breast-feeding	Safe

CALCIUM CHANNEL ANTAGONISTS

Clinical Review of Calcium Antagonists

Calcium channel antagonists (Table 9.3) achieve their antihypertensive effect through both vasodilation and negative inotropic action. Nifedipine, which has a predominant effect on the peripheral vasculature, was introduced as an antihypertensive agent in pregnancy 15 years ago (45). However, the calcium antagonists have not gained as much widespread acceptance as the β-adrenergic blockers for this indication. A survey of European obstetricians in the early 1990s showed that only 16% of obstetricians use calcium antagonists in pregnancy (46). Calcium antagonists are particularly suitable for severe hypertension in pregnancy because of their rapid onset of action. One randomized trial showed a calcium antagonist (nicardipine) to have pregnancy outcomes similar to those of a β-adrenergic blocker (metoprolol) in the treatment of mild hypertension in pregnancy (47). Nifedipine is the most commonly recommended calcium antagonist in pregnancy. However, there has been recent interest in urapidil for treatment of hypertension in pregnancy (48), and one randomized trial suggested it to be superior to dihydralazine (because of equivalent blood pressure control but fewer side effects) (49).

Once again, use of nifedipine in the treatment of mild hypertension is controversial. Although one trial showed nifedipine to be associated with better renal function compared with a placebo in mild PET (50), at least two other randomized controlled trials demonstrated no advantage of nifedipine over no treatment when used in this setting (51,52). However, nifedipine is a very useful agent in the treatment of severe hypertension in pregnancy. Its rapid action, short half-life, and considerable efficacy in reducing high systemic blood pressures lend itself to use in this clinical scenario. A significant decrease in blood pressure is observed 5 to 10 minutes after nifedipine administration, the peak effect is at between 30 and 60 minutes after administration, and the duration of action is approximately 6 hours (53,54). Randomized trials studying severe hypertension in pregnancy showed nifedipine to be as effective as hydralazine (55) and more effective than dihydralazine (56) in controlling blood pressure, with no discernible disadvantages to the mother or the fetus. One randomized study showed nifedipine to be more effective than hydralazine with fewer side effects (57). It should be noted that one of the more common side effects of nifedipine is headache, which should not be confused with headache resulting from severe PET. Caution should be exercised if nifedipine is prescribed in addition to a beta blocker because the cumulative negative inotropic action can precipitate heart failure (58).

Adverse Effects of Calcium Antagonists

Although nifedipine has been shown to be at least as effective as other medications when used in the treatment of hypertension in pregnancy, concerns about its safety have discouraged some practitioners from using it. The primary concern is that the rapid action of nifedipine will result in uteroplacental insufficiency secondary to maternal hypotension. Indeed, experimental work in sheep demonstrated reduced uteroplacental blood flow and impairment of fetal oxygenation (59) and even death (60). However, these findings have not been reproduced in the human. Doppler ultrasound studies of the uterine arteries or umbilical arteries in the human are unaffected by the use of calcium antagonists (61,62). An experimental study using indium 113m showed that there is no reduction in uteroplacental blood flow when sublingual nifedipine is administered (63). Despite these reassuring findings in clinical studies of calcium antagonists in pregnant humans, clinicians have remained cautious about their use for hypertension in pregnancy. Conventional wisdom has led us to believe that sublingual administration of nifedipine can precipitously lower systemic blood pressure, whereas oral administration is less likely to. This has led practitioners to use oral rather than sublingual administration in the belief that this will avoid sudden uncontrolled hypotension and resultant uteroplacental insufficiency. In fact, even when nifedipine is administered sublingually, the absorption is mainly through the intestinal route, with almost no buccal absorption (64). Sublingual administration delays the attainment of nifedipine peak plasma concentration (65,66). Sublingual nifedipine has been associated with sudden death in a predominantly elderly male population with underlying cardiovascular disease (67). To date, there still remains only one reported case of severe hypotension and accompanying fetal distress in the hypertensive gravid patient treated with nifedipine alone (68). Hypotension, resulting from nifedipine, is

therefore rare in pregnant women without preexisting risk factors. At least one similar clinical situation was reported with labetalol in PET (44), but such anxiety has not been associated with its administration in pregnancy. It is of note that in a review of the published literature on use of nifedipine in obstetrics, it was found to be a safe medication in pregnancy, including its use as an antihypertensive agent (69).

Several serious complications of calcium antagonists have been reported in nonpregnant patients, including an increased risk of myocardial infarction (70). A recent metaanalysis also reported a dose-dependent association between the use of nifedipine and sudden death (71). Until recently, these complications were restricted to the nonpregnant population; however, there is a recent report of myocardial infarction in a young healthy pregnant woman treated with nifedipine for preterm labor (72). Although extremely rare, the severity of these complications is likely to heighten physician's anxiety about the use of calcium antagonists in pregnancy, and, as a result, prescribing practices are unlikely to change.

VASODILATORS

Clinical Review of Hydralazine

Hydralazine (Table 9.4) is an antihypertensive agent that achieves its effect through peripheral vasodilation. It acts directly to relax arterial wall smooth muscle. As such, it affects the vessels involved in peripheral resistance rather than capacitance and is therefore a rapid-acting agent.

TABLE 9.4. *Vasodilators*

Agent	Hydralazine
Trade name	Apresoline
Class	Peripheral vasodilator
Dosage	10–50 mg p.o. q.i.d., IV bolus 10 mg every 15–20 min to maximum of 30 mg
Preparation	Tablet or solution
Contraindications	Hydralazine hypersensitivity, CAD, history of CVD (note acetylator status drives response)
Adverse effects	False-positive ANA test, lupus syndrome, tachycardia, peripheral neuropathy
Common drug interactions	None
Breast-feeding	Safe

CAD, coronary artery disease; CVD, cardiovascular disease.

Uteroplacental blood flow and maternal renal blood flow do not change with hydralazine administration (73), confirming a predisposition for peripheral vasculature. Although available in an oral preparation, its most common use in pregnancy is as an intravenous agent in the treatment of hypertensive emergencies. When used in this application, it is an attractive agent because of its ease of administration, relative safety, and, in many cases, lack of need for invasive blood pressure monitoring. Although hydralazine has been used in the treatment of mild chronic hypertension (17–19), its efficacy in this setting remains unclear. Intravenous hydralazine (or dihydralazine) is the preferred agent of many practitioners in severe hypertension in pregnancy. Hydralazine has been compared with nifedipine in a randomized fashion and has been found to have a similar efficacy in several trials (55,74). However, two trials showed hydralazine to be less effective than nifedipine (56,57). Perhaps caution in the prescription of nifedipine in pregnancy (as explained above) and familiarity with hydralazine have led to many practitioners preferring hydralazine to nifedipine for this indication. Evidence is inconclusive from randomized clinical trials that compared hydralazine with labetalol for the management of severe hypertension in pregnancy. Two randomized trials found hydralazine to be the better agent (31,34), whereas two found labetalol to be preferable for this indication (32,33).

Adverse Effects of Hydralazine

Although hydralazine is a popular drug for the treatment of severe hypertension in pregnancy, its use is not without disadvantages. Hypotensive episodes with fetal distress, headaches, tachycardia, systemic lupus-type syndrome, and tachyphylaxis have all been reported (74–76).

NITRATES (NITROPRUSSIDE AND NITROGLYCERIN)

Clinical Review of Sodium Nitroprusside

Sodium nitroprusside (Table 9.5) is a potent vasodilator. This agent has a rapid onset and a short duration of action. Hypotensive effects are found within 2 minutes of infusion and disappear within 5 minutes (77). Nitroprusside is therefore a potent and fast-acting agent. As such, its use should be accompanied by intraarterial blood pressure monitoring. The potency of this agent and the need for invasive monitoring in an intensive care setting have severely limited its use. Nitroprusside causes arterial and venous dilation. In addition to decreasing peripheral resistance, it therefore also causes venous pooling, which, in turn, reduces left ventricular preload. This leads to reduction of pulmonary congestion (77). This combination of actions makes sodium nitroprusside a particularly good agent for the treatment of severe hypertension in the setting of acute congestive heart failure and pulmonary edema. Its use has been described in this situation in pregnancy (78). Sodium nitroprusside is light sensitive. The intravenous delivery system should therefore be wrapped in opaque material. When sodium nitroprusside is used, care should be taken to ensure that the patient is well hydrated to prevent episodes of profound hypotension.

TABLE 9.5. *Nitrates: sodium nitroprusside*

Agent	Sodium nitroprusside
Trade names	Nipride, Nitropress
Class	Vasodilator
Dosage	0.25 μg/kg/min (increase by 0.25 μg/kg/min every 5 min)
Preparation	Solution
Contraindications	Evidence of decreased cerebral perfusion, arteriovenous shunts, coarctation of the aorta
Adverse effects	Cyanide formation, hypotension, headache, dizziness, drowsiness, abdominal cramps, nephrotoxicity
Common drug interactions	Sildenafil (Viagra)
Breast-feeding	Not applicable

TABLE 9.6. *Nitrates: nitroglycerin*

Agent	Nitroglycerin
Trade names	Nitrostat, Nitro-Bid, Tridil
Class	Vasodilator
Dosage	IV infusion starting at 10 μg/min (double dose every 5 min)
Preparation	Solution
Contraindications	Hypersensitivity, severe anemia, glaucoma, hypotension
Adverse effects	Aspirin (increase nitrates), alcohol, calcium channel antagonists, heparin (decreases efficacy of heparin)
Common drug interactions	Methemoglobinemia, dizziness, drowsiness, abdominal cramps, nephrotoxicity
Breast-feeding	Not applicable

Adverse Effects of Sodium Nitroprusside

Sodium nitroprusside is usually reserved for obstetric hypertensive crises, usually in the peripartum period. Its use before delivery is limited because of the potential for fetal cyanide toxicity. Arterial blood gases should be monitored for the occurrence of metabolic acidosis as this may be an early sign of cyanide toxicity. Sodium nitroprusside has also been associated with fetal bradycardia (79), and if used when the patient is still pregnant, continuous fetal surveillance should be instituted.

NITROGLYCERIN

Clinical Review of Nitroglycerin

Nitroglycerin (Table 9.6) is a vasodilator that primarily relaxes the venous system but, like nitroprusside, also affects the arteriolar system. It therefore decreases both peripheral resistance, and right atrial preload. This effect is dose related. At low doses, nitroglycerin decreases preload and at high doses, it decreases afterload (80). This dual effect lends itself to the treatment of severe hypertension complicated by pulmonary edema, and it has been recommended in this role in a published case series (81). Like sodium nitroprusside, it has a rapid potent action and short half-life. It has been noted that for smooth control of blood pressure, prevasodilator hydration is required (82). Again like nitroprusside, when used, care should be taken to ensure that the patient is adequately hydrated to prevent precipitous drops in blood pressure. However, again, the rarity of need, intensive care requirement, and physicians' inexperience with

this medication make for infrequent use of this drug in obstetric care.

Adverse Effects of Nitroglycerin

A significant side effect of higher doses of intravenous nitroglycerin is the potential occurrence of methemoglobinemia. A methemoglobin level of greater than 3% is diagnostic for toxicity and may impair fetal oxygenation. Evidence for methemoglobinemia should be sought in any patient who appears cyanotic on intravenous nitroglycerin.

CLONIDINE

Clinical Review of Clonidine Hydrochloride

Clonidine hydrochloride (Table 9.7) is an effective central-acting antihypertensive agent (similar to methyldopa). Clonidine also acts directly on the vagal nuclei to cause slowing of the maternal heart rate (22). Clonidine has a more rapid onset of action than methyldopa and is available in oral parenteral and transcutaneous preparations. In direct comparison with methyldopa in a randomized, double-blind, controlled trial as an antihypertensive agent in pregnancy, there was no significant difference in antihypertensive effect or maternal side effects between the two agents (22). Clonidine has been compared with placebo in a randomized fashion in the treatment of mild hypertension of pregnancy and was reported to prolong pregnancy (83). However, reports in the literature of this agent in this application are sparse. If use of this agent is considered, it is reassuring to note that a series of 82 hypertensive pregnant

TABLE 9.7. *Clonidine*

Agent	Clonidine
Trade names	Catapres, Duraclon
Class	Central α-adrenergic inhibitor
Dosage	0.2–0.6 mg/day p.o.
Preparation	Solution for injection, tablet, or transdermal patch
Contraindications	Clonidine hypersensitivity, conduction defects, bleeding disorders
Adverse effects	Central nervous system depression, orthostasis, dry mouth
Common drug interactions	Tricyclic antidepressants, beta-blockers
Breast-feeding	Unknown

mothers treated with clonidine reported no significant drug-related effects to mothers or babies (84).

Adverse Effects of Clonidine Hydrochloride

A potential association exists between clonidine use in pregnancy and Roberts syndrome (85). Known side effects in the nonpregnant individual include lethargy, dizziness, and dry mouth.

KETANSERIN

Clinical Review of Ketanserin

Ketanserin (Table 9.8) has been recommended for the treatment of PET (86–88). Ketanserin is a serotonin receptor antagonist. The rationale for use of this drug in PET is based on the observation that patients with PET have a greater pressor response to angiotensin II and have lower platelet levels. Serotonin augments the angiotensin II pressor response and also causes platelet aggregation. A randomized controlled

trial reported ketanserin to be as effective as hydralazine in lowering blood pressure in PET (86). This trial suggested ketanserin to be safer in that it caused less unforeseen hypotension. However, at this time, this agent is still investigational.

DIURETICS

Diuretics are not recommended as a first-line antihypertensive agent in pregnancy. However, women with chronic hypertension may present at their initial prenatal visit with well-controlled blood pressure on a diuretic. In such patients, it is reasonable to continue low-dose diuretics for the duration of the pregnancy. Traditional practice is not to commence diuretic therapy in pregnancy because of early experimental findings suggesting a decrease in intravascular volume and subsequent diminished uteroplacental perfusion (14). However, in that report, the dose of furosemide (Table 9.9) was far higher than would be routinely used in long-term management of hypertension in pregnancy (40 mg intravenous bolus). It is reasonable to assume that long-term

TABLE 9.8. *Ketanserin*

Agent	Ketanserin
Trade name	Not commercially marketed
Class	Serotonin antagonist
Dosage	10 mg IV every 20 min
Preparation	Solution
Contraindications	Maternal heart block, prescription of maternal antiarrhythmic agents
Adverse effects	Hypotension, dizziness
Common drug interactions	Increases levels of propranolol
Breast-feeding	Unknown (ketanserin is secreted in breast milk)

TABLE 9.9. *Furosemide*

Agent	Furosemide
Trade name	Lasix
Class	Loop diuretic
Dosage	20–80 mg p.o., o.d. or b.i.d.
Preparation	Tablet
Contraindications	Hypersensitivity to furosemide, patients with anuria or depleted blood volume
Adverse effects	Profound diuresis with water and electrolyte depletion, skin sensitivity to exposure to sunlight, hyperuricemia and gout, exacerbation of systemic lupus erythematosus, abdominal cramping, diarrhea, tinnitus, dizziness, pancratitis, and cholestasis
Common drug interactions	Aminoglycoside antibiotic levels may be increased, ethnacrynic acid, tubocurarine, lithium, and sucralfate
Breast-feeding	Safe

use of smaller doses, owing to the mechanism of action of diuretics, may lead to electrolyte imbalance and volume depletion. Because of the wide acceptance of this tenet, the use of diuretics has been avoided in pregnancy. It is of note that a recent report suggested that it is appropriate to use a diuretic as an additional therapeutic agent in early severe hypertension in pregnancy (15). However, with alternative safe antihypertensive agents, it is unlikely for this traditional avoidance of diuretics in pregnancy to change.

Hydrochlorothiazide

It should be noted that hydrochorothiazide (Table 9.10) (and all the thiazide-derived diuretics) are pregnancy class D, and with so many alternative

safe therapies, we do not recommend their use in pregnancy.

ACE INHIBITORS

Angiotension-converting enzyme inhibitors (Table 9.11) are pregnancy class D [they have been associated with fetal hypocalvaria, renal failure, oligohydramnios, and fetal and neonatal death, especially in the second trimester (89,90)]. Use of these agents is contraindicated in pregnancy.

ANGIOTENSIN RECEPTOR ANTAGONISTS

These agents (Table 9.12) are also pregnancy class D, and with so many alternative safe

TABLE 9.10. *Hydrochlorothiazide*

Agent	Hydrochlorothiazide
Trade name	HydroDiuril
Class	Loop diuretic
Dosage	25–50 mg p.o., o.d.
Preparation	Tablet
Contraindications	Anuria, renal disease, liver disease, systemic lupus erythematosus, hypersensitivity to hydrochlorothiazide or other sulfonamide-derived drugs
Adverse effects	Weakness, hypotension, pancreatitis, cholestasis, anemia, allergic reactions, electrolyte disturbance, hyperglycemia, hyperuricemia, dizziness, renal dysfunction
Common drug interactions	Alcohol, barbiturates, antidiabetic drugs, cholestyramine, corticosteroids, tubocurarine
Breast-feeding	Risk remote; however, there are concerns about potential thrombocytopenia in infant

TABLE 9.11. *Angiotensin-converting enzyme inhibitors*

Agent	Enalapril
Trade names	Vaseretic, Vasotec
Class	Angiotensin-converting enzyme inhibitor
Dosage	10–40 mg/day p.o., o.d., or b.i.d. IV, 1.25 mg given over 5 min every 6 h (maximum 5 mg/dose)
Preparation	Tablet, solution
Contraindications	Pregnancy
Adverse effects	Anaphylaxis, neutropenia, agranulocytosis, hepatic failure, cholestatic jaundice, fulminant hepatic necrosis
Common drug interactions	Diuretics, lithium
Breast-feeding	Safe

therapies, we do not recommend their use in pregnancy.

TERATOLOGY

The antihypertensive agents as a group of drugs are relatively safe in pregnancy. The adverse effects of each class of drug are discussed above. In the drugs recommended thus far, there are no known teratogenic effects. This is not true for all antihypertensive agents. It is important to recognize antihypertensive agents that are contraindicated in pregnancy, especially as women with preexisting chronic hypertension may present already on these medications. Angiotensin-converting enzyme inhibitors (and angiotensin receptor blockers) are not teratogenic per se but have been associated with fetal hypocalvaria, renal failure, oligohydramnios, and fetal and neonatal death, especially in the second trimester (89,90). Minoxidil has been associated with hypertrichosis and other congenital anomalies (91). Such medications should therefore be discontinued before, or as early as possible, in pregnancy to avoid these potential effects.

An interesting footnote is the fact that any antihypertensive agent that produces severe hypotension in the period of organogenesis could theoretically lead to teratogenic effects. Transverse limb defects were reported in a fetus and an infant born to mothers treated for hypertension (92). The fetus in this report also had a cleft lip and hypoxic renal damage. It was suggested that the antihypertensive agents caused maternal hypotension that led to reduced uteroplacental blood flow, fetal hypotension, and hypoxia and that the anomalies were secondary to these events.

CONCLUSION

Antihypertensive agents, with the exceptions of ACE inhibitors and angiotensin receptor agonists, are relatively safe in pregnancy. However, this should not lead to complacency in their prescription. There are significant adverse effects associated with all these agents. The varying presentation of hypertension in pregnancy necessitates that care is taken in the selection of an antihypertensive agent according to degree of effect, speed of action, and ease of administration. Hypertension in pregnancy lends itself to a stepwise approach to therapy (Tables 9.13 and 9.14), in which a first-line agent can be prescribed in increasing doses until another agent is necessary. Primary concern when prescribing in pregnancy should be given to safety and efficacy. Finally, a good therapeutic regimen should be integrated with careful and adequate surveillance of both mother and baby.

TABLE 9.12. *Angiotensin receptor antagonists*

Agent	Losartan
Trade name	Cozaar
Class	Angiotensin receptor antagonist
Dosage	25–100 mg/day p.o., o.d. or b.i.d.
Preparation	Tablet
Contraindications	Pregnancy
Adverse effects	Diarrhea, dyspepsia, cramps, myalgia, dizziness, insomnia, cough sinusitis
Common drug interactions	None known
Breast-feeding	Unknown

TABLE 9.13. *Protocol for nonemergent treatment of severe hypertension in pregnancy*

Clinical scenario	Management	Dosing schedule	Contraindications	Clinical notes
Consistent BP ≥160/105 on at least 2 occasions	Alpha methyldopa (some clinicians prefer to use a beta-blocker as first-line agent)	Commence at 250 mg p.o. t.i.d. Allow 24–48 h for optimal effect.[a] Increase to cumulative maximum dose of 2 g/day (q.i.d. dosing may be used for more steady-state effect)	History of hepatitis or autonomic dysfunction, patient on monoamine oxidase inhibitor	Maternal surveillance with regular BP, lab tests, and clinical review. Regular fetal surveillance assessing fetal well-being, and fetal growth and Doppler studies of umbilical artery
BP not adequately controlled with above regimen (after adequate time for methyldopa to become therapeutic)	Labetalol	Commence at 100 mg p.o. b.i.d. Increase to maximum cumulative dose of 2,400 mg/day. Use q.i.d. if required. Pulse may be used as indicator of beta-blockade	Asthma, heart failure, bradycardia	—
BP not adequately controlled with above regimen	Consider delivery, nifedipine	Commence at 10 mg p.o. t.i.d. Increase to maximum of cumulative daily dose of 90 mg/day	Congestive heart failure	Extreme caution should be exercised using 2 agents with negative inotropic effects
BP not adequately controlled with above regimen	Delivery	—	—	—

[a] Another agent may be used as an interim agent while methyldopa is becoming therapeutic (e.g., beta-blocker or calcium antagonist).
BP, blood pressure.

TABLE 9.14. Protocol for management of hypertensive crisis in pregnancy

Clinical scenario	Management	Dosing schedule	Contraindications	Clinical notes
Consistent BP ≥160/105 on at least 2 occasions with emergent presentation	Labetalol (hydralazine may be used as an alternative first-line agent)	5–10 mg IV first dose, then double it every 15 min to cumulative maximum dose of 300 mg	Asthma, heart failure, bradycardia	Maternal surveillance with regular BP every 10 min, lab tests, and clinical review, continuous fetal monitoring
BP not adequately controlled with above regimen	Hydralazine	10 mg IV every 10–15 min to a cumulative maximum dose of 300 mg	Extreme care if history of cardiovascular disease	—
	Nifedipine may be used as an alternative agent dose	10 mg p.o. every 15–20 min to a cumulative maximum dose of 90 mg		
BP not adequately controlled with above regimen. Consider team management with intensivist and maternal fetal medicine specialist	Consider delivery. sodium nitroprusside	0.25 μg/kg/min (increase by 0.25 μg/kg/min every 5 min to a maximum of 10 μg/kg/min)	Clinical evidence of cerebral hypoperfusion	Should be in intensive care setting with intraarterial BP monitoring and continuous fetal monitoring. Monitor for cyanide toxicity
BP not adequately controlled with above regimen	Delivery	—	—	—

BP, blood pressure.

REFERENCES

1. ACOG Technical Bulletin. 1996;219:1.
2. Sibai BM. Diagnosis and management of chronic hypertension in pregnancy. *Obstet Gynecol* 1991;78:451–461.
3. Sibai BM, Abdella TN, Anderson GD. Pregnancy outcome in 211 patients with mild chronic hypertension. *Obstet Gynecol* 1983;61:571–576.
4. Sibai BM, Mercer BM, Schiff E, et al. Aggressive versus expectant management of severe preeclampsia at 28–32 weeks' gestation: a randomized controlled trial. *Am J Obstet Gynecol* 1994;171:818–822
5. Serra-Serra V, Kyle PM, Chandran R, et al. The effect of nifedipine and methyldopa on maternal cerebral circulation. *Br J Obstet Gynaecol* 1997;104:532–537.
6. Nyrop M, Zweifler AJ. Platelet aggregation in hypertension and the effects of hypertensive treatment. *J Hypertens* 1988;6:262–269.
7. Redman CWG, Bonnar J, Beilin LJ. Early platelet consumption in pre-eclampsia. *BMJ* 1978;1:467–469.
8. Larkin JG, Butler E, Brodie MJ. Nifedipine for epilepsy? A pilot study. *BMJ* 1988;296:530–531.
9. The Cochrane Pregnancy and Childbirth Database. Cochrane Collaboration Group. Internet On Line. 1998.
10. Redman CWG. Hypertension in pregnancy. In: de Sweit M, ed. *Medical disorders of pregnancy*. London: Blackwell Scientific, 1989:249–305.
11. Steyn DW, Odendal HJ. Randomised controlled trial of ketanserin and aspirin in prevention of pre-eclampsia. *Lancet* 1997;350:1267–1271.
12. Steyn DW, Odendal HJ. Dihydralazine or ketanserin for severe hypertension in pregnancy? Preliminary results. *Eur J Obstet Gynecol Reprod Biol* 1997;75:155–159.
13. Trudinger BJ, Parik I. Attitudes to management of hypertension in pregnancy: a survey of Australian fellows. *Aust NZ J Obstet Gynaecol* 1982;22:191–197.
14. Gant NF, Madden JD, Siiteri PK, et al. The metabolic clearance rate of dehyroisandosterone sulfate IV. Acute effects of induced hypertension, hypotension, and naturesis in normal and hypertensive pregnancies. *Am J Obstet Gynecol* 1976;124:143–148.
15. Hall DR, Odendaal HJ. The addition of a diuretic to anti-hypertensive therapy for early severe hypertension in pregnancy. *Int J Gynaecol Obstet* 1998;60:63–64.
16. Cockburn J, Moar VA, Ounsted M, et al. Final report of study on hypertension during pregnancy: the effect of specific treatment on the growth and development of the children. *Lancet* 1986;i:647–649.
17. Leather HM, Humphreys DM, Baker PB, et al. A controlled trial of hypotensive agents in hypertension in pregnancy. *Lancet* 1968;2:488–490.
18. Redman CWG. Fetal outcome in trial of hypertensive outcome in pregnancy. *Lancet* 1976;2:753–756.
19. Arias F, Zamora J. Antihypertensive treatment and pregnancy outcome in patients with mild chronic hypertension. *Obstet Gynecol* 1979;53:489–494.
20. Sibai BM, Mabie WC, Shamsa F, et al. A comparison of no medication versus methyldopa or labetalol in chronic hypertension in pregnancy. *Am J Obstet Gynecol* 1990;162;960–967.
21. Plouin PF, Breart G, Llado J, et al. A randomized comparison of early with conservative use of antihypertensive drugs in the management of pregnancy-induced hypertension. *Br J Obstet Gynaecol* 1990;97:134–141.
22. Horvarth JS, Phippard A, Korda A, et al. Clonidine hydrochloride—a safe and effective hypertensive agent in pregnancy. *Obstet Gynecol* 1985;66:634–638.
23. Fidler J, Smith V, Fayers P, et al. Randomized controlled comparative study of methyldopa and oxprenolol in treatment of hypertension in pregnancy. *BMJ* 1983;286:1927–1930.
24. Smith GN, Piercy WN. Methyldopa hepatotoxicity in pregnancy: a case report. *Am J Obstet Gynecol* 1995;172:222–224.
25. Rubin PC, Butters L, Clark DM, et al. Placebo-controlled trial of atenolol treatment of pregnancy associated hypertension. *Lancet* 1983;i:431–434.
26. Hogstedt S, Lindeberg S, Axelsson O, et al. A prospective controlled trial of metoprolol-hydralazine treatment in hypertension during pregnancy. *Acta Obstet Gynecol Scand* 1985;64:505–510.
27. Ellenbogen A, Jaschevatsky O, Davidson A, et al. Management of pregnancy-induced hypertension with pindolol—comparative study with methyldopa. *Int J Gynecol Obstet* 1986;24:3–7.
28. Wichman K, Ryden G, Karlberg BE. A placebo controlled trial of metoprolol in the treatment of hypertension in pregnancy. *Scand J Clin Lab Invest Suppl* 1984;169:90–95.
29. Pickles CJ, Symonds EM, Broughton Pipkin F. The fetal outcome in a randomized double-blind controlled trial of labetalol versus placebo in pregnancy-induced hypertension. *Br J Obstet Gynaecol* 1989;96:38–43.
30. Montan S, Ingermarsson I, Marsal K, et al. Randomized controlled trial of atenolol and pindolol in human pregnancy: effects on fetal hemodynamics. *BMJ* 1992;304:946–949.
31. Mabie WC, Gonzalez AR, Sibai BM, et al. A comparative trial of labetalol and hydralazine in the acute management of severe hypertension complicating pregnancy. *Obstet Gynecol* 1987;70:328–333.
32. Garden A, Davey DA, Dommisse J. Intravenous labetalol and intravenous dihydralazine in severe hypertension in pregnancy. *Clin Exp Hypertens* 1982;1:371–383.
33. Michael GA. Intravenous labetalol and intravenous diazoxide in severe hypertension complicating pregnancy. *Aust N Z J Obstet Gynaecol* 1986;26:26–29.
34. Ashe RG, Moodley J, Richards AM, et al. Comparison of labetalol and dihydralazine in hypertensive emergencies of pregnancy. *S Afr Med J* 1987;71:354–356.
35. Lieberman BA, Stirrat GM, Cohen SL, et al. The possible adverse effect of propranolol on the fetus in pregnancies complicated by severe hypertension. *Br J Obstet Gynaecol* 1978;85:678–83.
36. Pruyn SC, Phelan JP, Buchanan GC. Long term propranolol therapy in pregnancy: maternal and fetal outcome. *Am J Obstet Gynecol* 1979;135:485–489.
37. Rubin PC, Butters L, Kennedy S. Atenolol in the management of essential hypertension during pregnancy. *BMJ* 1990;301:587–589.
38. Rubin PC, Butters L, Clark DM, et al. Obstetric aspects of the use in pregnancy-associated hypertension of the beta-adrenoreceptor agonist atenolol. *Am J Obstet Gynecol* 1984;150:389–392.
39. Sibai BM, Gonzalez AR, Mabie WC, et al. A comparison of labetalol plus hospitalization versus hospitalization alone in the management of pre-eclampsia remote from term. *Obstet Gynecol* 1987;70:323–327.

40. Reynolds B, Butters L, Evans L, et al. First year of life after use of atenolol in pregnancy associated hypertension. *Arch Dis Child* 1984;59:1061–1063.

41. MacPherson M, Broughton Pipkin F, Rutter N. The effect of maternal labetalol on the newborn infant. *Br J Obstet Gynaecol* 1986;93:539–542.

42. Crooks BN, Deshpande SA, Hall C, et al. Adverse neonatal effects of maternal labetalol treatment. *Arch Dis Child Fetal Neonatal Ed* 1998;79:150–151.

43. Klarr JM, Bhatt-Mehta V, Donn SM. Neonatal adrenergic blockade following single dose maternal labetalol administration. *Am J Perinatol* 1994;11:91–93.

44. Olsen KS, Beier-Holgersen R. Hemodynamic collapse following labetalol administration in preeclampsia. *Acta Obstet Gynecol Scand* 1992;71:151–152.

45. Walters BNJ, Redman CWG. Treatment of severe pregnancy-associated hypertension with the calcium antagonist nifedipine. *Br J Obstet Gynaecol* 1984;91:330–336.

46. Wide-Swensson D, Montal S, Ingemarsson I. How Swedish obstetricians manage hypertensive disorders in pregnancy. A questionnaire study. *Acta Obstet Gynecol Scand* 1994;73:619–624.

47. Jannet D, Carbonne B, Sebban E, et al. Nicardipine versus metoprolol in the treatment of hypertension during pregnancy: a randomized comparative trial. *Obstet Gynecol* 1994;84:354–359.

48. Dooley M, Goa KL. Urapidil. A reappraisal of its use in the management of hypertension. *Drugs* 1998;56:929–955.

49. Wacker J, Werner P, Walter-Sack I, et al. Treatment of hypertension in patients with pre-eclampsia: a prospective parallel-group study comparing dihydralazine with urapidil. *Nephrol Dial Transplant* 1998;13:318–325.

50. Ismail AAA, Medhat I, Tawfic TAS, et al. Evaluation of calcium antagonist (nifedipine) in the treatment of pre-eclampsia. *Int J Gynecol Obstet* 1993;40:39–43.

51. Sibai BM, Barton JR, Akl S, et al. A randomized prospective comparison of nifedipine and bed rest versus bed rest alone in the management of pre-eclampsia remote from term. *Am J Obstet Gynecol* 1992;167:879–884.

52. Gruppo di Studio Ipertensione in Gravidanza. Nideipine versus expectant management in mild to moderate hypertension in pregnancy. *Br J Obstet Gynaecol* 1998;105:718–722.

53. Bauer JH, Reams GP. The role of calcium entry blockers in hypertensive emergencies. *Circulation* 1987;75:174–180.

54. Beer N, Gallegos I, Cohen A, et al. Efficacy of sublingual nifedipine in the acute treatment of systemic hypertension. *Chest* 1981;79:571–574.

55. Martins-Costa S, Ramos JG, Barros E, et al. Randomized controlled trial of hydralazine versus nifedipine in pre-eclamptic women with acute hypertension. *Clin Exp Hypertens* 1992;11:25–44.

56. Seabe SJ, Moodley J, Becker P. Nifedipine in acute hypertensive emergencies in pregnancy. *S Afr Med J* 1989;76:248–250.

57. Fenakel K, Fenakel G, Appelman Z, et al. Nifedipine in the treatment of severe pre-eclampsia. *Obstet Gynecol* 1991;77:331–337.

58. Robson RH, Vishwaneth MC. Nifedipine and beta-blockade as a cause of cardiac failure. *BMJ* 1982;284:104.

59. Harake B, Gilbert RD, Ashwal S, et al. Nifedipine: effects on fetal and maternal hemodynamics in pregnant sheep. *Am J Obstet Gynecol* 1987;157:1003–1008.

60. Parisi VM, Salinas J, Stockmar EJ. Fetal vascular responses to maternal nicardipine administration in the hypertensive ewe. *Am J Obstet Gynecol* 1989;161:1035–1039.

61. Hanretty KP, Whittle MJ, Howie CA, et al. Effect of nifedipine on Doppler flow velocity waveforms in severe pre-eclampsia. *BMJ* 1989;299:1205–1206.

62. Mari G, Kirshon B, Moise KJ, et al. Doppler assessment of the fetal and uteroplacental circulation during nifedipine therapy for preterm labor. *Am J Obstet Gynecol* 1989;161:1514–1518.

63. Lindow SW, Davies N, Davey DA, et al. The effect of sublingual nifedipine on uteroplacental blood flow in hypertensive pregnancy. *Br J Obstet Gynaecol* 1988;95:1276–1281.

64. Van Harten J, Burggraf K, Danhof M, et al. Negligible sublingual absorption of nifedipine. *Lancet* 1987;2:1363–1365.

65. McAllister RG. Kinetics and dynamics after oral and sublingual doses. *Am J Med* 1986;81:2–5.

66. Diker E, Erturk S, Akgun G. Is sublingual nifedipine administration superior to oral administration in the active treatment of hypertension? *Angiology* 1992;43:477–481.

67. Grosman E, Messerli FH, Grodzicki T, et al. Should a moratorium be placed on sublingual nifedipine capsules given for hypertensive emergencies and pseudoemergencies? *JAMA* 1996;276:1328–1331.

68. Impey L. Severe hypotension and fetal distress following sublingual administration of nifedipine to a patient with severe pregnancy induced hypertension at 33 weeks. *Br J Obstet Gynaecol* 1993;100:959–961.

69. Childress CH, Katz VL. Nifedipine and its indications in obstetrics and gynecology. *Obstet Gynecol* 1994;83:616–624.

70. Psaty BM, Heckbert SR, Koepsell TD, et al. The risk of myocardial infarction associated with antihypertensive drug therapies. *JAMA* 1995;274:620–625.

71. Furberg CD, Psaty BM, Meyer JV. Nifedipine: dose-related increase in mortality in patients with coronary heart disease. *Circulation* 1995;92:1326–1331.

72. Oei SG, Oei SK, Rolmann HAM. Myocardial infarction during nifedipine therapy for preterm labor. *N Engl J Med* 1999;340:154.

73. Duggan PM, McCowan LME, Stewart AW. Antihypertensive drug effects on placental flow velocity waveforms in pregnant women with severe hypertension. *Aust N Z J Obstet Gynaecol* 1992;32:335–338.

74. Derham RJ, Robinson J. Severe preeclampsia: is vasodilatation therapy with hydralazine dangerous for the preterm fetus? *Am J Perinatol* 1990;7:239–244.

75. Overgaard J, Skinhoj E. A paradoxical cerebral hemodynamic effect of hydralazine. *Stroke* 1975;7:402–404.

76. Lin M-S, McNay JL, Shepperd AMM, et al. Increased plasma norepinephrine accompanies persistent tachycardia after dihydralazine. *Hypertension* 1983;5:257–263.

77. Guiha NH, Cohn JN, Mikulic E, et al. Treatment of refractory heart failure with infusion of nitroprusside. *N Engl J Med* 1974;291:587.

78. Stempel JE, O'Grady JP, Morton MJ, et al. Use of sodium nitroprusside in complications of gestational hypertension. *Obstet Gynecol* 1982;60:533–538.

79. Donchin Y, Amirav B, Sahar A. Sodium nitroprusside for aneurysm surgery in pregnancy. *Br J Anaesth* 1978;50:849–851.

80. Herling IM. Intravenous nitroglycerin: clinical pharmacology and therapeutic considerations. *Am Heart J* 1984;108:141–149.

81. Cotton DB, Jones MM, Longmire S, et al. Role of intravenous nitroglycerin in the treatment of severe pregnancy induced hypertension complicated by pulmonary edema. *Am J Obstet Gynecol* 1986;154:91–93.

82. Cotton DB, Longmire S, Jones MM, et al. Cardiovascular alterations in severe pregnancy-induced hypertension: effects of intravenous nitroglycerin coupled with blood volume expansion. *Am J Obstet Gynecol* 1986;154:1053–1059.

83. Phippard AF, Fischer WE, Horvath JS, et al. Early blood pressure control improves pregnancy outcome in primigravid women with mild hypertension. *Med J Aust* 1991;54:378–382.

84. Tuimala R, Punnonen R, Kauppila E. Clonidine in the treatment of hypertension during pregnancy. *Ann Chir Gynaecol Suppl* 1985;197:47–50.

85. Stoll C, Levy JM, Beshara D. Robert's syndrome and clonidine. *J Med Genet* 1979;16:486–487.

86. Rossouw HJ, Howarth G, Odendaal HJ. Ketanserin and hydralazine in hypertension in pregnancy—a randomized double blind trial. *S Afr Med J* 1995;85:525–528.

87. Bolte AC, van Eyck J, Strack van Schijndel RJ, et al. The haemodynamic effects of ketanserin versus dihydralazine in severe early-onset hypertension in pregnancy. *Br J Obstet Gynaecol* 1998;105:723–731.

88. Weiner CP, Socol ML, Vairub N. Control of pre-eclamptic hypertension by ketanserin, a new receptor antagonist. *Am J Obstet Gynecol* 1984;149:496–500.

89. Barr M, Cohen MM. Ace inhibitors fetopathy and hypocalvaria: the kidney-skull connection. *Teratology* 1991;44:485–495.

90. Hanssens M, Keirse MJNC, Vankelcom F, et al. Fetal and neonatal effects of treatment with angiotensin-converting enzyme inhibitors in pregnancy. *Obstet Gynecol* 1991;78:128–135.

91. Kaler SG, Patrinos ME, Lambert GH, et al. Hypertrichosis and congenital anomalies associated with maternal use of minoxidil. *Pediatrics* 1987;79:434–436.

92. Hurst JA, Houlston RS, Roberts A, et al. Transverse limb deficiency, facial clefting and hypoxic renal damage: an association with treatment of maternal hypertension. *Clin Dysmorphol* 1995;4:359–363.

10

Analgesic Use in Pregnancy

Mary E. Norton

*Department of Obstetrics, Gynecology, and Reproductive Sciences, University of California,
San Francisco, San Francisco, California*

Analgesics are among the most commonly used medications in pregnancy, in both prescription and over-the-counter formulations. It is therefore important that the prescribing physician have a good understanding of the relative risks of these agents and that patients are carefully counseled about use of these medications (Table 10.1).

NONSTEROIDAL ANTIINFLAMMATORY AGENTS

Aspirin

Aspirin is a nonsteroidal antiinflammatory agent that acts by irreversible inhibition of the enzymes necessary for the synthesis of prostaglandins. Although aspirin is a commonly used over-the-counter medication, data on the fetal effects of this medication have resulted in caution in its use during pregnancy.

Aspirin readily crosses the placenta in all animals (1–3). Although some studies suggested an association between aspirin and fetal malformations (4,5), the Collaborative Perinatal Project followed 5,128 pregnancies in which aspirin was consumed during the first 16 weeks with no detected increase in fetal malformations (6). Late in pregnancy, aspirin has been shown to lead to constriction of the ductus arteriosus in rats, rabbits, and sheep (7,8). When given near term, higher concentrations are found in the neonate than in the mother (9).

Several more recent reports suggested an association between aspirin exposure and gastroschisis (10,11). In the Spanish Collaborative Study of Congenital Malformations, first-trimester exposure to aspirin was associated with an increased risk of gastroschisis after controlling for potential effects of maternal age and smoking [odds ratio (OR), OR (3.33, 95% CI 1.05, 9.80)] (11). In a large case-control study of risk factors for gastroschisis, aspirin use was found to be associated with an increased risk [OR, 4.7; confidence interval (CI), 1.2 to 18.1] (10). Two other earlier studies had suggested this same association, further increasing the likelihood that this is not a spurious finding (12,13).

Aspirin decreases platelet adhesiveness and aggregation, and infants born after recent aspirin exposure appear to have an increased risk of bleeding complications. Stuart et al. (14) found minor bleeding complications (such as petechiae and cephalohematoma) in nine of 10 infants whose mothers had ingested 1 g or more of aspirin daily in the 5 days before birth, but found no such tendency if aspirin was ingested more than 6 days before birth. Premature babies whose mothers took aspirin within 1 week of delivery have been found to have an increased incidence of intracranial hemorrhage (15).

Like other prostaglandin synthetase inhibitors, aspirin exposure near term has been shown to cause constriction of the fetal ductus arteriosus with resultant pulmonary hypertension (16). High aspirin consumption during pregnancy may also produce adverse effects on the mother, including anemia, antepartum and/or postpartum hemorrhage, prolonged gestation, and prolonged labor (1).

Recently, it was suggested that the use of low-dose aspirin (60 to 100 mg) might decrease the

TABLE 10.1. *Relative safety of various analgesics in pregnancy and lactation*

Medication	Pregnancy risks[a]	Lactation risks[b]
Full-strength aspirin	4	4
Low-dose (baby) aspirin	1	1
Indomethacin		3
1st trimester	1	—
2nd trimester	3	—
3rd trimester[c]	4	—
Ibuprofen		1
1st trimester	3	—
2nd trimester	3	—
3rd trimester	4	—
Acetaminophen	2	1
Codeine	1[d]	2 (<240 mg/day)
Meperidine		2 (see text)
1st trimester	2	
2nd, 3rd trimesters	1[d]	
Oxycodone	1[d]	2

[a]Pregnancy risks: 1, no evidence of adverse fetal effects; 2, potential fetal effects described, unlikely to be of clinical significance; 3, adverse fetal effects described, recommend careful assessment of risk/benefit ratio and consideration of alternative treatment; 4, avoid during pregnancy.
[b]Lactation risks: 1, safe for lactating women; 2, safe with caveats concerning dosage; 3, safety unknown, although likely to be safe; 4, should be avoided during lactation.
[c]Avoid within 48 hours of preterm delivery.
[d]4 for multiple doses within a week of delivery.

incidence of preeclampsia and intrauterine growth restriction in women at risk. In these studies, exposed neonates were found to have significantly reduced levels of platelet cyclooxygenase (63%), but enzyme levels were not completely suppressed. These findings were interpreted to suggest that low doses of aspirin may permit normal hemostatic competence in the fetus and newborn (14,17). In a prospective randomized trial of women in the third trimester of pregnancy treated until delivery with as much as 80 mg per day of aspirin, platelet aggregation was not inhibited, and there was no excess of cephalohematomas, gastrointestinal bleeding, or purpura (18). All infants in this study had normal echocardiograms. Other studies confirmed that low-dose aspirin therapy during pregnancy does not increase neonatal bleeding complications (19) and has a negligible effect on the ductus arteriosus and other vascular smooth muscle (20).

Breast-feeding

Aspirin and other salicylates are excreted into breast milk in low concentrations. After single or repeated oral doses, peak milk levels occur at approximately 3 hours representing a milk:plasma ratio of 0.03:0.08 (21). Salicylates are eliminated more slowly from milk than from plasma, and the ratio increases to 0.34 at 12 hours. The reduced clearance of salicylates by neonates may result in drug accumulation and toxic effects, even when repeated exposures are small (9,22). Because of these concerns, the WHO Working Group on Human Lactation classified the salicylates as unsafe for use by nursing women (23). However, the American Academy of Pediatrics Committee on Drugs categorizes aspirin as being "associated with significant effects on some nursing infants and should be given to nursing mothers with caution" based on a single case report of a neonate that developed metabolic acidosis (24).

Indomethacin

Indomethacin is a nonsteroidal antiinflammatory agent used in the treatment of disorders such as rheumatoid arthritis, ankylosing spondylitis, and osteoarthritis, as well as in the treatment of preterm labor. Unlike aspirin, which causes an irreversible inhibition of the cyclooxygenase enzyme necessary for prostaglandin synthesis, indomethacin results in a competitive and reversible inhibition of this enzyme.

Oral administration of indomethacin has been found to result in *in utero* constriction of the ductus arteriosus. This response has been reported with doses as low as 1 mg/kg orally (25), and the effect increases with increasing gestational age (26). The effect is also increased when indomethacin is combined with betamethasone, which is often administered to aid in fetal lung maturation during tocolysis for preterm labor (27). In rats and sheep, chronic fetal ductal constriction has been shown to lead to persistent pulmonary hypertension in the newborn (28,29).

Data on first-trimester exposure in humans suggest no increased incidence in malformations. Aselton et al. (30) reported only one congenital anomaly in the offspring of 50 women who had taken indomethacin during pregnancy. A large surveillance study in Michigan of 229,101 pregnancies from 1985 to 1992 reported seven major birth defects in 114 newborns who had been exposed to indomethacin (five expected) (31).

Indomethacin has been used in the treatment of preterm labor since 1974. In the second half of pregnancy, this agent crosses the placenta and reaches concentrations in the fetus equal to those in the mother (32). In the fetus, indomethacin has been reported to cause constriction of the ductus arteriosus (33) and decreased urine output (34), frequently resulting in oligohydramnios (35). In the neonate born after indomethacin exposure, reported complications have included pulmonary hypertension (36), persistent ductus arteriosus (37), necrotizing enterocolitis (37,38), ileal perforation (39), intracranial hemorrhage (37,40), cystic brain lesions (41), and renal dysfunction (42). The likelihood of these complications is influenced in part by the timing of indomethacin administration. The ductus arteriosus becomes more responsive later in pregnancy, and at before 27 weeks, only 5% to 10% of fetuses will have ductal constriction after indomethacin exposure, whereas at after 34 weeks, 100% will demonstrate this response (26). The risk of neonatal complications, such as necrotizing enterocolitis, patent ductus arteriosus, and possibly intracranial hemorrhage, appears to be increased when this medication is administered within the 48 hours just before delivery (37,38).

Breast-feeding

Data on breast-feeding and indomethacin are very limited. One study reported that milk concentrations were similar to maternal plasma levels. The American Academy of Pediatrics classified indomethacin as compatible with breast-feeding (24).

Ibuprofen

Ibuprofen is a nonsteroidal antiinflammatory agent. In human pregnancies, ibuprofen use has been associated with an increased risk of gastroschisis in some studies (10), although others have found no association (13). There has also been a suggestion of an association of congenital heart disease with maternal use of ibuprofen (43,44).

Like other agents in this class, ibuprofen has been associated with third-trimester pregnancy complications such as oligohydramnios and premature closure of the ductus arteriosus with resultant pulmonary hypertension (45).

Breast-feeding

Ibuprofen does not enter breast milk in significant quantities. In a study of lactating women taking 400 mg ibuprofen every 6 hours, ibuprofen was undetectable in breast milk (46). The American Academy of Pediatrics considers ibuprofen compatible with breast-feeding (24).

Acetaminophen

Acetaminophen is widely used during pregnancy. Acetaminophen can cross the placenta (47), but is considered safe when taken in the normally recommended dosage, and is now taken much more frequently during pregnancy than aspirin (48). Acetaminophen is routinely used during all stages of pregnancy to relieve pain and lower elevated body temperature.

Acetaminophen appears to work by inhibiting prostaglandin synthesis in the central nervous system. Although this agent has been shown to increase the incidence of sister-chromatid exchanges and chromatid breaks in human peripheral lymphocytes, it is unlikely that these findings are of clinical significance (49). While cases of malformations in humans after prenatal exposure to acetaminophen exist, ascertainment bias, as well as exposure to numerous other agents, limits these reports (50–52). The Collaborative Perinatal Project did not find an association between the use of acetaminophen during pregnancy and congenital anomalies in the offspring (53). In a study of 697 women with first-trimester exposure to acetaminophen, no increase in malformations was identified (30). A case-control study of risk factors for gastroschisis suggested an increased risk of borderline significance with first-trimester maternal acetaminophen exposure [relative risk (RR), 2.1; CI, 1.0 to 2.9] (13). A second study did not find maternal acetaminophen use to be associated with an increased risk of gastroschisis (12). A study of IQ and attention deficit disorder found that first-trimester aspirin exposure had a detrimental effect, whereas maternal acetaminophen use was not significantly related to child IQ or attention (54).

There have been many reported cases of acetaminophen overdose during pregnancy. Although such overdoses have not been demonstrated to lead to an increased risk of congenital anomalies in offspring, there have been reports of fetal hepatotoxicity with spontaneous abortion and stillbirth (55–57). Many cases of acetaminophen overdose during pregnancy with normal outcomes for the offspring have also been reported (58–60). Prompt use of N-acetylcysteine after acetaminophen overdose appears to improve outcome for both mother and fetus.

Unlike aspirin, acetaminophen does not affect platelet function, and there is no increased risk of hemorrhage if the drug is given to the mother at term (7). Studies in rats and sheep demonstrated that acetaminophen can, like other prostaglandin synthetase inhibitors, cause constriction of the fetal ductus arteriosus (61). These effects were much milder than those that occur with aspirin, ibuprofen, or indomethacin, however, and are less likely to be clinically significant.

Breast-feeding

Acetaminophen is excreted into breast milk in small amounts. Based on available data, a nursing infant ingests a maximum of 4% of the weight-adjusted maternal dose; this corresponds to approximately 4% of the therapeutic dose that is used in infants. The American Academy of Pediatrics Committee on Drugs (24) and the WHO Working Group on Drugs and Human Lactation (62) concluded that the use of this drug during breast-feeding is safe.

Opioid Analgesics

Many narcotic preparations are available, but their pharmacologic properties and observed effects are similar. All narcotics easily cross the placenta. Central nervous system depression of the fetus is a concern when these medications are given around the time of delivery, as respiratory efforts and neurobehavioral adjustments may be delayed. Neonatal respiratory depression is usually mild and transient.

Epidemiologic studies have not detected a statistically significant association between the use of opioid analgesics and abnormal morphologic development in the human fetus (53).

Codeine

A large case-control study of 141 infants with cardiac malformations did not find any association with first trimester use of codeine (63). Although a number of retrospective studies of human pregnancies have associated codeine with a variety of anomalies, the lack of a consistent pattern of malformations makes it unlikely that codeine was a causative agent in these abnormalities (53,64,65). Neonatal withdrawal has been described in infants born to women taking codeine before delivery (66,67).

Breast-feeding

Small amounts of codeine and its metabolite, morphine, are transferred to breast milk (68). If the maternal dose is less than 240 mg per day, the quantity of these compounds ingested by a suckling infant is not considered sufficient to contraindicate breast-feeding (24,68).

Meperidine (Demerol)

Meperidine is one of the most commonly used opioid analgesics. In humans, epidemiologic studies have not detected a statistically significant association between the use of meperidine during the first trimester and abnormal morphologic development (53).

Meperidine readily crosses the placenta and enters the fetal circulation (69,70). Systemically administered meperidine has been documented to produce respiratory depression in the neonate when administered up to several hours before delivery (71). Neonatal metabolism of meperidine is much slower than that of adults (72), and behavioral and electroencephalographic changes have been observed in exposed newborns 72 hours after delivery (73). Clinical studies have not uncovered lasting impairments of neonatal function or correlated variations in neurologic performance during the first 6 weeks of development with meperidine exposure during labor (74).

Breast-feeding

Meperidine is excreted into breast milk in small amounts (75). In one study, the peak concentration of meperidine in breast milk was 0.13 μg/mL 2 hours after administration of a 50-mg intramuscular dose, and adverse effects on nursing infants were not identified. Because the possibility of accumulation of meperidine in suckling infants has not been studied, the WHO Working Group on Human Lactation concluded that although breast-feeding after one dose of meperidine is probably safe, recommendations cannot be made on repeated use of this drug during lactation (76).

Oxycodone (Percocet)

Oxycodone is a narcotic analgesic that is used most commonly in combination with aspirin (Percodan) or acetaminophen (Percocet). Although there are relatively few data available on the use of this agent in pregnancy, there are no reports linking this agent to congenital birth defects. The Collaborative Perinatal Project followed 50,282 mother-infant pairs, of whom eight had had first-trimester exposure to oxycodone (53). There was no evidence of an increased incidence of birth defects in this very limited number of patients. Likewise, a large surveillance study of Michigan Medicaid recipients identified 281 newborns who had been exposed to oxycodone during the first trimester. A total of 13 (4.6%) major birth defects were observed in this population in which a baseline rate of 12 birth defects was expected. There was no consistent pattern of anomalies, indicating that it is unlikely there was any association between the exposure and the observed birth defects (77).

Breast-feeding

Oxycodone is excreted into human breast milk with a large degree of variability. Peak milk concentrations occur 1.5 to 2 hours after the first dose, and at varying times after multiple doses. The mean milk:plasma ratio averages 3.4:1, with no reported adverse effects in nursing infants (78).

SUMMARY

1. Several studies have associated therapeutic doses of aspirin with an increased risk of gastroschisis when taken in the first trimester.

2. Later in gestation, aspirin can lead to ductal constriction and bleeding complications.

3. Concerns about accumulation in the infant have led to the recommendation that aspirin be avoided during lactation.

4. These complications have not been seen with low dose (80 mg per day) aspirin. Therefore, full-strength aspirin should be avoided by pregnant and lactating women.

5. Indomethacin does not appear to have significant adverse fetal effects when given in the first half of pregnancy. Later in pregnancy, several adverse consequences of this medication have been demonstrated, including ductal constriction and oligohydramnios. In addition, preterm infants born after recent

indomethacin exposure may have an increased risk of neonatal complications. It is therefore suggested that indomethacin be avoided in the third trimester of pregnancy and that it be used judiciously in the second trimester with use limited to patients who do not seem likely to deliver within 48 hours of exposure. If indomethacin is used after 24 weeks of gestation, surveillance for evidence of ductal constriction or development of oligohydramnios is reasonable.

6. It has been suggested that ibuprofen exposure in early pregnancy may increase the risk of gastroschisis in the infant. Later in pregnancy, this medication has been associated with oligohydramnios and premature closure of the ductus arteriosus. It is therefore suggested that this medication be avoided at all stages of pregnancy, although it does appear to be safe for use by lactating women.

7. Acetaminophen appears to have the best safety profile of the prostaglandin synthetase inhibitors. However, this medication shares activity with other agents in this class, and there are some data implying similar, although lower, risks of gastroschisis and possibly adverse effects on the ductus arteriosus. As with any medication, acetaminophen should only be taken during pregnancy when clearly indicated. Acetaminophen does appear to be safe for use during lactation.

8. There has been no association of codeine with any pattern of birth defects in humans, and this drug is not considered teratogenic. As with other narcotics, codeine should be used cautiously near term and in lactating women, to avoid sedating effects and withdrawal in the infant.

9. There has been no association of meperidine with any pattern of birth defects in humans, and this drug is not considered teratogenic. Meperidine should be used cautiously near term, in labor, and in lactating women to avoid sedating effects and withdrawal in the infant.

10. There is no evidence of any adverse effects of oxycodone in either pregnant or lactating women, although there are very few data available on studies of potential effects. The fact that other agents in this class have not been demonstrated to be teratogenic is reassuring with regard to oxycodone use in early pregnancy. As with other narcotics, this agent should be used cautiously near term, when neonatal withdrawal becomes an issue. Likewise, the medication should be used judiciously by lactating women.

REFERENCES

1. Schoenfeld A, Bar Y, Merlob P, et al. NSAIDs: Maternal and fetal considerations. *Am J Reprod Immunol* 1992;28:141–147.
2. Levy G, Garrettson LK. Kinetics of salicylate elimination by newborn infants of mothers who ingested aspirin before delivery. *Pediatrics* 1974;53:202–210.
3. Palmisano PA, Cassady G. Salicylate exposure in the perinate. *JAMA* 1969;209:556–558.
4. Saxen I. Associations between oral clefts and drugs taken during pregnancy. *Int J Epidemiol* 1975;4:37–46.
5. Nelson MM, Forfar JO. Associations between drugs administered during pregnancy and congenital abnormalities of the newborn. *BMJ* 1971;1:523–525.
6. Slone D, Heinonen OP, Kaufman DW, et al. Aspirin and congenital malformations. *Lancet* 1976;1:1373–1375.
7. Rudolph AM. Effects of aspirin and acetaminophen in pregnancy and in the newborn. *Arch Intern Med* 1981;141:358–363.
8. Sharp GL, Larsson KS, Thalme B. Studies on closure of the ductus arteriosus. XII. In utero effect of indomethacin and sodium salicylate in rats and rabbits. *Prostaglandins* 1975;9:585–596.
9. Levy G. Salicylate pharmacokinetics in the human neonate. In: Morselli PL, Garattini S, Sesreni F, eds. *Basic and therapeutic aspects of perinatal pharmacology.* New York: Raven Press, 1975:319–329.
10. Torfs CP, Katz EA, Bateson TF, et al. Maternal medications and environmental exposures as risk factors for gastroschisis. *Teratology* 1996;54:84–92.
11. Martinez-Frias ML, Rodriguez-Pinilla E, Prieto L. Prenatal exposure to salicylates and gastroschisis: a case-control study. *Teratology* 1997;56:241–243.
12. Drongowski RA, Smith RK Jr, Coran AG, et al. Contribution of demographic and environmental factors to the etiology of gastroschisis: a hypothesis. *Fetal Diagn Ther* 1991;6:14–27.
13. Werler MM, Mitchell AA. First trimester maternal medication use in relation to gastroschisis. *Teratology* 1992;45:361–367.
14. Stuart MJ, Gross SJ, Elrad H, et al. Effects of acetylsalicylic acid ingestion on maternal and neonatal hemostasis. *N Engl J Med* 1982;307:909–912.
15. Rumack CM, Guggenheim MA, Rumack BH, et al. Neonatal intracranial hemorrhage and maternal use of aspirin. *Obstet Gynecol* 1981;58[Suppl]:52S–56S.
16. Levin DL, Fixlet DE, Morriss FC, et al. Morphologic analysis of the pulmonary vascular bed in infants exposed in utero to prostaglandin synthetase inhibitors. *J Pediatr* 1978;92:478–483.
17. Ylikorkala D, Makila U, Kaapa P, et al. Maternal ingestion of acetylsalicylic acid inhibits fetal and neonatal

prostacyclin and thromboxane in humans. *Am J Obstet Gynecol* 1986;155:345–349.

18. Sibai BM, Mirro R, Chesney CM, et al. Low-dose aspirin in pregnancy. *Obstet Gynecol* 1989;74:551–557.

19. Sibai BM, Caritis SN, Thom E, et al. Prevention of preeclampsia with low dose aspirin in healthy nulliparous pregnant women. *N Engl J Med* 1993;329:1213–1218.

20. Veille J-C, Hanson R, Sivakoff M, et al. Effects of maternal ingestion of low-dose aspirin on the fetal cardiovascular system. *Am J Obstet Gynecol* 1993;168: 1430–1437.

21. Findlay JWA, De Angelis RL, Kearney MF, et al. Analgesic drugs in breast milk and plasma. *Clin Pharmacol Ther* 1981;29:625–633.

22. McNamara PJ, Burgio D, Yoo SD. Pharmacokinetics of acetaminophen, antipyrine, and salicylic acid in the lactating and nursing rabbit, with model predictions of milk to serum concentration ratios and neonatal dose. *Toxicol Appl Pharmacol* 1991;109:149–160.

23. The WHO Working Group on Human Lactation. Salicylates. In: Bennet PN, ed. *Drugs and human lactation*. New York: Elsevier, 1988:325–326.

24. American Academy of Pediatrics Committee on Drugs. The transfer of drugs and other chemicals into human milk. *Pediatrics* 1994;93:137–150.

25. Arishima K, Yamamoto M, Takizawa T, et al. Onset of the constrictive effect of indomethacin on the ductus arteriosus in fetal rats. *Acta Anat* 1991;142:231–235.

26. Moise K. Effect of advancing gestational age on the frequency of fetal ductal constriction in association with maternal indomethacin use. *Am J Obstet Gynecol* 1993;168:1350–1353.

27. Momma K, Takao A. Increased constriction of the fetal ductus arteriosus with combined administration of indomethacin and betamethasone in fetal rats. *Pediatr Res* 1989;25:69–75.

28. Momma K, Takao A. Right ventricular concentric hypertrophy and left ventricular dilatation by ductal constriction in fetal rats. *Circ Res* 1989;64:1137–1146.

29. Morin FC III. Ligating the ductus arteriosus before birth causes persistent pulmonary hypertension in the newborn lamb. *Pediatr Res* 1989;25:245–250.

30. Aselton PA, Jick H, Milunsky A, et al. First trimester drug use and congenital disorders. *Obstet Gynecol* 1985;65:451–455.

31. Briggs GG, Freeman RK, Yaffe SJ, eds. *Drugs in pregnancy and lactation,* 5th ed. Baltimore: Williams & Wilkins, 1998:538–547.

32. Moise KJ, Ou C-N, Kirshon B, et al. Placental transfer of indomethacin in the human pregnancy. *Am J Obstet Gynecol* 1990;162:549–554.

33. Moise KJ, Huhta JC, Sharif DS, et al. Indomethacin in the treatment of premature labor: effects on the fetal ductus arteriosus. *N Engl J Med* 1988;319:327–331.

34. Hickok DE, Hollenback KA, Reilley SF, et al. The association between decreased amniotic fluid volume and treatment with nonsteroidal anti-inflammatory agents for preterm labor. *Am J Obstet Gynecol* 1989;160:1525–1531.

35. Bivins HA, Newman RB, Fyfe DA, et al. Randomized trial of oral indomethacin and terbutaline sulfate for the long-term suppression of preterm labor. *Am J Obstet Gynecol* 1993;169:1065–1070.

36. Manchester D, Margolis HS, Sheldon RE. Possible association between maternal indomethacin therapy and primary pulmonary hypertension of the newborn. *Am J Obstet Gynecol* 1976;126:467–469.

37. Norton ME, Merrill J, Cooper BAB, et al. Neonatal complications after the administration of indomethacin for preterm labor. *N Engl J Med* 1993;329:1602–1607.

38. Major CA, Lewis DF, Harding JA, et al. Tocolysis with indomethacin increases the incidence of necrotizing enterocolitis in the low-birth-weight neonate. *Am J Obstet Gynecol* 1994;170:102–106.

39. Vanhaesebrouck P, Thiery M, Leroy JG, et al. Oligohydramnios, renal insufficiency and ileal perforation in preterm infants after intrauterine exposure to indomethacin. *J Pediatr* 1988;113:738–743.

40. Iannucci TA, Besinger RE, Fisher SG, et al. Effect of dual tocolysis on the incidence of severe intraventricular hemorrhage among extremely low-birth-weight infants. *Am J Obstet Gynecol* 1996;175:1043–1046.

41. Baerts W, Fretter WP, Hop WC, et al. Cerebral lesions in preterm infants after tocolytic indomethacin. *Dev Med Child Neurol* 1990;32:910–918.

42. Buderus S, Thomas B, Fahnenstich H, et al. Renal failure in two preterm infants: toxic effect of prenatal maternal indomethacin treatment? *Br J Obstet Gynecol* 1993;100:97–98.

43. Loffredo CA, Ferencz C, Lurie IW, et al. Are major cardiovascular malformations defects of a single developmental field? *Teratology* 1995;51:190.

44. Correa-Villasenor A, Ferencz C, Loffredo C. Atrioventricular septal defects: heterogeneity risk factors in cases with and without Down's syndrome. *Teratology* 1995;51:164.

45. Turner GR, Levin DL. Prostaglandin synthesis inhibition in persistent pulmonary hypertension of the newborn. *Clin Perinatol* 1984;11;581–589.

46. Townsend RJ, Bendetti TJ, Erickson S, et al. Excretion of ibuprofen into breast milk. *Am J Obstet Gynecol* 1984;149:184–186.

47. Levy G, Garrettson LK, Soda DM. Evidence of placental transfer of acetaminophen. *Pediatrics* 1975;55:895.

48. Rayburn W, Wible-Kant J, Bledsoe P. Changing trends in drug use during pregnancy. *J Reprod Med* 1982;27:569–575.

49. Hongslo JK, Christensen T, Brunborg G, et al. Genotoxic effects of paracetamol in V79 Chinese hamster cells. *Mutat Res* 1988;204:333–341.

50. Golden SM, Perman KI. Bilateral clinical anophthalmia: drugs as potential factors. *South Med J* 1980;73:1404–1407.

51. Williams DA, Weiss T, Wade E, et al. Prune perineum syndrome: report of a second case. *Teratology* 1983;28:145–148.

52. Golden NL, King KC, Sokol RJ. Propoxyphene and acetaminophen: possible effects on the fetus. *Clin Pediatr* 1982;21:752–754.

53. Heinonen OP, Slone D, Shapiro S. *Birth defects and drugs in pregnancy*. Littleton, MA: Publishing Sciences Group, 1977:286–295.

54. Streissguth AP, Treder RP, Barr HM, et al. Aspirin and acetaminophen use by pregnant women and subsequent child IQ and attention decrements. *Teratology* 1987;35:211–219.

55. Haiback H, Akhter JE, Muscato MS, et al. Acetaminophen overdose with fetal demise. *Am J Clin Pathol* 1984;82:240–242.

56. Kurzel RB. Can acetaminophen excess result in maternal and fetal toxicity? *South Med J* 1990;83:953–955.

57. Wang P-H, Yang M-J, Lee W-L, et al. Acetaminophen poisoning in late pregnancy: a case report. *J Reprod Med* 1997;42:367–371.

58. Stokes IM. Paracetamol overdose in the second trimester of pregnancy: case report. *Br J Obstet Gynaecol* 1984; 91:286–288.

59. Rosevear SK, Hope PL. Favourable neonatal outcome following maternal paracetamol overdose and severe fetal distress: case report. *Br J Obstet Gynaecol* 1989;96:491–493.

60. McElhatton PR, Sullivan FM, Volans GN, et al. Paracetamol poisoning in pregnancy: an analysis of the outcomes of cases referred to the Teratology Information Service of the National Poisons Information Service. *Hum Exp Toxicol* 1990;9;147–153.

61. Peterson RG. Consequences associated with nonnarcotic analgesics in the fetus and newborn. *Fed Proc* 1985;44:2309–2312.

62. The WHO Working Group on Human Lactation. Acetaminophen. In: Bennet PN, ed. *Drugs and human lactation.* New York: Elsevier, 1988:327–328.

63. Shaw GM, Malcoe LH, Swan SH, et al. Congenital cardiac anomalies relative to selected maternal exposures and conditions during early pregnancy. *Eur J Epidemiol* 1992;8:757–760.

64. Bracken MB, Holford TR. Exposure to prescribed drugs in pregnancy and association with congenital malformations. *Obstet Gynecol* 1981;58:336–344.

65. Saxen I. Associations between oral clefts and drugs taken during pregnancy. *Int J Epidemiol* 1975;4:37–44.

66. Mangurten HH, Benawra R. Neonatal codeine withdrawal in infants of nonaddicted mothers. *Pediatrics* 1980;65:159–160.

67. Khan K, Chang J. Neonatal abstinence syndrome due to codeine. *Arch Dis Child Fetal Neonatal Ed* 1997;76:59–60.

68. Meny RG, Naumburg EG, Alger LS, et al. Codeine and the breastfed neonate. *J Hum Lact* 1993;9:237–240.

69. Crawford JS, Rudofsky S. The placental transmission of pethidine. *Br J Anaesth* 1965;37:929–933.

70. Szeto HH, Zervoudakis IA, Cederqvist LL, Inturrisi CE. Amniotic fluid transfer of meperidine from maternal plasma in early pregnancy. *Obstet Gynecol* 1978;52:59–62.

71. Morrison JC, et al. Metabolites of meperidine related to fetal depression. *Am J Obstet Gynecol* 1973;115:1132–1137.

72. Hodgkinson R, Husain FJ. The duration of effect of maternally administered meperidine on neonatal neurobehavior. *Anesthesiology* 1982;56:51–52.

73. Borgstedt AD, Rosen MG. Medication during labor correlated with behavior and EEG of the newborn. *Am J Dis Child* 1968;115:21–24.

74. Belsey EM, Rosenblatt DB, Lieberman BA, et al. The influence of maternal analgesia on neonatal behavior. I. Pethidine. *Br J Obstet Gynaecol* 1981;88:398–406.

75. Von Peiker G, Muller B, Ihn W, et al. Excretion of pethidine in mother's milk. *Zentralbl Gynaekol* 1980;102:537–541.

76. The WHO Working Group on Lactation. Meperidine. In: Bennet PN, ed. *Drugs and human lactation.* New York: Elsevier, 1988:317.

77. Briggs GG, Freeman RK, Yaffe SJ, eds. *Drugs in pregnancy and lactation,* 5th ed. Baltimore: Williams & Wilkins, 1998:814–815.

78. Marx CM, Pucino F, Carlson, JD, et al. Oxycodone excretion in human milk in the puerperium. *Drug Intell Clin Pharm* 1986;20:474(abst).

11

Psychotropic Drugs in Pregnancy and Lactation

Alexander D. Allaire* and Jeffrey A. Kuller†

*Department of Obstetrics and Gynecology, National Capitol Uniformed Services,
National Naval Medical Center, Bethesda, Maryland.
†Department of Obstetrics and Gynecology, University of North Carolina at Chapel Hill,
Chapel Hill, North Carolina

Psychiatric illness is very common during the childbearing years. Major depression and schizophrenia are among the most common psychiatric illnesses in reproductive age women with incidences of 15% and 8% to 10%, respectively (1–4). Although all psychotropic medications readily cross the placenta, most seem to be safe for use during pregnancy and lactation (5–7). Several psychiatric disorders may worsen during pregnancy and the peripartum period (6).

When the pregnant women requires pharmacologic management of a psychiatric illness in pregnancy, concerns include teratogenesis, neonatal toxicity and/or withdrawal, lactation, and long-term adverse neurobehavioral effects. It is also important to recognize the potential harm to the mother and fetus posed by discontinuation of a much needed psychotropic agent because of concern for fetal exposure. As with any medication in pregnancy, one must weigh the risk of fetal exposure against the consequences of untreated psychiatric illness (7,8).

This chapter reviews the safety of the most frequently prescribed psychotropic medications. For many drugs, there are few or no data concerning use in pregnancy, making an assessment of their safety during pregnancy difficult. Recommendations for pharmacologic management of common specific psychiatric disorders appear at the end of the chapter.

ANTIDEPRESSANT MEDICATIONS

Tricyclic Antidepressants

Antidepressant medications are listed in Table 11.1. The most commonly prescribed tricyclic agents are amitriptyline and imipramine. These agents are most commonly used to treat major depression, but other uses include anxiety disorders, obsessive-compulsive disorder, migraines, chronic pain, and urinary incontinence (5). Tricyclic antidepressants were initially thought to be associated with congenital anomalies, including heart defects and limb reduction defects. More recent evidence suggests that these agents are not teratogenic (5,9). A recent summation of 14 studies assessing the effect of exposure of the fetus to tricyclics evaluated more than 300,000 births (only 414 cases included first-trimester exposure) (6). When pooled or viewed individually, no significant association between fetal exposure to tricyclic antidepressants and congenital malformations was found (6). In a surveillance study of Michigan Medicaid recipients involving 229,101 completed pregnancies between 1985 and 1992, 467 newborns had been exposed to amitriptyline and 75 newborns had been exposed to imipramine during the first trimester (F. Rosa, US Food and Drug Administration, personal communication, 1994). A total of 25 (5.4%) major birth defects were observed (20 expected) in those exposed to

TABLE 11.1. *Antidepressants*

Medication	Pregnancy use recommendation	Lactation use recommendation
Nortriptyline	1	1
Desipramine	1	1
Amitriptyline	2	2
Imiprimine	2	2
Fluoxetine	2	3
Clomipramine	3	3
Doxepin	3	3
Paroxitine	3	3
Sertraline	3	3
Fluvoxamine	3	3
Bupropion	3	3
St. John's wort	3	3
Amphetamines	4	4
Methylphenidate	4	4
Pamoline	4	4

1, Primary recommended agent; 2, recommended if currently using or primary agent contraindicated; 3, limited data to support or proscribe use, best avoided, if clinically possible; 4, not recommended for use.

amitriptyline, and a total of six (1.39%) major birth defects were observed (three expected). These data do not support an association between tricyclics and congenital anomalies.

The use of tricyclic antidepressants has been associated with withdrawal symptoms in the newborn. Withdrawal symptoms attributed to tricyclics include jitteriness, irritability, colic, cyanosis, rapid breathing, and convulsions (10–16). These studies were poorly controlled, making associations with adverse outcome speculative. Anticholinergic effects of tricyclics have also been reported in newborns after maternal exposure. These include functional bowel obstruction and urinary retention (17,18). In addition, there do not appear to be any adverse long-term behavioral or neurodevelopmental changes in children followed up for 7 years (19,20).

Both amitriptyline (and its active metabolite nortriptyline) and imipramine (and its active metabolite desipramine) are excreted into breast milk (5,8). The serum:milk ratio of both amitriptyline and imipramine is approximately 1.0 (8,21). Neither amitriptyline nor imipramine nor their metabolites have been detected in the serum of breast-feeding infants of women taking amytriptiline (21–25). The American Academy of Pediatrics classifies amitriptyline and imipramine as drugs whose effects on the nursing infant are unknown but may be of concern (26). The evidence to date does not suggest any potential adverse effects on the breast-fed infant with the maternal use of amitriptyline or imipramine, but the existing evidence is based on case series and case reports; therefore, a small effect cannot be excluded.

Other tricyclic agents such as clomipramine and doxepin have been less well studied, and information concerning their effects in pregnant or lactating women are limited to case reports and case series (5,8). Similar to other tricyclics, there are several reports of withdrawal symptoms in infants after maternal exposure to clomipramine but no long-term adverse effects have been reported (27–32).

If tricyclic agents are used in pregnancy, it is prudent to select those agents for which more data have accumulated, such as amitriptyline and imipramine. When a pregnant or lactating woman already on a tricyclic agent presents for consultation, the risk of changing or stopping medication should be weighed against the unknown or theoretical risk to the fetus or infant. An example of this risk is evident in a report describing five women who stopped their tricyclic medication because they were breast-feeding (19). Two of these women required hospitalization and three required outpatient treatment with suicide precautions. The risk of development of major depression in the mother usually outweighs the risk tricyclics are thought to pose to infants.

Selective Serotonin Reuptake Inhibitors (SSRIs)

The SSRIs include sertraline, paroxetine, and fluoxetine. Pastuszak et al. (33) reported 128 women treated with fluoxetine for depression during the first trimester and compared them with 128 controls treated with agents classified as known nonteratogens. No significant difference was noted in the rates of major birth defects or any other pregnancy outcome measured in the fluoxetine-exposed group compared with the control group. When compared with an age-matched set of subjects taking tricyclics, there were also no significant differences in the percentage of infants with major congenital anomalies or other adverse pregnancy outcome.

Using Michigan Medicaid data, it was found that 142 newborns had been exposed to fluoxetine (109 during the first trimester) and only two (1.8%) had major birth defects diagnosed (five expected) (F. Rosa, US Food and Drug Administration, personal communication, 1994). A major malformation rate of 3.4% and a spontaneous abortion rate of 15.9% among those exposed to fluoxetine was reported in a prospectively collected database of 1,103 pregnancies (34). This was not different from the expected rate. In a follow-up study, outcomes of 796 pregnancies with confirmed first-trimester fluoxetine exposure were reported (35). Spontaneous abortions were reported in 110 pregnancies (13.8%) and of the 686 continuing, 34 (5.0%) displayed malformations, deformations, or disruptions. These outcomes are similar to what would be expected using historical controls (34,35).

In a prospectively collected series of women who telephoned a teratogen hotline, 228 women who were taking fluoxetine during pregnancy and 254 controls who were taking agents not thought to be teratogenic were evaluated for adverse pregnancy outcome (36). The rate of spontaneous pregnancy loss and the rate of major structural anomalies were not different in women taking fluoxetine (36). In contrast, among the 97 infants exposed to fluoxetine who were evaluated for minor anomalies, the incidence of three or more minor anomalies was significantly higher than anomalies among 153 similarly examined control infants (15.5% versus 6.5%, $p = 0.03$). Infants who were exposed to fluoxetine in the third trimester were compared with those exposed only in the first trimester. Interestingly, those exposed in the third trimester had a greater incidence of perinatal complications compared with those treated only in the first trimester. These perinatal complications included prematurity, admission to special care nurseries, poor neonatal adaptation, lower mean birth weight, shorter length, and a higher proportion of full-term infants with birth weights at or below the 10th percentile. Although these results cause concern, their long-term clinical significance is unknown. It must

also be noted that this was a prospective cohort study. The study group was a group of women with psychiatric illness who called the California Teratogen Information Service and Clinical Research Program out of concern for exposure to fluoxetine and the control group was a group of women who called with questions concerning nonteratogenic exposures (e.g., acetaminophen use), suggesting self-selection bias. In addition, not all infants were examined (approximately half), which could introduce selection bias. The comparison of women continuing to take medication into the third trimester with those with only first- and second-trimester exposure again may introduce selection bias. Patients requiring continued medication may have had more severe psychiatric illness and associated risk factors for a worse perinatal outcome. Many potential confounding factors were adjusted for using multivariate logistic regression, but psychiatric disorders themselves are associated with prematurity, admission to special care nursery, and poor neonatal adaptation (37–39).

To study the cognitive and language development and behavior in children exposed *in utero* to antidepressants, Nulman et al. (20) studied 55 children whose mothers received fluoxetine during pregnancy, 80 children whose mothers received a tricyclic during pregnancy, and 84 children whose mothers had not been exposed during pregnancy to any agent known to affect the fetus adversely. The authors found that *in utero* exposure to either tricyclics or fluoxetine did not affect global IQ, language development, or behavioral development in children followed to preschool.

The use of fluoxetine during pregnancy does not appear to increase the risk of major congenital anomalies. One study suggests that fluoxetine use during pregnancy may increase the risk of minor congenital anomalies, but this study is plagued by methodologic concerns and the clinical significance of these minor anomalies is uncertain (36). This same study suggested an increased risk of perinatal complications in women taking fluoxetine in the third trimester. Before discontinuing medication in a depressed pregnant woman, the potential adverse consequences of worsening depression must be considered.

Fluoxetine and its active metabolite norfluoxetine are present in breast milk at 20% to 25% of the levels in maternal plasma (40). There have been reports of adverse events related to use of fluoxetine during lactation. Lester et al. (41) reported an infant with serum concentrations in the adult therapeutic range in a breast-feeding infant of a women receiving fluoxetine. The adverse affects included increased crying, irritability, decreased sleep, vomiting, and watery stools. These effects resolved with discontinuation of the drug. The long-term effects of SSRIs during lactation have not been investigated. In 1994, the US Food and Drug Administration advised the manufacturer to revise the labeling of fluoxetine to caution against its use in lactating mothers (42). The American Academy of Pediatrics considers the SSRIs as a group of drugs whose effects on the infant are unknown but may be of concern (26). It is important to consider the risk of withholding medication in a woman with major depression who is adamant about breast-feeding. In addition, it is important to consider the risks to the infant of not receiving the benefits of breast-feeding. Therefore, SSRIs are not considered to be contraindicated during lactation. The decision whether to breast-feed during their use is complex and should be made by a woman and her obstetrician, pediatrician, and psychiatrist or psychologist (43).

The newer SSRIs include fluvoxamine, paroxetine, and sertraline. In a prospective, multicenter, cohort study, 267 women exposed to the new SSRIs during the first trimester (146 used sertraline, 97 used paroxetine, and 26 used fluvoxamine) were compared with 267 controls (44). Exposure to SSRIs was not associated with either increased major malformations or higher rates of miscarriage, stillbirth, or prematurity. No data are available concerning the safety of these agents to the nursing infant.

Other Antidepressants

The safety of monoamine oxidase inhibitors (MAOIs) during pregnancy is currently unknown. There have been no epidemiologic studies of these agents in pregnancy. Similarly, no data are available concerning the safety of

bupropion, a combined SSRI and dopaminergic agent, during pregnancy or lactation. Given the lack of data concerning their safety, these agents are ideally avoided in pregnancy.

Extracts of the plant *Hypericum perforatum* (St. John's wort) is an herbal agent commonly used in Europe and enjoying current popularity in the United States as an antidepressant. A recent metaanalysis of 15 placebo-controlled trials and eight trials with other antidepressants as controls suggests that this agent is superior to placebo and equally effective as standard antidepressants with fewer side effects (45). No data on the safety or efficacy of St. John's wort in pregnancy are available in the medical literature. Because of this, it is recommended that St. John's wort not be used by pregnant or lactating women.

Psychostimulants

Psychostimulants such as amphetamines, methylphenidate, and pamoline are often prescribed for depressive disorders (46). Most of the human studies investigating the use of central stimulants in pregnancy involve women who were abusing these agents and, therefore, are possibly confounded by coexisting risk factors for adverse pregnancy outcome. Several reports associated fetal anomalies with amphetamine exposure (47–51). Reported anomalies include acrania, congenital heart disease, biliary defects, palatal defects, microcephaly, mental retardation, and motor dysfunction. In a matched case-control study of 458 women who delivered infants with major or minor congenital anomalies and 911 controls, it was found that appetite suppressants were consumed during pregnancy by significantly more women delivering infants with congenital abnormalities than by controls (3.9% versus 1.1%, $p < 0.01$) (52). This was a retrospective study based on patient drug histories suggesting the possibility of recall bias.

A subsequent prospective study of 1,824 white women who were ingesting anorectic drugs (primarily amphetamines) during pregnancy and 8,989 controls showed no significant differences in severe congenital malformations (53). Long-term effects of maternal amphetamine abuse in children include an increase in neonatal irritability, shrill crying, jerking movements, lassitude, and apnea, as well as an increase in violent behavior (47,54–56).

No adverse effects have been reported in nursing mothers who were taking amphetamines (8,57,58). Amphetamine is concentrated in breast milk with milk:plasma ratios varying between 2.8 and 7.5 (57). Because of this, the American Academy of Pediatrics considers amphetamines to be contraindicated during breast-feeding (26).

In conclusion, the use of psychostimulants in pregnancy has not conclusively been shown to be teratogenic. However, withdrawal symptoms have been observed in neonates, and long-term adverse behavioral effects have been suggested. Because of these concerns, stimulants should be avoided during pregnancy and lactation.

MOOD STABILIZERS

Mood stabilizers are listed in Table 11.2. Lithium is the most commonly used psychotropic agent for the treatment of bipolar disorder. The International Register of Lithium Babies includes women with histories of first-trimester exposure to lithium (59,60). These early reports suggested that first-trimester lithium use was associated with a fivefold increased risk of congenital cardiovascular malformations, and a 400-fold increased risk of Ebstein's anomaly (a rare cardiac anomaly consisting of malattachment of the tricuspid leaflets leading to tricuspid regurgitation, right ventricular dilation, and occasionally a ventricular septal defect) (59–62). These studies are limited by the fact that they are potentially biased by overreporting of anomalous infants.

More recent epidemiologic studies were done that question the reported strong association between lithium exposure and congenital cardiac abnormalities. Two cohort studies investigating

TABLE 11.2. *Mood stabilizers*

Medication	Pregnancy use recommendation	Lactation use recommendation
Lithium	2	3
Valproic acid	4	3
Carbamazepine	4	3

See footnote to Table 11.1

the incidence of congenital anomalies in women exposed prenatally to lithium have been reported. In a cohort study linking the Swedish Birth Registry with the records of bipolar women, 59 infants were found whose mothers were treated with lithium early in pregnancy (63). Four (6.8%) of the 59 infants exposed to lithium had congenital heart disease compared with two infants (0.9%) of 228 bipolar women not exposed [relative risk (RR), 7.7; 95% confidence interval (CI), 1.5 to 41.2; $p < 0.05$]. None of the infants had Ebstein's anomaly. In a prospective cohort study of 148 women treated with lithium during the first trimester and 148 controls not exposed to any known teratogens, there were no statistically significant differences in the incidence of major congenital anomalies or cardiac malformations (64), although one lithium-exposed infant did have Ebstein's anomaly. If the data are pooled, these two cohort studies do not suggest a statistically significant risk in congenital malformations or cardiac malformations in women exposed to lithium during pregnancy [RR, 1.95; 95% CI, 0.88 to 4.33 and RR, 3.55; 95% CI, 0.86 to 14.66, respectively, using STATA 5 statistical software (Stata Corporation, College Station, TX)]. Four case-control studies were identified that investigate the relationship between lithium exposure and Ebstein's anomaly (65–68). None of the cases was found to have had exposure to lithium, suggesting that the prior initial estimate of the strength of the association was exaggerated. Although the risk for congenital malformations associated with *in utero* lithium exposure is likely to be lower than previously reported, an absence of risk cannot be assumed from the available data. The two available cohort studies indicate that the risk of all types of congenital anomalies in fetuses exposed to lithium in the first trimester is 4% to 12% and the risk of cardiac malformations is 0.9% to 6.8% (62). This risk may not be significantly different in unexposed women. No increase in long-term behavioral abnormalities in children exposed *in utero* to lithium was observed in 60 children in 5 years of follow-up compared with 57 of their siblings not exposed to lithium (69).

Polyhydramnios has also been associated with lithium therapy during pregnancy (70,71). There are at least two case reports of pregnant women with bipolar disorder taking lithium whose pregnancy was complicated by polyhydramnios (70,710. The pathogenesis of polyhydramnios in these two cases was thought to be fetal diabetes insipidus and resulting fetal polyuria. One of the infants had symptoms suggestive of lithium toxicity: asphyxia, apnea, cardiac decompensation, respiratory distress, hypoglycemia, hypotonia, thrombocytopenia, and diabetes insipidus (70).

Little information exists in the literature regarding the use of lithium during lactation. Lithium has been detected in breast milk at levels 10% to 50% of that found in maternal serum (72,73). Although no toxic effects in infants exposed to lithium through breast milk have been reported, long-term effects have not been studied. Thus, the American Academy of Pediatrics considers lithium to be contraindicated during breast-feeding (26).

Alternatives to lithium for patients requiring mood stabilizers include the anticonvulsant agents valproic acid (and its salt form sodium valproate) and carbamazepine. Valproic acid and valproate readily cross the placenta and have a reported rate of neural tube defect in first trimester exposed fetuses of 1% to 5%, a 15-fold increase from baseline (47,74). A pattern of minor malformations associated with valproic acid includes craniofacial abnormalities, abnormalities in digits, urogenital abnormalities, low birth weight, and psychomotor retardation (8,75–77). Similarly, carbamazepine has also been associated with neural tube defects. Among Michigan Medicaid recipients who had taken carbamazepine, a 0.9% incidence of neural tube defects was seen for *in utero* exposure (F. Rosa, US Food and Drug Administration, personal communication, 1994). In a prospective study of 35 live-born children exposed to carbamazepine, there was an 11% incidence of craniofacial defects, a 26% incidence of fingernail hypoplasia, and a 20% incidence of developmental delay (79). It is important to note that the existing studies investigating the teratogenic potential of anticonvulsants were in women with seizure disorders, not in women requiring mood stabilizers. This distinction is critical because seizure disorders themselves have been associated with

a higher rate of congenital malformations than that seen in the general population (80). Although these studies are flawed by lack of control groups and poor selection of controls, these agents should generally be avoided for use as mood stabilizers in pregnancy given the potential for teratogenesis (78,79). No adverse effects of valproic acid or carbamazepine have been reported in children of lactating mothers and the American Academy of Pediatrics considers them to be compatible with breast-feeding (8,26).

ANTIANXIETY AGENTS

Antianxiety agents are listed in Table 11.3. Benzodiazepines are the most commonly used anxiolytic agents. These agents are also used as anticonvulsants and for alcohol withdrawal. The use of benzodiazepines during the first trimester may be associated with an increased risk of cleft lip and palate (47,81). A recent review, based on three studies with similar study design, calculated a pooled risk of oral clefting after first-trimester exposure to benzodiazepines (6,83–85). The resulting odds ratio was 2.4 (95% CI, 1.40 to 4.03) for the development of oral clefts. This odds ratio groups the effects of diazepam and alprazolam. Although these reports suggest an increased risk of cleft lip after exposure, the baseline risk for this anomaly is only 0.06% (6). Therefore, the absolute risk of oral clefting after *in utero* drug exposure is small.

Other reports do not suggest an increase in congenital abnormalities with fetal exposure to benzodiazepines. In a case-control study of 611 infants with cleft lip or cleft palate and 2,498

TABLE 11.3. *Antianxiety agents*

Medication	Pregnancy use recommendation	Lactation use recommendation
Alprazolam	3	3
Lorazepam	3	3
Midazolam	3	3
Orazepam	3	3
Oxazepam	3	3
Buspirone	3	3
Diazepam	4	4

See footnote to Table 11.1.

controls with other birth defects, no association between diazepam and cleft palate was found; the odds ratios after adjustment for potential confounders were 0.8 for cleft lip with or without cleft palate (95% CI, 0.4 to 1.7) and 0.8 for cleft palate alone (95% CI, 0.2 to 2.5) (84). In a study of Michigan Medicaid recipients from 1980 to 1983, 80 of 104,000 pregnant women were found to have received 10 or more prescriptions for benzodiazepines during their pregnancy. Neonatal outcomes were assessed from health claims 6 to 9 years after delivery. Among these 80 women, three deaths occurred, and eight women had babies with congenital anomalies. This increased rate of teratogenesis was likely the result of associated heavy alcohol and illicit drug use in these women (85). A more recent study of 460 women exposed to benzodiazepines during pregnancy compared with 424 control pregnancies found no difference in the incidence of congenital anomalies (3.1% versus 2.6%) (86).

The use of benzodiazepines during labor or late in pregnancy has been associated with effects in the newborn infant. Several reports suggest a floppy infant syndrome consisting of neonatal apnea, hypotonia, lethargy, and poor suckling (87–91). In addition, a neonatal withdrawal syndrome has been described, the symptoms of which include tremors, hypertonicity, diarrhea, vomiting, irritability, and vigorous suckling (8,92–95). Given these concerns, benzodiazepines are best avoided in the peripartum period.

Benzodiazepines are secreted into breast milk (96,97). There is concern that use of these agents could result in toxicity in infants in the first 1 to 2 weeks of life when their metabolic systems are immature and could result in withdrawal symptoms after abrupt weaning or discontinuation of breast-feeding (5,97–99). Reported breast milk:maternal plasma ratios for diazepam and oxazepam and their metabolites range from 0.08 to 0.28 (100–103), for alprazolam 0.36 (104), and for lorazepam 0.15 to 0.26 (105). The calculated doses of benzodiazepines for breast-feeding infants in women taking benzodiazepines are likely below the therapeutic range for most infants. However, the slow neonatal metabolism of benzodiazepines may lead to accumulation of drug in infant plasma with chronic maternal use

(5,99,101,103–107). The American Academy of Pediatrics considers the effects of benzodiazepines on the breast-fed infant to be unknown but possibly of concern (26). There are no studies of long-term effects of maternal use of benzodiazepines on breast-fed infants. If these agents must be used in a lactating woman, it is recommended that short-acting agents with inactive metabolites be selected such as oxazepam, lorazepam, orazepam, alprazolam, and midazolam (5). The infant should be monitored for signs of sedation during use and withdrawal symptoms after stopping the medication or after discontinuation of breast-feeding.

Buspirone is an oral anxiolytic agent that is chemically unrelated to benzodiazepines. Among pregnant Michigan Medicaid recipients between 1985 and 1992, 42 newborns had been exposed to buspirone during the first trimester (8). Only one (2.4%) had a major birth defect (two expected) (F. Rosa, US Food and Drug Administration, personal communication, 1994). Despite no reported teratogenesis, use of this agent during pregnancy and lactation is not recommended because of the paucity of information concerning effects on the fetus and newborns.

ANTIPSYCHOTIC AGENTS

Butyrophenones

Antipsychotic agents are listed in Table 11.4. The majority of antipsychotic agents, including the phenothiazines and butyrophenones, are dopamine antagonists. These agents are associated with several unpleasant side effects including sedation, dry mouth, constipation, extrapyramidal symptoms, and orthostatic hypotension

TABLE 11.4. *Antipsychotics*

Medication	Pregnancy use recommendation	Lactation use recommendation
Haloperidol	1	1
Chlorpromazine	2	3
Thioridazine	3	3
Thiothixene	3	3
Fluphenazine	3	3
Clozapine	3	3

See footnote to Table 11.1.

(108–128). These agents are also commonly used in pregnancy for their antiemetic properties in hyperemesis gravidarum and in conjunction with narcotics for their sedative properties.

Haloperidol is a commonly used butyrophenone antipsychotic. Early reports of infant exposure to haloperidol *in utero* noted cases of limb reduction defects (8,110,111). However, a causative effect cannot be inferred from these reports. In a cohort study of 98 pregnant women treated in the first trimester with a lower dose of haloperidol than that used for psychosis (0.6 mg twice daily), no adverse effects or congenital abnormalities were found (112). Among pregnant Michigan Medicaid recipients (F. Rosa, US Food and Drug Administration, personal communication, 1994), 56 infants had been exposed to haloperidol in the first trimester. Three (5.4%) major birth defects were noted (two expected). There is no evidence that haloperidol is a teratogen at therapeutic doses. Thus, it is not contraindicated in pregnancy. Given the seriousness of psychosis, patients controlled on haloperidol should generally have their medication continued.

Haloperidol is excreted into breast milk (5). No adverse effects of this agent on nursing infants have been reported. The American Academy of Pediatrics considers haloperidol an agent whose effect on the nursing infant is unknown but may be of concern (26).

Phenothiazines

Psychotic illness itself has been associated with higher rates of congenital malformations, confounding the evaluation of the effects of agents to treat psychosis (113–115). A recent metaanalysis compiled the data from five studies investigating the rate of congenital anomalies after first-trimester exposure to low-potency phenothiazines for nausea and vomiting (14,116–120). This metaanalysis evaluated 2,591 first-trimester exposures in 74,337 live births. The pooled odds ratio was 1.21 (95% CI, 1.01 to 1.45). These pooled data suggest a small increased risk in congenital anomalies after first-trimester exposure to phenothiazines in the treatment of hyperemesis gravidarum. The authors of the

metaanalysis point out that with a baseline risk of congenital anomalies of 2.0%, phenothiazine use may increase the incidence to 2.4%. No specific pattern of malformations was identified.

Other smaller series of pregnant women exposed to various phenothiazines not included in the above metaanalysis have been reported. Two series of women exposed to chlorpromazine during the first trimester, including 140 and 263 subjects, failed to find an increase in congenital malformations among *in utero* exposed newborns (121,122). In 63 women exposed to perphenazine during the first trimester, no increased frequency of congenital malformations was noted (121). Similarly, in a series of 23 patients exposed to thioridazine, no increased incidence of congenital defects was observed (123). Among pregnant Michigan Medicaid recipients (F. Rosa, US Food and Drug Administration, personal communication, 1994), phenothiazine exposures in the first trimester had no apparent increase in congenital malformations: thioridazine, 63 exposures with two (3.2%) major birth defects; thiothixene, 38 exposures with one (2.6%) major birth defect; fluphenazine, 13 exposures with one (7.7%) major birth defect; perphenazine, 140 exposures with five (3.6%) major birth defects. All these series either have too few patients to comment on any potential teratogenic risk or suggest no increased risk over baseline rate of congenital malformations in the population.

The phenothiazines are excreted into breast milk (5). The calculated infant dose is 0.15% of the usual maternal dose (124). There is no reported contraindication to the use of phenothiazines during lactation (5,125).

Clozapine

Clozapine is a relatively new antipsychotic medication that is not a dopamine antagonist. Several case reports of diverse adverse pregnancy outcomes have been reported for this agent, but given the absence of denominator data, an increased risk of congenital anomalies cannot be assumed. No other data are available concerning the safety of this agent in pregnancy or lactation (8).

SUMMARY AND RECOMMENDATIONS

The decision to prescribe, continue, or stop a pharmacologic agent for a pregnant woman with a psychiatric illness should be a joint decision between the patient, her obstetrician, and her psychiatrist. The inclusion of a psychiatrist in the decision process is especially important in pregnant women because of the many nonpharmacologic treatments such as counseling, electroconvulsive therapy, and light therapy. These modalities could pose less risk to the developing fetus. Many women have fears (which they may not easily volunteer) of taking medication during pregnancy that could potentially affect compliance. The risk of the psychiatric illness on the mother and fetus must also be considered when deciding on the appropriate therapy. Attention must be paid to altered drug pharmacokinetics in pregnancy, which may necessitate a higher dose of certain medications. At the same time, it is desirable to use the lowest effective dose for the shortest period of time to minimize fetal drug exposure (41).

Suggested starting doses for selected psychotropic medications are given in Table 11.5.

DEPRESSION

Many common somatic symptoms seen in pregnancy can mimic depression, thus making the diagnosis difficult. These include change in appetite, fatigue, loss of energy and libido, and sleep disturbance (47). Some specific markers of depression in pregnancy include lack of interest in

TABLE 11.5. *Starting dosages for psychotropic medications in pregnancy*

Medication	Dosage
Amitriptyline	25–50 mg q.h.s.
Chlorpromazine	100 mg once or twice daily
Desipramine	25–50 mg q.h.s.
Fluoxetine	10–20 mg q.h.s.
Haloperidol	5–10 mg/day
Imiprimine	25–50 mg q.h.s.
Lithium	0.6–2.1 g/day in 3 divided doses
Nortriptyline	10–25 mg q.h.s.

the pregnancy, guilty ruminations, and profound anhedonia (126).

Women with mild depression who are pregnant or attempting conception may benefit from nonpharmacologic interventions (126). If a woman is already taking an antidepressant, a trial of drug tapering or discontinuation is appropriate in women with mild depression (47,126). In women with moderate to severe depression (suicidal, psychosis, or anorexia), the use of antidepressants is generally warranted during pregnancy and during the preconception period, especially if prior attempts at tapering the medication have failed (47,126).

Although no antidepressant has been proven to be completely safe in pregnancy and lactation, the tricyclic antidepressants and the SSRI fluoxetine are relatively well studied and should be the first-line agents if pharmacotherapy is considered necessary. Among the tricyclics, desipramine and nortriptyline are preferred because they are least likely to cause orthostatic hypotension (47). Fluoxetine may be used if there is no response to the other agents. The new SSRIs, MAOIs, St. John's wort, and bupropion are less optimal treatments for depression because of the paucity of information concerning their safety in pregnancy.

Because the incidence of postpartum depression in women with a history of depression in pregnancy is high (approximately 25%), these agents may be continued through the third trimester and lactation (127,128). Although there have been isolated reports of irritability, restlessness, functional bowel obstruction, decreased sleep, vomiting, and watery stools with antidepressant use in late pregnancy and lactation, the potential for recurrent or worsening major depression during a period of increased risk seems to outweigh these potential adverse side effects (10–18,41,47).

BIPOLAR DISORDER

There is a reported worsening of bipolar disorder during the puerperium. The rates of relapse during this period range from 20% to 50% (126). In addition, during the first month, postpartum admissions for bipolar disorder are eight times more common than during nonpregnancy-related periods (47). It especially important to note that the rate of relapse is high with abrupt discontinuation of lithium and approaches 50% within 6 months of lithium discontinuation (47,126). In women with severe bipolar disorder, in whom discontinuation of medication poses a risk of increased morbidity, it is reasonable to leave patients on this medication because the benefits likely outweigh the small risk of teratogenesis. Reproductive risk counseling should be offered, as well as prenatal diagnosis by fetal echocardiography at 18 to 22 weeks' gestation. Conversely, in less severely affected women with long periods of well-being infrequently interrupted by affective instability, tapering and discontinuation of lithium before or during early pregnancy may be attempted with reintroduction in the second and third trimesters if needed (62). Given the high rate of puerperal worsening of this disorder, lithium should not generally be discontinued in the postpartum period. The American Academy of Pediatrics considers lithium to be contraindicated during lactation (26). In the woman who insists on nursing her infant, lithium therapy can be continued with close monitoring of the infant (5,73).

Alternative mood stabilizers, including carbamazepine and valproate, are of concern during pregnancy because of their high rate of reported congenital malformations (8,75–79,80). However, these agents can be used during lactation (8,26).

ANXIETY DISORDERS

Patients with anxiety disorders maintained on benzodiazepines who are pregnant or desire to become pregnant should ideally have these agents tapered slowly under the supervision of a psychiatrist. If tapering is unsuccessful, reinstitution of benzodiazepines may be required. Although the use of benzodiazepines may be associated with orofacial clefting, the absolute risk seems to be less than 1% (47). Therefore, the severity of the underlying psychiatric disorder and the potential for adverse consequences worsening the psychiatric condition should be carefully weighed against the small risk of congenital malformations. Alternatively, patients with panic

disorder or obsessive compulsive disorder may be treated with tricyclic antidepressants or fluoxetine (47,126). Behavioral therapy (cognitive-behavioral therapy) is an effective nonpharmacologic treatment for anxiety disorders (47,126). These agents should also be avoided in the peripartum period and during lactation given reports suggesting a floppy infant syndrome and a neonatal withdrawal syndrome (8,87–95).

PSYCHOSIS

Psychosis during pregnancy can be a life-threatening emergency to a woman and her fetus. In addition, psychosis may impair a woman's ability to obtain adequate prenatal care. A pregnant woman experiencing any psychotic symptoms requires immediate psychiatric consultation. If a patient has a history of psychosis or experiences new onset psychosis in pregnancy, treatment with antipsychotic agents is often necessary and should not be withheld because of pregnancy or lactation. Haloperidol is the agent of choice for first-line treatment because there is no evidence of teratogenesis with this agent. The phenothiazines may also be used if needed, but data concerning their use in pregnancy are more limited. The use of antipsychotic agents during lactation should generally be avoided until more data are available (5). The use of clozapine or other new antipsychotic agents should generally be avoided in pregnancy and lactation because of the lack of data concerning their safety.

REFERENCES

1. American College of Obstetricians and Gynecologists. Depression in women. ACOG technical bulletin no. 182. Washington: American College of Obstetricians and Gynecologists, 1992.
2. Pickar D. Prospects for pharmacotherapy of schizophrenia. *Lancet* 1995;345:557–562.
3. Myers JK, Weissman MM, Tischler GL, et al. Six-month prevalence of psychiatric disorders in three communities; 1980 to 1982. *Arch Gen Psychiatry* 1984;41;959–967.
4. McGrath E, Ketia GP, Strickland BR, et al. Women and depression: risk factors and treatment issues. Washington: American Psychological Association, 1990.
5. Chisolm CA, Kuller JA. A guide to the safety of CNS-active agents during breastfeeding. *Drug Saf* 1997;17:127–142.
6. Altshuler LL, Cohen L, Szuba M, et al. Pharmacologic management of psychiatric illness during pregnancy:

dilemmas and guidelines. *Am J Psychiatry* 1996; 153:592–606.

7. Kuller JA, Katz VL, McMahon MJ, et al. Pharmacologic treatment of psychiatric disease in pregnancy and lactation: fetal and neonatal effects. *Obstet Gynecol* 1996;87:789–794.

8. Briggs GG, Freeman RK, Yaffe SJ, eds. *Drugs in pregnancy and lactation*, 5th ed. Baltimore: Williams & Wilkins, 1998.

9. Goldberg HL, Nissim R. Psychotropic drugs in pregnancy and lactation. *Int J Psychiatry Med* 1994;24:129–149.

10. Eggermont E. Withdrawal symptoms in neonates associated with maternal imipramine therapy. *Lancet* 1973;2:680.

11. Schimmell MS, Katz EZ, Shaag Y, et al. Toxic neonatal effects following maternal clomipramine therapy. *Clin Toxicol* 1991;29:479–484.

12. Cowe L, Lloyd DJ, Dawling S. Neonatal convulsions caused by withdrawal from maternal clomipramine. *BMJ* 1982;284:1837–1838.

13. Webster PAC. Withdrawal symptoms in neonates associated with maternal antidepressant therapy. *Lancet* 1973;2:318–319.

14. Altshuler LL, Szuba MP. Course of psychiatric disorders in pregnancy: dilemmas in pharmacologic management. *Neurol Clin* 1994;12:613–635.

15. Hill RM. Will this drug harm the unborn infant? *South Med J* 1977;67:1476–1480.

16. Shrand H. Agoraphobia and imipramine withdrawal? *Pediatrics* 1982;70:825.

17. Falterman LG, Richardson DJ. Small left colon syndrome associated with maternal ingestion of psychotropic drugs. *J Pediatr* 1980;97:100–110.

18. Shearer WT, Schreiner RL, Marshall RE. Urinary retention in a neonate secondary to maternal ingestion of nortriptyline. *J Pediatr* 1972;81:570–572.

19. Misri S, Sivertz K. Tricyclic drugs in pregnancy and lactation: a preliminary report. *Int J Psychiatry Med* 1991;21:157–171.

20. Nulman I, Rovert J, Stewart DE, et al. Neurodevelopment of children exposed in utero to antidepressant drugs. *N Engl J Med* 1997;336:258–362.

21. Bader TF, Newman K. Amitriptyline in human breast milk and the nursing infants serum. *Am J Psychiatry* 1980;137:855–856.

22. Sovner R, Orsulak PJ. Excretion of imipramine and desipramine in human breast milk. *Am J Psychiatry* 1979;136:451–452.

23. Breyer-Pfaff U, Nill K, Entenmann KN, et al. Secretion of amitriptyline and metabolites into breast milk [Letter]. *Am J Psychiatry* 1995;5:812–813.

24. Brixen-Rasmussen L, Halgrener J, Jorgensen A. Amitriptyline and nortriptyline excretion in human breast milk. *Psychopharmacology* 1982;76:94–95.

25. Stancer HC, Reed KL. Desipramine and 2-hydroxydesipramine in human breast milk and the nursing infant's serum. *Am J Psychiatry* 1986;143:1597–1600.

26. Committee on Drugs, American Academy of Pediatrics. The transfer of drugs and other chemical into human milk. *Pediatrics* 1994;93:137–150.

27. Ben Muza A, Smith CS. Neonatal effects of maternal clomipramine therapy. *Arch Dis Child* 1979;54:405.

28. Ostergaard GZ, Pedersen SE. Neonatal effects of maternal clomipramine treatment. *Pediatrics* 1982;69:233–234.

29. Cowe L, Lloyd DJ, Dawling S. Neonatal convulsions caused by withdrawal from maternal clomipramine. *BMJ* 1982;284:1837–1838.

30. Schimmell MS, Katz EZ, Shaag Y, et al. Toxic neonatal effects following maternal clomipramine therapy. *J Toxicol Clin Toxicol* 1991;29:479–484.

31. Singh S, Gulati S, Narang A, et al. Non-narcotic withdrawal syndrome in a neonate due to maternal clomipramine therapy. *J Pediatr Child Health* 1990; 26:110.

32. Bromiker R, Kaplan M. Apparent intrauterine fetal withdrawal from clomipramine hydrochloride. *JAMA* 1994;272:1722–1723.

33. Pastuszack A, Schick-Boschetto B, Zuber C, et al. Pregnancy outcome following first-trimester exposure to fluoxetine (Prozac). *JAMA* 1993;269:2246–2248.

34. Goldstein DJ, Marvel DE. Psychotropic medications during pregnancy: risk to the fetus. *JAMA* 1993;270: 2177.

35. Goldstein DJ, Corbin LA, Sundell KL. Effects of first-trimester fluoxetine exposure on the newborn. *N Engl J Med* 1997;89:713–718.

36. Chambers CD, Johnson KA, Dick LM, et al. Birth outcomes in pregnant women taking fluoxetine. *N Engl J Med* 1996;335:1010–1015.

37. Robert E. Treating depression in pregnancy. *N Engl J Med* 1996;351:1056–1058.

38. Kinney DK, Yurgelun-Todd DA, Levy DL, et al. Obstetrical complications in patients with bipolar disorder and their siblings. *Psychiatry Res* 1993;48:47–56.

39. Kallen B, Tandberg A. Lithium and pregnancy: a cohort study on manic-depressive women. *Acta Psychiatr Scand* 1983;68:134–139.

40. Isenberg KE. Excretion of fluoxetine in human breast milk. *J Clin Psychiatry* 1990;51:169.

41. Lester BM, Cucca J, Andreozzi L, et al. Possible association between fluoxetine hydrochloride and colic in an infant. *J Am Acad Child Adolesc Psychiatry* 1993;32:1253–1255.

42. Nightingale SL. Fluoxetine labeling revised to identify phenytoin interaction and to recommend against use in nursing mothers. *JAMA* 1994;271:1067.

43. Wisner KL, Perel JM, Findling RL. Antidepressant treatment during breast-feeding. *Am J Psychiatry* 1996; 153:1132–1137.

44. Kulin NA, Pastuszack A, Sage SR, et al.. Pregnancy outcome following maternal use of the new selective serotonin reuptake inhibitors: a prospective controlled multicenter study. *JAMA* 1998;279:609–610.

45. Linde K, Ramirez G, Mulrow CD, et al. St John's wort for depression—an overview and meta-analysis of randomised clinical trials. *BMJ* 1996;313:253–238.

46. Chiarello RJ, Cole JO. The use of psychostimulants in general psychiatry: a reconsideration. *Arch Gen Psychiatry* 1987;30:205–215.

47. Altshuler LL, Szuba MP. Course of psychiatric disorders in pregnancy: dilemmas in pharmacologic management. *Neurol Clin* 1994;12:613–635.

48. Matera RF, Zabala H, Jimenez AP. Bifid exencephalia: teratogen action of amphetamine. *Int Surg* 1968;50:79–85.

49. Gilbert EF, Khoury GH. Dextroamphetamine and congenital cardiac malformations. *J Pediatr* 1970;76:638.

50. Levin JN. Amphetamine ingestion with biliary atresia. *J Pediatr* 1971;79:130–131.

51. McIntire MS. Possible adverse drug reaction. *JAMA* 1966;197:62–63.
52. Nelson MM, Forfar JO. Associations between drugs administered during pregnancy and congenital abnormalities of the fetus. *BMJ* 1971;1:523–527.
53. Milkovich L, Van den Berg BJ. Effects of antenatal exposure to anorectic drug. *Am J Obstet Gynecol* 1977; 129:637–642.
54. Ramer CM. The case history of an infant born to an amphetamine addicted mother. *Clin Pediatr* 1974;13:596–597.
55. Oro AS, Dixon SD. Perinatal cocaine and methamphetamine exposure: maternal and neonatal correlates. *J Pediatr* 1987;111:571–578.
56. Eriksson M, Billing L, Steneroth G, et al. Health and development of 8-year old children whose mothers abuse amphetamine during pregnancy. *Acta Paediatr Scand* 1989;78:944–949.
57. Steiner E, Villen T, Hallberg M, et al. Amphetamine secretion in breast milk. *Eur J Clin Pharmacol* 1984; 27:123–124.
58. Ayd FJ Jr. Excretion of psychotropic drugs in human breast milk. *Int Drug Ther News Bull* 1973;8:33–40.
59. Weinstein MR. The International Register of Lithium Babies. *Drug Infor J* 1976;1094–1101.
60. Schou M, Goldfield MD, Weinstein MR, et al. Lithium and pregnancy, I: report from the Register of Lithium Babies. *BMJ* 1973;2:135–136.
61. Nora JJ, Nora AH, Toews WH. Lithium, Ebstein's anomaly and other congenital heart defects. *Lancet* 1974;1:594–595.
62. Cohen LS, Friedman JM, Jefferson JW, et al. A reevaluation of risk of in utero exposure to lithium. *JAMA* 1994;271:146–150.
63. Kallen B, Tandberg A. Lithium and pregnancy: a cohort study on manic-depressive women. *Acta Psychiatr Scand* 1983;68:134–139.
64. Jacobson SJ, Jones K, Johnson X, et al. Prospective multicenter study of pregnancy outcome after lithium exposure during the first trimester. *Lancet* 1992;339:530–533.
65. Zalzstein E, Koren G, Einarson T, et al. A case control study on the association between first trimester exposure to lithium and Ebstein's anomaly. *Am J Cardiol* 1990;65:817–818.
66. Kallen B. Comments on teratogen update: lithium. *Teratology* 1988;38:597.
67. Edmonds LD, Oakley GP. Ebstein's anomaly and maternal lithium exposure during pregnancy. *Teratology* 1990;41:551–522.
68. Sipek A. Lithium and Ebstein's anomaly. *Cor Vasa* 1989;31:149–156.
69. Schou M. What happened to the lithium babies? A follow-up study of children born without malformations. *Acta Psychiatr Scand* 1976;54:193–197.
70. Krause S, Ebbesen F, Lange AP. Polyhydramnios with maternal lithium treatment. *Obstet Gynecol* 1990;75:504–506.
71. Ang MS, Thorp JA, Parisi VM. Maternal lithium therapy and polyhydramnios. *Obstet Gynecol* 1990;76:517–519.
72. Sykes PA, Quarrie J, Alexander FW. Lithium carbonate and breastfeeding. *BMJ* 1976;2:1299.
73. Schou M, Amdisen A. Lithium and pregnancy. III: lithium ingestion by children breast-fed by women in lithium treatment. *BMJ* 1973;2:138.
74. Delgado-Escueta AV, Janz D. Consensus guidelines: preconception counseling, management, and care of pregnant woman with epilepsy. *Neurology* 1992; 42[Suppl 5]:149–160.
75. Jager-Roman E, Deichl A, Jakob S, et al. Fetal growth, major malformations, and minor anomalies in infants born to women receiving valproic acid. *J Pediatr* 1986;108:997–1004.
76. DiLiberti JH, Farndon PA, Dennis NR, et al. The fetal valproate syndrome. *Am J Med Genet* 1984;19:473–481.
77. Ardinger HH, Atkin JF, Blackston RD, et al. Verification of the fetal valproate syndrome phenotype. *Am J Med Genet* 1988;29:171–185.
78. Gaily E, Granstrom ML. Minor anomalies in children of mothers with epilepsy. *Neurology* 1992;42(Suppl 5):128–131.
79. Aarskog D. Association between maternal intake of diazepam and oral clefts. *Lancet* 1975;2:921.
80. Jones KL, Lacro RV, Johnson KA, et al. Pattern of malformations in the children of women treated with carbamazepine during pregnancy. *N Engl J Med* 1989;320:1661–1666.
81. Rosa FW. Spina bifida in infants of women treated with carbamazepine during pregnancy. *N Engl J Med* 1991;324:674–647.
82. Saxen I, Saxen L. Association between maternal intake of diazepam and oral clefts. *Lancet* 1975;2:498.
83. St. Clair SM, Schirmer RG. First-trimester exposure to alprazolam. *Obstet Gynecol* 1992;80:843–846.
84. Rosenberg L, Mitchell AA, Parsells JL, et al. Lack of relation of oral clefts to diazepam use during pregnancy. *N Engl J Med* 1983;309:1282–1285.
85. Bergman U, Rosa FW, Baum C, et al. Effects of exposure to benzodiazepines during fetal life. *Lancet* 1992;340:694–696.
86. Ornoy A, Arnon J, Shectman S, et al. Is benzodiazepine use during pregnancy really teratogenic? *Reprod Toxicol* 1998;12:511–515.
87. Fisher JB, Edgren BE, Mammel MC, et al. Neonatal apnea associated with maternal clonazepam therapy; a case report. *Obstet Gynecol* 1985;66[Suppl]:34S–35S.
88. Gillberg C. "Floppy infant syndrome" and maternal diazepam. *Lancet* 1977;2:244.
89. Haram K. "Floppy infant syndrome" and maternal diazepam. *Lancet* 1977;2:612–613.
90. Speight AN. Floppy-infant syndrome and maternal diazepam and/or nitrazepam. *Lancet* 1977;1:878.
91. Whitelaw AGL, Cummings AJ, McFadyen IR. Effect of maternal lorazepam on the neonate. *BMJ* 1981;282:1106–1108.
92. Mazzi E. Possible neonatal diazepam withdrawal: a case report. *Am J Obstet Gynecol* 1977;129:586–587.
93. Rementeria JL, Bhatt K. Withdrawal symptoms in neonates from intrauterine exposure to diazepam. *J Pediatr* 1977;90:123–126.
94. Backes CR, Cordero L. Withdrawal symptoms in the neonate from presumptive intrauterine exposure to diazepam: report of case. *J Am Osteopath Assoc* 1980;79:584–585.
95. Barry WS, St. Clair SM. Exposure to benzodiazepines in utero. *Lancet* 1987;1:1436–1437.

96. Gaudreault P, Guay J, Thivierge RL, et al. Benzodiazepine poisoning: clinical and pharmacological considerations and treatment. *Drug Saf* 1991;6:247–265.

97. Ananth J. Side effects in the neonate from psychotropic agents excreted through breast feeding. *Am J Psychiatry* 1978;135:801–805.

98. Anderson PO. Therapy review: drug use during breast-feeding. *Clin Pharm* 1991;10:594–624.

99. Mandelli M, Morselli PL, Nordio S, et al. Placental transfer of diazepam and its disposition in the newborn. *Clin Pharmacol Ther* 1975;17:564–572.

100. Erkkola R, Kanto J. Diazepam and breast-feeding. *Lancet* 1972;1:1235–1236.

101. Brandt R. Passage of diazepam and desmethyldiazepam into breast milk. *Arzneimittelforschung* 1976;25:454–457.

102. Dusci LJ, Good SM, Hall RW, et al. Excretion of diazepam and its metabolites in human milk during withdrawal from combination high dose diazepam and oxazepam. *Br J Clin Pharmacol* 1990;29:123–126.

103. Cole AP, Hailey DM. Diazepam and active metabolite in breast milk and their transfer to the neonate. *Arch Dis Child* 1975;50:741–742.

104. Oo CY, Kuhn RJ, Desai N, et al. Pharmacokinetics in lactating women: prediction of alprazolam transfer into milk. *Br J Clin Pharmacol* 1995;40:231–236.

105. Summerfield RJ, Nielson MS. Excretion of lorazepam into breast milk. *Br J Anaesth* 1985;57:1042–1043.

106. Wretlind M. Excretion of oxazepam in breast milk. *Eur J Clin Pharmacol* 1987;29:123–126.

107. Reider J, Wendt G. Pharmacokinetics and metabolism of the hypnotic nitrazepam. In: Garattini S, Mussini E, Randall LO, eds. *The benzodiazepines.* New York: Raven, 1973:99–127.

108. Goldaber KG. Psychotropics. *Semin Perinatol* 1997;21:154–159.

109. Dielangard P, Coignet J, Vidal JC. Sur un cas d'ectrophocomelie peut-etre d'origine medicamenteuse. *Bull Fed Gynecol Obstet* 1966;18:85–87.

110. Kopelman AE, McCullar FW, Heggeness L. Limb malformations following maternal use of haloperidol. *JAMA* 1975;231:62–64.

111. Van Waes A, Van de Veld E. Safety evaluation of haloperidol in the treatment of hyperemesis gravidarum. *J Clin Pharmacol* 1969;9:224–227.

112. Elia J, Katz IR, Simpson GM. Teratogenicity of psychotherapeutic medications. *Psychopharmacol Bull* 1987;28:531.

113. Rieder RO, Rosenthal D, Wender P, et al. The offspring of schizophrenics: fetal and neonatal deaths. *Arch Gen Psychiatry* 1975;32:200–211.

114. Sobel DE. Fetal damage due to ECT, insulin coma, chlorpromazine or reserpine. *Arch Gen Psychiatry* 1960;2:606–611.

115. Moriarty AJ, Nance NR. Trifluoperazine and pregnancy. *Can Med Assoc J* 1963;88:375–376.

116. Milkovich L, van den Berg BJ. An evaluation of the teratogenicity of certain antinauseant drugs. *Am J Obstet Gynecol* 1976;125:244–248.

117. Rumeau-Rouquette C, Goujard J, Huel G. Possible teratogenic effects of phenothiazines in human beings. *Teratology* 1977;15:57–64.

118. Slone D, Siskind V, Heinonen OP, et al. Antenatal exposure to the phenothiazines in relation to congenital malformations, perinatal mortality rate, birth weight, and intelligence quotient score. *Am J Obstet Gynecol* 1977;128:486–488.

119. Edlund MJ, Craig TJ. Antipsychotic drug use and birth defects: an epidemiologic reassessment. *Compr Psychiatry* 1984;25:32–38.

120. Heinonen OP, Slone D, Shapiro S. *Birth defects and drugs in pregnancy.* Littleton, MA: Publishing Sciences Group, 1977.

121. Farkus VG, Farkus G. Teratogenic action of hyperemesis in pregnancy and of medication used to treat it. *Zentrabl Gynakol* 1971;10:325.

122. Scanlon FJ. The use of thioridazine during the first trimester. *Med J Aust* 1972;1:1271.

123. Oleson OV, Bartel SA, Paulsen JH. Perphenazine in breast milk and serum. *Am J Psychiatry* 1996;147:1378–1379.

124. Maitra R, Menkes DB. Psychosomatic drugs and lactation. *N Z Med J* 1996;109:217–219.

125. Cohen LS, Rosenbaum F. Psychotropic drug use during pregnancy: weighing the risks. *J Clin Psychiatry* 1998;59[Suppl 2]:18–28.

126. Gotlib IH, Whiffen VE, Mount JH, et al. Prevalence rates and demographic characteristics associated with depression in pregnancy and the post partum. *J Consult Clin Psychol* 1989;57:269–274.

127. O'Hara MW, Neunaber DH, Zekoski EM. Prospective study of postpartum depression: prevalence, course, and predictive factors. *J Abnorm Psychol* 1984;93:158–171.

128. Suppes T, Baldessarini RJ, Faedda GL, et al. Risk of recurrence following discontinuation of lithium treatment in bipolar disorder. *Arch Gen Psychiatry* 1991;48:1082–1088.

12

Licit and Illicit Drug Use in Pregnancy:

Epidemiology, Amphetamines, LSD, PCP, and "Ts and Blues"

Melissa H. Fries

*Program Director, OB/GYN Residency, 81 MSGS/SGCG, Keesler Medical Center,
Keesler Air Force Base, Mississippi*

Illicit drug use in pregnancy cuts across demographic lines to affect any prenatal practice. Often considered to be a problem only in inner city populations, drug use has been reported in 7.5% to 15% of all pregnant women (1,2). Such information is rarely volunteered. The challenge for the obstetrician is to identify patients at risk and to provide the optimal care during pregnancy, with needed psychosocial support after delivery. This chapter focuses on the epidemiology of drug use in pregnancy; the means to identify high-risk patients; the specific details of prenatal exposure risk to hallucinogenic drugs, amphetamines and "designer drugs," phencyclidine, and "Ts and blues,"; and the nature of care needed during pregnancy and afterward for the drug-using mother and exposed infant.

EPIDEMIOLOGY

A 1990 Institute of Medicine report suggests that there are approximately 5.5 million people, or approximately 2.7% of the US population over the age of 12 who clearly (2.4 million) or probably (3.1 million) need treatment for drug-use disorders (3). Drug use is associated with a significant increase in morbidity and mortality; approximately 100,000 deaths each year occur in association with alcohol or drug use, with two thirds of these in cocaine or heroin addicts. More than one third of all new acquired immunodeficiency

syndrome cases occur in abusers of intravenous drugs and their sexual contacts, and more than half of the cases of domestic violence occur in the presence of illicit drugs or alcohol. Twenty percent to 90% of substance abusers may also manifest other significant forms of psychopathology (4). Countless more individuals have casual or infrequent exposure to illicit drugs, short of frank dependence or addiction.

Despite the magnitude of drug exposure, it is often difficult to obtain an accurate assessment of the severity of the problem in pregnant patients. In the absence of universal testing at every prenatal visit, estimates of drug use are based on patient self-report, urine drug testing at the first prenatal visit, urine drug testing on mother and infant at delivery, and testing of infant hair or meconium. Urine testing will reflect recent drug use within the past 3 to 5 days (5). Hair and meconium testing has been used principally for cocaine assay; hair studies demonstrate recent and sequential use depending on the area of hair assayed (6) and meconium studies demonstrate exposure up to several weeks before delivery (7).

Anonymous testing of urine in patients presenting for delivery in Rhode Island hospitals (not limited to inner city) in 1989 showed that 7.5% of the 465 women tested were positive for cocaine, marijuana, opiates, or amphetamines (1). Women with public insurance coverage were four times more likely to be positive than were women with private insurance. Another population-based study of pregnant patients in public health or private obstetrical services in Pinellas County, Florida, showed 13.3% positive urine testing for opiates, cocaine, or cannabinoids (2). Both studies indicated that cocaine use was more common in nonwhite patients; marijuana use alone was more common in white patients. Urine testing at presentation for prenatal care of predominantly white, rural patients from small towns in Missouri showed 11% positivity for illicit drugs, 85% of which was marijuana (8).

Self-reporting is typically unreliable. A report of urine testing for cocaine metabolites in patients presenting for prenatal care in a large urban hospital in the southeast United States indicated that 76% of patients were willing to be tested, of which 5% were positive for cocaine metabolites; only 47% of those who were positive admitted cocaine use in the previous 6 months (9). Urine assays for cocaine and marijuana in inner city women at presentation for care and at delivery showed that 17% used cocaine and 28% used marijuana at least once in their pregnancy (10). Of the cocaine users, 24% denied use in interviews but had positive urinary testing, 23% reported use and had positive urine, and 51% reported use but did not have positive tests; 15% of marijuana users denied use.

Infant testing has shown varied amounts of exposure. A review in *Morbidity and Mortality Weekly Report* of prenatal exposure to cocaine in infants born in Georgia at more than 31 weeks of gestation and more than 1,500 g using assays from Guthrie spots gave a prevalence of 4.9 positive infants per 1,000 newborns (11). However, anonymous meconium screening of all birth weight and age infants delivered at a tertiary perinatal center in Detroit, Michigan, showed 30.5% were positive for cocaine, 20.2% were positive for opiates, and 11.4% were positive for cannabinoid; 16.2% of infants were positive for two or more drugs (12).

The social profile of mothers who use illicit drugs in pregnancy can be stratified by type of drug used, age, or ethnicity. Among a study of pregnant adolescents in public health programs in North Carolina, 60.4% reported tobacco use, 32.2% reported marijuana use, and 3.6% reported use of other drugs; use of all drugs was higher in white adolescents, who also reported earlier age of onset of drug use, but were also more likely to be married and not in school (if aged 15 to 17) (13). In an interview study of patients presenting for prenatal care in Galveston, Texas, white (7%) and Mexican-American (5%) patients younger than 18 years of age were more likely to report illicit drug use than patients of similar ethnicity older than 21 years; black patients older than 21 reported the highest rate of current illicit drug use (9%) (14). Other reports of inner city cocaine users (ascertained by patient report and drug testing) indicated that users were significantly more likely to be black, have a lower prepregnant weight and pregnancy weight gain and lower hematocrit, have at least one episode of sexually transmitted disease before pregnancy, have given birth to a low birth weight infant, report one or more previous spontaneous abortions, and have undergone one or more previous elective abortions (10). Cocaine users were also more likely to be heavy users of tobacco and alcohol. A report of cocaine-using pregnant patients (ascertained by interview and urine studies) also found that drug-using patients were significantly older, had more children, presented later for prenatal care, were less likely to be employed, and more than twice as likely to use tobacco. Users were also more likely to have a family history of drug or alcohol use/abuse, to have been introduced to drugs by a male partner who was still using, to be depressed, to have less social support, and to have lived in a shelter in the past year (15).

These demographics lead to several pertinent conclusions about identifying drug use in pregnancy. Although patient self-identification is not reliable enough to be used exclusively, many patients will admit drug use in pregnancy if asked. Any patient from any age group in any ethnicity may use drugs. Cigarette smoking may be a marker for concomitant drug use; a retrospective analysis of pregnant adolescents taken from the 1988 National Maternal and Infant Health Survey indicated that smokers were four times more likely to use alcohol or cocaine than nonsmokers when other socioeconomic variables were controlled (16). Screening patients who admit to drug or alcohol use and smokers who deny drug use with urine drug testing may be helpful. Understanding the nature of the population served and maintaining a high index of suspicion in general may be the most useful approach.

These studies also underscore two critical issues about drug use in pregnancy. First, it is rarely isolated to a single agent. Polydrug use, including alcohol, tobacco, cocaine, marijuana, and amphetamines, is common and compounds concerns about fetal exposure. Second, drug use is often reflective of coexistent problems of poverty, lack of education, minimal social support, and general life stress (17); identifying fetal outcomes only in terms of drug exposure clearly underestimates the other critical aspects of environment that may be equally as damaging.

AMPHETAMINES

Amphetamines are artificially derived stimulant drugs initially developed for the treatment of narcolepsy or for use as decongestants. The chemical structure of amphetamine resembles that of norepinephrine; however, it differs in the lack of hydroxyl groups and the presence of an additional methyl group. These changes render the molecule more lipid soluble and prevent its metabolism by monoamine oxidases, leading to a wide distribution and long duration of action. Minor changes in the structure of the molecule lead to significant variations in drug effect: methamphetamine ("crystal" or "ice"), which can be dissolved in water for injection; STP (serenity, tranquility, and peace), which is the most potent psychostimulant; trimethoxyamphetamine, which resembles mescaline; and designer amphetamines such as methylenedioxymethamphetamine or Ecstasy and methylenedioxyethamphetamine or Eve (18). Creation of such designer drugs is not complicated and forms the subject of easily available books, leading to a high likelihood for continued drug development and use (19).

Amphetamines are typically taken orally or nasally, with their actions being dose dependent, initially yielding stimulation, alertness, decreased fatigue, sleeplessness, euphoria, and exhilaration. The amphetamine leads to the release of norepinephrine, serotonin, and dopamine, creating subsequent effects of hypertension, dilated pupils, agitation, and visual and audial hallucinations. An additional characteristic is the development of anorexia, which has led to their popularity as diet pills, although this effect seems to diminish with continued use (18). Many of these effects are similar to those of cocaine, which acts to prevent the reuptake of norepinephrine. Side effects of paranoia, sleep problems, and panic attacks are not uncommon (20). Ecstasy is often used as a "dance drug" at "raves," where it is typically taken with large volumes of water as an "antidote"; this may lead to dilutional hyponatremia and SIADH (syndrome of inappropriate secretion of antidiuretic hormone), with the potential for renal failure, seizures, and hepatitis (21,22).

Maternal-Fetal Effects

Maternal amphetamine use has been associated with an increase in prematurity, although, unlike cocaine, this has not been associated with preterm rupture of membranes, abruptio placentae, or placenta previa (23,24). A case of amphetamine use in late pregnancy was interpreted as eclampsia because of associated seizures, hypertension, and proteinuria (25). Reports of fetal anomalies associated with amphetamine use have been inconclusive. Although cardiac anomalies and other congenital anomalies were reported in association with dexamphetamine use in early studies (26,27), later studies have not confirmed these findings but have indicated an increased frequency of oral clefting (28). No significant increase in congenital anomalies was observed in a prospective study of intravenous methamphetamine- (as well as tobacco-, marijuana-, and cocaine-) using mothers compared with controls, although a significant reduction in fetal body weight, length, and head circumference was observed (29). In a report of narcotic- or amphetamine-using mothers (no cocaine use), a 10-fold increase in the frequency of fetal cleft lip/palate was identified (30). It is not clear whether this increased frequency of clefting is a causative action of the amphetamine or reflects an alteration in maternal diet as a result of drug action, leading to a decrease in folic acid intake, which may be a common pathway for the development of many anomalies.

Longitudinal follow-up of Swedish children exposed prenatally to amphetamines demonstrated below average weight, height, and head circumference at birth and at ages 1 and 4 years; these findings reached statistical significance in girls (31). When followed to 8 years of age, psychometric testing suggested an increase in aggressive behavior and adjustment, which was also correlated with maternal psychiatric treatment, alcohol abuse, and number of custodians (32). After 14 years of follow-up, more exposed children were one grade below that expected for their age and had significantly lower scores in math, language, and sports. Girls continued to be smaller at ages 10 and 14 than the average, although boys by age 14 were significantly taller and heavier (33).

These findings suggest that maternal amphetamine use constitutes a high-risk state in pregnancy, principally for the development of maternal illness unrelated to pregnancy, poor fetal and childhood growth (particularly in girls), and a potential for fetal facial clefting.

LYSERGIC ACID DIETHYLAMIDE

Lysergic acid diethylamide (LSD) is a synthetic hallucinogen frequently used in association with other illicit drugs. LSD and peyote (mescaline) are the archetypal drugs used to induce hallucinogenic or trance-like dream states, which may be associated with vivid, bizarre, and occasionally frightening images. Pure LSD is rarely sold but is adulterated with other products, often amphetamines. This has clouded the literature regarding the fetal effects of LSD, which has focused on concerns for chromosome breakage and congenital anomalies. No specific perinatal complications have been attributed to isolated LSD use, although hallucinogenic behavior in labor may hinder adequate maternal response, particularly in the second stage. Chromosomal breakage was first reported after the addition of LSD to cell culture in 1967 (34) and observed more frequently in hospitalized psychiatric patients with a drug history of LSD exposure. However, in chromosomal studies of patients before and after LSD use, there was no increase in chromosomal breaks, or, if observed, the pattern was transient. Likewise, no increase in chromosomal breakage was seen in human male and female meiosis or in that of rhesus monkeys. Monkey fetuses exposed prenatally to LSD likewise did not show an increase in chromosomal breakage; normal-appearing human infants did show an increased frequency of chromosome breaks, but this paralleled that of their mothers (35). Rare congenital anomalies reported after LSD use include limb reduction anomalies (some similar to amniotic band syndrome), extrophy of the bladder, megacolon, and ophthalmologic abnormalities (36,37). Animal studies of mice, rabbits, and rhesus monkeys did not demonstrate any similar anomalies (35). Given these rare findings, a confirmed pattern of teratogenicity can not be established for LSD.

PHENCYCLIDINE

Phencyclidine or 1-phenylcyclohexyl piperidine is typically referred to as PCP or "angel dust." It was initially developed as an anesthetic agent similar to ketamine but lost favor because of the persistent delirium, agitation, and hallucinations seen in patients emerging from anesthesia (38). It is easily manufactured and was a common street drug in the 1970s and 1980s, before the popularity of crack cocaine. It can be absorbed orally, nasally, or transdermally and has an extremely long duration of action, leading to confusion, bizarre, often violent behavior, and hallucinations. Maternal PCP and marijuana use has been associated with a single report of a premature birth of an abnormal infant with dysmorphic facies, spastic quadriparesis, and dislocated hip (39); postnatal irritability, jitteriness, and poor feeding were described in two other cases. These abnormal behaviors, however, had resolved by 2 years of age, when mental and psychomotor development were thought to be similar to unexposed infants (40). Maternal PCP use is probably underrecognized because few drug screens measure its levels; however, its use should be considered in confused, violent patients with otherwise negative drug screens.

Ts AND BLUES

"Ts and Blues" is the street name for the combination of the narcotic analgesic pentazocine (Talwin) and the over-the-counter antihistamine tripelennamine (Pyribenzamine). It has been used as a cheap substitute for heroin and because of this is typically injected to induce euphoria, relaxation, and to decrease agitation. Several reports of infants born to mothers using intravenous Ts and Blues describe decreased birth weight, length, and head circumference relative to unexposed controls; daily or weekly exposure was associated with neonatal withdrawal symptoms characterized by irritability, excessive sucking, and feeding difficulties (41). These findings were confirmed in a later report, which also reported one ventricular septal defect (VSD), one case of cardiomegaly, and one hypospadias in infants of 23 Ts and Blues users; the significance of these anomalies is confounded by a concomitant use of alcohol and cocaine (42).

OVERVIEW

It becomes apparent that most illicit drug exposure in pregnancy is not associated with any well-defined teratogenic syndrome. Although numerous anomalies have been seen in infants of drug-using mothers, these have not been consistent, except for the common observation of growth retardation. Preterm delivery appears to be the most common perinatal complication. Postnatal developmental delays are subtle and may relate to the combined effect of polydrug exposure and the disadvantaged environment seen with continued parental drug use. However, the cost of care for drug-exposed infants is escalating, potentially 10-fold higher for the cost of caring for cocaine-exposed infants than unexposed (43). In today's dollar-conscious health environment, the greatest risk created by maternal drug exposure may be the excessive cost of maternal and infant care.

OBSTETRIC AND NEONATAL MANAGEMENT

Providers who identify a drug-using patient in pregnancy often feel a mixed sense of frustration and anger toward the patient, largely based on perceptions of poor outcome for the fetus. Filled with the media-emphasized thoughts of hopelessly impaired cocaine babies, physicians have an unrealistically high perception of teratogenic risk associated with drug use, which is echoed in the patient herself. In a study of physicians, control patients, and cocaine-using pregnant women, all perceived cocaine to be teratogenic (13.4% average perceived teratogenic risk by physicians, 56.5% perceived teratogenic risk by control patients, and 37.5% perceived teratogenic risk by using patients). Fifty-six percent of physicians and 70% of controls had a greater than 50% tendency toward pregnancy termination (44). This indicates an important general need for education in this area, emphasizing that in most circumstances, early recognition of drug use with subsequent discontinuation will lead to a healthy pregnancy and infant. Using cocaine as an example, for light to moderate users, early cessation of drug use has been shown to lead to pregnancy outcomes that do not differ significantly from those of nonusers (45). Such an emphasis may decrease undesired pregnancy terminations and support continued avoidance of drugs. Many patients may view themselves as "doomed" to have an abnormal infant because of their early use and thus see no reason to stop—much the same as lung cancer patients see no reason to stop smoking once they have already developed cancer.

Once identified, patients benefit from a comprehensive approach to their care that should include personalized, sensitive, culturally competent, nonjudgmental care; referral to rehabilitation programs, with hospitalization and psychiatric services if indicated; and supportive counseling about the risks of returning to drug use (46). In large urban areas, this may require a special prenatal clinic, although any regular prenatal care for drug-using women has been shown to result in the birth of infants with greater weight and larger head circumferences (47). If identified early enough, patients may benefit from maternal serum screening and targeted ultrasounds for anomalies, as well as dietary counseling to encourage maternal weight gain. Patients should be educated about the signs and symptoms of early labor, preterm rupture of membranes, and abruptio placentae. Repeated urine drug screening throughout pregnancy and at delivery may help reinforce compliance, although patients may also view this as punitive and distrustful. If poor fetal growth is identified, regular fetal monitoring may detect early signs of fetal distress.

Frank drug addiction, however, increases the need for prenatal care while decreasing the likelihood that it will be obtained (48). In such addicted patients, fetal outcomes may be worsened not only because of drug effects but because of the hazards of poor parenting and lack of attachment. Studies of dyads of drug-using mothers and prenatally exposed children indicate that the children's behaviors were subject to environmental control and depended on specific maternal behaviors within the interaction (49). Postnatal social services or home nursing may be needed to provide individual maternal training with the child as well as to teach overall parenting skills. Even if drug use cannot be stopped, this parental education may make a significant improvement in childhood growth and development. Education and social support by family, friends, neighborhood, or government services are vital in assisting socioeconomically disadvantaged women to decrease drug use and improve their overall health and that of their children (50).

REFERENCES

1. Anonymous. Statewide prevalence of illicit drug use by pregnant women—Rhode Island. *MMWR Morb Mortal Wkly Rep* 1981;39:225–227.
2. Chasnoff IJ, Landress HJ, Barrett ME. The prevalence of illicit-drug of alcohol use during pregnancy and discrepancies in mandatory reporting in Pinellas County, Florida. *N Engl J Med* 1990;322:1202–1206.
3. Institute of Medicine. *Broadening the base of treatment for alcohol problems*. Washington: National Academy Press, 1990.
4. Anonymous. Practice guidelines for the treatment of patients with substance use disorders: alcohol, cocaine, opioids. *Am J Psychiatry* 1995;152[Suppl 11]:1–59.
5. Osterloh JD, Lee BL. Urine drug screening in mothers and newborns. *Am J Dis Child* 1989;143:791–793.
6. Graham K, Koren G, Klein J, et al. Determination of gestational cocaine exposure by hair analysis. *JAMA* 1989;262:3328–3330.
7. Ostrea EM, Brady M, Gause S, et al. Drug screening of newborns by meconium analysis: a large scale, prospective, epidemiologic study. *Pediatrics* 1992;89:107.
8. Sloan LB, Gay JW, Snyder SW, et al. Substance abuse during pregnancy in a rural population. *Obstet Gynecol* 1992;79:245–248.
9. Lindsay MK, Carmichael S, Peterson H, et al. Correlation between self-reported cocaine use and urine toxicology in an inner-city prenatal population. *J Natl Med Assoc* 1997;89:57–60.
10. Frank DA, Zuckerman BS, Amaro H, et al. Cocaine use during pregnancy: prevalence and correlates. *Pediatrics* 1988;82:888–895.
11. Anonymous. Population-based prevalence of perinatal exposure to cocaine—Georgia, 1994. *MMWR Morb Mortal Wkly Rep* 1996;45:887–891.
12. Ostrea E, Ostrea AR, Simpson P. Mortality within the first 2 years in infants exposed to cocaine, opiate, or cannabinoid during gestation. *Pediatrics* 1997;100:79–83.
13. Teagle SE, Brindis CD. Substance use among pregnant adolescents: a comparison of self-reported use and provider perception. *J Adolesc Health* 1998;22;229–238.
14. Wiemann CM, Berenson AB, San Miguel VV. Tobacco, alcohol, and illicit drug use among pregnant women–age and racial/ethnic differences. *J Reprod Med* 1994;39:769–776.
15. Hutchins E, Dipietro J. Psychosocial risk factors associated with cocaine use during pregnancy: a case-control study. *Obstet Gynecol* 1997;90:142–147.
16. Archie CL, Anderson MM, Gruber EL. Positive smoking history as a preliminary screening device for substance use in pregnant adolescents. *J Pediatr Adolesc Gynecol* 1997;10:13–17.
17. Hanna EZ, Faden VB, Dufour MC. The motivational correlates of drinking, smoking, and illicit drug use during pregnancy. *J Subst Abuse* 1994;6:155–167.
18. Plessinger MA. Prenatal exposure to amphetamines—risk and adverse outcomes in pregnancy. *Obstet Gynecol Clin North Am* 1998;25:119–138.
19. Fester, Uncle Fester. *Secrets of methamphetamine manufacture including recipes for Mda, Ecstasy, and other psychedelic amphetamines*, 4th ed. New York: Lompanics Unlimited, 1997.
20. Williamson S, Gossop M, Powis B, et al. Adverse effects of stimulant drugs in a community sample of drug users. *Drug Alcohol Depend* 1997;44:87–94.
21. Cohen RS, Cocores J. Neuropsychiatric manifestations following the use of 3,4-methylenedioxymethamphetamine (MDMA; "Ecstasy"). *Prog Neuropsychopharmacol Biol Psychiatry* 1997;21:727–734.
22. Dykhuizen RS, Brunt PW, Atkinson P, et al. Ecstasy induced hepatitis. *Gut* 1995:36:939–941.
23. Oro AS, Dixon SP. Perinatal cocaine and methamphetamine exposure: maternal and neonatal correlates. *J Pediatr* 1987:111:571–578.
24. Eriksson M, Larsson G, Winbladh B, et al. The influence of amphetamine addiction on pregnancy and the newborn infant. *Acta Paediatr Scand* 1978;67:95–99.
25. Elliott RH, Rees GB. Amphetamine ingestion presenting as eclampsia. *Can J Anaesth* 1990;337:130–133.
26. Nora JJ, Vargo TA, Nora AH, et al. Dexamphetamine: a possible environmental trigger in cardiovascular malformations. *Lancet* 1970;1:1290.
27. Nelson MM, Forfar JO. Associations between drugs administered during pregnancy and congenital anomalies of the fetus. *BMJ* 1971;1:523–527.
28. Milkovich L, Van der Berg BJ. Effects of antenatal exposure to anorectic drugs. *Am J Obstet Gynecol* 1977;129:637–642.

29. Little BB, Snell LM, Gilstrap LC. Methamphetamine abuse during pregnancy: outcome and fetal effects. *Obstet Gynecol* 1988;72:541–544.

30. Thomas DB. Cleft palate, mortality and morbidity in infants of substance abusing mothers. *J Paediatr Child Health* 1995;31:457–460.

31. Eriksson M, Jonsson B, Steneroth G, et al. Cross-sectional growth of children whose mothers abused amphetamines during pregnancy. *Acta Paediatr* 1994;83:612–617.

32. Billing L, Eriksson M, Jonsson B, et al. The influence of environmental factors on behavioural problems in 8-year-old children exposed to amphetamine during fetal life. *Child Abuse Negl* 1994;18:3–9.

33. Cernerud L, Eriksson M, Jonsson B, et al. Amphetamine addiction during pregnancy: 14-year follow-up of growth and school performance. *Acta Paediatr* 1996;85:204–208.

34. Cohen MM, Hirschorn K, Frosch WA. In vivo and in vitro chromosomal damage induced by LSD-25. *N Engl J Med* 1967;277:1043–1049.

35. Long SY. Does LSD induce chromosomal damage and malformations? A review of the literature. *Teratology* 1972;6:75–90.

36. Chan CC, Fishman M, Egbert PR. Multiple ocular anomalies associated with maternal LSD ingestion. *Arch Ophthalmol* 1978;96:282–284.

37. Margolis S, Martin L. Anophthalmia in an infant of parents using LSD. *Ann Ophthalmol* 1980;12:1378–1381.

38. Petrucha RA, Kaufman KR, Pitts FN. Phencyclidine in pregnancy—a case report. *J Reprod Med* 1983;27:301–303.

39. Golden NL, Sokol RJ, Rubin IL. Angel dust: possible effects on the fetus. *Pediatrics* 1980;65:18–20.

40. Chasnoff IJ, Burns KA, Burns WJ, et al. Prenatal drug exposure: effects on neonatal and infant growth and development. *Neurobehav Toxicol Teratol* 1980;8:357–362.

41. Chasnoff IJ, Hatcher R, Burns WJ, Schnoll SH. Pentazocine and tripelennamine (T's and blue's): effects on the fetus and neonate. *Dev Pharmacol* 1983;6:162–169.

42. Little BB, Snell LM, Breckenridge JD, et al. Effects of T's and blues abuse on pregnancy outcome and infant health status. *Am J Perinatol* 1990;7:359–362.

43. Plessinger MA, Woods JR. Cocaine in pregnancy—recent data on maternal and fetal risks. *Obstet Gynecol Clin North Am* 1998;25:99–118.

44. Koren G, Gladstone D, Robeson C, et al. The perception of teratogenic risk of cocaine. *Teratology* 1992;46:567–571.

45. Richardson GA, Day NL. Maternal and neonatal effects of moderate cocaine use during pregnancy. *Neurotoxicol Teratol* 1991;13:455–460.

46. Carrington BW, Loftman PO, Jones K, et al. The special prenatal clinic: one approach to women and substance abuse. *J Women Health* 1998;7:189–193.

47. Berenson AB, Wilkinson GS, Lopez LA. Effects of prenatal care on neonates born to drug-using women. *Subst Use Misuse* 1996;31:1063–1076.

48. McCalla S, Minkoff HL, Feldman J, et al. The biologic and social consequences of perinatal cocaine use in an inner-city population: results of an anonymous cross-sectional study. *Am J Obstet Gynecol* 1991;164:625–630.

49. Heller MC, Sobel M, Tanaka-Matsumi J. A functional analysis of verbal interactions of drug-exposed children and their mothers: the utility of sequential analysis. *J Clin Psychol* 1996;52:687–697.

50. Sun WY, Chen W. The impact of maternal cocaine use on neonates in socioeconomic disadvantaged population. *J Drug Educ* 1997;27:389–396.

13

Licit and Illicit Drugs: Tobacco, Alcohol, and Opioids

Gail Best and James R. Woods, Jr.

Department of Obstetrics and Gynecology, University of Rochester, Strong Memorial Hospital, Rochester, New York

Drug use can begin at any point in one's lifetime. The consequences of this risky behavior never are of more concern than they are during pregnancy. Outcomes of pregnancies that are complicated by drug use have far-reaching consequences, not only for the woman and her child, but also for the public as a whole. Perinatal outcomes, not only of illicit drug users but of smokers as well, are poorer. There is a great deal of evidence supporting the fact that there is an increased incidence of neonatal morbidity and mortality among newborns born to women who abuse these substances.

Of growing concern are the long-term results. What are the life-time effects of growth retardation, congenital malformations, and prematurity? How is neurologic development affected? If development is influenced by the woman's use of drugs during her pregnancy, what are the consequences when these children grow into adults?

Despite a general acknowledgment among the public of the dangers of using drugs, use of harmful licit and illicit substances continues. In the 1992 National Household Survey on Drug Abuse, 22.6% of women age 18 to 25 and 14.4% of women aged 26 to 34 reported having used an illicit drug. In those same age groups, 40% and 36% of women, respectively, reported smoking (1). Additionally, during pregnancy, illicit drug, alcohol, and tobacco use is not discontinued, although there may be a decrease in the amounts used. In the 1992–1993 National Pregnancy and Health Survey by the National Institute on Drug Abuse, 221,000 women (of 4 million who gave

birth) reported using illegal drugs during their pregnancies. Marijuana use was most prevalent; cocaine use was second in predominance. Alcohol and tobacco use were even more extensive (2). In the general population, alcohol and cigarettes also are used more commonly than are illicit drugs. Of illicit drugs, marijuana is used most and cocaine, second most often (1,3).

Studying these substances and their effects on pregnancy can be difficult for a variety of reasons. Often times, more than one substance is used, making the establishment of cause and effect complex. Some substances actually are a combination of multiple compounds, present in varying amounts. Again, this makes analysis difficult. Additionally, environmental and psychosocial factors may play a role (4).

This chapter provides an overview of tobacco, alcohol, and opiates. Their impact on pregnancy is reviewed. Although long-term outcomes have yet to be determined with certainty, findings to date are discussed.

TOBACCO

Epidemiology

Although a great deal of attention has been paid to the impact of illicit drug and alcohol use in pregnancy, the effects of cigarette smoking are numerous and can be as devastating or even more devastating than those of illicit substances. In one study, 15% of cases of low birth weight could have been prevented if not for smoking during pregnancy (5). The importance of urging pregnant patients to stop smoking cannot be overstated because of the serious consequences of smoking. In recent years, attempts to educate women about the hazards of tobacco use have been successful, and, in fact, there has been a decline in smoking during pregnancy (6). Certain segments of the population, however, require additional emphasis in this area.

According to a study by the National Center of Health Statistics (Smoking During Pregnancy, 1990–96), the overall rate of smoking during pregnancy declined by 26% during that period. In 1990, 20% of women reported smoking during pregnancy. This decreased to 14% in 1996 (6). The decline in rates of smoking was reported across all races with varying rates of decline among different races. Native American women had the smallest decrease in the rate of tobacco use and still have the highest rate at 21%. Smoking rates of non-Hispanic white mothers dropped 20% but were still high at 17%. The rates for Hispanic and African American women declined by 35%. The lowest rate of smoking is among Asian and Pacific Islander women at 3%, a decrease of 40% (6).

Despite the decline in the overall rate of smoking cigarettes during pregnancy, the rate among pregnant teenagers is still high. The most recent report shows that this rate actually has increased. For young women who are between the ages of 15 and 19, the rate increased to 17.2%. Before 1995, the rate among pregnant teens had been declining. Non-Hispanic white teenagers have the highest rate of smoking while pregnant at 29% (6).

Pharmacokinetics

Tobacco smoke contains more than 4,000 compounds. Most studies on the effects of smoking in pregnancy, however, have focused on nicotine.

Nicotine is lipid soluble and has a rapid and wide distribution. Most metabolism of nicotine occurs in the liver, and nicotine is excreted by the kidneys. The primary metabolite of nicotine is cotinine, which is metabolized in the liver as well with approximately 15% of cotinine being excreted by the kidneys. The half-life of nicotine is 1 to 2 hours, whereas that of cotinine is 15 to 20 hours (7–10). As a result of this longer half-life, cotinine provides a better measure of nicotine exposure than does nicotine itself.

Fetal exposure occurs as a result of passage across the placenta. Maternal levels of both nicotine and cotinine generally are lower than those in the fetus and amniotic fluid (8,11–14). Amniotic-fluid nicotine concentrations have been reported as being as much as 54% higher than maternal levels (12,14). Effects on the fetus occur as a result of direct influence on maternal hemodynamics and placental blood flow, as well as through ingestion of the nicotine and cotinine as the fetus swallows amniotic fluid.

Antepartum Effects

Adverse perinatal outcomes have been found to be associated strongly with cigarette use in pregnancy. There are several complications of pregnancy that are well established as occurring more frequently among smokers. Thus, unlike some negative outcomes, prevention is possible in some cases if smoking ceases.

Uteroplacental Effects

The data in several studies suggest that nicotine causes a reduction in uteroplacental blood flow. Direct studies have been conducted in animals, but only indirect measurements have been made in humans. The effects of nicotine on the human fetus have been presumed to be the result of decreases in uterine blood flow. This is based on the direct measurements taken in animal models and Doppler ultrasound examinations that have been used to measure the effects of smoking on uterine and umbilical blood flow velocities in humans. In two studies using Doppler examinations, maternal smoking was found to be associated with increased maternal blood pressure and heart rate as well as increases in fetal heart rate. In addition, umbilical artery S/D ratios increased, whereas uterine artery S/D ratios did not change (8,15,16).

Preterm Birth

Preterm delivery continues to be a major cause of perinatal morbidity and mortality. Smoking increases the risk of preterm birth; however, whether there is an increased rate of preterm labor has not been determined. The perinatal and neonatal mortality rate increases 33% in women who smoke during pregnancy (8,17). The increased rate of perinatal morbidity and mortality among smokers is associated with many factors. There is a well-established risk of low birth weight in women who smoke. Both the increased rates of preterm delivery and low birth weight may be consequences of other complications of smoking in pregnancy, those being placental abruption, placenta previa, and preterm premature rupture of membranes (PPROM). In addition, there is a significant positive correlation between smoking and intrauterine fetal death (18–25).

The frequency of PPROM is greater for smokers, and the incidence of this is dose related. The incidence of PPROM in nonsmokers was found to be 0.3% in one study, whereas in smokers it was 0.6% to 1.4%. The increased frequency correlated with an increase in the amount smoked (12,26,27). Additionally, there is evidence that chorioamnionitis occurs more frequently in smokers. In one study of pregnant teenagers, those diagnosed with chorioamnionitis were more likely to be smokers than nonsmokers (28,29). Both complications affect morbidity and mortality and contribute to the increased rate of preterm delivery.

Placental abruption is more common in women who smoked during pregnancy. This risk has been found to be increased in all smokers except those who smoke fewer than 10 cigarettes per day for fewer than 6 years or those who stop smoking early in pregnancy. The duration of smoking is correlated positively with risk of abruption (30,31). Placental abruption is reported to occur in 0.5% to 4% of all deliveries regardless of smoking status. In several studies, a 2.5-fold increased risk of abruption, over the general population risk, was found in patients who smoked (30,32).

The risk of placenta previa, which occurs in the general population at a rate of one in every 100 to 200 pregnancies, also increases significantly in smokers. The odds ratio for placenta previa among smokers varies in reports from 2% to 4.4% (33–35). In some studies, as with placental abruption, the incidence correlated positively with frequency and duration of smoking. This was not reported in all studies, however. Cessation of smoking in pregnancy has been found to have the same effect on placenta previa as on abruption. It does decrease the incidence of placenta previa to the same as that for nonsmokers (30,31). This risk remains the same regardless of whether smoking ceased during pregnancy. The relationship to the amount and duration of tobacco use, however, is not certain.

Low Birth Weight

Newborns of smoking mothers weigh on average 200 g less than those born to nonsmoking mothers at the same gestational age (36–39). In one study by Lindsay et al. (36), this low birth weight was found to be the result of a decrease in fat-free mass. The effect of smoking involves long bone growth rather than causing a difference in percentage of body fat. The evidence indicates that these findings are independent of and not a result of maternal nutritional status. Infants of malnourished mothers generally have a decrease in both fat and fat-free mass. This is in contrast to the infants of smokers in this and other studies of newborn body composition, who were found to have a decrease in long bone growth (36,38). The component in tobacco that contributes to low birth weight is uncertain. Uterine blood flow, as discussed, has been shown to be decreased by nicotine. Oxygen and nutrient supply to the fetus is thus presumed to be affected. Carbon monoxide, found in tobacco, also decreases oxygen delivery to the fetus. It has a stronger affinity for fetal hemoglobin than adult hemoglobin and results in a shift of the oxygen–hemoglobin saturation curve. Delivery and release of oxygen to the fetus therefore are decreased (8,36,40).

Postpartum and Long-Term Effects

Sudden Infant Death Syndrome

The effects of smoking during pregnancy unfortunately do not end with delivery. Complications as a result of prenatal tobacco exposure often are long-lasting. There are many investigations in which maternal smoking was found to be a critical risk factor for sudden infant death syndrome

(SIDS), and this risk was found to be dose dependent (19,41,42). It has been postulated that maternal nicotine use may result in poor fetal nutrition secondary to decreased uteroplacental blood flow. Chronic fetal hypoxia and an accumulation of carboxyhemoglobin, which has been found to cause impairment of fetal brain development in rats, have both been implicated in SIDS (19,43–45).

The relationship between tobacco use in pregnancy and SIDS is not an independent one. Other risk factors have an impact on the effect of maternal smoking on SIDS. In one study, preterm birth, low birth weight, and few prenatal visits were found to be important predictors in women who smoked heavily (43). In another investigation, there was no evidence of growth restriction in babies with SIDS born to nonsmoking mothers (12,43). The incidence of low birth weight in preterm infants with SIDS was considerably higher for smokers than that for nonsmokers. Smoking in pregnancy is an important risk factor for SIDS. Additionally, those infants who are preterm and with a low birth weight are at even greater risk (19,43).

Lung Function

The effects of smoking on adults are well known. What does this mean for the infant of a mother who smoked during pregnancy? Are there any effects of maternal smoking, and, if so, are they similar to those on the mother's lungs? It has been hypothesized that maternal smoking may adversely affect the development of the fetal lung. Some data do indicate that this indeed is the case. In one study of pregnant rats, the lungs of the neonate showed a decreased number of type I pneumocytes, but an increase in type II pneumocytes. The morphology of the type II pneumocytes was abnormal, however (8,46). In a study by Wuenschell et al. (47) embryonic mouse lung buds were exposed to nicotine and compared to controls. It was reported that the nicotine exposure stimulated an increase in the branching of the lung buds when compared to those of the controls.

It has been thought that maternal smoking may contribute to the development of persistent pulmonary hypertension in the newborn (PPHN). There has been some evidence that the pulmonary vascular changes found in infants with PPHN are similar to those seen in animals exposed to *in utero* hypoxemia. Maternal smoking does cause fetal hypoxemia. There also is some evidence that there may be an association between PPHN and smoking (48–50). In one study, infants with PPHN were more likely to have cotinine in their blood. This increase in the presence of cotinine in infants with PPHN included those exposed to smoke *in utero* from maternal active smoking and from passive exposure (51).

In addition to the possible association of maternal smoking and PPHN, the effects on general lung function have been considered. It is known that exposure to smoke in early childhood adversely affects respiratory function. One investigation attempted to define the effects on lung function in childhood as a result of *in utero* exposure only. This study was conducted within the first 9 days of life. It was found that tidal breathing parameters (time to reach peak expiratory flow to total expiratory time and volume to reach peak expiratory flow to total expiratory volume) were lower in children whose mothers smoked during pregnancy. These parameters were inversely related to the amount of smoking (52). Although the long-term effects of these findings have not been determined, this does indicate that there may be some change in lung function in childhood as a result of *in utero* exposure to smoke.

Carcinogenesis

Concern has been raised regarding transplacental cigarette smoke exposure and its contribution to childhood cancers. There are several carcinogens in tobacco smoke, and this smoke has been found to induce reactive oxygen species and cause oxidative DNA damage. Of importance is whether this oxidative damage occurs in fetal tissues when mothers smoke during pregnancy. Sipowicz et al. (53) found that transplacental exposure to 4(methyl-nitrosamino)-1-(2-pyridyl)-1-butanone (NNK) did cause oxidative damage to maternal and fetal tissues after multiple doses. Fetal DNA damage occurred to a lesser extent than did maternal DNA damage. In another study, however, 8-hydroxy-2′-deoxyguanosine, a marker for oxidative stress, was not found to be increased in smokers compared with nonsmoking women. In that same study, however, it was shown that there may be a protective role of vitamin E against the formation of this DNA adduct in placental DNA, a possible explanation for the previously described findings (54). At this point, there is no conclusive evidence that *in utero* tobacco exposure increases the risk of childhood cancer; however, there is cause for concern.

Cognitive Development

The long-term effects of maternal smoking include those on the cognitive development of the child. In one study of 9- to 12-year-old children, there was a negative association between smoking during pregnancy and the reading function of the child, especially reading function that is auditory related. The association was correlated positively to amount of *in utero* cigarette smoke exposure (55–61). Others found more behavioral problems as well as auditory deficits in children of smokers, although this has not been reported in all studies. There are many data to suggest that smoking has an effect on the cognitive functioning of these children, and smoking in the latter part of pregnancy is associated with an increase in the prevalence of mental retardation (62).

Prenatal exposure to lead adversely affects cognitive development of the fetus and child. The relationship of cigarette smoking during pregnancy and lead levels in newborns was examined as a potential cause of cognitive deficits. In one study, it was found that maternal cigarette smoking and cord blood lead levels are correlated positively. Even for women who stopped smoking during pregnancy, their newborns had higher blood lead levels compared with nonsmokers or those who quit before pregnancy (63). This suggests that maternal smoking may be related to lead toxicity.

Nicotine Replacement

Given the substantial risks to the fetus as a result of maternal smoking, the importance of smoking cessation cannot be overstated. The difficulty of quitting smoking can be formidable. Pregnant women, however, may have more motivation. The advice to stop smoking, therefore, is crucial, although not sufficient to be successful in many cases. Heavier smokers are even less likely to be able to quit smoking despite counseling. In many cases, nicotine replacement therapies may be beneficial because they reduce tobacco withdrawal symptoms. Nicotine replacement systems have been found to be particularly helpful among heavier smokers and can improve cessation rates (64–66).

Concerns have been raised regarding the effects on the fetus of these nicotine replacement systems. These systems, however, have not been proved to increase adverse outcomes (67). In fact, they should present less of a risk theoretically, given that tobacco smoke delivers not only nicotine but hundreds of other potentially, as well as proven, dangerous chemicals, including carbon monoxide, to the fetus. Cigarette smoking has been shown to provide higher nicotine concentrations to the mother and fetus, and these concentrations are delivered at more rapid rates than are those in nicotine replacement systems (64,68–70). In one study, although long-term outcomes were not measured, there were no differences in measures of fetal well-being measured before and after transdermal nicotine replacement was administered on a short-term basis (71). There also is evidence that the cardiovascular effects of both intravenous nicotine and cigarette smoking are similar to the effects of either alone. This indicates that there should be no change in cardiovascular effect if a patient decides to smoke while using a nicotine replacement product (64,72).

Although long-term studies of the effects on pregnancy of these relatively new drugs have yet to be completed, there is evidence that short-term pregnancy outcomes are not adversely affected. Heavier smokers are at even greater risk for poor outcomes in pregnancy. It is this same group that is most likely to benefit from replacement systems as an adjunct to behavioral therapy in smoking cessation (64,73). The benefits of these therapies thus appear to far outweigh the risks of continued smoking in pregnancy.

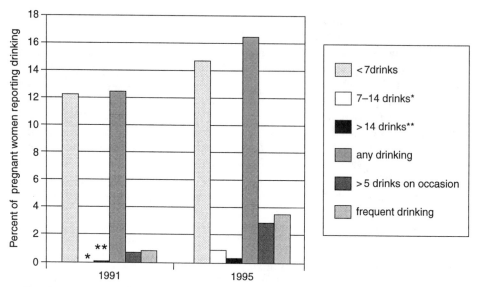

FIG. 13.1. Weekly alcohol consumption reported by pregnant women. *There were too few observations in 1991 among pregnant women drinking seven to 14 drinks per week. **The number of pregnant women drinking more than 14 drinks per week in 1991.

The above chart is based on figures reported by the CDC in its *Morbidity and Mortality Weekly Report* of 4/25/97.

ALCOHOL

Epidemiology

Alcohol use during pregnancy has been associated with many adverse effects. No specific amount has been deemed a safe level of consumption, and alcohol universally is not recommended for use during pregnancy. Despite this fact, many women continue to consume alcohol while pregnant. In fact, between 1991 and 1995, the prevalence of alcohol use during pregnancy increased.

A survey of women of ages 18 to 44 analyzed by the Centers for Disease Control and Prevention demonstrated that there was a substantial increase in alcohol use by pregnant women during the aforementioned time period. All levels of use were found to have increased among pregnant women. The number of women of childbearing age who reported any drinking and those who reported frequent drinking remained essentially the same in a comparison of the two time periods. In 1991, 49.4% of all women reported some drinking and 12.4% reported frequent drinking. By 1995, those numbers had increased to 50.6% and 12.6%, respectively. Among pregnant women, however, the prevalence of any drinking

and frequent drinking increased dramatically, from 12.4% and 0.8% (1991) to 16.3% and 3.5% (1995), respectively (74,75) (Fig. 13.1).

Pharmacokinetics

Blood alcohol level depends on the alcohol concentration in the beverage, the type of beverage, and individual gastrointestinal function. Most of the absorption of ethanol occurs within 0.5 to 1 hour. Ethanol is both water and lipid soluble. It rapidly crosses the placenta and distributes throughout the fetal circulation. Ethanol is converted to acetaldehyde. It is the acetaldehyde that causes the effects seen with alcohol consumption. Acetaldehyde is oxidized in the liver to acetate, and this in turn is oxidized in the bloodstream (76,77). Alcohol has been shown, in both human and animal studies, to cross the placenta readily (78–81).

Cellular Effects

The exact mechanisms of the teratogenic effects of alcohol remain unknown. It has been found that ethanol may affect embryonic cells differently during the preimplantation period than it affects postimplantation fetal cells. Several studies showed that embryos during the preimplantation period are not affected adversely by ethanol toxicity and, in fact, embryonic development is accelerated. During fetal development, however, those cells that are in the process of differentiating, rather than dividing, are affected by alcohol exposure, and this creates malformations (76,82). Human neurons appear to be sensitive to these effects; the resulting injuries depend on the timing of the exposure. This is of particular interest, given the long-term consequences of central nervous system (CNS) impairment from ethanol use in pregnancy.

Spontaneous Abortion

Studies on the risk of spontaneous abortion with consumption of alcohol have yielded conflicting results. In several studies, the risk of spontaneous abortion was found to increase with increasing levels of alcohol use. In other studies done in Europe and Australia, there was no association found between the two (83–85). In addition, as mentioned previously, some studies showed that exposure of preimplantation embryos to ethanol in culture enhances their development. The limitation of this is that the effects on the embryo of the maternal system in association with alcohol are unknown. A safe level of consumption has not been established, as these studies are based on women's reports of their alcohol consumption and underreporting may occur for a variety of reasons.

Fetal Alcohol Syndrome

Fetal alcohol syndrome (FAS) is a distinct set of birth defects found to be associated with the consumption of alcohol by the mother during pregnancy. The overall pattern involves growth restriction, CNS abnormalities, and craniofacial anomalies. Growth restriction can occur either in the prenatal or postnatal period or both. Infants with FAS eventually may reach normal growth, but not all do. CNS involvement includes cognitive impairment, developmental delay, and/or neurologic abnormalities. Some of the craniofacial abnormalities are microcephaly, microphthalmia, flat nasal bridge, and a thin vermilion border on the upper lip. Not all these features are present in every infant with FAS. In some cases, only a few of the features of FAS are identifiable (77,86,87). The term *fetal alcohol effects* is used for neonates with two or fewer of the characteristics of FAS (77). Alcohol-related birth defects and alcohol-related neurodevelopmental disorder are other terms that are used. These apply to maternal alcohol ingestion during pregnancy, which leads to the presence in the resulting offspring of anomalies or behavioral abnormalities associated with prenatal ethanol exposure (87).

As has been stated, there is no known safe level of alcohol consumption in pregnancy. Heavier drinkers are more likely to have children with FAS, however. Of women who are alcoholics, 2.5% to 10% have a child with FAS. Approximately one to three infants per 1,000 live births have FAS (77,87–90). FAS occurs when six or more drinks are consumed per day. The risk of FAS is not increased with two drinks per day, although fetal alcohol effects or alcohol-related birth defects and alcohol-related neurodevelopmental disorder have been found to occur in women consuming fewer than two drinks per day (87,91).

It is accepted that heavy maternal alcohol consumption is associated with serious adverse outcomes in the child. Moderate alcohol consumption, however, is yet to be defined, as are its effects. Many women do not realize that they are pregnant initially and continue to consume alcohol unknowingly after conception. A meta-analysis of alcohol consumption during the first trimester found no increased risk of major fetal malformations upon examination of such babies at or soon after birth. This particular study did not address the risk of spontaneous abortion or the risk of other adverse outcomes associated with alcohol consumption during pregnancy (92).

Neurologic Impairment

Although FAS is a known consequence of heavy maternal alcohol use during pregnancy, prenatal alcohol consumption at varying levels can produce fetal damage. Yet the babies of some heavily drinking women may not meet the criteria for a diagnosis of FAS. There is a broad spectrum of neurologic abnormalities in children that are associated with maternal prenatal ethanol use, and these can occur at levels below those accepted as causing FAS (93). Moderate alcohol intake during pregnancy produces behavioral rather than physical abnormalities (94–96). Although all dysmorphic features of FAS are not present in every case of fetal alcohol exposure, long-term outcomes can be profound nonetheless. The influence of alcohol on the developing nervous system produces damage that results in long-term deficits in these children. Cognitive and behavioral difficulties have been associated with even social drinking (97). In addition, destructive effects occur on sensory functions, resulting in impairments in the visual and auditory systems, which in turn affect hearing and language development (98–101).

Neurobehavioral and Cognitive Effects

There is a wide spectrum of neurobehavioral effects of prenatal alcohol exposure. Hyperactivity and attention deficits commonly are seen. Hyperkinetic disorders persist throughout childhood and can occur with no cognitive impairment (102–105). This has been found in long-term follow-up studies of children with FAS and in those who do not meet the criteria for the diagnosis of FAS. Studies in rats also have found effects on activity levels as a result of prenatal alcohol exposure (102). Higher rates of attention deficit disorders have been found in children of mothers who consumed alcohol during pregnancy (102,106–108).

In addition to the behavioral effects of prenatal alcohol exposure, cognitive impairment occurs as well, although either disorder can be present alone. Levels of cognitive function vary, and different learning disorders occur (103,109,110). Impairment can occur even in the absence of other features of FAS (109). Mental retardation, however, is more likely to occur in those children who are more severely affected with FAS (104). As the dose and length of alcohol abuse during pregnancy increase, behavioral and cognitive disturbances increase as well, in both frequency and severity (103). Behavioral and cognitive impairment occurs in adolescence even in cases of maternal prenatal social drinking, and there does appear to be a dose–response relationship

in these circumstances (97). Psychopathology is prevalent among children with FAS as well (104). It is unknown whether these effects are the result solely of the teratogenicity of alcohol or whether environmental factors play a substantial role in the development of behavioral, cognitive, and psychological deficits.

Neuroanatomical Abnormalities

The effects of alcohol on the developing fetal CNS depends on the timing of the insult. There are different stages of development during which all teratogens exert their effects. It has been found that ethanol has an influence on all stages of brain development, which accounts for the wide range of cognitive and behavioral deficits that result from prenatal alcohol exposure (94). In addition, different regions in the brain have differing levels of adverse effects of ethanol. Some regions are more susceptible to the effects of alcohol than others (111). Behavioral deficits have been found to result from injury by alcohol exposure to the neocortex, hippocampus, and cerebellum (94,111–113).

Neuronal migration also has been found to be adversely affected by prenatal alcohol exposure. Development of neurotransmitter function may be modified as well. Several studies showed that neurotransmitter systems do not form normally in the babies of alcohol-consuming pregnant women. The neurotransmitter content, the number of uptake sites, and some classes of receptors in different regions are decreased after prenatal alcohol exposure (94,114).

Hearing and Vestibular Disorders

Hearing disorders are frequently present among children with FAS. There are four different types of hearing disorders that can occur as a result of *in utero* ethanol exposure: developmental delay in maturation of the auditory system, congenital sensorineural hearing loss, intermittent conductive hearing loss as a result of recurrent serous otitis media, and central hearing loss. The consequence of this hearing loss will be impaired speech and language function. Hearing loss also contributes to the behavioral problems that are seen in children with FAS. Hearing loss can aggravate hyperactivity and attention deficit disorders. Learning disabilities are compounded if the diagnosis of hearing loss and intervention do not occur before the speech and language development stage, which will be affected detrimentally by the hearing loss. Although speech pathologies also can be caused by craniofacial abnormalities, they are most likely the result of a combination of the effects of both in children with FAS. When physical anomalies are present in addition to hearing loss, speech problems tend to last longer than those that are the result of hearing loss alone (98–100)

The effects of prenatal alcohol exposure on vestibular function are uncertain. Children with FAS can exhibit balance and gait abnormalities. Studies on both animal and human brain tissue have shown that cerebellar dysfunction is more likely (98,99,115–118).

Identification of Alcohol Use in Women

Alcohol is a very widely used drug and a teratogen. Despite its well-publicized, broad range of devastating effects on both the user and the offspring of users, alcohol use remains common among pregnant women. The number of pregnant women who drink alcohol, at any level of consumption, rose in the period from 1991 to 1995. A safe level of exposure has yet to be determined, as well as a safe pattern of use. It is not clear what

difference exists between chronic prenatal alcohol exposure and sporadic consumption of large amounts of alcohol.

Binge drinking, defined as the consumption of five or more alcoholic beverages on one occasion, results in a high blood alcohol concentration. The outcomes of a single heavy exposure of ethanol on the fetus are unknown. Studies have shown, however, that blood alcohol concentration is a good predictor of teratogenic effect. It has yet to be determined with certainty that neurologic deficits occur as a result of this type of exposure, although there are data to suggest that such an effect occurs in both primates and humans as a result of heavy, single exposures to alcohol (118–120). The real concern is in the number of unplanned pregnancies that occur as a consequence of unexpected sexual activity that results from binge drinking (121). Continued alcohol consumption can occur until the woman realizes that she is pregnant. What, if any, effect this will have on the developing embryo/fetus has not been determined with certainty.

Screening of pregnant women who use alcohol is the first step toward preventing teratogenic effects. In one study by Chang et al. (122), a screening questionnaire was found to be sensitive for assessing alcohol consumption. The questionnaire consists of four items and can be self-administered (Fig. 13.2). The questions asked are about tolerance to alcohol, annoyance at others'

T-ACE Questionnaire

1) **This first question is related to Tolerance. How many drinks does it take to make you high? Or how many drinks can you hold?**

2) **Do you feel Annoyed by people complaining about your drinking?**

3) **Do you feel the need to Cut down?**

4) **Do you ever drink an Eye-opener in the morning?**

FIG. 13.2. T-ACE questionnaire. Scoring is as follows: Two points are given for an answer of 2 or more to the first question. One point is given for each affirmative answer to the other three questions. The result is considered positive if the total score is 2 or more (123).

comments regarding alcohol use, thoughts about attempting to cut down, and the need for an "eye-opener" drink. In this study, the questionnaire was a sensitive screen for identifying women with an alcohol use disorder and for flagging those patients who drink during pregnancy. This screening method has been more effective in determining which patients consumed alcohol than staff assessment of risk. It also has demonstrated that prenatal alcohol use is not based on socioeconomics (122,123).

OPIOIDS

Pharmacology

Multiple opioid receptors have been identified in the CNS. The exhilaration effects are, for the most part, mediated through activation of the receptors. Other effects produced are analgesia, respiratory depression, constipation, and meiosis (124). Short-term actions include a "rush," flushing of the skin, dry mouth, and heavy extremities. Subsequently, users alternate between a state of wakefulness and drowsiness (125). Long-term use results in tolerance of analgesic and euphoric effects, as well as physical dependence and withdrawal symptoms if the drug is discontinued (124). Other long-term consequences of opiate use or related activities are medical complications including myocarditis, endocarditis, cellulitis, liver disease, human immunodeficiency virus/acquired immunodeficiency syndrome, and pulmonary disease (125).

Morphine is the drug typically used as the prototype opioid. With oral use, bioavailability is 30% as a result of the first-pass mechanism. The half-life is approximately 2 hours. It is metabolized by the liver, with morphine-3-glucuronide being the major metabolite, although it is mostly inactive. Another metabolite is morphine-6-glucuronide, which has more analgesic effect and causes less nausea, sedation, and respiratory depression. Morphine and all its metabolites are found in urine (7,126).

Heroin's analgesic potency is double that of morphine. It is hydrolyzed to 6-mono-acetylmorphine (MAM) and then to morphine. Most of the effects of heroin are owing to morphine. The presence of MAM in a urine screen is specific for heroin use. Heroin is injected, smoked the base in a cigarette, or inhaled after vaporization of the heroin base (7). The greatest intensity and quickest onset of euphoria occurs with intravenous injection, usually within 7 to 8 seconds. Onset of euphoria is slower with intramuscular injection, usually occurring in 5 to 8 minutes. When heroin is inhaled or smoked, the effects are felt within 10 to 15 minutes (125,127). All three forms of administration are addictive.

Methadone

The bioavailability of methadone is greatly increased over that of morphine and is 80% (7). There are large individual variations in the half-life of methadone. The range has been reported to be 13 to 58 hours, and this varies even more so during pregnancy. In studies of rats during pregnancy, the acute lethal dose has been found to be lowered (128). Methadone is highly protein bound. It distributes rapidly but eliminates slowly and has high lipid solubility. As a result, it has the ability to accumulate and penetrates the CNS quickly (7).

Methadone is used to prevent withdrawal symptoms and to block the euphoric effects and cravings associated with discontinuation of heroin use by producing a steady plasma level (129). It is given long term, in tapering doses, to discourage heroin use.

The dose of methadone used during pregnancy has been questioned because of concerns regarding collateral fetal effects. In addition, as pregnancy progresses, some women display withdrawal symptoms that were not present before (130–133). Such patients require higher doses of methadone to maintain a steady plasma level. Women who received methadone maintenance before pregnancy should be continued at their prepregnancy doses. Pregnant women who were not treated for opioid dependence before pregnancy should be hospitalized to begin a methadone program until determination of the appropriate maintenance dose (131,134).

Initial methadone doses of 10 to 20 mg are administered orally with additional doses of 5 to 10 mg given every 4 to 6 hours for withdrawal symptoms. On day 2, patients are then given the total dose received the day before, with supplemental doses given as needed. The mean maintenance dose is 50 mg (range, 10 to 90 mg) (124,135,136). As pregnancy progresses, a higher dose may be needed. Some clinicians have recommended using a split-dose regimen. There have been no studies to date on the effects on maternal plasma levels with this type of dosing (131). However, a study by Wittman and Segal (132) showed no change in fetal effects with a split-dose regimen compared with once daily dosing.

During labor, the usual dosage of methadone should be continued. If the patient exhibits withdrawal symptoms, an additional dose of 10 to 20 mg can be administered either orally or intramuscularly. Narcotics with agonist–antagonist properties should not be used because they may cause acute withdrawal. Other narcotics can be used for analgesia, and spinal and epidural anesthesia may be given, as well, During the postpartum period, the prepregnancy dose should be resumed. If the patient's methadone maintenance was begun during pregnancy, then half the dose is needed (131,135). Breast-feeding is not contraindicated if the mother is in a methadone maintenance program as long as other illicit drugs are not being used (137).

Opioid Effects on Pregnancy

Both intrauterine growth restriction (IUGR) and intrauterine fetal death (IUFD) are more common for women who use opiates during pregnancy. Methadone use is not associated with an increased incidence of IUFD, however (131,138,139). The incidence of low birth weight is increased in infants born to mothers who use heroin during pregnancy. This is true for those in methadone maintenance programs also and has been shown in animal studies as well (140). Those patients who do not use additional heroin or other illicit drugs do show an improvement in birth weight (138,141). There is some evidence that long-term growth is not adversely affected. Within 12 months, infant weight is improved, although still in the lower percentiles. In one study, persistent growth restriction was found at

12 months in infants of mothers maintained only on higher doses of methadone (142).

Other obstetric complications found in opioid-dependent women include increased risk of spontaneous abortion, preterm labor and delivery, premature rupture of membranes, placental insufficiency, placental abruption, preeclampsia, and meconium passage during narcotic withdrawal (131,143,144).

In view of the increased incidence of IUGR with opioid use in pregnancy, early sonography to establish estimated date of confinement is recommended. Additional ultrasonography to monitor fetal growth may be indicated. Given the risk for placental insufficiency and IUFD, weekly nonstress tests (NSTs) are indicated for intravenous opioid users. For those women in methadone-maintenance programs, NSTs are recommended only when IUGR is present as the incidence of IUFD is not increased in these women (131,139,145). Assessment of fetal well-being in methadone-maintained pregnancies presents a challenge. There is a higher incidence of nonreactive NSTs, and longer intervals are required for NSTs to become reactive in these patients. Although biophysical profile scores generally are not changed in these pregnancies, in one study, the time to complete the test was increased. These findings are believed to be the result of a change in response in fetal CNS neurotransmitters with the administration of methadone (131,146,147). In one reported case of narcotic withdrawal, fetal testing improved after methadone treatment. An umbilical artery Doppler flow study showed absent end diastolic flow velocity until the administration of methadone, which was used to treat the patient's withdrawal symptoms. After this treatment, diastolic flow returned, and the S/D ratio was normal (143).

Neonatal Effects of Methadone

Concerns about the use of methadone during pregnancy include the risk of neonatal withdrawal. Some of a baby's symptoms are similar to those seen in adults during withdrawal. Characteristic signs and symptoms are CNS hyperirritability, gastrointestinal dysfunction, respiratory distress, and autonomic symptoms such as yawning, tremors, and mottling. The disorder typically begins within 72 hours after birth. Approximately 60% of infants who are born to women receiving methadone will experience neonatal withdrawal. The severity of the symptoms has been found in some studies to correlate with the dose of methadone that the mother received, whereas in others, no such relationship has been found (124,128,148–150).

Some physicians have advocated using lower doses of methadone during pregnancy to prevent withdrawal in neonates (124). Determination of the dose should be made with discretion. Lowering the dose may cause maternal plasma levels to be less than that needed to prevent maternal withdrawal symptoms, and this may encourage other drug use. Among women who use heroin during pregnancy, severe withdrawal in their neonates occurs more frequently than among women who are on methadone maintenance throughout pregnancy. Additionally, women in methadone maintenance programs deliver infants with increased birth weights compared with the newborns of those women who have used heroin (124).

Although this may be attributed to improved prenatal care for those who are enrolled in programs, use of methadone will prevent the changing opioid levels found in heroin users (138,151). This should be of benefit to the fetus because repeated withdrawal episodes, which are associated with fetal distress, thus can be avoided (131,152). No uniform long-term effects of methadone have been detected, although developmental delay is more common in children whose mothers required methadone maintenance during pregnancy (88,153).

CONCLUSION

Prenatal care can play an important role in limiting adverse perinatal outcomes associated with drug use. Berenson et al. (154) found that birth weight was improved in women who received prenatal care. Other investigators previously found that gestational age at delivery also was enhanced (155). These are two examples of why intervention in the pregnant woman's drug use during pregnancy can improve outcomes and benefit the offspring of the drug-abusing patient.

Recognition of risk factors and behaviors is key. Counseling patients on the seriousness of their actions and the effects on their children is the first step in helping them.

REFERENCES

1. Kandel DB, Warner LA, Kessler RC. *The epidemiology of substance use and dependence among women.* In: Wetherington NIDA Drug Addiction Research & the Health of Women CL, ed. Washington, D.C.: National Institutes of Health, 1998.
2. National Institute on Drug Abuse. *Pregnancy and drug use trends.* National Institutes of Health, 1999.
3. Young N. Alcohol and other drugs: the scope of the problem among pregnant and parenting women in California. *J Psychoactive Drugs* 1997;29:3–22.
4. Landry SH, Whitney JA. The impact of prenatal cocaine exposure: studies of the developing infant. *Semin Perinatol* 1996;20:99–106.
5. Shiono PH, Klebanoff MA, Nugent RP, et al. The impact of cocaine and marijuana use on low birth weight and preterm birth: a multicenter study. *Am J Obstet Gynecol* 1995;172:19–27.
6. National Center for Health Statistics, Health and Human Services Centers for Disease Control and Prevention. *Smoking during pregnancy,* 1996.
7. Quinn DI, Wodak A, Day RO. Pharmacokinetic and pharmacodynamic principles of illicit drug use and treatment of illicit drug users. *Clin Pharmacokinet* 1997;33:344–400.
8. Lambers DL, Clark KE. The maternal and fetal physiologic effects of nicotine. *Semin Perinatol* 1996;20:115–126.
9. Busto U, Bendayan R, Sellers EM. Clinical pharmacokinetics of non-opiate abused drugs. *Clin Pharmacokinet* 1989;16:1–26.
10. Benowitz NL. Pharmacologic aspects of cigarette smoking and nicotine addition. *N Engl J Med* 1988; 319:1318–1330.
11. Huisman M, Risseeuw B, van Eyck J, et al. Nicotine and caffeine, influence on prenatal hemodynamics; and behavior in early twin pregnancy. *J Reprod Med* 1997;42:731–734.
12. Lee M. Marihuana and tobacco use in pregnancy: substance abuse in pregnancy. *Obstet Gynecol Clin North Am* 1998;25:65–97.
13. Koren G. Fetal toxicology of environmental tobacco smoke. *Curr Opin Pediatr* 1995;7:128–131.
14. Luck W, Nau H, Hansen R, et al. Extent of nicotine and cotinine transfer to the human fetus, placenta and amniotic fluid of smoking mothers. *Dev Pharmacol Ther* 1985;8:384–395.
15. Morrow RJ, Ritchie JW, Bull SB. Maternal cigarette smoking: the effects on umbilical and uterine blood flow velocity. *Am J Obstet Gynecol* 1988;159:1069–1071.
16. Bruner JP, Forouzan I. Smoking and buccally administered nicotine: acute effect on uterine and umbilical vascular resistance. *J Reprod Med* 1991;36:435–440.
17. Walsh RA. Effects of maternal smoking on adverse pregnancy outcomes: examination of the criteria of causation. *Hum Biol* 1994;66:1059–1092.

18. Ogunyemi D, Jackson U, Buyske S, et al. Clinical and pathologic correlates of stillbirths in a single institution. *Acta Obstet Gynecol Scand* 1998;77:722–728.

19. Schellscheidt J, Jorch G, Menke J. Effects of heavy maternal smoking on intrauterine growth patterns in sudden infant death victims and surviving infants. *Eur J Pediatr* 1998;157:246–251.

20. Ahiborg G Jr, Bodin L. Tobacco smoke and pregnancy outcome among working women: a prospective study at prenatal care centers in Orebo County, Sweden. *Am J Epidemiol* 1991;133:338–347.

21. Schauer GM, Kalousek DK, Magee IF. Genetic causes of stillbirth. *Semin Perinatol* 1992;16:341–351.

22. Little RE, Weinberg CR. Risk factors for antepartum and intrapartum stillbirth. *Am J Epidemiol* 1993;137:1177–1189.

23. Raymond EG, Cattingius S, Kiley JL. Effects of maternal age, parity and smoking on the risk of stillbirth. *Br J Obstet Gynaecol* 1994;101:201–206.

24. Curry CJR. Pregnancy loss, stillbirth, and neonatal death. *Pediatr Clin North Am* 1992;39:157–192.

25. Alessandri LM, Stanley FJ, Read AW. A case control study of intrapartum deaths. *Br J Obstet Gynaecol* 1992;99:719–723.

26. Perrson P, Grennert L, Gennser G, et al. A study of smoking and pregnancy with special reference to fetal growth. *Acta Obstet Gynecol Scand* 1978;78:33–39.

27. Harger JH, Hsing AW, Tuomala RE, et al. Risk factors for preterm premature rupture of fetal membranes: a multicenter case controlled study. *Am J Obstet Gynecol* 1990;169:460–462.

28. Rickert VI, Wemann CM, Hankins GD, et al. Prevalence and risk factors of chorioamnionitis among adolescents. *Obstet Gynecol* 1998;92:254–257.

29. Newton ER. Chorioamnionitis and intraamniotic infection. *Clin Obstet Gynecol* 1993;36:795–808.

30. Andres RL. The association of cigarette smoking with placenta previa and abruptio placentae. *Semin Perinatol* 1996;20:154–159.

31. Naeye R. Abruptio placentae and placenta previa: frequency, perinatal mortality and cigarette smoking. *Obstet Gynecol* 1980;55:701–704.

32. Spinillo A, Capuzzo E, Colonna C, et al. Factors associated with abruptio placentae in preterm deliveries. *Acta Obstet Gynecol Scand* 1994;73:307–312.

33. Williams MA, Mittendorf R, Lieberman E, et al. Cigarette smoking during pregnancy in relation to placenta previa. *Am J Obstet Gynecol* 1991;165:28–32.

34. Kramer MD, Taylor V, Hickok DR, et al. Smoking and placenta previa. *Epidemiology* 1991;2:221–223.

35. Monica G, Lilja C. Placenta previa, maternal smoking and recurrence risk. *Acta Obstet Gynecol Scand* 1995;74:341–345.

36. Lindsay CA, Thomas AJ, Catalano PM. The effect of smoking tobacco on neonatal body composition. *Am J Obstet Gynecol* 1997;177:1124–1128.

37. Nordentoft M, Lou HC, Hansen D, et al. Intrauterine growth retardation and premature delivery: the influence of maternal smoking and psychosocial factors. *Am J Public Health* 1996;86:347–354.

38. Harrison GG, Branson RS, Vaucher YE. Association of maternal smoking with body composition of the newborn. *Am J Clin Nutr* 1983;38:757–762.

39. Cornelius MD, Taylor PM, Geva D, et al. Prenatal tobacco and marijuana use among adolescents: effects on offspring gestational age, growth, and morphology. *Pediatrics* 1995;95:738–743.

40. Kretchmer N, Schumacher LB, Silliman K. Biological factors affecting intrauterine growth. *Semin Perinatol* 1989;13:169–179.

41. Blair PS, Fleming PJ, Bensley D, et al. Smoking and the sudden infant death syndrome: results from 1993–5 case-control study for confidential inquiry into stillbirths and deaths in infancy. *BMJ* 1996;313:195–198.

42. Schellscheidt J, Jorch G. Epidemiologic features of sudden infant death (SID) after a German intervention campaign in 1992. *Eur J Pediatr* 1997;156:655–660.

43. Schellscheidt J, Oyen N, Jorch G. Interactions between maternal smoking and other prenatal risk factors for sudden infant death syndrome (SIDS). *Acta Paediatr* 1997;86:857–863.

44. Bulterys MG, Greenland S, Kraus JF. Chronic fetal hypoxia and sudden infant death syndrome: interaction between maternal smoking and low hematocrit during pregnancy. *Pediatrics* 1990;86:535–540.

45. Krous HF, Campbell GA, Fowler MW, et al. Maternal nicotine administration and fetal brain stem damage: a rat model with implications for the fetus. *Am J Obstet Gynaecol* 1981;140:743–746.

46. Maritz GS, Thomas RA. Maternal nicotine exposure: response of type II pneumocytes of neonatal rat pups. *Cell Biol Int* 1995;19:323–331.

47. Wuenschell CW, Zhao J, Tefft JD, et al. Nicotine stimulates branching and expression of SP-A and SP-C mRNAs in embryonic mouse lung culture. *Am J Physiol* 1998;274:L165–L170.

48. Van Marter LJ, Leviton A, Allred EN, et al. Persistent pulmonary hypertension of the newborn and smoking and aspirin and nonsteroidal antiinflammatory drug consumption during pregnancy. *Pediatrics* 1996;97:658–663.

49. Goldberg SJ, Levy RA, Siassi B, et al. The effects of maternal hypoxia and hyperoxia upon the neonatal pulmonary vasculature. *Pediatrics* 1971;48:528–533.

50. Gersony WM, Morishima HO, Daniel SS, et al. The hemodynamic effects of intrauterine hypoxia: an experimental model in newborn lambs. *J Pediatr* 1976;89:631–635.

51. Bearer C, Emerson RK, O'Riordan MA, et al. Maternal tobacco smoke exposure and persistent pulmonary hypertension of the newborn. *Environ Health Perspect* 1997;105:202–206.

52. Lodrup Carlsen KC, Jaakkola JJK, Nafstad P, et al. In utero exposure to cigarette smoking influences lung function at birth. *Eur Respir J* 1997;10:1774–1779.

53. Sipowicz MA, Amin S, Desai D, et al. Oxidative DNA damage in tissues of pregnant female mice and fetuses caused by the tobacco-specific nitrosamine, 4-(methyl-nitrosamino)-1-(3-pyridyl)-1-butanone (NNK): *Cancer Lett* 1997;117:87–91.

54. Daube H, Scherer G, Riedel K, et al. DNA adducts in human placenta in relation to tobacco smoke exposure and plasma antioxidant status. *J Cancer Res Clin Oncol* 1997;123:141–151.

55. Fried PA, Watkinson B, Siegel LS. Reading and language in 9 to 12 year old prenatally exposed to cigarettes and marijuana. *Neurotoxicol Teratol* 1997;19:171–183.

56. Butler NR, Goldstein H. Smoking in pregnancy and subsequent child development. *BMJ* 1973;4:573–575.

57. Naeya RL, Peters EC. Mental development of children whose mothers smoked during pregnancy. *Obstet Gynecol* 1984;64:601–607.

58. Fried PA, Watkinson B. 12 and 24 month neurobehavioral follow-up of children prenatally exposed to marijuana, cigarettes and alcohol. *Neurotoxicol Teratol* 1988;10:305–313.

59. Makin J, Fried PA, Watkinson B. 60- and 72-month follow-up of children prenatally exposed to marijuana, cigarettes, and alcohol. *J Dev Behav Pediatr* 1992;13: 383–391.

60. Abel AL. Smoking during pregnancy: a review of effects on growth and development of offspring. *Hum Biol* 1980;42:593–625.

61. Weitzman M, Gortmaker S, Sobel A. Maternal smoking and behavior problems of children. *Pediatrics* 1992;90:342–349.

62. Drews CD, Murphy CC, Yeargin-Allsopp M, et al. The relationship between idiopathic mental retardation and maternal smoking during pregnancy. *Pediatrics* 1996;97:547–553.

63. Rhainds M, Levallois P. Effects of maternal cigarette smoking and alcohol consumption on blood lead levels of newborns. *Am J Epidemiol* 1997;145:250–257.

64. Benowitz NL. Nicotine replacement therapy during pregnancy. *JAMA* 1991;266:3174–3177.

65. Tonnesen P, Fryd V, Hansen M, et al. Effect of nicotine chewing gum in combination with group counseling on the cessation of smoking. *N Engl Med* 1988;318:15–18.

66. Tonnesen P, Norregaard J, Simonsen K, et al. A double-blind trial of 16-hour transdermal nicotine patch in smoking cessation. *N Engl J Med* 1991;325:311–315.

67. Jimenez Ruiz C, Kunze M, Fagerstrom KO. Nicotine replacement: a new approach to reducing tobacco-related harm. *Eur Respir J* 1998;11:473–479.

68. Benowitz NL. Pharmacologic aspects of cigarette smoking and nicotine addiction. N Engl J Med 1988; 319:1318–1330.

69. Benowitz NL, Jacob P III, Savanapridi C. Determinants of nicotine intake while chewing nicotine polacrilex gum. *Clin Pharmacol Ther* 1987;41:467–473.

70. Benowitz NL, Chan K, Denaro CP, et al. Stable isotope methodology for studying transdermal drug absorption: the nicotine patch. *Clin Pharmacol Ther* 1991;50:286–293.

71. Wright LN, Thorp JM, Kuller JA, et al. Transdermal nicotine replacement in pregnancy: maternal pharmacokinetics and fetal effects. *Am J Obstet Gynecol* 1997;176:1090–1094.

72. Benowitz NL, Jacob P III. Intravenous nicotine replacement suppresses nicotine intake from cigarette smoking. *J Pharmacol Exp Ther* 1990;254:1000–1005.

73. Slotkin TA. Fetal nicotine or cocaine exposure: which one is worse? *J Pharmacol Exp Ther* 1998;285:931–945.

74. Centers for Disease Control and Prevention. *MMWR Morb Mortal Wkly Rep* 1997;46:345–350.

75. Centers for Disease Control and Prevention. *MMWR Morb Mortal Wkly Rep* 1995;44:249–264.

76. Armant DR, Saunders DE. Exposure of embryonic cells to alcohol: contrasting effects during preimplantation and postimplantation development. *Semin Perinatol* 1996;20:127–139.

77. Kopecky EA, Koren G. Maternal drug abuse: effects on the fetus and neonate. In: Polin RA, Fox WW, eds. *Fetal and neonatal physiology*. Philadelphia: WB Saunders, 1998;203–219.

78. Little BB, Van Beveren TT. Placental transfer of selected substances of abuse. *Semin Perinatol* 1996;20:147–153.

79. Blakley PM, Scott WJ Jr. Determination of the proximate teratogen of the mouse fetal alcohol syndrome. 2. Pharmacokinetics of the placental transfer of ethanol and acetaldehyde. *Toxicol Appl Pharmacol* 1984;72:364–371.

80. Kuhnert BR, Kuhnert PM. Placental transfer of drugs, alcohol, and components of cigarette smoke and their effects on the human fetus [review]. *NIDA Res Monogr* 1985;60:98–109.

81. Singh SP, Snyder AK, Pullen GL. Maternal alcohol ingestion inhibits fetal glucose uptake and growth. *Neurotoxicol Teratol* 1989;11:215–219.

82. Miller MW. *Development of the central nervous system: effects of alcohol and opiates.* New York: Wiley-Liss, 1991.

83. Windham GC, Von Behren J, Fenster L, et al. Moderate maternal alcohol consumption and risk of spontaneous abortion. *Epidemiology* 1997;8:509–514.

84. Harlap S, Shiono PH. Alcohol, smoking and incidence of spontaneous abortions in the first and second trimester. *Lancet* 1980;2:173–176.

85. Kline J, Shrout P, Stein Z, et al. Drinking during pregnancy and spontaneous abortion. *Lancet* 1980;2:176–180.

86. Zuckerman B. Developmental consequences of maternal drug use during pregnancy. *NIDA Res Monogr* 1985;59:96–106.

87. Sampson PD, Streissguth AP, Bookstein FL, et al. Incidence of fetal alcohol syndrome and prevalence of alcohol related neurodevelopmental disorder. *Teratology* 1997;56:317–326.

88. Sokol RJ, Miller SI, Reed G. Alcohol abuse during pregnancy: an epidemiologic study. *Alcohol Clin Exp Res* 1980;4:135–145.

89. Abel EL, Sokol RJ. A revised conservative estimate of the incidence of FAS and its economic impact. *Alcohol Clin Exp Res* 1991;15:514–524.

90. Young NK. Effects of alcohol and other drugs on children. *J Psychoactive Drugs* 1997;29:23–42.

91. Streissguth AP, Barr HM, Simpson PD. IQ at age 4 in relation to maternal alcohol use and smoking during pregnancy. *Dev Psychol* 1989;25:3–11.

92. Polygenis D, Wharton S, Malmberg C, et al. Moderate alcohol consumption during pregnancy and the incidence of fetal malformation: a meta-analysis. *Neurotoxicol Teratol* 1998;20:61–67.

93. Larroque B, Kaminski M. Prenatal alcohol exposure and development at preschool age: main results of a French study. *Alcohol Clin Exp Res* 1998;22:295–303.

94. Guefri C. Neuroanatomical and neurophysiological mechanisms involved in central nervous system dysfunctions induced by prenatal alcohol exposure. *Alcohol Clin Exp Res* 1998;22:304–312.

95. Streissguth AP, Barr HM, Sampson PD. Moderate prenatal alcohol exposure: effects on child IQ and learning problems at age 7 1/2 years. *Alcohol Clin Exp Res* 1990;14:662–669.

96. Streissguth AP, Sampson PD, Olson HC, et al. Maternal drinking during pregnancy: attention and short term memory in 14 year old offspring: a longitudinal prospective study. *Alcohol Clin Exp Res* 1994;18:202–218.

97. Olson HC, Streissguth AP, Sampson PD, et al. Association of prenatal alcohol exposure with behavioral and learning problems in early adolescence. *J Am Acad Child Adolesc Psychiatry* 1997;36:1187–1194.

98. Church MW, Kaltenbach A. Hearing, speech, language, and vestibular disorders in the fetal alcohol syndrome: a literature review. *Alcohol Clin Exp Res* 1997;21:495–512.

99. Church MW, Abel EL. Fetal alcohol syndrome: hearing, speech, language, and vestibular disorders. *Obstet Gynecol Clin North Am* 1998;25:85–98.

100. Church MW, Eldis F, Blakley BW, et al. Hearing, speech, language, vestibular and dentofacial disorders in the fetal alcohol syndrome (FAS). *Alcohol Clin Exp Res* 1997;21:227–237.

101. Church MW, Gerkin KP. Hearing disorders in children with fetal alcohol syndrome: findings from case reports. *Pediatrics* 1988;82:147–154.

102. Mattson SN, Riley EP. A review of the neurobehavioral deficits in children with fetal alcohol syndrome or prenatal exposure to alcohol. *Alcohol Clin Exp Res* 1998;22:279–294.

103. Aronson M, Hagberg B. Neuropsychological disorders in children exposed to alcohol during pregnancy: a followup study of 24 children to alcoholic mothers in Goteborg, Sweden. *Alcohol Clin Exp Res* 1998;22:321–324.

104. Steinhausen H-C, Spohr H-L. Long term outcome of children with fetal alcohol syndrome: psychopathology, behavior, and intelligence. *Alcohol Clin Exp Res* 1998;22:334–338.

105. Hanson JW, Jones KL, Smith DW. Fetal alcohol syndrome: experience with 41 patients. *JAMA* 1976;235:1458–1460

106. Aronson M, Hagberg B, Gillberg C. Attention deficits and autistic spectrum problems in children exposed to alcohol during gestation: a followup study. *Dev Med Child Neurol* 1997;39:583–587.

107. Bond NW, DiGiusto EL. Avoidance conditioning and Hebb-Williams maze performance in rats treated prenatally with alcohol. *Psychopharmacology* 1978;58:69–71.

108. Ulug S, Riley EP, The effect of methylphenidate on overactivity in rats prenatally exposed to alcohol. *Neurobehav Toxicol Teratol* 1983;5:35–39.

109. Mattson SN, Riley EP, Gramling L, et al. Heavy prenatal alcohol exposure with or without physical features of fetal alcohol syndrome leads to IQ deficits. *J Pediatr* 1997;131:718–721.

110. Jacobson SW. Specificity of neurobehavioral outcomes associated with prenatal alcohol exposure. *Alcohol Clin Exp Res* 1998;22:313–320.

111. Roebuck TM, Mattson SN, Riley EP. A review of the neuroanatomical findings in children with fetal alcohol syndrome or prenatal exposure to alcohol. *Alcohol Clin Exp Res* 1998;22:339–344.

112. Mattson SN, Riley EP, Jernigan TL, et al. A decrease in the size of the basal ganglia following prenatal alcohol exposure: a preliminary report. *Neurotoxicol Teratol* 1994;16:283–289.

113. Mattson SN, Riley EP, Jernigan TL, et al. Fetal alcohol syndrome: A case report of neuropsychological, MRI, EEG assessment of two children. *Alcohol Clin Exp Res* 1992;16:1001–1003.

114. Druse MJ. Effects of in utero ethanol exposure on the development of neurotransmitter system. In: Watson RR, ed. *Development of the central nervous system: effects of alcohol and opiates.* New York: Wiley-Liss, 1992:139–167.

115. Sowell ER, Mattson SN, Riley EP, et al. A reduction in the area of the anterior cerebellar vermis in children exposed to alcohol prenatally. *Alcohol Clin Exp Res* 1995;19:53A(abst).

116. Clarren SK. Recognition of fetal alcohol syndrome. *JAMA* 1981;245:2436–2439.

117. Meyer LS, Kotch LE, Riley EP. Neonatal ethanol exposure: functional alterations associated with cerebellar growth retardation. *Neurotoxicol Teratol* 1990;12:15–22.

118. Gladstone J, Nulman I, Koren G. Reproductive risks of binge drinking during pregnancy. *Reprod Toxicol* 1996;10:1–11.

119. Pierce DR, West JR. Blood alcohol concentration: a critical factor for producing fetal alcohol effects. *Alcohol* 1986;3:269–272.

120. West JR, Goodlett CR, Bonthius DJ, et al. Manipulating peak blood alcohol concentrations in neonatal rats: review of an animal model for alcohol-related developmental effects. *Neurotoxicology* 1989;10:347–365.

121. Gladstone J, Levy M, Nulman I, Koren G. Characteristics of pregnant women who engage in binge alcohol consumption. *Can Med Assoc J* 1997;156:789–794.

122. Chang G, Wilkins Haug L, Berman S, et al. Alcohol use and pregnancy: improving identification. *Obstet Gynecol* 1998;91:892–898.

123. Rostenberg PO. *Alcohol and other drug screening of hospitalized trauma patients.* SAMHSA Center for Substance Abuse Treatment. Washington D.C.: U.S. Department of Health, 1995.

124. Warner EA, Kosten TR, O'Connor PG. Pharmacotherapy for opioid and cocaine abuse. *Med Clin North Am* 1997;81:909–925.

125. *Heroin.* National Institute on Drug Abuse, National Institutes of Health, 1999.

126. Sawe J. High-dose morphine and methadone in cancer patients: clinical pharmacokinetic considerations of oral treatment. *Clin Pharmacokinet* 1986;11:87–106.

127. *Heroin: abuse and addiction.* NIDA Research Report, NIH publication no. 97-4165, 1997.

128. Hutchings DE. Prenatal opioid exposure and the problem of causal inference. *NIDA Res Monogr* 1985;59:6–19.

129. Kreek MJ. Opiate and cocaine addictions: challenge for pharmacotherapies. *Pharmacol Biochem Behav* 1997;57:551–569.

130. Schnoll SH, Weaver MF. Pharmacology: gender specific considerations in the use of psychoactive medications. In: Wetherington CL, Roman AB, eds. *NIDA Drug Addict Res Health Women.* Washington, D.C.: National Institutes of Health, 1998:223–228.

131. Kaltenbach K, Berghella V, Finnegan L. Opioid dependence during pregnancy: effects and management. *Obstet Gynecol Clin North Am* 1998;25:139–152.

132. Wittman BK, Segal SA. A comparison of the effects of single- and split-dose methadone administration on the fetus: ultrasound evaluation. *Int J Addict* 1991;26:213–218.

133. Pond SM, Kreek MJ, Tong TG, et al. Altered methadone pharmacokinetics in methadone-maintained pregnant women. *J Pharmacol Exp Ther* 1985;233:1–6.

134. Jarvis MA, Schnoll SH. Methadone use during pregnancy. *NIDA Res Monogr* 1995;149:58–77.

135. Finnegan LP, Wapner RJ. Narcotic addiction in pregnancy. In: Niebyl JR, ed. *Drug use in pregnancy.* Philadelphia: Lea and Febiger, 1987.

136. Kaltenbach K, Silverman N, Wapner RJ. Methadone maintenance during pregnancy. State methadone treatment guidelines. Rockville, MD: Center for Substance Abuse Treatment, U.S. Department of Health and Human Services, 1992:85–93.

137. Kreek MJ, Schenter A, Gutjahr Cl, et al. Analyses of methadone and other drugs in maternal and neonatal body fluids: use in evaluation of symptoms in neonate of mother maintained on methadone. *Am J Drug Alcohol Abuse* 1974;1:409–419.

138. Poland Lake M, Fry McComish J, Ager J. Predictors of prenatal substance use and birth weight during outpatient treatment. *J Subst Abuse Treat* 1997;14:359–366.

139. Newman R, Bashkow S, Calko D. Results of 313 consecutive live births of infants delivered to patients in the New York City methadone treatment program. *Am J Obstet Gynecol* 1975;121:233–237.

140. Barr GA, Zmitrovich A, Hamowy AS, et al. Neonatal withdrawal following pre- and postnatal exposure to methadone in the rat. *Pharmacol Biochem Behav* 1998;60:97–104.

141. Hulse GK, Milne E, English DR, et al. The relationship between maternal use of heroin and methadone and infant birth weight. *Addiction* 1997;92:1571–1579.

142. Vance JC, Chant DC, Tudehope DI, et al. Infants born to narcotic dependent mothers: physical growth patterns in the first 12 months of life. *J Paediatr Child Health* 1997;33:504–508.

143. Wong WM, Lao TT. Abnormal umbilical artery flow velocity waveform–a sign of fetal narcotic withdrawal? *Aust N Z J Obstet Gynaecol* 1997;37:358–359.

144. Blinick G, Wallach RC, Ferez E. Pregnancy in narcotics addicts treated by medical withdrawal. The methadone detoxification program. *Am J Obstet Gynecol* 1969;105:997–1003.

145. Briggs G, Bodendorfer T, Freeman R, et al. *Drugs in pregnancy and lactation*. Baltimore: Williams & Wilkins, 1993.

146. Anyaegbunam A, Tran T, Jadali D, et al. Assessment of fetal well being in methadone maintained pregnancies: abnormal nonstress tests. *Gynecol Obstet Invest* 1997;43:25–28.

147. Archie CL, Lee MI, Sokol RJ, et al. The effects of methadone treatment on the reactivity of the nonstress test. *Obstet Gynecol* 1989;74:254–255.

148. Rosen TS, Johnson HL. Long term effects of prenatal methadone maintenance. *NIDA Res Monogr* 1985;59:73–83.

149. Doberczak TM, Kandall SR, Friedmann P. Relationship between maternal methadone dosage, maternal neonatal methadone levels, and neonatal withdrawal. *Obstet Gynecol* 1993;81:936–940.

150. Blinick G, Jerez E, Wallach RC. Methadone maintenance, pregnancy and progeny. *JAMA* 1973;225:477–479.

151. Jarvis MA, Schnoll SH. Methadone treatment during pregnancy. *J Psychoactive Drugs* 1995;26:155–161.

152. Zuspan FP, Gumpel JA, Mejia-Zelaya A, et al. Fetal stress from methadone withdrawal. *Am J Obstet Gynecol* 1975;122:43–46.

153. Chasnoff LF, Hatcher R, Burno WJ. Polydrug and methadone addicted newborns: a continuum of impairment? *Pediatrics* 1982;70:210.

154. Berenson AB, Wilkinson GS, Lopez LA. Effects of prenatal care on neonates born to drug using women. *Subst Use Misuse* 1996;31:1063–1076.

155. MacGregor SN, Keith LG, Bachicha JA, et al. Cocaine abuse during pregnancy: correlation between prenatal care and perinatal outcome. *Obstet Gynecol* 1989;74:882–885.

14

Licit and Illicit Drugs: Marijuana and Cocaine

Melissa H. Fries*, Gail Best[†], and James R. Woods, Jr.[‡]

*Program Director, Obstetrics and Gynecology, Clinical Geneticist, Air Force Medical Genetics
Center, 81st Medical Group, Keesler Medical Center, Keesler Air Force Base, Missisipi;
[†]Department of Obstetrics and Gynecology, University of Rochester, Strong Memorial Hospital,
Rochester, New York;
[‡]Strong Memorial Hospital, Division of Maternal/Fetal Medicine, Rochester, New York

MARIJUANA

Marijuana is a substance that originates from the plant *Cannabis sativa* (also known as the hemp plant) which is the source of several illicit drug products. Its fibrous stems are still legally used for making rope and cloth; the dried leaves and flowers are the source of marijuana, or pot, and the extract of its resinous juices is called hashish (1). The major psychoactive component is delta-9-tetrahydrocannabinol (THC) available as dronabinol for controlling nausea and vomiting during chemotherapy. This is one of 61 chemicals contained in cannabis that are known as cannabinoids (2,3). The effects caused by marijuana, in addition to its psychoactive properties, are attention and memory impairment and cognitive impairment. The desired effects of its users are euphoria, excitement, hallucinations, and hypnosis (3).

Pharmacokinetics

Most illicitly used cannabis is smoked or occasionally eaten because THC is lipid soluble and readily absorbed through the lungs or gastrointestinal tract. When inhaled, the onset of its effects is rapid, usually occurring within 6 to 12 minutes, and maximum effects are experienced at 15 to 30 minutes. Acute effects are dose dependent, lasting 2 to 4 hours (4). As a result of its affinity for lipids, marijuana will accumulate in adipose tissue. Despite its presence, it produces no long-lasting psychoactive effects but will result in positive urine drug tests for as long as 10 days after exposure (2,3,5).

Two receptors for cannabis have been identified: one in the central nervous system, which responds directly to THC, and a peripheral receptor in the spleen, which may involve pain and anxiety control (6). In the lungs and the liver, THC is converted to 11-hydroxy-THC (11-OH-THC), which is an active metabolite (2,3,7). In the liver, this compound is converted to inactive metabolites and then is excreted by the kidneys (3,5). THC appears to freely cross the placenta (8–10).

In addition to euphoria and relaxation, marijuana's effects include improvement in appetite and energy, reduction in nausea, and reduction in general anxiety. Adverse effects may relate to age of the user. In adolescents, cannabis intoxication has an adverse effect on learning and cognitive function and behavior, and dependency and, rarely, psychosis can develop (11). In adults, significant differences in speed of psychomotor performance, estimation of moderate distances and time intervals, short-term memory, and visuomotor coordination have been described in chronic marijuana users compared with nonusing controls (12). Infrequent social smoking of marijuana is not associated with detectable pulmonary impairment in healthy young men, although heavy use may lead to early components of obstructive airway disease (13). The greatest concerns for marijuana use continue to be its potential for concomitant use with other drugs, such as alcohol, tobacco, and crack cocaine.

Effects on Pregnancy

Marijuana use in pregnancy has been the subject of a Maternal Health Practices and Child Development Project I. Based on intake interviews of equal numbers of low income black and white women attending a prenatal clinic at 4 months of gestation, 30% reported marijuana use during the first trimester, although a significant decline was noted in use throughout gestation, from 24% in the first month to 12% in the second month to 7% in the third trimester. Heavy users were least likely to discontinue their use. Those who continued to use during pregnancy were more likely to be black, single, of lower socioeconomic status, less educated, and younger; in addition, they were also more likely to use alcohol, tobacco, and other illicit drugs. No specific effects of prenatal marijuana exposure in terms of length of gestation, labor, or delivery complications were identified (14). Adolescents who used marijuana were more likely to deliver at lower gestational age than controls, although no significant increase in prematurity was noted. This finding was observed at marijuana use levels less than that described in adult studies, suggesting that young maternal age may have an increased negative effect in association with marijuana (15). Animal concerns for increased stillbirths or embryo toxicity related to marijuana exposure have not been borne out in human studies, in which no increase in spontaneous abortions was seen in a large study of more than 500 women using marijuana in the first trimester of pregnancy compared with 2,000 nonusing controls (16). A study of fetal body proportionality in infants exposed prenatally to cocaine or marijuana did not demonstrate decrease in birth weight, although detection of marijuana metabolites in maternal urine at least once during pregnancy or postpartum was associated with a decreased mean arm muscle circumference and nonfat area of the arm (17). This was thought to reflect a hypoxic effect on growth, which might have been confounded by tobacco

use. In a comparison of carboxy and oxyhemoglobin levels in pregnant ewes, tobacco smoke exposure was associated with a greater increase in carboxyhemoglobin than marijuana smoke exposure, although greater and more prolonged declines in oxyhemoglobin were noted after marijuana smoke exposure (18).

No increase in minor or major anomalies has been observed in infants of marijuana-using mothers (19,20). In Jamaica, where marijuana use is common but not typically associated with cocaine, no increase in anomalies has been described, even among heavy daily users (21).

There are several problems with interpretation of studies of marijuana use in pregnancy. It is difficult to determine whether any poor outcomes are the consequence of direct effects of the drug itself or a secondary result of maternal physical and behavioral changes from THC use. For example, is low birth weight owing to drug exposure or the outcome expected of a pregnant woman who has decreased her food intake because of marijuana use (2,22,23)? Drug exposure is difficult to measure as a result of varying smoking techniques. In addition, other substances are present in varying amounts in blends of marijuana cigarettes, and therefore the effect of each component cannot be determined (2).

Studies of fetal growth in women who use marijuana during pregnancy have not produced consistent results. Some show a negative effect on fetal growth, others show no effect, and still others have found children to be both taller and heavier. There has been some evidence that there may be an association of growth restriction with heavier and regular marijuana use (2,22,24–28).

Differing study populations may explain, in part, the inconsistent findings. The simultaneous use of tobacco presents another limitation to these studies. Tobacco often is used by those who smoke marijuana. The association of maternal tobacco use with intrauterine growth restriction is well established. Therefore, when growth restriction is present, it is difficult to establish whether it is the result of tobacco or marijuana use or both. There are other factors to consider as well. Cannabis mixtures often contain tobacco, and therefore it is difficult to measure exposure to marijuana. Differing smoking techniques, as previously mentioned, make comparisons difficult (22,24,25).

Postnatal Effects

There is no evidence that marijuana has teratogenic effects. A clear picture of outcomes in the long term, however, has not been established. There have been some conflicting results among the different studies. Some have shown negative effects on certain areas of development, but these findings were not consistent. This again brings up the question of whether a poor outcome is the direct effect of *in utero* exposure or the result of poor child care by a parent who uses marijuana (2,9,11,29).

Marijuana use throughout pregnancy has been associated with some mild withdrawal symptoms in the newborn (30,31) that typically do not require treatment. No increased frequency of sudden infant death syndrome (SIDS) has been observed (32). The acoustic characteristics of the cries of the infants of marijuana users in Jamaica have been noted to differ from nonusers in higher frequency, but shorter length with higher proportion of disphonation, suggesting an effect on neurophysiologic integrity (33).

One study found that infants of mothers who used marijuana during pregnancy responded less frequently to visual stimuli and also had more tremors (34,35). The question arises, as it does with other illicit substances, as to the long-term effects on the neurobehavioral function of these children and the consequences when they are adults. Longitudinal studies of infants with a history of prenatal tobacco or marijuana exposure at 12 and 24 months did not demonstrate a decline in motor, mental, or language variables relative to controls, although this was seen with tobacco exposure (36). However, the same infants studied at 36 and 48 months did demonstrate some significantly lower scores in verbal and memory domains, even after adjustment for confounding socioeconomic variables (37). When studied at 9 and 12 years of age, however, no differences were noted in reading, language, or WISC-III for the marijuana-exposed

children, although some deficiencies were noted in executive function tasks, impulse control, and visual analysis/hypothesis testing (29,38). Another longitudinal study of school-age children exposed prenatally to alcohol and marijuana did not disclose any negative effects on gross motor development (39).

Prenatal and postnatal exposure to marijuana (as well as other mind-altering drugs) has also been associated epidemiologically with an increased risk for the development of acute non-lymphoblastic leukemia in the exposed child (40). It has been shown that marijuana smokers have a higher frequency of mutations in the *hprt* gene. Although a relatively small number of offspring were tested in one study, it was shown that children of marijuana smokers also had a higher frequency of these mutations than did children of nonsmokers (41).

To summarize, isolated prenatal marijuana exposure does not seem to be linked with perinatal or fetal abnormalities beyond mild growth delay. However, long-term follow-up studies do suggest some subtle cognitive findings in exposed children as well as a potential increase in a rare childhood leukemia.

COCAINE

Pharmacologic Actions

Cocaine is an alkaloid extracted from the leaves of the coca or *Erythroxylon* plant grown in the Andes Mountains of South America. When treated with hydrochloric acid, the cocaine (or benzoylmethylecogonine) becomes soluble cocaine hydrochloride salt, which can be readily absorbed by nasal and mucous membranes or injected intravenously or intramuscularly. Freebase cocaine and crack cocaine are alkaloid derivatives. Freebase cocaine is extracted with ether, which later evaporates, and smoked; the persistence of ether remnants leads to the volatility of this process and the potential for severe burns. Crack cocaine is made by dissolving the cocaine hydrochloride in water and treatment with baking soda; the base settles out as a soft mass that hardens into the "rocks" of crack after drying. Crack is typically smoked either in a pipe or mixed with tobacco or marijuana (42).

Its derivations have a wide variety of actions on multiple systems in the body. Although cocaine does have clinical applications, its most widely recognized use is as a psychostimulant. The three general pharmacologic actions are release of catecholamines, blockade of reuptake of amine neurotransmitters, and local anesthesia (43–47).

Central Nervous System

In the central nervous system (CNS), cocaine acts as a stimulant, producing feelings of profound euphoria, alertness, and enhanced self-esteem. Drives are heightened and cocaine users experience increased sexual interest and become uninhibited and hyperactive. There are increased self-confidence and loss of fear within seconds or minutes. Heavy users become anxious and suspicious, and there is tolerance to the euphoria. With increased amounts of cocaine, central stimulation is followed by depression, and respiratory failure can occur. Other CNS reactions to an acute overdose are seizures and strokes (44,45,47).

Cardiovascular System

There also are effects on the cardiovascular system from cocaine use. Small doses produce a slowing of the heart rate, whereas larger doses cause an increased heart rate. The increased heart rate is the result of central sympathetic stimulation and effects on the sympathetic nervous system. Tachycardia and vasoconstriction produce elevated blood pressure. The consequence of the actions on the cardiovascular system can be death when cocaine is administered intravenously in a large dose. Death results from arrhythmias, myocardial infarction, and cardiac failure (45).

Temperature

Cocaine causes an elevation in body temperature. The pyrogenic effect is secondary to increased muscle activity from stimulation. There is an enhancement of body heat production. Additionally, heat loss is limited as a result of the cardiovascular change of vasoconstriction. A rise in body temperature also may be the result of CNS activity. Heat-regulating centers may be stimulated directly by cocaine (45).

Sympathetic Nervous System

Cocaine causes organs that are sympathetically innervated to have a heightened response to norepinephrine. Cocaine blocks the uptake of catecholamines at adrenergic nerve endings (45).

Local Anesthetic Actions

Cocaine can be used clinically because of its ability after local application to block the initiation and conduction of the nerve impulse (45).

Other Physiologic Effects

Pulmonary complications, gastrointestinal ulceration and perforation, and acute renal failure are also well described (42).

Pregnancy

The effects of cocaine in pregnancy are theorized to be the result of vasoconstriction of arterial beds (46,48–50). This is believed to be the result of the blockade of the reuptake of norepinephrine at nerve terminals. This results in accumulation in these regions, followed by distribution to other areas. There is enhanced cardiovascular activity in pregnancy with cocaine use, which is caused by the elevated levels of norepinephrine in the circulation (46,48,51,52). It is not known whether this increase in cardiovascular response differs during the three trimesters of pregnancy (51). It has been concluded that fetal oxygenation is decreased as a result of vasoconstriction that leads to uterine ischemia. Oxygen content and uterine blood flow have been found to be decreased and uterine vascular resistance increased in studies of cocaine use in pregnant sheep (46,53).

Cocaine Withdrawal

Symptoms of withdrawal from cocaine are neuropsychological rather than physiologic because decreasing levels of cocaine produce dysphoria. Other withdrawal symptoms include depression, fatigue, sleep pattern changes, and cravings for cocaine (44,54).

Pharmacokinetics

There are three common modes of delivery of cocaine: inhalation of smoked preparations, intravenous injection, and intranasal inhalation of cocaine. Cocaine is rapidly absorbed regardless of its route of use, the rate of distribution is rapid, and the volume of distribution is large. The most rapid delivery is through smoked cocaine, with a lung-to-CNS transit time of 6 to 8 seconds. CNS exposure occurs within 12 to 16 seconds with intravenous injection, and the effects are felt within 2 to 5 minutes when cocaine is snorted. The limiting factor with snorting cocaine is the rate of absorption by the nasal mucosa, where vasoconstriction occurs as a result of cocaine use (43,55–57).

The half-life of cocaine ranges from 30 to 80 minutes. Cocaine is metabolized to several metabolites, including ecgonine methyl ester, ecgonine, benzoylecgonine, and norcocaine. The half-life of its major metabolites, which are inactive, is 4 to 6 hours. Route of delivery does affect the half-life. Nasal administration has a longer half-life than smoking or intravenous use. Consumption of alcohol with cocaine prolongs the euphoria because of the transformation of cocaine to cocaethylene, which has a half-life of almost 3 hours (42). Norcocaine has a variable half-life. This metabolite may be responsible for some of the adverse effects exhibited after cocaine use (43,48,57,58).

Transfer across the placenta is very rapid (46,59,60). Because plasma cholinesterase activity is decreased in fetuses and pregnant women, cocaine levels may actually be higher in the fetus than in the mother (61).

The actions of cocaine are achieved by blocking the uptake and removal of catecholamines, particularly norepinephrine, dopamine, and serotonin, from the presynaptic nerve terminals, with the resultant accumulation of catecholamines in the synaptic cleft and stimulus of the cell receptors.

It also has a substantial local anesthetic effect through blockage of fast sodium channels in the nerves, decreasing conduction of nerve impulses in peripheral nerves as well as cardiac channels (42).

Treatment of the acutely intoxicated individual may involve lowering the blood pressure with clonidine or labetalol; use of benzodiazepines is helpful in dealing with agitation and seizure prevention (62). Patients withdrawing from cocaine in treatment programs have benefited to some extent by treatment with amantadine or bromocriptine for reduction of symptoms of craving and subsequent use (62).

Metabolism of cocaine is quicker in women than in men. The rise to peak drug concentration is more rapid, and the peak concentration is higher in men than in women. There appears to be a hormonal effect because there is a difference in peak drug concentration during the different parts of the menstrual cycle (43,63,64).

Epidemiology of Cocaine Use

The number of women using cocaine during pregnancy is difficult to establish accurately. In one large multicenter study of drug use during pregnancy, the prevalence of cocaine use was 2.3%. Screening using biochemical markers of metabolites has shown lower prevalence rates of 1.1%. The difficulty in establishing accurate data results from the inconsistent testing of patients and from patient knowledge of drug testing. Many cocaine users are familiar with the fact that urine drug screening will usually give negative results after 72 hours of use. Thus, in many cases, they know when they can alter their use patterns, based on their prenatal appointments and expected testing times. Moreover, many caregivers do not ask everyone about drug use and only test certain patients. Therefore, reports of prevalence of use are inaccurate (48,65,66).

Smoking status, family history of alcohol and/or other drug problems, drug use by a current male partner, depression, and unstable living situation were found in one study to be predictors of cocaine use during pregnancy (67). Other studies found that the drug use is correlated with multiple social and psychological problems (68).

Antepartum Effects

The relatively low cost of crack cocaine, general ease of cocaine use, and its rapid mood-elevating effects create a high potential for addiction. Its means of use, in tobacco or marijuana cigarettes as well as with alcohol, lead to an almost obligatory polydrug status for those exposed. Although the perinatal effects of maternal cocaine exposure have been largely attributed to its cardiovascular effects of hypertension and vasoconstriction, these clearly interact with other socioeconomic concerns and polydrug exposure (48). Burkett et al. (69) report that less than half of the prior pregnancies in cocaine-using women delivering in a high-risk institution actually resulted in term liveborn infants. This may be related to an increased potential for spontaneous abortions, an increased use of therapeutic abortions instead of contraception, and the actual use of cocaine as a putative abortifacient (70).

The cardiovascular effects of cocaine during pregnancy include a pronounced increase in maternal heart rate and blood pressure, with decreased blood flow to the heart, brain, and uterus. Fetal blood pressure, heart rate, and fetal cerebral blood flow are increased, but fetal intestinal blood flow is decreased (46). The risk of placental abruption has been reported widely as being increased among pregnant women who use cocaine. It is believed that the cardiovascular changes secondary to cocaine use are related to the increased incidence of placental abruption (48,71,72). A 4.5 adjusted relative risk has been noted for placental abruption (73), which was also confirmed in a metaanalysis that found a pooled odds ratio for abruptio placentae and maternal cocaine use of 3.92 [95% confidence interval (CI) 2.77 to 5.46] (74).

Studies of isolated myometrial strips have also shown a dose-dependent increase in the frequency, duration, and force of spontaneous contractions with cocaine exposure (75,76). These findings may contribute to the increased frequency of preterm labor (as high as 50%) reported in chronic cocaine users (77).

The incidence of preterm premature rupture of membranes (PPROM) is increased in some populations with cocaine use, with Delaney et al. (78) reporting earlier gestational age at rupture and longer latency despite more advanced cervical dilatation in cocaine-positive patients compared with nonusers. There are conflicting results regarding the latency period (length of time from rupture of membranes to labor) in those who have PPROM associated with cocaine use. In one study, latency was decreased, whereas in another, it was increased. The increased latency period may be explained by the fact that, in that study, PPROM tended to occur at an earlier gestational age (78,79). PPROM may result from the same factor that plays a role in preterm labor, increased contractile activity (48,78).

Epidemiologic studies showed an association between maternal cocaine exposure and low birth weight (80–83). A retrospective cohort study of perinatal outcome for substance abuse or use in pregnancy compared with nonusing controls showed a 2.4 adjusted relative risk for prematurity, a 2.8 adjusted relative risk for low birth weight, and a 2.1 adjusted relative risk for perinatal death (73). In many of these studies, however, maternal tobacco use was not adjusted for. Tobacco use in pregnancy has an established association with low birth weight. In many cases, there are other factors, in addition to smoking, that are related to cocaine use that may contribute to low birth weight. Poor nutritional status, low socioeconomic status, and polydrug use frequently are present in these populations. In studies that have controlled for confounding variables, cocaine use was found to be associated with a higher risk of fetal growth restriction, and this appears to be dose dependent (84–87). Additionally, there have been findings of a smaller head circumference among infants of cocaine users (80,82).

Maternal cocaine use has also been identified as an independent risk factor for placenta previa, particularly in association with prior cesarean delivery, elective abortion, and multiparity (all of which may be increased as well with a history of chronic cocaine use) (88). Cesarean deliveries in cocaine-using women are most commonly for fetal distress and placental abruption (89).

Maternal Effects

In addition to the cardiovascular and other complications noted earlier, pulmonary complications are prevalent in those who inhale cocaine. These include asthma, pulmonary hypertension, chronic cough, respiratory infections, and pneumothorax (90,91). Although there is no increased risk of alveolar rupture in pregnancy owing to inhalation of cocaine, there is an increased risk of hypoxia owing to pneumothorax. This is the result of changes in oxygen consumption that occur during pregnancy. Spontaneous pneumothorax in pregnancy is rare; there have been case reports of pneumothorax in pregnancy that was associated with cocaine use (90).

Some case reports suggest an association between thrombocytopenia and cocaine use in pregnancy. One retrospective study of an inner city population did find a possible relationship between cocaine use and transient thrombocytopenia. This relationship was determined after exclusion of patients who either were human immunodeficiency virus–positive or had other medical conditions known to be associated with thrombocytopenia. Although further investigation is needed, it is important, however, to keep these findings in mind when caring for pregnant patients who recently have used cocaine (91,92).

Fetal/Teratogenic Effects

There have been many reports of congenital abnormalities associated with cocaine exposure in pregnancy. A definite connection has not been established, however, as some studies have not demonstrated a significant increased risk (93–95). It is believed that, as a result of increased uterine vascular resistance, fetal hypoxemia is present. Damage then occurs as a result of vasoconstriction and reperfusion. It has been found that the defects produced by hypoxia in animal studies are similar to those reported to occur in humans after cocaine exposure (48,86,93).

Numerous congenital anomalies have been reported in human fetuses after maternal cocaine exposure. These can be characterized as (i) genitourinary anomalies, (ii) cardiac anomalies, (iii) CNS anomalies, (iv) ophthalmologic abnormalities, and (v) limb anomalies/vascular disruptions. Genitourinary anomalies, including hypospadias, hydronephrosis, ambiguous genitalia in a female with anal atresia and absent uterus and ovaries, prune belly syndrome in males and masculinization of the female genitalia, and a cloacal anomaly have been reported in infants born to cocaine- and polydrug-using mothers (96,97). An increase in cardiac abnormalities, including peripheral pulmonic stenosis, patent ductus arteriosus, ventricular septal defects, and atrial septal defects, has been observed in infants of cocaine- and polydrug-using mothers, as high as a rate of 65 per 1,000 livebirths in infants positive for cocaine metabolites on neonatal urine toxicology (98,99). CNS abnormalities reported after maternal cocaine use include acute infarctions, hydranencephaly, holoprosencephaly, porencephaly, hypoplastic corpus callosum, intraparenchymal hemorrhage, cerebral infarction, and encephalomalacia (100–102). Optic nerve abnormalities, including unilateral and bilateral optic nerve hypoplasia, severe bilateral optic atrophy, and microphthalmia with coloboma, as well as delayed visual maturation, retinal hemorrhages, persistent hypoplastic primary vitreous, and eyelid edema have been reported in infants with positive urine toxicology for cocaine (103–106). The findings of marked periorbital and eyelid edema, low nasal bridge with transverse crease short nose, lateral soft tissue nasal build up, prominent glabella, large fontanels, small toenails, and neurologic irritability have been described as distinctive for a potential "fetal cocaine" facies (107), although other researchers failed to substantiate these findings with consistency (108). Fetal vascular disruption has been suggested as the common pathogenesis for many of these specific findings, particularly congenital limb reduction abnormalities, such as unilateral terminal transverse limb reduction defects, atypical ectrodactyly, radial ray anomalies, and the Poland anomaly, which have also been described in association with prenatal cocaine exposure (49). Vascular compromise, either through the development of hemorrhage after an increase in fetal blood pressure or vasoconstriction with resultant hypoperfusion and hypoxia, is postulated to lead to disruption of existing structures and altered morphogenesis of developing structures. Such disruption is thought to be responsible for the development of some cases of limb defects, porencephaly, gastroschisis, hypoglossi, intestinal atresia/stenosis, and renal anomalies such as renal agenesis/dysgenesis. However, a review of the frequency of these anomalies from 1968 to 1989 (the time period of greatly increased cocaine use) in the Metropolitan Atlanta Congenital Defects Program showed no increase in the frequency of these anomalies (109). An odds ratio of 1.58 for cocaine exposure and vascular disruption (95% CI, 0.55 to 4.47) has been calculated based on a review of more than 68,000 deliveries at a large urban referral hospital, supporting this mechanism for fetal injury as a relatively small contributor to the actions of cocaine (110). Fetal growth retardation, however, is a consistent observation, typically with low birth weight for fetal age. In a comparison of the effects of marijuana and cocaine, prenatal cocaine use was associated with a decrease in fetal fat (111). Meta-analysis of studies of cocaine effects on birth weight concluded that maternal cocaine use caused low birth weight and that the effect was greater for heavier use (85). Although birth weight and length are significantly reduced in cocaine-exposed infants compared with unexposed, this finding is not always persistent after adjusting for the concomitant effects of marijuana, alcohol, and tobacco. However, the combined effect of tobacco use and cocaine exposure has been shown to lead to a significant but not dramatic decrease in fetal head and chest circumference (82). Poor fetal growth is common, but no consistent cocaine embryopathy can be clearly demonstrated.

Neurobehavioral Effects

In addition to physical effects on the offspring of cocaine users, there have been many reports of adverse effects on the behavioral and cognitive development of newborns. The resulting long-term outcomes are of concern (112). It is difficult to assess the development of these children and relate findings to a direct effect of cocaine. Other factors may have a role in cognitive and behavioral maturation. Polysubstance abuse is not uncommon. Therefore, adverse consequences could be owing to the other drugs used.

Long-term studies of the behavior of cocaine-exposed children are ongoing and have yielded conflicting results. A blinded study of infants of cocaine-using Caucasian mothers who also used marijuana, alcohol, or tobacco showed that cocaine-exposed newborns were developmentally at risk using the Neonatal Neurobehavioral Risk Summary Score (81). Early studies of cocaine exposure also suggested an increased frequency of SIDS (113). However, a 2-year follow-up of infants who tested positive for drugs on meconium assay (30% positive for cocaine) did not reveal an overall increase in mortality or incidence of SIDS in this time period, despite a high perinatal morbidity. A significantly higher mortality rate was observed among infants with birth weights of less than 2,500 g who were positive for both cocaine and opiates (114). Assessment of controls and cocaine-exposed infants and their mothers using the Neonatal Behavioral Assessment Scale and the Nursing Child Assessment of Feeding Scale could not detect any clinically meaningful effects of cocaine exposure on behavior or maternal-child interaction (115). However, subsequent studies of infants of women identified prenatally as cocaine users and nonusers who were administered the Brazelton Neonatal Behavioral Assessment Scale did demonstrate a dose- and time of exposure–related decline in exposed infants' scores in state regulation (the ability to maintain alertness), attention, and responsiveness (116).

Longitudinal follow-up of the developmental competence of children exposed to cocaine, marijuana, and alcohol prenatally compared with unexposed children and those exposed only to marijuana and alcohol demonstrated catch-up growth by 18 months of age, although the height at 2 years of both exposed groups was significantly shorter than that of the unexposed groups. At all ages, the exposed infants had lower mean head circumferences than the unexposed infants; head size correlated significantly with the Bayley Mental Development scale. However, at age 2 years, the mean developmental scores did not differ significantly between groups, although more cocaine-exposed than unexposed infants scored more than 1 standard deviation below the mean on the Bayley Scale of Infant Development (117). In a later study, *in utero* cocaine-exposed and control children from an inner city cohort were administered the Wechsler Preschool and Primary Scale of Intelligence–Revised at age 4 years. IQ scores did not differ significantly between the groups, although 93% of cocaine-exposed children and 96% of control children scored below the mean IQ (118). Similarly, a masked study of cocaine-exposed and unexposed children of low socioeconomic status to assess early language development at 2.5 years of age did not identify any differences between groups in language scores (119). Other studies, using the Sequenced Inventory of Communicative Development–Revised and the Bayley Scales of Infant Development, demonstrated significant differences between control and prenatal drug- (including cocaine) exposed children aged 14 to 50 months who had been living in stable, drug-free foster home environments (120). However, other reports that assessed the development of school-age children (age 6) who were prenatally exposed to light to moderate cocaine use *in utero* compared with nonexposed controls did not demonstrate any significant effects on growth, intellectual ability, academic achievement, or teacher-related classroom behaviors in the exposed children, although deficiencies were observed in sustaining attention (121). Earlier, more sensitive tests of infant information processing such as the FTII or novelty preference test and the visual expectancy paradigm showed decreased cognitive function in prenatal cocaine-exposed infants, suggesting that some standardized testing may not detect subtle cognitive findings (83).

Although several studies concentrated on the development and function of the CNS after birth as a result of *in utero* cocaine exposure, there have been no conclusive findings of permanent cognitive deficits. This may be owing to study limitations (122). What has been found is that there is some effect on neurobehavioral development that occurs in the neonatal period or early childhood. Adverse outcomes later in life have not been demonstrated conclusively (123).

Despite the limitations of studies conducted, adverse neurobehavioral effects certainly have been found in children exposed to cocaine *in utero* and postnatally. Newborns have been found to have poorer state regulation, increased excitability and motor activity, signs of CNS stress, and decreased attention span. Reflexes and tone are exaggerated in these neonates as well. These findings were dose related (80,81,116,124–127). The findings, however, were not consistent with respect to timing of occurrence of these effects. Richardson et al. (127) found that poor autonomic stability and increased tone and reflexes were present at days of life 1 and 2, but not at day 3. Tronick et al. (80) found that increased excitability and poor state regulation were not present at days 2 to 3 but were present when the infants were tested at 3 weeks of age (80). Of note is that plasma norepinephrine levels in babies who are exposed to cocaine and marijuana have been found to be elevated. These correlate with some abnormal findings in cocaine-exposed neonates on the Neonatal Behavioral Assessment Scale in the early neonatal period but not at 2 weeks of age (128). Jacobson et al. (83) found that newborn infants had difficulty habituating, needed more frequent stimulation, and had poorer visual recognition during memory tasks.

Behavioral problems have been identified in children exposed to cocaine *in utero*. In one study, at the ages of 1 and 3 years, these children were more likely to be described as having more difficult personalities and to be characterized as fussy by their mothers. Memory deficits were found among these same children at 3 years of age (125). School-age children have been found to have decreased attention spans, language delay, and lower IQs (122,129,130). Chasnoff et al. (131) reported that in their study, the IQ, behavioral effects, and global cognitive function in school-age children were affected adversely by environmental factors as a result of parental cocaine use. They also found that it was their *in utero* cocaine exposure that negatively affected their behavior during the period from 4 to 6 years of age.

There are a number of limitations thus far in the studies of neurobehavioral effects of cocaine. Nevertheless, the findings cannot be ignored. The implications can be far-reaching and devastating. The possible long-term effects are of critical importance to society as a whole.

In summary, the overall effects of cocaine exposure in pregnancy are multiple, with the most common being perinatal concerns, manifested by preterm labor, preterm rupture of membranes, abruptio placentae, placenta previa, and fetal growth retardation. Although no frank "fetal cocaine" syndrome has been confirmed, numerous anomalies have been reported after cocaine exposure, although these findings may well be confounded by polydrug exposure. Postnatally, cocaine-exposed children appear to improve in growth, although they may manifest subtle cognitive and behavioral findings. These children may be at risk for these problems both from the drug exposure and many environmental variables such as poverty, low socioeconomic class, persistent drug exposure, and poor parenting. Parenting is a critical issue because cocaine-using mothers may characteristically overestimate their infant's mental and physical development (132) and underutilize preventive health maintenance and immunization services (133). The "environmental" impact of parents' use of cocaine after birth may markedly effect a child's growth (122,131).

REFERENCES

1. Doyle E, Spense AA. Cannabis as a medicine? *Br J Anaesth* 1995;74:359–361.
2. Lee M. Marihuana and tobacco use in pregnancy: substance abuse in pregnancy. *Obstet Gynecol Clin North Am* 1998;25:65–97.
3. Taylor HG. Analysis of their medical use of marijuana and its societal implications. *J Am Pharm Assoc (Wash)* 1998;38:220–227.
4. Lemberger L, Weiss J, Watanabe A, et al. Delta-9-tetrahydrocannabinol: temporal correlation of the psychological effects and blood levels after various routes of administration. *N Engl J Med* 1972;286:685–688.
5. Agurell S, Halldin M, Jan-Erik L, et al. Pharmacokinetics and metabolism of delta-1-tetrahydrocannabinol and other cannabinoids with emphasis on man. *Pharmacol Rev* 1986;38:21–43.
6. Musty RE, Reggio P, Consroe P. A review of recent advances in cannabinoid research and the 1994 International Symposium on cannabis and the cannabinoids. *Life Sci* 1995;56:1933–1940.
7. Hollister L, Reaven G. Delta-9-tetrahydrocannabinol and glucose tolerance. *Clin Pharmacol Ther* 1974;16:297–302.
8. Woods JR. Adverse consequences of prenatal illicit drug exposure. *Curr Opin Obstet Gynecol* 1996;8:403–411.
9. Little BB, VanBeveren TT. Placental transfer of selected substances of abuse. *Semin Perinatol* 1996;20:147–153.
10. Fisher SE, Atkinson M, Chang B. Effect of delta-9-tetrahydrocannabinol on the in vitro uptake of alpha-amino isobutyric acid by term human placental slices. *Pediatr Res* 1987;21:104–107.
11. Court JM. Cannabis and brain function. *J Paediatr Child Health* 1998;34:1–5.
12. Soueif MI. Chronic cannabis users: further analysis of objective test results. *Bull Narc* 1975;27:1–26.
13. Tashkin DP, Shapiro BJ, Lee YE, et al. Subacute effects of heavy smoking on pulmonary function in healthy men. *N Engl J Med* 1976;294:125–129.
14. Richardson GA, Day NL, McGauhey PJ. The impact of prenatal marijuana and cocaine use on the infant and child. *Clin Obstet Gynecol* 1993;36:302–318.
15. Cornelius MD, Taylor PM, Geva D, et al. Prenatal tobacco and marijuana use among adolescents: effects on offspring gestational age, growth, and morphology. *Pediatrics* 1995;95:738–743.
16. Kline J, Hutzler M, Levin B, et al. Marijuana and spontaneous abortion of known karyotype. *Paediatr Perinat Epidemiol* 1991;5:320–332.
17. Frank DA, Bauchner H, Parker S, et al. Neonatal body proportionality and body composition after in utero exposure to cocaine and marijuana. *J Pediatr* 1990;117:622–626.
18. McTiernan MJ, Burchfield DJ, Abrams RM, et al. Carboxy- and oxyhemoglobin in pregnant ewe and fetus after inhalation of marijuana, marijuana placebo and tobacco cigarette smoke. *Life Sci* 1988;43:2043–2047.
19. O'Connell CM, Fried PA. An investigation of prenatal cannabis exposure and minor physical anomalies in a low risk population. *Neurobehav Toxicol Teratol* 1984;6:345–350.
20. Astley SJ, Clarren SK, Little RE, et al. Analysis of facial shape in children gestationally exposed to marijuana, alcohol, and/or cocaine. *Pediatrics* 1992;89:67–77.
21. Dreher MC, Nugent K, Hudgins R. Prenatal marijuana exposure and neonatal outcomes in Jamaica: an ethnographic study. *Pediatrics* 1994;93:254–260.
22. Abel EL. Effects of prenatal exposure to cannabinoids. *NIDA Res Monogr* 1985;59:20–35.
23. Hutchings D, Dow-Edwards D. Animal models of opiate, cocaine, and cannabis use. *Clin Perinatol* 1991;18:1–22.
24. Tennes K, Avitable N, Blackard C, et al. Marijuana: Prenatal and postnatal exposure in the human. *NIDA Res Monogr* 1985;59:48–60.
25. English DR, Hulse GK, Milne E, et al. Maternal cannabis use and birth weight: a meta-analysis. *Addiction* 1997;92:1553–1560.
26. Hingson R, Alpert J, Day N, et al. Effects of maternal drinking and marijuana use on fetal growth and development. *Pediatrics* 1982;70:539–546.
27. Linn S, Schoenbaum R, Monson, R, et al. The association of marijuana use with outcome of pregnancy. *Am J Public Health* 1983;72:1161–1164.
28. Hatch E, Bracken M. Effects of marijuana use in pregnancy on fetal growth. *Am J Epidemiol* 1986;124:986–993.
29. Fried PA, Watkinson B, Siegel LS. Reading and language in 9- to 12-year olds prenatally exposed to cigarettes and marijuana. *Neurotoxicol Teratol* 1997;19:171–183.

30. Fried PA. Prenatal exposure to marihuana and tobacco during infancy, early and middle childhood: effects and an attempt at synthesis. *Arch Toxicol* 1995;17:233–260.
31. Musty RE, Reggio P, Consroe P. Neonatal neurological status in a low-risk population after prenatal exposure to cigarettes, marijuana, and alcohol. *J Dev Behav Pediatr* 1987;8:318–326.
32. Ostrea EM, Ostrea AR, Simpson PM. Mortality within the first 2 years in infants exposed to cocaine, opiate, or cannabinoid during gestation. *Pediatrics* 1997;100:79–83.
33. Lester BM, Dreher M. Effects of marijuana use during pregnancy on newborn cry. *Child Dev* 1989;60:765–771.
34. Zuckerman B. Developmental consequences of maternal drug use during pregnancy. *NIDA Res Monogr* 1985;59:96–106.
35. Fried PA. Marijuana use by pregnant women: neurobehavioral effects on neonates. *Alcohol Depend* 1980;6:415–424.
36. Fried PA. Cigarettes and marijuana: are there measurable long-term neurobehavioral teratologic effects? *Neurotoxicology* 1989;10:577–583.
37. Fried PA, Watkinson B. 36- and 48-month neurobehavioral follow-up of children prenatally exposed to marijuana, cigarettes, and alcohol. *J Dev Behav Pediatr* 1990;11:49–58.
38. Fried PA, Watkinson B, Gray R. Differential effects on cognitive functioning in 9- to 12-year olds prenatally exposed to cigarettes and marijuana. *Neurotoxicol Teratol* 1998;20:293–306.
39. Chandler LS, Richardson GA, Gallagher JD, et al. Prenatal exposure to alcohol and marijuana: effects on motor development of preschool children. *Alcohol Clin Exp Res* 1996;20:455–461.
40. Children's Cancer Study Group. Maternal drug use and risk of childhood nonlymphoblastic leukemia among offspring. *Cancer* 1989;63:1904–1911.
41. Ammenheuser MM, Berenson AB, Babiak AE, et al. Frequencies of hprt mutant lymphocytes in marijuana-smoking mothers and their newborns. *Mutat Res* 1998;403:55–64.
42. Bodhadadi MS, Henning RJ. Cocaine: pathophysiology and clinical toxicology. *Heart Lung* 1997;26:466–485.
43. Quinn DI, Wodak A, Day RO. Pharmacokinetic and pharmacodynamic principles of illicit drug use and treatment of illicit drug users. *Clin Pharmacokinet* 1997;33:344–400.
44. Warner EA, Kosten TR, O'Connor PG. Pharmacotherapy for opioid and cocaine abuse. *Med Clin North Am* 1997;81:909–925.
45. Ritchie JM, Greene NM. *Local anesthetics, the pharmacological basis of therapeutics.* New York: Pergamon Press, 1990;311–331.
46. Chao CR. Cardiovascular effects of cocaine during pregnancy. *Semin Perinatol* 1996;20:107–114.
47. Benowitz NL. Clinical pharmacology and toxicology of cocaine. *Pharmacol Toxicol* 1992;72:3–12.
48. Plessinger MA, Woods JR Jr. Cocaine in pregnancy: recent data on maternal and fetal risks. *Obstet Gynecol Clin North Am* 1998;25:99–118.
49. Hoyme HE, Jones KL, Dixon SD, et al. Prenatal cocaine exposure and fetal vascular disruption. *Pediatrics* 1990;85:743–747.

50. Jones KL. Developmental pathogenesis of defects associated with prenatal cocaine exposure: fetal vascular disruption. *Clin Perinatol* 1991;18:139–146.
51. Woods JR. Maternal and transplacental effects of cocaine. *Ann N Y Acad Sci* 1998;846:1–11.
52. Woods JR Jr, Plessinger MA. Pregnancy increases cardiovascular toxicity to cocaine. *Am J Obstet Gynecol* 1990;162:529–533.
53. Woods JR, Plessinger MA. Effect of cocaine on uterine blood flow and fetal oxygenation. *JAMA* 1987;257:957–961.
54. Gawin FH. Cocaine addiction: psychology and neurophysiology. *Science* 1991;251:1580–1586.
55. Foltin RW, Fischman MW. Self-administration of cocaine by humans: choice between smoked and intravenous cocaine. *J Pharmacol Exp Ther* 1992;261:841–849.
56. Jones RT. The pharmacology of cocaine smoking in humans. *NIDA Res Monogr* 1990;99:30–41.
57. Javaid JI, Musa MN, Fischman M, et al. Kinetics of cocaine in humans after intravenous and intranasal administration. *Biopharm Drug Dispos* 1983;4:9–18.
58. Busto U, Bendayan R, Sellers EM. Clinical pharmacokinetics of non-opiate abused drugs. *Clin Pharmacokinet* 1989;16:1–26.
59. Biley DN. Cocaine and cocaethylene binding to human placenta in vitro. *Am J Obstet Gynecol* 1997;177:527–531.
60. Roe BS, Little BB, Bawdon RE, et al. Metabolism of cocaine by human placentas: implications for exposure. *Am J Obstet Gynecol* 1990;163:715–718.
61. Rizk B, Atterbury JL, Groome LJ. Reproductive risks of cocaine. *Hum Reprod Update* 1996;2:43–55.
62. Anonymous. Practice guidelines for the treatment of patients with substance use disorders: alcohol, cocaine, opioids. *Am J Psych* 1995;152[Suppl 11]:1–59.
63. Morishima HO, Whittington RA. Species-, gender-, and pregnancy-related differences in the pharmacokinetics and pharmacodynamics of cocaine. *NIDA Res Monogr* 1995;158:2–21.
64. Lukas SE, Sholar MB, Fortin M, et al. Gender and menstrual cycle influences on cocaine's effects in human volunteers. In: Harris LS, ed. *56th Annual Scientific Meeting: The College on Problems of Drug Dependence.* Rockville, MD: NIH (publication no. 95-3883), 1994:490.
65. Shiono PH, Klebanoff MA, Nugent RP, et al. The impact of cocaine and marijuana use on low birth weight and preterm birth: a multicenter study. *Am J Obstet Gynecol* 1995;172:19–27.
66. Lindsay MK, Carmichael S, Peterson H, et al. Correlation between self reported cocaine use and urine toxicology in an inner-city prenatal population. *J Natl Med Assoc* 1997;89:57–60.
67. Hutchins E, Dipietro J. Psychosocial risk factors associated with cocaine use during pregnancy: a case-control study. *Obstet Gynecol* 1997;90:142–147.
68. Young N. Alcohol and other drugs: the scope of the problem among pregnant and parenting women in California. *J Psychoactive Drugs* 1997;29:3–22.
69. Burkett G, Yasin S, Palow D. Perinatal implications of cocaine exposure. *J Reprod Med* 1990;35:35–42.
70. Bandstra ES, Burkett G. Maternal-fetal and neonatal effects of *in utero* cocaine exposure. *Semin Perinatol* 1991;15:288–301.

71. Plessinger MA, Woods JR Jr. Maternal, placental, and fetal pathophysiology of cocaine exposure during pregnancy. *Clin Obstet Gynecol* 1993;36:267–278.

72. Acher D, Sachs BP, Tracey KJ, et al. Abruptio placentae associated with cocaine use. *Am J Obstet Gynecol* 1983;146:220–221.

73. Handler A, Kistin N, Davis F, et al. Cocaine use during pregnancy: perinatal outcomes. *Am J Epidemiol* 1991; 133:818–825.

74. Hulse GK, Milne E, English DR, et al. Assessing the relationship between maternal cocaine use and abruptio placentae. *Addiction* 1997;92:1547–1551.

75. Monga M, Weisbrodt NW, Andres RL, et al. The acute effect of cocaine exposure on pregnant human myometrial contractile activity. *Am J Obstet Gynecol* 1993;169:782–785.

76. Monga M. The effect of cocaine on myometrial contractile activity: basic mechanisms. *Semin Perinatol* 1996;20:140–146.

77. Cherkuri R, Minkoff H, Feldman J, et al. A cohort study of alkaloidal cocaine ("crack") in pregnancy. *Obstet Gynecol* 1988;72:147–151.

78. Delaney DB, Larrabee KD, Monga M. Preterm premature rupture of the membranes associated with recent cocaine use. *Am J Perinatol* 1997;14:285–288.

79. Dinsmoor MJ, Irons SJ, Christmas JT. Preterm rupture of the membranes associated with recent cocaine use. *Am J Obstet Gynecol* 1994;171:305–309.

80. Tronick EZ, Frank DA, Cabral H, et al. Late dose response effects of prenatal cocaine exposure on newborn neurobehavioral performance. *Pediatrics* 1996;98:76–83.

81. Martin JC, Barr HM, Martin DC, et al. Neonatal neurobehavioral outcome following prenatal exposure to cocaine. *Neurotoxicol Teratol* 1996;18:617–625.

82. Eyler FD, Behnke M, Conlon M, et al. Birth outcome from a prospective, matched study of prenatal crack/cocaine use: 1. Interactive and dose effects on health and growth. *Pediatrics* 1998;101:229–237.

83. Jacobson SW, Jacobson JL, Sokol RJ, et al. New evidence for neurobehavioral effects of *in utero* cocaine exposure. *J Pediatric* 1996;129:581–590.

84. Sprauve ME, Lindsay MK, Herbert S, et al. Adverse perinatal outcome in parturients who use crack cocaine. *Obstet Gynecol* 1997;89:674–678.

85. Hulse GK, English DR, Milne E, et al. Maternal cocaine use and low birth weight newborns: a meta-analysis. *Addiction* 1997;92:1561–1570.

86. Church MW, Crossland WJ, Holmes PA, et al. Effects of prenatal cocaine on hearing, vision, growth, and behavior. *Ann N Y Acad Sci* 1998;846:12–28.

87. Church MW, Dintcheff BA, Gessner PK. The interactive effects of alcohol and cocaine on maternal and fetal toxicity in the Long-Evans rat. *Neurotoxicol Teratol* 1988;10:355–361.

88. Macones GA, Sehdev HM, Parry S, et al. The association between maternal cocaine use and placenta previa. *Am J Obstet Gynecol* 1997;177:1097–1100.

89. Kain ZN, Mayes LC, Ferris C, et al. Cocaine-abusing parturients undergoing cesarean section: a cohort study. *Anesthiology* 1996;85:1028–1035.

90. Chan L, Hoangmai P, Reece EA. Pneumothorax in pregnancy associated with cocaine use. *Am J Perinatol* 1997;14:385–388.

91. Kain ZN, Mayes LC, Pakes J, et al. Thrombocytopenia in pregnant women who use cocaine. *Am J Obstet Gynecol* 1995;173:885–890.

92. Abramowicz JS, Sherer DM, Woods JR Jr. Acute transient thrombocytopenia associated with cocaine abuse in pregnancy. *Obstet Gynecol* 1991;78:499–501.

93. Buehler BA, Conover B, Andres RL. Teratogenic potential of cocaine. *Semin Perinatol* 1996;20:93–98.

94. Lutiger B, Graham K, Einarson TR, et al. Relationship between gestational cocaine use and pregnancy outcome: a meta-analysis. *Teratology* 1991;44:405–414.

95. Zuckerman B, Frank DA, Hingson R, et al. Effects of maternal marijuana and cocaine use on fetal growth. *N Engl J Med* 1989;320:762–768.

96. Chasnoff IJ, Chisum GM, Kaplan WE. Maternal cocaine use and genitourinary tract malformations. *Teratology* 1988;37:201–204.

97. Greenfield SP, Rutigliano E, Steinhardt G, et al. Genitourinary tract malformation and maternal cocaine use. *Urology* 1991;37:455–459.

98. Bingol N, Fuchs M, Diaz V, et al. Teratogenicity of cocaine in humans. *J Pediatr* 1987;110:93–96.

99. Lipshultz SE, Frassica JJ, Orav EJ. Cardiovascular abnormalities in infants prenatally exposed to cocaine. *J Pediatr* 1991;118:44–51.

100. Chasnoff IJ, Bussey ME, Savich R, et al. Perinatal cerebral infarction and maternal cocaine use. *J Pediatr* 1986;108:456–459.

101. Rais-Bahrami K, Naqvi M. Hydranencephaly and maternal cocaine use: a case report. *Clin Pediatr* 1990;29:729–730.

102. Kobori JA, Ferreiro DM, Golabi M. CNS and craniofacial anomalies in infants born to cocaine abusing mothers.*Proc Greenwood Genet Cen* 1990;9:67A(abstract).

103. Good WV, Ferreiro DM, Golabi M, et al. Abnormalities of the visual system in infants exposed to cocaine. *Ophthalmology* 1992;9:341–346.

104. Teske MP, Trese MT. Retinopathy of prematurity-like fundus and persistent hyperplastic primary vitreous associated with maternal cocaine use. *Am J Ophthalmol* 1987;103:719–720.

105. Silva-Araujo AL, Tavares MA, Patacao MH, et al. Retinal hemorrhages associated with *in utero* exposure to cocaine. *Retina* 1996;16:411–418.

106. Block SS, Moore BD, Emigh Scharre J. Visual anomalies in young children exposed to cocaine. *Optom Vis Sci* 1997;74:28–36.

107. Fries MH, Kuller J, Norton M, et al. Facial features of infants exposed prenatally to cocaine. *Teratology* 1993;48:413–420.

108. Little BB, Wilson GN, Jackson G. Is there a cocaine syndrome? Dysmorphic and anthropometric assessment of infants exposed to cocaine. *Teratology* 1996;54:145–149.

109. Martin ML, Khoury MJ, Cordero JF, et al. Trends in rates of multiple vascular disruption defects, Atlanta, 1968–1989: is there evidence of a cocaine teratogenic epidemic? *Teratology* 1992;45:647–653.

110. Hume RF, Martin LS, Bottoms SF, et al. Vascular disruption birth defects and history of prenatal cocaine exposure: a case-control study. *Fetal Diagn Ther* 1997;12:292–295.

111. Frank DA, Bauchner H, Parker S, et al. Neonatal body proportionality and body composition after *in utero* exposure to cocaine and marijuana. *J Pediatr* 1990;117:622–626.

112. Romano AG, Harvey JA. Prenatal cocaine exposure: long-term deficits in learning and motor performance. *Ann N Y Acad Sci* 1998;846:89–108.

113. Chasnoff IJ, Burns K, Burns W. Cocaine use in pregnancy: perinatal morbidity and mortality. *Neurotoxicol Teratol* 1987;9;291–293.

114. Ostrea E, Ostrea AR, Simpson P. Mortality within the first 2 years in infants exposed to cocaine, opiate, or cannabinoid during gestation. *Pediatrics* 1997;100:79–83.

115. Neuspiel DR, Hamel SC, Hochberg E, et al. Maternal cocaine use and infant behavior. *Neurotoxicol Teratol* 1991;13:229–233.

116. Eyler FD, Behnke M, Conlon M, et al. Birth outcome from a prospective, matched study of prenatal crack/cocaine use: II. Interactive and dose effects on neurobehavioral assessment. *Pediatrics* 1998;101:237–241.

117. Frank DA, Bresnahan K, Zuckerman BS. Maternal cocaine use: impact on child health and development. *Curr Prob Pediatr* 1996;Feb:52–69.

118. Hurt H, Malmud E, Betancourt L, et al. Children with *in utero* cocaine exposure do not differ from control subjects on intelligence testing. *Arch Pediatr Adolesc Med* 1997;151:1237–1241.

119. Hurt H, Malmud E, Betancourt L, et al. A prospective evaluation of early language development in children with *in utero* cocaine exposure and control subjects. *J Pediatr* 1997;130:310–312.

120. Johnson JM, Seikel JA, Madison CL, et al. Standardized test performance of children with a history of prenatal exposure to multiple drugs/cocaine. *J Commun Disord* 1997;30:45–73.

121. Richardson GA, Conroy ML, Day NL. Prenatal cocaine exposure: effects on the development of school-age children. *Neurotoxicol Teratol* 1996;18:627–634.

122. Koren G, Nulman I, Rovet J, et al. Long-term neurodevelopmental risks in children exposed *in utero* to cocaine. *Ann N Y Acad Sci* 1998;846:306–313.

123. Landry SH, Whitney JA. The impact of prenatal cocaine exposure: studies of the developing infant. *Semin Perinatol* 1996;20:99-106.

124. Chiriboga CA. Neurological correlates of fetal cocaine exposure. *Ann N Y Acad Sci* 1998;846:109–125.

125. Richardson GA. Prenatal cocaine exposure, a longitudinal study of development. *Ann N Y Acad Sci* 1998;846:144–152.

126. Napiorkowskii BS, Lester BM, Freier MC, et al. Effects of *in utero* substance exposure on infant neurobehavior. *Pediatrics* 1996;98:71–75.

127. Richardson GA, Hamel SC, Goldschmidt L, et al. The effects of prenatal cocaine use on neonatal neurobehavioral status. *Neurotoxicol Teratol* 1996;18:519–528.

128. Mirochnick M, Meyer J, Frank, DA, et al. Elevated plasma norepinephrine after *in utero* exposure to cocaine and marijuana. *Pediatrics* 1997;99:555–559.

129. Richardson GA, Conroy ML, Day NL. Prenatal cocaine exposure: effects on the development of school-age children. *Neurotoxicol Teratol* 1996;18:627–634.

130. Mayes LC, Grillon C, Granger R, et al. Regulation of arousal and attention in preschool children exposed to cocaine prenatally. *Ann N Y Acad Sci* 1998;846:126–143.

131. Chasnoff IJ, Anson A, Hatcher R, et al. Prenatal exposure to cocaine and other drugs, Outcome at four to six years. *Ann N Y Acad Sci* 1998;846:314–328.

132. Seagull FN, Mowery JL, Simpson PM, et al. Maternal assessment of infant development: associations with alcohol and drug use in pregnancy. *Clin Pediatr* 1996;Dec:621–628.

133. Forsyth BW, Leventhal JM, Qi K, et al. Health care and hospitalizations of young children born to cocaine-using women. *Arch Pediatr Adolesc Med* 1998;152:177–184.

15

Multivitamin and Mineral Supplementation in Pregnancy

Stephen D. Ratcliffe

Department of Family and Preventive Medicine, University of Utah, Salt Lake City, Utah

This chapter addresses the use of multivitamins and minerals in pregnancy in the context of routine supplementation, deficiency states, and special populations in which the incidence of deficient states is greater. Whenever possible, evidence-based sources such as randomized controlled trials (RCTs) or metaanalyses of RCTs are used to support recommendations.

PERICONCEPTIONAL MULTIVITAMIN SUPPLEMENTATION

There is strong RCT evidence that the periconceptional use of multivitamins containing at least 0.4 mg folic acid can reduce the incidence of first-time neural defects and that 4 mg prevents repeat neural tube defects (NTDs) (1). Periconception is defined as the period beginning 30 days before conception and extending to 90 days after conception.

A recent case-control study demonstrated a relationship between periconceptional multivitamin use and a reduction in conotruncal defects (2). Another case control study (3) and a retrospective cohort study (4) demonstrated an association between periconceptional multivitamin use and a reduction in low birth weight and small for gestational age infants. A RCT in Hungary showed a reduction in urinary and cardiovascular defects with the use of periconceptional multivitamin supplements (5). These studies should be viewed as hypothesis generating and should lead to further RCTs to answer these questions.

Implications for Practice

1. Multivitamins that contain at least 0.4 mg folic acid can reduce the incidence of first-time and recurrent NTDs.
2. Additional RCTs are needed to determine whether the use of periconceptional multivitamins reduce the incidence of other congenital anomalies or improve subsequent birth outcomes.

ROUTINE SUPPLEMENTATION WITH MULTIVITAMINS DURING PREGNANCY

A recent review provides an excellent summary of this area for the interested reader (6). Table 15.1 summarizes the recommended daily allowance of vitamins and minerals during pregnancy and lactation. The National Research Council and a special subcommittee of the Institute of Medicine both concluded that a woman having a singleton pregnancy who eats a balanced diet should be able to consume these recommended nutrients during pregnancy with the exception of folate and iron (7).

Recent evidence underscores the importance of consuming at least 0.4 mg folic acid before and during pregnancy. An average American diet contains roughly half this amount of folic acid, perhaps 0.3 mg since food fortification began. These groups also concluded that the average diet would not provide sufficient iron and recommended that women receive 30 mg of supplemental iron during the second and third trimesters of

TABLE 15.1. *Recommended dietary allowances for women*

Nutrient	Nonpregnant 15–18 yr	Nonpregnant 25–50 yr	Pregnant	Lactating	Dietary sources
Vitamin A (RE)	800	800	800	1,300	Dark green, yellow, or orange fruits and vegetables
Vitamin B_1 (thiamine) (mg)	1.1	1.1	1.5	1.6	Enriched grains, pork
Vitamin B_2 (riboflavin) (mg)	1.3	1.3	1.6	1.8	Meats, liver, enriched grains
Vitamin B_3 (niacin) (mg)	15	15	17	20	Meats, nuts, legumes
Vitamin B_6 (pyridoxine) (mg)	1.5	1.6	2.2	2.1	Meats, liver, enriched grains
Vitamin B_{12} (μg)	2.0	2.0	2.2	2.6	Meats
Folic acid (μg)	180[a]	180[a]	400	240	Leafy vegetables, liver
Vitamin C (mg)	60	60	70	95	Citrus fruits, tomatoes
Vitamin D (IU)	400	200	400	400	Fortified dairy products
Calcium (mg)	1,200	800	1,200	1,200	Dairy products
Iodine (μg)	150	150	175	200	Iodized salt, seafood
Iron (mg)	15	15	30	15	Meats, eggs, seafood
Magnesium (mg)	300	280	320	355	Seafood, legumes, grains
Zinc (mg)	12	12	15	19	Meats, seafood, eggs
Protein (g)	44	50	60	65	Meats, fish, poultry, dairy

[a]1992 recommendations of the Centers for Disease Control and Prevention is 400 μg daily.
From Menard M. Vitamin and mineral supplement prior to and during pregnancy. *Obstet Gynecol Clin North Am* 1997;24:479–498, with permission.

pregnancy. The evidence to support routine iron supplementation is addressed later in this chapter.

Every clinician provides prenatal care for women who do not meet the above criteria for adequate nutritional intake. Table 15.2 summarizes many of the groups who are at increased nutritional risk during pregnancy (6,8).

Although it is not recommended that healthy, well-nourished women receive prenatal multivitamin/mineral supplements, it is routine practice for these supplements to be prescribed by maternity care providers. It is important to note that deficiencies in dietary intake of vitamin and minerals are common among middle class women, as noted in several recent large nutritional surveys (9). Thus, routine multivitamin/mineral supplementation may serve a purpose. It is an

unfortunate paradox that those women with the greatest need for these supplements (lower income African American, single) consume these agents 75% as much as their white, middle-income, married counterparts (10). There is additional evidence that the use of these supplements in these at-risk populations improves infant morbidity and mortality (11).

Implications for Practice

1. Clinicians should conduct a basic nutritional assessment for each prenatal patient and use multivitamin/mineral supplements in at-risk populations and targeted vitamin or mineral supplements in other groups identified in Table 15.2.

TABLE 15.2. *Groups at increased nutritional risk*

Group/condition	Associated deficiency
Eating disorders (bulimia or anorexia nervosa)	Folic acid, iron
Adolescents	Folic acid, vitamin B_6, iron, calcium
Vegetarians	Iron, B_{12}
Poverty	Folic acid, calcium, zinc, iron; vitamins B_6, D, and E
Smoking	Vitamin C
Substance abuse	Vitamins C, B_6, D, E; calcium, zinc, iron
Alcoholism	Vitamin C
Lactose intolerance	Calcium
Epilepsy (receiving anticonvulsant therapy)	Vitamin K
Receiving chronic heparin therapy	Vitamin D
Multiple gestation	Vitamin B_6, C, iron

2. Women with singleton pregnancies who eat a balanced diet do not require multivitamin/mineral supplementation. It is recommended that they receive supplemental folic acid (0.4 mg) before and during pregnancy and 30 mg of elemental iron in the second and third trimesters.

SPECIAL INDICATIONS AND PRECAUTIONS FOR VITAMIN USE DURING PREGNANCY

Vitamin A

Vitamin A is a fat-soluble vitamin found in many vegetable food groups. Its presence is required for the maintenance of normal bone, vision, and reproduction. The recommended daily allowance (RDA) set by the US Food and Drug Administration for pregnancy is 800 retinol equivalents that are equivalent to 2,700 international units (IU). Most prenatal multivitamin supplements contain 4,000 to 5,000 IU of vitamin A, which exceeds the RDA. Because most diets provide this amount of vitamin A, routine supplementation is not recommended.

It is well documented that excessive doses of vitamin A taken in the periconceptional period or in pregnancy are teratogenic. Until recently, the threshold for vitamin A toxicity was thought to be 25,000 to 50,000 IU daily. There is now evidence that this threshold may be as low as 10,000 IU in causing an increase in cranial neural crest anomalies (12).

Implications for Practice

1. Routine supplementation with vitamin A during pregnancy is not recommended.
2. If supplementation is used, it should not exceed 5,000 IU daily; patients should not take additional over-the-counter vitamin A supplements because of the increased risk of birth defects.

Vitamin B$_6$

Vitamin B$_6$ (pyridoxine and related compounds) is a water-soluble vitamin that is required for protein, carbohydrate, and lipid metabolism (6).

There is increased need for B$_6$ during pregnancy, and various groups are at increased risk of deficiency during pregnancy as summarized in Table 15.2.

There is RCT evidence that vitamin B$_6$ has therapeutic potential for the treatment of nausea and vomiting in the first trimester at a dose of 25 mg three times daily for 3 days (13–15). Extensive safety data have not been compiled, and there is no evidence to support the routine use of vitamin B$_6$ supplementation during pregnancy (16).

FOLIC ACID: ITS USE IN THE PERICONCEPTION PERIOD AND DURING PREGNANCY

Additional information is given in the chapter on folic acid in the prevention of birth defects.

Natural History and Mechanism of Action

Folic acid is one of the B vitamins and plays an important role in nucleoprotein synthesis and in the production of red blood cells. Folic acid deficiency is common during pregnancy and occurs because of decreased maternal intake, malabsorption, and depletion of maternal stores by the fetus (17).

Folic acid deficiency in pregnancy is associated with NTDs and other anomalies. Placental abruption, intrauterine growth restriction, and premature delivery may be increased in patients with folate deficiency, although these are possibly owing to other associated conditions and not deficiency of the vitamin (3,17). The use of certain antiepileptic medications (phenytoin and phenobarbital) is associated with an increased incidence of folic acid deficiency in pregnancy (17). This association is not seen with carbamazepine or valproate acid. A small retrospective study found that the periconceptional folic acid supplementation (2.5 to 5.0 mg per day) appeared to be effective in lowering the risk of NTDs in patients on these anticonvulsant agents (18).

Folic acid, when taken in adequate amounts (0.4 mg per day) in the periconceptional period, reduces the incidence of first-time NTDs (1). Periconceptional use of folic acid taken in quantities of 4 mg per day decreases the recurrence of

NTDs for women with a history of a NTD. Note that the periconceptional administration of multivitamins that do not contain folic acid does not reduce the incidence of NTDs. The exact mechanism of action is unknown, although it is thought to be related to the gene-mediated regulation of homocystine and methionine metabolism (4).

Folic acid and iron help to ensure the adequate production of hemoglobin and prevention of anemia in pregnancy. Routine folic acid supplementation during pregnancy is effective in preventing anemia at the time of delivery, although there is little evidence at this time that this intervention has any effect, positive or negative, on maternal or fetal outcome (19).

Health Care Policy Implications

In September 1992, the Public Health Service recommended that all women of childbearing age consume 0.4 mg folic acid per day. Despite this recommendation, approximately 80% of women in Georgia were not consuming this recommended amount (20). Accordingly, in January 1998, the United States initiated a requirement that folic acid be added to enriched cereal grain products such as flours, corn meals, pasta, and rice. Breakfast cereals may be fortified with as much as 0.4 mg folic acid per serving (21).

A recent study concluded that only 33% of multivitamin products met US Pharmacopeia specifications for folic acid release (22). At a time when there is evidence of the effectiveness of folic acid in the prevention of NTDs, this disturbing finding needs further investigation. If this finding is confirmed, corrective steps should be undertaken.

Implications for Practice

1. Reproductive-age women should take at least 0.4 mg folic acid per day to lessen the risk of NTDs in their offspring. This should begin at least 1 month before conception. It appears that the most effective manner to achieve this intake involves taking a folic acid supplement or consuming foods that are fortified with additional folate (23).

2. Women who have a history of a child with a NTD should take approximately 4 mg folic acid per day in the periconceptional period.
3. Folic acid supplementation (0.4 mg per day) beyond the first trimester lessens the incidence of maternal anemia at delivery without impacting perinatal outcomes. There is, at present, no evidence to argue for or against its routine use.
4. Periconceptional folic acid supplementation at a dose of 2.5 to 5.0 mg/day should be given to epileptic women who are treated with phenytoin and phenobarbital.

MINERAL USE IN PREGNANCY

Iron

Most women demonstrate hematologic changes of iron deficiency as pregnancy advances (16). There is strong evidence from numerous RCTs that routine iron supplementation (100 mg of elemental iron per day) prevents anemia at the time of delivery and at 6 weeks postpartum. The number needed to treat (NNT) to prevent anemia at the time of delivery is 4 and the NNT to prevent anemia at 6 weeks after childbirth is 14. These hematologic improvements have not translated into other improvements in perinatal outcomes (24).

The bioavailability of iron in prenatal vitamin preparations varies. Two enhancers of iron absorption are organic acids, such as ascorbic acid, and animal tissues. Iron absorption is inhibited by salt formation with phosphates, phytic acids, caffeine, and antacids. Other minerals, such as calcium, magnesium, zinc, and copper, compete with iron for absorption in the small intestine (25). Iron preparations can cause gastrointestinal side effects such as epigastric discomfort, a metallic taste, or constipation. They may need to be taken with food or with stool softeners to mitigate these side effects.

Implications for Practice

1. Supplementation with 100 mg of elemental iron per day in pregnancy does serve to improve a woman's hematologic status at the

time of delivery and at the 6-week postpartum follow-up visit.
2. In developing countries where iron deficiency is both more common and severe, this supplementation may play even greater protective and preventive roles.

Calcium

In some studies, calcium supplementation of 1 g per day is associated with a decreased incidence of gestational hypertension (26). This effect is greatest among women at increased risk of hypertension (relative risk, 0.35; confidence interval, 0.21 to 0.57) and those with low baseline dietary calcium (relative risk, 0.49; confidence inteval, 0.38 to 0.62). Calcium supplementation at this level is also associated with a similar decrease in preeclampsia, particularly in some subgroups. A recent RCT that did not demonstrate this association studied women at low risk of hypertension who had adequate dietary calcium intake (27).

A major cause of inadequate calcium intake is lactose intolerance. This condition is commonly seen in women of color. Clinicians serving Native American, black, and Hispanic populations should be particularly attuned to identifying women with inadequate calcium intake because of lactose intolerance and poverty-related conditions. Every attempt should be made to enroll these women in nearby Women, Infant, and Children Nutritional Programs.

Implications for Practice

1. Calcium supplementation of 1 g per day may result in a decrease in gestational hypertension and preeclampsia in women with inadequate dietary calcium intake and those at increased risk of gestational hypertension.

Magnesium

Magnesium is an essential mineral found in a wide variety of foods, including dairy products, breads and cereals, vegetables, and meats. Magnesium works with many enzyme systems to regulate body temperature and protein synthesis

(28). Retrospective studies demonstrated an association between magnesium-deficient states and an increased risk of intrauterine growth restriction and preeclampsia (29,30). This led to several recent RCTs to determine whether routine magnesium supplementation in pregnancy led to improved perinatal outcomes.

A metaanalysis of the six RCTs show that oral magnesium supplementation resulted in a lower incidence of preterm birth, fewer maternal hospitalizations during pregnancy, and a decreased incidence of low birth weight and small for gestational age infants. Unfortunately, five of the six studies used poor randomization techniques. The only high-quality trial did not show the improved outcomes noted above (31).

Implications for Practice

1. Dietary magnesium supplementation during pregnancy is not recommended at the current time. Further studies are needed to resolve the question of the need for magnesium supplementation, particularly as it pertains to at-risk populations.

Zinc

Low serum zinc levels have been associated with adverse pregnancy outcomes such as small for gestational age infants and labor abnormalities (32,33). As a result of these associations, several RCTs were done to determine whether routine supplementation with zinc (20 to 62 mg elemental zinc) improves perinatal outcome. A metaanalysis of these studies demonstrated that routine supplementation with zinc did not show any effect, positive or negative, on pregnancy outcome (34). However, women with zinc deficiency or those judged to be at high risk of this deficiency do appear to benefit from zinc supplementation. The main benefit for this subset of women is a decrease in low birth weight infants by decreasing prematurity rates and the incidence of small for gestational age infants (35). A recent RCT confirmed the finding that zinc supplementation of 25 mg per day in women with low plasma zinc concentrations is associated with increased infant birth weights and head circumferences (36). This association was strongest in women with a body mass index less than 26 kg/m^2.

Implications for Practice

1. Routine zinc supplementation in the general US population does not affect perinatal outcome.
2. There is preliminary evidence that zinc supplementation of 25 mg per day for women at increased risk of zinc deficiency is associated with increased birth weight and head circumference. This association is primarily in women with a body mass index less than 26 kg/m^2.

SUMMARY

Periconceptional folate supplementation can reduce the risk of first-time and recurrent NTDs. Women should be encouraged to maintain an adequate intake of dietary folate or be offered supplementation in the periconceptional period. Iron supplementation can reduce the risk of anemia at delivery and postpartum, and therefore women should be offered such supplementation. Multivitamin use may or may not have any benefit but can be offered to pregnant women. Megadose supplementation should be avoided in pregnancy because of unknown effects or the known teratogenic effects of some vitamins such as vitamin A.

REFERENCES

1. Lumley J, Watson L, Watson M, et al. Periconceptional supplementation with folate and/or multivitamins to prevent neural tube defects (Cochrane Review). In: *The Cochrane Library,* Issue 4. Oxford: Update Software, 1998.
2. Botto L, Khoury M, Mulinare J, et al. Periconceptional multivitamin use and the occurrence of conotruncal heart defects: results from a population-based, case-control study. *Pediatrics* 1996;98:911–917.
3. Scholl T, Hediger M, Schall J, et al. Dietary and serum folate: their influence on the outcome of pregnancy. *Am J Clin Nutr* 1996;63:520–525.
4. Shaw G, Liberman R, Todoroff K, et al. Low birth weight, preterm delivery, and periconceptional vitamin use [Letter]. *J Pediatr* 1997;130:1013–1014.
5. Creizel A. Reduction of urinary tract and cardiovascular defects by periconceptional multivitamin supplementation. *Am J Med Genet* 1996;62:179–183.
6. Menard MK. Vitamin and mineral supplement prior to and during pregnancy. *Obstet Gynecol Clin North Am* 1997;24:479–498.
7. Institute of Medicine, Committee on Nutritional Status During Pregnancy and Lactation, Food and Nutrition Board. *Nutrition during pregnancy: part I, weight gain: part II, nutrition supplements.* Washington: National Academy Press, 1990.
8. Higgenbottom M, Sweetman L, Nyhan W. A syndrome of methemoglobinuria, homocystinuria, megaloblastic anemia, and neurologic abnormalities in a vitamin B12 deficient infant of a strict vegetarian. *N Engl J Med* 1978;299:317–319.
9. Block G, Abrams B. Vitamin and mineral status of women of childbearing potential. *Ann N Y Acad Sci* 1993;678:244–254.
10. Yu S, Kepel K, Singh G, et al. Preconceptional and prenatal multivitamin-mineral supplement use in the 1988 National Maternal and Infant Health Survey. *Am J Public Health* 1996;86:240–242.
11. Scholl T, Hediger M, Bendich A, et al. Use of multivitamin/mineral prenatal supplements: influence on the outcome of pregnancy. *Am J Epidemiol* 1997;146:134–141.
12. Rothman K, Moore L, Singer M, et al. Teratogenicity of high vitamin A intake. *N Engl J Med* 1995;333:1369–1373.
13. Scholl R, Hediger M, Schall J, et al. Dietary and serum folate: their influence on the outcome of pregnancy. *Am J Clin Nutr* 1996;63:520–525.
14. Sahakian V, Rouse D, Sipes S, et al. Vitamin B6 is effective therapy for nausea and vomiting of pregnancy: a randomized, double-blind, placebo-controlled trial. *Am J Obstet Gynecol* 1995;173:881–884.
15. Jewell D, Young G. Interventions for nausea and vomiting in early pregnancy (Cochrane Review). In: *The Cochrane Library,* Issue 1. Oxford: Update Software, 1999.
16. Mohamed K, Gulmezoglu AM. Pyridoxine (vitamin B6) supplementation in pregnancy (Cochrane Review). In: *The Cochrane Library,* Issue 1. Oxford: Update Software, 1999.
17. Briggs G, Freeman R, Yaffe S. *Drugs in pregnancy and lactation,* 5th ed. Baltimore: Williams & Wilkins, 1998:456–470.
18. Biale Y, Lewenthal H. Effect of folic acid supplementation on congenital malformations due to anticonvulsive drugs. *Eur J Obstet Gynecol Reprod Biol* 1984;18:211–216.
19. Mahomed K. Routine iron and folate supplementation in pregnancy (Cochrane Review). In: *The Cochrane Library,* Issue 4. Oxford: Update Software, 1998.
20. Centers for Disease Control. Knowledge about folic acid and use of multivitamins containing folic acid among reproductive-aged women–Georgia. *MMWR Morb Mortal Wkly Rep* 1996;45:793–795.
21. Centers for Disease Control. Knowledge and use of folic acid by women of childbearing age–United States, 1997. *JAMA* 1997;278:892–893.
22. Hoag S, Ramachandruni H, Shangraw F. Failure of prescription prenatal vitamin products to meet USP standards for folic acid dissolution. *J Am Pharm Assoc* 1997;NS37:397–400.
23. Cuskelly G, McNulty H, Scott J. Effect of increasing dietary folate on red-cell folate: implications for prevention of neural tube defects. *Lancet* 1996;347:657–759.

24. Mahomed K. Routine iron supplementation during pregnancy (Cochrane Review). In: *The Cochrane Library,* Issue 4. Oxford: Update Software, 1998.

25. Dawson D, Dawson R. Iron in prenatal multivitamin/multimineral supplements. *J Reprod Med* 1998;43:133–140.

26. Atallah A, Hofmeyr G, Duley L. Calcium supplementation during pregnancy to prevent hypertensive disorders and related adverse outcomes (Cochrane Review). In: *The Cochrane Library,* Issue 4. Oxford: Update Software, 1998.

27. Levine R for the CPEP Study Group. Calcium for preeclampsia prevention (CPEP): a double-blind, placebo-controlled trial in healthy nulliparas. *Am J Obstet Gynecol* 1997;176:S2.

28. Makrides M, Crowther CA. Magnesium supplementation during pregnancy (Cochrane Review). In: *The Cochrane Library,* Issue 1. Oxford: Update Software, 1999.

29. Conradt A, Weidinger H, Algayer H. On the role of magnesium fetal hypotrophy, pregnancy induced hypertension and pre-eclampsia. *Magnes Bull* 1984;6:68–76.

30. Doyle W, Crawford M, Wynn A, et al. Maternal magnesium intake and pregnancy outcome. *Magnes Res* 1989;2:205–210.

31. Sibai B, Villar M, Bary E. Magnesium supplementation during pregnancy: a double-blind randomized controlled clinical trial. *Am J Obstet Gynecol* 1989;161:115–119.

32. Prema K, Ramalagshmi B, Neelakumari S, et al. Serum copper and zinc in pregnancy. *Ind Med Res* 1980;71:547–553.

33. Kiilholma P, Gronroos M, Erkkola P, et al. The role of calcium, iron, copper and zinc in preterm delivery and premature rupture of membranes. *Gynecol Obstet Invest* 1984;17:194–201.

34. Mahomed K. Zinc supplementation in pregnancy (Cochrane Review). In: *The Cochrane Library,* Issue 4. Oxford: Update Software, 1998.

35. Simmer K, Lort-Phillips L, James C, et al. A double blind trial of zinc supplementation in pregnancy. *Eur J Clin Nutr* 191;45:139–144.

36. Goldenberg R, Tamura T, Neggers Y, et al. The effect of zinc supplementation on pregnancy outcome. *JAMA* 1995;274:463–468.

16

Folic Acid Supplementation for Prevention of Birth Defects

Jerome Yankowitz and Jennifer R. Niebyl

Department of Obstetrics and Gynecology, University of Iowa Hospitals and Clinics, Iowa City, Iowa

PREVENTION OF NEURAL TUBE DEFECTS

The Centers for Disease Control (CDC) of the United States recommended in 1991 that women who have had a pregnancy complicated by a fetal neural tube defect (NTD) take 4 mg folic acid per day before conception and through the first 3 months of pregnancy to reduce the risk of a recurrence (1). In 1992, the CDC recommended that all women consume 0.4 mg folic acid to reduce the risk of primary occurrence of NTDs (2).

These recommendations were based on data accumulated over a 30-year period linking folate deficiency or deranged folate metabolism to NTDs and protection from such defects with vitamin or folic acid supplements. Thiersch (3) described the occurrence of a large meningoencephalocele in a fetus that had survived an attempt to induce abortion with a folic acid antagonist. Although such early studies are difficult to interpret owing to problems in accurately dating the pregnancy and thus the time of exposure to the abortifacient, they are often cited as the initial clue to the role of folate in the development of the neural axis.

Smithells and colleagues (4–9) extensively studied the role of vitamins, and specifically folic acid, in protecting against the occurrence of NTDs in high-risk pregnancies. Hibbard and Smithells (4) compared 98 women who had delivered fetuses with anomalies with 54 matched controls. Women delivering anomalous infants were five times more likely to have an abnormality in folate metabolism as assessed by a forminiminoglutamic acid excretion test. Similar results were obtained when the mothers of infants with central nervous system anomalies were considered separately (4). Subsequently, it was shown that among 900 women tested in the first trimester for serum folate, red-cell folate, and other vitamin levels, women who delivered infants with NTDs had significantly lower red-cell folate levels than women who delivered normal infants (5). Other studies revealed that women who had at least one pregnancy complicated by a NTD and took a vitamin supplement containing 0.36 mg folic acid had a significantly reduced rate of recurrence: approximately 5.0% in the unsupplemented group versus only 0.6% recurrence in the supplemented group (6–9). The apparent protection was not dependent on other socioeconomic or demographic factors. An apparent protective effect of periconceptional multivitamin use in preventing the occurrence of NTDs had been reported in the Atlanta Birth Defects Case-Control Study (10), but multivitamin users were markedly different from nonusers in demographic, health-related, and lifestyle characteristics.

NTDs may result from an unknown etiology, may be secondary to a definable genetic influence, or may result from environmental effects such as nutritional deficiency or drugs. Because there may be a certain irreducible minimum of genetic factors involved, the effect of supplementation may be highest in high-prevalence areas.

A genetic disorder in folic acid metabolism may be overcome by supplementation (11,12).

The geographic distribution of NTDs also supports folic acid deficiency as an etiology because NTDs are more prevalent in colder, darker climates with less availability of fresh fruits and vegetables. For example, the prevalence in Maine is twice that in southern California (13), and in the northern provinces in China, it is 3 to 5 per 1,000 compared with 1 to 3 per 1,000 in the south (14). There is no clear correlation with serum folate and NTDs (15,16) because a difference was found in only one of seven studies. Two studies showed lower levels of red-cell folate in mothers of children with NTDs (11,16). This is presumably because serum folate fluctuates more rapidly with food intake, whereas red-cell folate is more slowly affected (11,15,16).

Three studies showed an association of levels of dietary folate intake and NTDs. In the Australian case-control study of intake in the first 6 weeks of pregnancy (17), there was a clear dose-related association with free folate intake and the risk of NTDs. An American study also found that a relatively high dietary intake of folate may reduce the risk (18). In another study, the relative risk of NTDs was 0.42 for those ingesting more than 0.1 mg per day compared with less than 0.1 mg per day of folate (19), but it was still 2.5 times higher than in those taking folic acid supplements. The increase in NTDs in Jamaica after hurricane Gilbert was associated with a significantly lower mean dietary folate intake in the periconceptional period in case subjects (0.154 mg per day) versus controls (0.254 mg per day) (20). In the United States, 92.5% of women consume less than 0.4 mg per day in their diets (21).

The richest sources of folate in foods are liver, green vegetables, legumes, dried beans, egg yolks, beets, whole wheat bread, and citrus fruits and juices. The most common sources of folate in the US diet are orange juice, bread or crackers, dried beans, green salads, and cold cereals (21). Folate dissolves with prolonged boiling and is significantly more bioavailable as folic acid than food folate. Folic acid is also found in several fortified cereals and in many multivitamin preparations.

In the first randomized, prospective, controlled, double-blind trial, Laurence et al. (22) used 4 mg folic acid per day to prevent recurrence of NTDs. Compliance was evaluated by testing serum folate levels. There were 0 in 44 recurrences in compliant patients, two in 16 recurrences in noncompliant patients, and four in 51 in the placebo group. This distribution showed a statistically significant protective effect by the ingestion of folic acid, although small numbers limited this study.

In the Atlanta birth defects case-control study (10), 347 mothers of infants with NTDs were compared with 2,829 controls. The odds ratio of the cases being periconceptional multivitamin users versus nonusers was 0.4. The folic acid doses were not specified.

In one study, patients were ascertained prospectively at the time of α-fetoprotein screening (19). The rate of NTDs in patients who never used multivitamins was 3.5 per 1,000 compared with 0.9 per 1,000 in multivitamin users, for an odds ratio of 0.27. The doses of folic acid varied, with 23% receiving 0.4 mg daily and 45% receiving 1 mg daily.

One major study reached a negative conclusion (23). The authors interviewed 571 mothers of infants with NTDs, 546 mothers of children with other defects, and 573 mothers of normal infants. The percentage of multivitamin use in each group was similar, suggesting no effect of folic acid in the prevention of NTDs. Of the patients in this study, 73% came from California, which may explain the lack of reduction in NTDs because the prevalence was low in all groups (0.9/1,000). This study was also criticized (19) as being subject to a recall bias.

The largest randomized, prospective trial was published by the Medical Research Council Vitamin Study Research Group in Great Britain in 1991 (24). Eighteen hundred women with a child affected with a NTD were randomized into one of four groups. One group received 4 mg folic acid daily, one group received seven other vitamins, one group received both the folic acid and the seven vitamins, and the fourth group received only iron and calcium. They started the supplementation at least 4 weeks before conception and continued until 12 weeks from the last menstrual period. There was a 72% reduction in affected pregnancies for a relative risk of 0.28 in both of the folic acid groups, but not in the other two groups.

Two subsequent studies (25,26) were reported from Hungary in low-risk women with no affected children. The first was a randomized, prospective trial with 0.8 mg folic acid per day given from 1 month preconception to the second missed menses. Of 2,104 women treated with 0.8 mg folic acid, no patients had infants with NTDs, and of 2,052 women in the control group, there were six NTDs, which was a statistically significant difference. This was the first trial demonstrating that periconceptional folic acid use decreases the first occurrence of neural tube defects. The Hungarian study also analyzed the risk of other major anomalies, excluding genetic syndromes and NTDs. In the group receiving folic acid, there were 9 per 1,000 defects detected at birth compared with 16.6 per 1,000 in the control group ($p < 0.03$). At 8 months, the difference was 14.7 per 1,000 compared with 28.3 per 1,000 ($p < 0.0025$). There was no difference noted in minor anomalies. Additional support for the protective effects of folic acid was found in studies from Cuba (27) and Ireland (28), where doses of 5 mg and 0.36 mg, respectively, were used.

More recently, the effect of folic acid supplementation on the rate of NTDs in an area of China with high rates of NTDs (northern region) versus one with low rates (southern region) was reported. It evaluated outcomes of pregnancy in women who were asked to take 0.4 mg folic acid daily from the time of their premarital examination until the end of their first trimester of pregnancy. Fetuses or neonates of 130,142 women who took folic acid and 117,689 who had not taken folic acid were studied. The authors identified 102 and 173 NTDs, respectively. The rates of NTDs were 4.8 per 1,000 pregnancies in the northern and 1.0 per 1,000 in the southern regions with no folic acid supplementation. The rates were 1.0 per 1,000 in the northern and 0.6 per 1000 in the southern regions with supplementation. Thus, supplementation in the amount suggested by the CDC reduced

the rated of NTDs in both high- and low-risk populations (29).

An intervention program along the Texas–Mexico border was also found to be effective in reducing recurrence risk of NTDs in this very high risk population (30).

In addition to the CDC recommendations for folate in pregnancy (1,2), the Clinical Teratology Committee of the Canadian College of Medical Geneticists (31) recommended in 1993 a minimum dosage of 0.8 mg folic acid per day, not to exceed 5.0 mg per day, for women who are at increased risk of having offspring with NTDs. They recommended that supplementation should begin before conception and continue to 10 to 12 weeks of gestation.

Although knowledge about the protective effects of folic acid in reducing NTDs is encouraging and raises hope that guidelines may provide public health benefits, the average intake of folate in the U.S. diet before food fortification was 0.2 mg per day (32); less than 10% of individuals ingest 0.4 mg or more folate in their diets (18,19,21). In areas where folate supplementation has been evaluated, the public health benefits in terms of reduced rates of NTDs have not been realized. Despite a recommendation for periconceptional folate supplementation in the United Kingdom since the early 1990s, no concurrent decline in NTDs has been observed by regional congenital anomaly registers. A clear decline in the 1980s shows that the registries are capable of detecting such a trend when it exists (33). Poor compliance with use of folic acid supplements along with poor folate intake remains a major problem, possibly accounting for these results (34).

A policy of supplementation with tablets may not reach many women because of poor compliance, unplanned pregnancy, or lack of knowledge. Thus, the FDA (35) began requiring cereal and grains (e.g. bread) to be fortified with 0.14 mg of folic acid per 100 g of grain as of January 1, 1998. This is estimated to add 0.1 mg/day of folic acid to the average diet. Mean daily folate intake for women in the United States is only 0.207 mg/day, so this level of fortification will not ensure that most women are adequately supplemented (36).

This fortification would affect older people also, who are at increased risk of pernicious anemia from achlorhydria and gastric atrophy (37). If the anemia is masked by increased folate intake, the neurologic manifestations of vitamin B_{12} deficiency may be irreversible by the time they are diagnosed. The dose level at which this might happen is not clear. However, folic acid supplementation of more than 1 mg per day may mask the diagnosis of vitamin B_{12} deficiency. Thus, 1 mg or more per day must be given by prescription. It does not appear that supplementation of less than 1 mg per day results in masking symptoms of pernicious anemia. The American College of Preventive Medicine supported a fortification policy of enriching foods with folic acid to reduce the occurrence of NTDs. They believed that at least 350 μg per day appears to be the most appropriate fortification level to maximize the prevention of NTDs while protecting the health of the general population (38). The Teratology Society also recommended that women of childbearing age take a daily vitamin supplement containing 0.4 mg folic acid and that fortification of enriched cereal grain products be carried out to a level that would provide 0.4 mg folic acid per day to at least 95% of reproductive-age women (39).

Whether the current level of fortification is appropriate is argued vehemently in the literature. Oakley (40) and others strongly believe that the suggested level is too low, whereas Mills (41), in outlining data concerning folate and NTDs and concerns about masking pernicious anemia, stated that until data are available, there should be no increase in fortification. Data from a North Carolina Birth Defects Monitoring Program showed no clear reduction in birth defects after fortification (42). These disappointing data may be related to CDC data (43) that showed that in 1997 only 30% of nonpregnant women were taking a multivitamin containing folic acid on a daily basis. Although this is an improvement over the 25% rate in 1995, it is still inadequate. These CDC data (43) highlighted the need for additional educational efforts targeted toward women aged younger than 25 years of age who account for approximately 39% of all births in the United States. No impact on occurrence of NTDs has yet been noted. Lack of proof that fortification is reducing the occurrence of NTDs is particularly disappointing as studies have shown that fortification of grain with folic acid could theoretically yield a substantial economic benefit (44).

Another mechanism of NTD formation may be an abnormality in homocysteine metabolism. In one study, mothers of infants with NTDs had higher serum homocysteine values than vitamin B_{12}–level matched controls (12). In another study, the homocysteine concentration in amniotic fluid was higher in infants affected with NTDs than in controls (45). The values of vitamin B_{12} and folate were in the normal range, suggesting a metabolic defect rather than a deficiency. However, the effect may be more marked with low vitamin B_{12} levels, and vitamin B_{12} supplementation could decrease the folic acid dose required (12). A thermolabile form of the enzyme 5,10 methylenetetrahydrofolate reductase (MTHFR) results in elevated plasma homocysteine levels. The thermolability is owing to a common mutation, 677C to T, in the *MTHFR* gene. It was shown that NTDs are much more common with fetal homozygosity for the 677C to T mutation (46). Others also showed a relationship between maternal and/or fetal homozygosity for the 677C to T mutation in populations in the Netherlands and Ireland (47,48).

Wenstrom et al. (49) hypothesized that the thermolabile variant of the enzyme MTHFR with its reduced activity leading to altered homocysteine metabolism can be overcome by folate supplementation. They found that approximately 38% of NTDs occur in fetuses with normal 677C to T alleles or that approximately two thirds occur in the presence of an abnormal allele. They also found that there were no higher rates of mutant alleles in cases of anencephaly and sacral defects, whereas there were in defects at the cervical and lumbar spine, leading to the hypothesis that the influence of the MTHFR mutation was site specific. The relationship between allele type and amniotic fluid homocysteine levels is complex, and the specific relationship between allele type, homocysteine levels, and production of NTDs awaits additional research (50).

The association between other adverse pregnancy-related outcomes and homocysteine levels suggests that folate supplementation could have more far-reaching effects. Homocysteine and folate levels were measured in 123 women who had at least two consecutive spontaneous early losses and were compared with 104 healthy controls. It was noted that the serum folate concentrations were significantly lower than those of controls. Both elevated fasting and afterload homocysteine levels were risk factors for recurrent early pregnancy loss (51). There is also a large body of evidence indicating that elevated plasma total homocysteine may be causally related to risk of coronary, cerebral, and peripheral arterial diseases. Increased levels may also be a marker for adverse outcomes in pregnancy such as increased risk of preeclampsia, premature delivery, very low birth weight, NTDs, and clubfoot (52). One hospital-based, case-control study in Zimbabwe of 33 pregnant women with eclampsia, 138 with preeclampsia, and 185 normotensive pregnant women was reported. Plasma homocysteine levels were measured postpartum. Significantly higher levels were seen in eclamptic and preeclamptic women (12.54 and 12.77 μmol/L, respectively) versus those in controls (9.93 μmol/L) (53). Homocysteine levels were normally significantly lower during all three trimesters than in nonpregnant controls and were directly correlated with albumin levels. Homocysteine concentrations were decreased in subjects taking folic acid supplementation (54).

Whether the occurrence of other anomalies is related to folate and homocysteine is not clear, but periconceptional multivitamin use has also been shown, in a case-control study, to reduce the risk of cleft lip/cleft palate (55). A relationship to homocysteine metabolism is hypothesized (56) but is not clear.

Studies including women on antiepileptic drugs who are known to be at increased risk of NTDs are lacking. It is known that blood folate levels decrease with increasing plasma levels of antiepileptic drugs and that folic acid supplementation can lower phenytoin levels (57). The recommendation for these women is to continue the folic acid supplementation and monitor plasma levels of the antiepileptic drugs (57,58). There is no clear proof that folic acid supplementation of as much as 1 mg per day is a problem, and this level was deemed safe in individuals with controlled epilepsy by the Folic Acid Subcommittee of the US Department of Health and Human Services (36). One study does indicate a reduced risk of congenital malformations in women who are using anticonvulsive drugs and receive folic acid supplementation versus those who do not receive folic acid supplementation (59). Recently, Hernandez-Diaz S et al (60) performed a case control study evaluating the ability of dihydrofolate reductastase inhibitors and certain anti-epileptic drugs to increase the risk of cardiovascular anomalies, urinary tract defects, or oral-facial clefts and whether use of multivitamin supplements containing folic acid could diminish any adverse effects of these drugs. The authors found that use of dihydrofolate reductastase inhibitors, such as aminopterin, methotrexate, sulfasalazine, pyrimethamine, triamterene, and trimethoprim increase the risks of cardiovascular defects and oral clefts. The risk of these defects was reduced back to the normal range if the mother gave a history of multi-vitamin use containing folic acid. The anti-epileptic drugs such as carbamazepine, phenytoin, primidone, and phenobarbital also caused an increase in cardiovascular defects, oral clefts, and urinary tract defects. Maternal use of multi-vitamins containing folic acid did not appear to reduce the increased risk of these malformations however. Clearly this is an area that will require additional evaluation. Other high-risk women such as diabetics have not been studied, but the "metabolic block" (12) theory would support the use of the 4-mg dose.

SUMMARY

In summary, birth defects are of several etiologies. Low folate intake has been associated with NTDs and a high level of dietary intake may be relatively protective. Folic acid supplementation can prevent most NTDs in high-risk populations. The daily recommended dose is 4 mg for all women with a previously affected child, and 0.4 mg daily is recommended for all women preconceptionally. Because folic acid supplementation does not eliminate all cases of NTDs, prenatal diagnosis should still be offered.

REFERENCES

1. Centers for Disease Control. Use of folic acid for prevention of spina bifida and other neural tube defects—1983–1991. *MMWR Morb Mortal Wkly Rep* 1991;40:513–516.
2. Centers for Disease Control. Recommendations for the use of folic acid to reduce the number of cases of spina bifida and other neural tube defects. *MMWR Morb Mortal Wkly Rep* 1992;41:1–7.
3. Thiersch JB. Therapeutic abortions with a folic acid antagonist, 4-amino-pteroylglutamic acid (4-amino P.G.A.) administered by the oral route. *Am J Obstet Gynecol* 1952;63:1298–1304.
4. Hibbard ED, Smithells RW. Folic acid metabolism and human embryopathy. *Lancet* 1965;i:1254.
5. Smithells RW, Sheppard S, Schorah CJ. Vitamin deficiencies and neural tube defects. *Arch Dis Child* 1976;51:944–950.
6. Smithells RW, Sheppard S, Schorah CJ, et al. Apparent prevention of neural tube defects by periconceptional vitamin supplementation. *Arch Dis Child* 1981;56:911–918.
7. Wild J, Read AP, Sheppard S, et al. Recurrent neural tube defects, risk factors and vitamins. *Arch Dis Child* 1986;61:440–444.
8. Smithells RW, Sheppard S, Schorah CJ, et al. Possible prevention of neural tube defects by periconceptional vitamin supplementation. *Lancet* 1980;i:339–340.
9. Smithells RW, Seller MJ, Harris R, et al. Further experience of vitamin supplementation for prevention of neural tube defect recurrences. *Lancet* 1983;i:1027–1031.
10. Mulinare J, Cordero JF, Erickson JD, et al. Periconceptional use of multivitamins and the occurrence of neural tube defects. *JAMA* 1988;260:3141–3145.
11. Yates JRW, Ferguson Smith MA, Shenkin A, et al. Is disordered folate metabolism the basis for the genetic predisposition to neural tube defects? *Clin Genet* 1987; 31:279–287.
12. National Institute of Child Health and Human Development, National Institutes of Health, Health Research Board of Ireland, et al. Homocysteine metabolism in pregnancies complicated by neural-tube defects. *Lancet* 1995;345:149–151.
13. Flood T, Brewster M, Harris J, et al. Spina bifida incidence at birth—United States, 1983–1990. *MMWR Morb Mortal Wkly Rep* 1992;41:497–500.
14. Chung Hua TSC. Epidemiology of neural tube defects in China. *Chinese J Med* 1989;69:189–191.
15. Mills JL, Tuomilehto J, Yu KF, et al. Maternal vitamin levels during pregnancies producing infants with neural tube defects. *J Pediatr* 1992;120:863–871.
16. Rush D. Periconceptional folate and neural tube defect. *Am J Clin Nutr* 1994;59[Suppl]:511S–516S.
17. Bower C, Stanley FJ. Dietary folate as a risk factor for neural tube defects: evidence from a case control study in western Australia. *Med J Aust* 1989;150:613–619.
18. Werler MM, Shapiro S, Mitchell AA. Periconceptional folic acid exposure and risk of occurrent neural tube defects. *JAMA* 1993;269:1257–1261.
19. Milunsky A, Jick H, Jick SS, et al. Multivitamin/folic acid supplementation in early pregnancy reduces the prevalence of neural tube defects. *JAMA* 1989;262:2847–2852.
20. Duff EMW, Cooper ES. Neural tube defects in Jamaica following Hurricane Gilbert. *Am J Public Health* 1994; 84:473–476.
21. Subar AF, Block G, James LD. Folate intake and food sources in the US population. *Am J Clin Nutr* 1989;50: 508–516.
22. Laurence KM, James N, Miller MH, et al. Double blind randomized controlled trial of folate treatment before conception to prevent recurrence of neural tube defects. *BMJ* 1981;282:1509–1511.
23. Mills JL, Rhoads GG, Simpson JL, et al. The absence of relation between the periconceptional use of vitamins and neural tube defects. *N Engl J Med* 1989;321:430–435.
24. MRC Vitamin Study Research Group. Prevention of neural tube defects: results of the Medical Research Council Vitamin Study. *Lancet* 1991;338:13–17.
25. Czeizel AE, Dudas I. Prevention of the first occurrence of neural tube defects by periconceptional vitamin supplementation. *N Engl J Med* 1992;327:1832–1835.
26. Czeizel AE. Prevention of congenital abnormalities by periconceptional multivitamin supplementation. *BMJ* 1993;306:1645–1648.
27. Vergel RG, Sanchez LR, Heredero BL, et al. Primary prevention of neural tube defects with folic acid supplementation: Cuban experience. *Prenat Diagn* 1990;10: 149–152.
28. Kirke PN, Daly LE, Elwood JH for the Irish Vitamin Study Group. A randomised trial of low dose folic acid to prevent neural tube defects. *Arch Dis Child* 1992;67;1442–1446.
29. Berry RJ, Li Z, Erickson JD, et al. Prevention of neural-tube defects with folic acid in China. China–U.S. Collaborative Project for Neural Tube Defect Prevention. *N Engl J Med* 1999;341:1485–1490.
30. Anonymous. From the Centers for Disease Control and Prevention. Neural tube defect surveillance and folic acid intervention—Texas-Mexico border, 1993–1998. *JAMA* 2000;283:2928–2930.
31. Van Allen M, Fraser FC, Dallaire L, et al. Recommendations on the use of folic acid supplementation to prevent the recurrence of neural tube defects. *Can Med Assoc J* 1993;149:1239–1243.
32. National Academy of Sciences. Nutrition during pregnancy. Institute of Medicine, Food and Nutrition Board. Washington: National Academy Press, 1990:365.
33. Abramsky L, Botting B, Chapple J, et al. Has advice on periconceptional folate supplementation reduced neural-tube defects? *Lancet* 1999;354:998–999.
34. Michie CA, Narang I, Rogers J, et al. Folate supplementation and neural-tube defects. *Lancet* 2000;355:147.
35. Nightingale SL. From the Food and Drug Administration: Proposals for folic acid fortification and labelling of certain foods to reduce the risk of neural tube defects. *JAMA* 1993;270:2283.
36. Lewis DP, Van Dyke DC, Stumbo PJ, et al. Drug and environmental factors associated with adverse pregnancy outcomes. Part III: folic acid: pharmacology, therapeutic recommendations, and economics. *Ann Pharmacother* 1998;32:1087–1095.
37. Wald NJ, Bower C. Folic acid, pernicious anaemia, and prevention of neural tube defects. *Lancet* 1994;343:307.

38. Bentley JR, Ferrini R, Hill LL. American College of Preventive Medicine public policy statement. Folic acid fortification of grain products in the U.S. to prevent neural tube defects. *Am J Prev Med* 1999;16:264–267.

39. Holmes L, Harris J, Oakley GP Jr, et al. Teratology Society Consensus Statement on use of folic acid to reduce the risk of birth defects. *Teratology* 1997;55:381.

40. Oakley GP Jr. Prevention of neural-tube defects. *N Engl J Med* 1999;341:1546.

41. Mills JL. Fortification of foods with folic acid—how much is enough?. *N Engl J Med* 2000;342:1442–1445.

42. Meyer RE, Oakley GP Jr. Folic acid fortification. *Lancet* 1999;354:2168.

43. Anonymous. From the Centers for Disease Control and Prevention. Knowledge and use of folic acid by women of childbearing age—United States, 1997. *JAMA* 1997;278:892–893.

44. Romano PS, Waitzman NJ, Scheffler RM, et al. Folic acid fortification of grain: an economic analysis. *Am J Public Health* 1995;85:667–676.

45. Steegers-Theunissen RP, Boers GH, Blom HJ, et al. Neural tube defects and elevated homocysteine levels in amniotic fluid. *Am J Obstet Gynecol* 1995;172:1436–1441.

46. Ou CY, Stevenson RE, Brown VK, et al. 5,10 methylenetetrahydrofolate reductase genetic polymorphism as a risk factor for neural tube defects. *Am J Med Genet* 1996;63:610–614.

47. van der Put N, Steegers-Theunissen R, Frosst P, et al. Mutated 5,10 methylenetetrahydrofolate reductase as a risk factor for spina bifida. *Lancet* 1995;346:1070–1071.

48. Whitehead AS, Gallagher P, Mills JL, et al. A genetic defect in 5,10 methylenetetrahydrofolate reductase in neural tube defects. *Q J Med* 1995;88:763–766.

49. Wenstrom KD, Johanning GL, Owen J, et al. Amniotic fluid homocysteine levels, 5,10-methylenetetrahydrafolate reductase genotypes, and neural tube closure sites. *Am J Med Genet* 2000;90:6–11.

50. Wenstrom KD, Johanning GL, Owen J, et al. Role of amniotic fluid homocysteine level and of fetal 5,10-methylenetetrahydrafolate reductase genotype in the etiology of neural tube defects. *Am J Med Genet* 2000;90:12–16.

51. Nelen WL, Blom HJ, Steegers EA, et al. Homocysteine and folate levels as risk factors for recurrent early pregnancy loss. *Obstet Gynecol* 2000;95:519–524.

52. Picciano MF. Is homocysteine a biomarker for identifying women at risk of complications and adverse pregnancy outcomes? *Am J Clin Nutr* 2000;71:857–858.

53. Rajkovic A, Mahomed K, Malinow MR, et al. Plasma homocyst(e)ine concentrations in eclamptic and preeclamptic African women postpartum. *Obstet Gynecol* 1999;94:355–360.

54. Walker MC, Smith GN, Perkins SL, et al. Changes in homocysteine levels during normal pregnancy. *Am J Obstet Gynecol* 1999;180:660–664.

55. Shaw GM, Larnmer EJ, Wasserman CR, et al. Risks of orofacial clefts in children born to women using multivitamins containing folic acid periconceptionally. *Lancet* 1995;345:393–396.

56. Wong WY, Eskes TK, Kuijpers-Jagtman AM, et al. Nonsyndromic orofacial clefts: association with maternal hyperhomocysteinemia. *Teratology* 1999;60:253–257.

57. Dansky LV, Rosenblatt DS, Andermann E. Mechanisms of teratogenesis: folic acid and antiepileptic therapy. *Neurology* 1992;42:32–42.

58. Berg MJ, Fischer LJ, Rivey MP, et al. Phenytoin and folic acid interaction: a preliminary report. *Ther Drug Monit* 1983;5:389–394.

59. Biale Y, Lewenthal H. Effect of folic acid supplementation on congenital malformations due to anticonvulsant drugs. *Europ J Obstet Gynec Reprod Biol* 1984;18:211–216.

60. Hernandez-Diaz S, Werler MM, Walker AM, Mitchell AA. Folic acid antagonist during pregnancy and the risk of birth defects. *N Engl J Med* 2000;343:1608–1614.

17

Treatment of Connective Tissue Disorders in Pregnancy

William F. Rayburn

Department of Obstetrics and Gynecology, The University of New Mexico Health Sciences Center, Albuquerque, New Mexico

Connective tissue disorders are immuno-pathologically mediated as a consequence of a variety of autoantibodies. Many of these disorders are encountered among reproduction-age women. Although the pathogenesis is not well understood, immunologically mediated tissue destruction of various organs (skin, joints, blood vessels, kidneys) is a common denominator. Such diseases that are occasionally encountered during pregnancy include systemic lupus erythematosus, rheumatoid arthritis, scleroderma, dermatomyositis, and a multitude of vasculitis syndromes.

Renal involvement is common in these diseases. As pregnancy is affected by glomerulopathology, a search for coexisting renal involvement is essential. Hypertension is also common, and either chronic or pregnancy-induced hypertension frequently requires preterm delivery. Antiphospholipid antibodies, formed in some of these immune-mediated diseases, can cause injury to the placenta and the fetus.

This chapter provides general information about precautions to take when prescribing during pregnancy. The literature is reviewed on representative drugs used for maintenance therapy of women with preexisting connective tissue disorders who either are anticipating childbearing or are already pregnant. Guidelines for counseling a nursing mother about each medication are also provided.

PRESCRIBING DURING PREGNANCY

Preconception counseling should include an evaluation for whether the drug is to be continued, whether another drug may be a safer substitute, and whether monotherapy is permissible when more than one drug is taken. Unfortunately, many women with medical disorders requiring medication conceive without having benefited from such counseling. Menstrual delays or dysfunctional uterine bleeding from impaired ovulation are often associated with chronic illness, especially when hormones or centrally acting drugs are ingested. Sexual impotence and reduced sperm count or motility may result from certain medications and are often reversible if discontinuation of medication is acceptable. It is assumed that most medications, when taken long term, can be transferred from the plasma to the seminal fluid and, with mating, transferred to females. The effect that this precopulatory treatment may have on early pregnancy loss is unknown but unlikely.

Drugs may be absorbed as easily during pregnancy as when nonpregnant, and the maternal serum concentration of albumin is lower for drug binding (1). Unless the unbound drug or active metabolite has a large spatial configuration or a large molecular weight, it should cross the placenta easily. Umbilical serum concentrations become comparable with the mother's with long-term exposure (1,2). The risk of newer drugs to the fetus may not have been fully explored. Drugs prescribed as maintenance therapy during pregnancy are, therefore, usually older and have a larger body of experience.

Fetal exposure may be divided into three periods: (i) ovum, from fertilization to implantation; (ii) embryo, from the second through the eighth week; and (iii) fetus, from the eighth completed week until term. The embryonic period encompasses the most critical time with respect to malformations. Some drugs, because of their mechanisms of action, may have detrimental fetal effects when taken after the eighth week. Craniofacial abnormalities, intrauterine growth restriction, temporary hematologic abnormalities, and transient immunosuppression are possible (3).

Limitations exist when considering which medication is safe to continue when pregnant. Comparative trials of drugs during gestation are uncommon because of a lack of sufficient case numbers. A control population is often not possible, making it difficult to distinguish between any additional risks from the medication and from the underlying disease. A case report about prenatal exposure to a particular drug is more likely to be published if a malformation is present rather than absent. Such reports may feature exposures to other agents, making any association between a malformation and a single causative agent unlikely. Interpretation of published findings is also limited when a higher dose and a different route of administration are used. For example, a lower dose given orally may be safer to the mother and to the fetus than a higher dose given intravenously.

Alternative therapies occasionally exist that are safer to a developing fetus. Any single drug or combination of medications should be altered, when possible, in the preconception period to include those drugs that have been most thoroughly assessed in human pregnancy and that have been determined to pose the lowest risk.

Principles of maintenance therapy are the same during gestation as when nonpregnant. Knowledge about one or two medications for each disorder is recommended. Symptoms of pregnancy, such as nausea, fatigue, edema, headaches, and gastrointestinal disturbance, may mimic side effects or toxic reactions to drugs. A challenge to

the rheumatologist and to the obstetrician is to choose that drug with the maximum therapeutic response to the mother and with the least adverse effect on the mother, fetus, and nursing infant.

SPECIFIC MEDICATIONS: PRECAUTIONS DURING PREGNANCY AND BREAST-FEEDING

Prednisone and Prednisolone

Prednisone, a glucocorticoid, is not biologically active until it is converted by the liver into prednisolone, an active metabolite. High doses of prednisone consistently cause teratogenic effects in rodents; however, such effects have not been reported during human pregnancy (4). Data from animal experiments and from clinical observations suggest that prenatal exposure to prednisone may restrict fetal growth and increase the incidence of low birth weight offspring (5,6). This outcome may be attributed to the underlying disease for which the glucocorticoid was given (7,8). Although an increased risk of stillbirth has been described among women treated with prednisolone, many other reports demonstrated successful pregnancies among women exposed to these agents before pregnancy and throughout gestation (9–11). Prednisone has not been shown to prevent recurrent fetal death in women with antiphospholipid antibody syndrome; instead it may worsen fetal outcome, especially when administered to asymptomatic women (12). Although immunosuppression lasting 15 weeks after birth was reported in one infant born to a woman receiving high doses of prednisone and azathioprine, lymphopenia and reduced immunoglobulin levels have not been commonly observed in similarly treated infants (13,14).

Small amounts of prednisone and prednisolone are secreted into breast milk (15). Even at 80 mg/dL, however, the amount of prednisone in breast milk is equivalent to less than 10% of a nursing infant's endogenous cortisol production. This dose would unlikely produce any clinically significant effects (15). The American Academy of Pediatrics classified prednisone and prednisolone as being compatible with breast-feeding (16).

Aspirin

Some case-control studies reported associations between aspirin use and human congenital malformations during early gestation, but a consistent adverse outcome attributable to drug use has not been uncovered. A prospective study of more than 50,000 pregnancies did not disclose any evidence of aspirin-induced teratogenicity, altered birth weight, or increase in perinatal deaths (17). Postterm pregnancy and a longer duration of pregnancy were more common among those who took aspirin (18). This observation is consistent with animal and human data for other aspirin-like drugs that decrease uterine contractions and prolong pregnancy (19,20).

Two case-control studies reported conflicting information that aspirin is associated with an increased risk of some heart defects in the offspring (21,22). The near-term use of aspirin and other prostaglandin synthetase inhibitors may cause constriction or closure of the fetal ductus arteriosus with resultant pulmonary hypertension (23,24). Aspirin also decreases platelet adhesiveness and aggregation, and premature infants exposed to aspirin within 1 week before delivery are at increased risk of intracranial hemorrhage (25). Available reports suggest that analgesic doses of aspirin may complicate delivery and adversely affect the newborn (26).

Several studies indicated that small daily doses of aspirin (60 to 100 mg) taken by women at high risk of preeclampsia may significantly reduce the incidence of pregnancy-induced hypertension (27–34). To address the many limitations of previous smaller studies, a multinational investigation involving more than 9,000 women was undertaken (35). Data from this prospective study did not support previously published observations that routine use of low-dose (60 mg per day) aspirin produced significant benefits for pregnancies at increased risk of preeclampsia or fetal growth restriction. Low-dose aspirin reduced fetal morbidity in a select population of women with early-onset preeclampsia. These women were typically those with preexisting disorders, such as chronic hypertension or renal disease, or those who developed preeclampsia before 32 weeks in a previous pregnancy. No significant adverse effects to the mother, fetus, or newborn were associated with use of low-dose aspirin (36).

For women with lupus anticoagulant and anticardiolipin antibodies, use of low-dose (60 to 80 mg per day) aspirin in conjunction with heparin may improve pregnancy outcomes and prevent most thrombotic events. One report did not find any benefit from the use of prednisone in conjunction with low-dose aspirin (37).

Newborns exposed *in utero* to a low dose, rather than a therapeutic dose, of aspirin have not been found to be at increased risk of bleeding abnormalities (27,28). Neonatal levels of 6-keto-prostaglandin $F_{1\alpha}$ and thromboxane B_2 were unaffected when the mother took as much as 80 mg per day (38). Platelet aggregation was not inhibited, all infants had normal echocardiograms, and no cephalhematomas, gastrointestinal bleeding, or purpura were evident (38).

Aspirin and other salicylates are transferred into breast milk (39,40). The reduced clearance of salicylates by neonates may result in drug accumulation and toxic effects even when repeated exposures are small (39,41). Because of this concern, the WHO Working Group on Human Lactation classified salicylates as being unsafe for chronic use by nursing women (42). Many pediatricians disagree with this classification.

Other Nonsteroidal Antiinflammatory Drugs

Ibuprofen

Use of ibuprofen (Motrin, Advil, Nuprin, Medipren) has been reported in small animals and in approximately 100 human pregnancies to not increase the risk of congenital anomalies (43–45). However, a case-control study on gastroschisis found affected pregnancies to be at significantly increased risk of this malformation after exposure to aspirin or ibuprofen (46).

Ibuprofen and other nonsteroidal antiinflammatory agents are reversible inhibitors of prostaglandin synthetase and are, therefore, used as tocolytics to inhibit preterm uterine contractions. The greatest concern with ibuprofen and other nonsteroidal antiinflammatory agents during the third trimester has been premature closure of the ductus with resultant pulmonary hypertension in the fetus and neonate. This reversible phenomenon has been demonstrated in rats and in several human cases (47–51). This potential toxicity from ibuprofen is the basis for the recommendation that nonsteroidal antiinflammatory drugs not be used during the third trimester. In addition, a reduction of amniotic fluid volume is associated with exposure to those drugs. A case report on a triplet gestation in which ibuprofen was taken as a tocolytic drug demonstrated a relationship between the administration of ibuprofen and oligohydramnios (52). This relationship, which is mediated by arginine vasopressin, was also found in a group of 30 women with preterm labor who received ibuprofen (53). Many clinicians have recommended that weekly or biweekly ultrasonographic examinations be performed to search for this possible complication if ibuprofen, or any prostaglandin synthetase inhibitor, is used as a tocolytic (52).

Nonsteroidal antiinflammatory agents are not transferred into breast milk in significant quantities (54,55). The American Academy of Pediatrics classified ibuprofen as being compatible with breast-feeding (16).

Indomethacin

Indomethacin crosses the human placenta easily (56). The reported number of exposed pregnancies is too small to conclude that indomethacin is safe during the first trimester. In a study of nine infants born after first-trimester exposure, one had hypospadias and the others were apparently normal (57).

Several cases of premature closure of the ductus arteriosus and subsequent pulmonary hypertension and pleural effusion have been reported with administration of this drug (58–64). This observation was evaluated in a more formal study that found fetal exposure to indomethacin was associated with a 5% to 10% rate of ductal constriction before 32 weeks of gestation with a rapid rise in response rate to 50% at 32 weeks and 100% at approximately 34 weeks (24). Minimal effects on ductal size have been reported when gestational age is less than 27 weeks (63). Moise

et al. (24,56,65) recommended weekly echocardiographic surveillance of any fetus exposed to this agent or to other drugs that may cause ductal constriction, although in their experience, ductal constriction is unusual in fetuses before 32 weeks of gestation.

Indomethacin has been associated with intraventricular hemorrhage, necrotizing enterocolitis, and sepsis in retrospective studies (65–68). In contrast to these reports, a review of 62 infants delivered prematurely after exposure to indomethacin between 24 and 32 weeks did not show an increased risk of any complications (69).

Fetal and neonatal renal function may be impaired by exposure to indomethacin (60,63). A decrease in renal perfusion has not been documented. Increases in the circulating levels of vasopressin and enhanced renal vasopressin effects explain the fetal oliguria and hypertension (69,70). Because of these renal effects, oligohydramnios is associated with maternal use of indomethacin (23,63,69). Scrutiny for adverse hemodynamic effects is especially necessary when indomethacin, or any other antiinflammatory drug, is used by hypertensive pregnant patients (53,71–75).

Indomethacin is transferred into breast milk (76). The American Academy of Pediatrics classified indomethacin as being compatible with breast-feeding (16).

Antimalarials

Hydroxychloroquine (Plaquenil) is a quinine derivative that shares many of the pharmacologic properties of chloroquine, an antimalarial and antiinflammatory agent. Antirheumatic doses of both hydroxychloroquine and chloroquine have been used safely during pregnancy by mothers with systemic lupus erythematosus (77–82). In a report on the outcome of 169 births in which 300 mg chloroquine were ingested once weekly throughout pregnancy, only two infants with anomalies were identified: one with tetralogy of Fallot and the second with congenital hypothyroidism (83). After exposure to larger antiinflammatory doses (250 to 500 mg per day), two cases of cochleovestibular paresis were reported (84). As with all drugs of this class, the possibility of hemolysis related to glucose-6-phosphate de-hydrogenase deficiency in the mother or fetus must be considered.

Small amounts of hydroxychloroquine are transferred into breast milk, and any harmful effects are considered to be unlikely (85). The WHO Working Group on Drugs and Human Lactation concluded that women using larger doses of this drug for treating connective tissue disorders should avoid breast-feeding (42). Potential problems would include the accumulation of this alkaline drug in breast milk and its probable reduced renal clearance by infants.

Gold Salts

Gold (Au), an element of atomic number 79 and atomic weight 197, is incorporated in several compounds used for arthritis treatment. Transplacental passage of this agent has been documented (42,86), and fetal serum concentrations of gold approach those in maternal serum. Outcomes of 10 gold-exposed pregnancies did not identify any abnormalities in the offspring attributable to the medication (87). Another study of 119 pregnancies exposed to gold during the first trimester found two pregnancies with minor fetal anomalies (one with a dislocated hip and one with acetabular flattening) (88). At this time, however, gold therapy is not contraindicated during pregnancy if necessary for maternal health (89).

Gold is excreted into breast milk and absorbed by the infant (90–93). Exposure to gold has been speculated to cause rashes, nephritis, hepatitis, and hematologic abnormalities, but these associations have not been proven (86–93). Close monitoring is recommended, although exposure to a relatively high dose of gold throughout gestation and during lactation appears to be well tolerated by exposed infants (86,93). The American Academy of Pediatrics classified gold salts as being compatible with breast-feeding (16).

Methotrexate

Methotrexate (Amethopterin) is a folic acid antagonist. Folic acid is important for the replication of nucleic acids and, because of its role in these processes, folic acid antagonism may result in abnormal development (94). It is not known how methotrexate treatment is compatible with normal reproduction. Toxicity to embryonic or trophoblastic tissues is clearly demonstrated by the use of this drug to terminate ectopic pregnancies and as an abortifacient (95–98).

Teratogenic effects from methotrexate have been identified in a small number of pregnancies (99). Malformations induced by methotrexate include a "clover-leaf" skull with a large head, swept-back hair, low-set ears, prominent eyes, and a wide nasal bridge. Limb defects, absent ossification centers, and central nervous system abnormalities (anencephaly, hydrocephaly, and meningomyelocele) have also been described (99). Findings from case reports suggest that maternal methotrexate produces developmental anomalies if more than 10 mg is taken per week (100). Given the small number of available case reports and the limited details on the timing of methotrexate exposures, any delineation of a narrow critical period for exposure (e.g., 6 to 8 weeks) should be considered tentative. The possibility exists that use of this agent during pregnancy will be associated with abnormal fetal growth and perhaps with transplacental carcinogenesis (101).

Methotrexate is excreted into breast milk in small quantities. Although the amount ingested daily through milk is less than 0.5% of the pediatric therapeutic dose (0.12 mg/kg) and has not been associated with adverse effects (102), methotrexate has been listed by the American Academy of Pediatrics as being contraindicated during breast-feeding (16).

Cyclophosphamide

Cyclophosphamide (Cytoxan, Neosar) is an alkylating agent used as an immunosuppressant in cancer chemotherapy. Based on various reports, the risk of malformation from cyclophosphamide has been estimated to be one in every six exposures (99). In human pregnancies, cyclophosphamide during the first trimester has been associated with skeletal and palate defects and with malformations of the limbs and eyes (103–109). Use of cyclophosphamide during the second and third trimesters is associated with a much smaller risk, but published studies indicate it may induce pancytopenia and may impair fetal growth (110,111). Transplacental carcinogenesis has not been described.

Cyclophosphamide is secreted into breast milk (112). One report indicates that the platelet and leukocyte counts of a nursing infant were reversibly depressed during maternal cyclophosphamide therapy (113). Cyclophosphamide has been classified as being contraindicated during breast-feeding by the American Academy of Pediatrics (16).

Azathioprine

Azathioprine (Imuran) is an antimetabolite used for immunosuppression. This drug and its metabolic, 6-mercaptopurine, are purine analogs that are cytotoxic. Although azathioprine is mutagenic in several bacterial test systems, it is unlikely to be a mutagen in humans (114). Successful pregnancies in patients using azathioprine and other immunosuppressants have been reported (99,112,115–118).

Many reports about azathioprine include the coadministration of other medications (especially prednisone) and involve women with serious medical illnesses such as renal failure. The role of the other agents or of the underlying medical conditions in producing azathioprine-associated reproductive toxicity is unclear (99–118). Because of its mechanism of action, azathioprine may be associated with fetal growth restriction and fetal immunosuppression and/or marrow toxicity. Increased rates of spontaneous abortions, birth defects, and stillbirths have not been described with prenatal exposure to this drug, although the number of reported cases with adequate follow-up is insufficient to detect a small increase in these rates or to detect late-occurring abnormalities.

Azathioprine is secreted into breast milk in small amounts (42,119,120). Reported studies of three breast-fed infants who were exposed to azathioprine did not find any abnormalities in their blood counts or in their growth rates (42,120). Despite these reports, breast-feeding while receiving azathioprine and its metabolite is not recommended by the WHO Working Group on Drugs and Human Lactation (42).

REFERENCES

1. Noschel H, Peiker G, Muller M, et al. Pharmacokinetics during pregnancy and delivery. *Biol Res Pregnancy* 1982;3:66–73.
2. Mirkin BL, Singh S. Placental transfer of pharmacologically active molecules. In: Mirkin BL, ed. *Perinatal pharmacology and Therapeutics*. New York: Academic Press, 1976:5770.
3. Livesey G, Rayburn W. Principles of perinatal pharmacology. In: Rayburn WF, Zuspan FP, eds. *Drug therapy in obstetrics and gynecology,* 3rd ed. St. Louis: Mosby–Year Book, 1992:5–7.
4. Fraser F, Sajoo A. Teratogenic potential of corticosteroids in humans. *Teratology* 1995;51:45–46.
5. Reinisch JM, Simon N, Karow W. Prenatal exposure to prednisone in humans and animals retards intrauterine growth. *Science* 1978;202:436–438.
6. Scott JR. Fetal growth retardation associated with maternal administration of immunosuppressive drugs. *Am J Obstet Gynecol* 1977;128:668–676.
7. Fine LG, Barnett E, Danovitch G, et al. Systemic lupus erythematosus in pregnancy. *Ann Intern Med* 1981;94:667–677.
8. Fitzsimons R, Greenberger P, Patterson R. Outcome of pregnancy in women requiring corticosteroids for severe asthma. *J Allergy Clin Immunol* 1986;78:349–353.
9. Warrell DW, Taylor R. Outcome for the fetus of mothers receiving prednisolone during pregnancy. *Lancet* 1968;1:117–118.
10. Brown JH, Maxwell AP, McGeown MG. Outcome of pregnancy following renal transplantation. *Ir J Med Sci* 1991;160:255–256.
11. Schardein JL. *Chemically induced birth defects,* 2nd ed. New York: Marcel Dekker, 1993:310.
12. Lockshin MD, Druzin M, Qamar T. Prednisone does not prevent recurrent fetal death in women with antiphospholipid antibody. *Am J Obstet Gynecol* 1989;160:439–443.
13. Cote CJ, Meuwissen H, Pickering R. Effects on the neonate of prednisone and azathioprine administered to the mother during pregnancy. *J Pediatr* 1974;85:324–328.
14. Cedeqvist LL, Merkatz I, Litwin S. Fetal immunoglobulin synthesis following maternal immunosuppression. *Am J Obstet Gynecol* 1977;129:687–690.
15. Ost L, Wettrell G, Bjorkhem I, et al. Prednisolone excretion in human milk. *J Pediatr* 1985;106:1008–1011.
16. Committee on Drugs, American Academy of Pediatrics. The transfer of drugs and other chemicals into human breast milk. *Pediatrics* 1994;93:137–150.
17. Slone D, Heinonen O, Kaufman D. Aspirin and congenital malformations. *Lancet* 1976;1:1373–1375.
18. Lewis RB, Schulman JD. Influence of acetylsalicylic acid, an inhibitor of prostaglandin synthesis, on the duration of human gestation and labor. *Lancet* 1973;2:1159–1163.
19. Powell JG Jr, Cochrane RL. The effects of a number of non-steroidal anti-inflammatory compounds on parturition in the rat. *Prostaglandins* 1982;23:469–488.
20. Fuchs F. Prevention of prematurity. *Am J Obstet Gynecol* 1976;126:809–820.

21. Zierler S, Rothman KJ. Congenital heart disease in relation to maternal use of Bendectin and other drugs in early pregnancy. *N Engl J Med* 1985;313:347–352.

22. Werler MM, Mitchell A, Shapiro S. The relation of aspirin use during the first trimester of pregnancy to congenital cardiac defects. *N Engl J Med* 1989;321:1639–1642.

23. Levin DL, Fixler D, Morris F, et al. Morphologic analysis of the pulmonary vascular bed in infants exposed *in utero* to prostaglandin synthetase inhibitors. *J Pediatr* 1978;92:478–483.

24. Moise KJ, Huhta J, Sharif D, et al. Indomethacin in the treatment of premature labor: effects on the fetal ductus arteriosus. *N Engl J Med* 1988;319:327–331.

25. Rumack CM, Guggenheim M, Rumack B, et al. Neonatal intracranial hemorrhage and maternal use of aspirin. *Obstet Gynecol* 1981;58:52S–56S.

26. Corby DG. Aspirin in pregnancy: maternal and fetal effects. *Pediatrics* 1978;62:930–945.

27. Schiff E, Peleg E, Goldenberg M, et al. The use of aspirin to prevent pregnancy-induced hypertension and lower the ratio of thromboxane A2 to prostacyclin in relatively high risk pregnancies. *N Engl J Med* 1989;321:351–356.

28. Trudinger BJ, Cook C, Thompson R, et al. Low-dose aspirin therapy improves fetal weight in umbilical placental insufficiency. *Am J Obstet Gynecol* 1988;159:681–685.

29. Beaufils M, Donsimoni R, Uzan S. Prevention of pre-eclampsia by early antiplatelet therapy. *Lancet* 1985;1:840–842.

30. Wallenburg HC, Makouitz J, Dekker G. Low-dose aspirin prevents pregnancy-induced hypertension and preeclampsia in angiotensin-sensitive primigravidae. *Lancet* 1986;1:1–3.

31. Benigni A, Gregorini G, Frusen T, et al. Effect of low-dose aspirin on fetal and maternal generation of thromboxane by platelets in women at risk for pregnancy-induced hypertension. *N Engl J Med* 1989;321:357–362.

32. Dekker GA, Sibai BM. Low-dose aspirin in the prevention of preeclampsia and fetal growth retardation: rationale, mechanisms and clinical trials. *Am J Obstet Gynecol* 1993;168:214–227.

33. Hauth JC, Goldenberg RL, Parker R Jr, et al. Low-dose aspirin therapy to prevent preeclampsia. *Am J Obstet Gynecol* 1993;168:1083–1093.

34. Sibai BM, Caritis SN, Thom E, et al. Prevention of preeclampsia with low-dose aspirin in healthy, nulliparous pregnant women. *N Engl J Med* 1993;329:1213–1218.

35. CLASP Collaborative Group. CLASP: a randomized trial of low-dose aspirin for the prevention and treatment of preeclampsia among 9364 pregnant women. *Lancet* 1994;343:619–625.

36. CLASP Collaborative Group. Low dose aspirin in pregnancy and early childhood development; follow up of the collaborative Low Dose Aspirin Study in Pregnancy. *Br J Obstet Gynaecol* 1995;102:861–868.

37. Silver RK, MacGregor SN, Sholl JS, et al. Comparative trial of prednisone plus aspirin versus aspirin alone in the treatment of anticardiolipin antibody-positive obstetric patients. *Am J Obstet Gynecol* 1993;169:1411–1417.

38. Sibai BM, Mirro R, Chesney CM, et al. Low-dose aspirin in pregnancy. *Obstet Gynecol* 1989;74:551–557.

39. Levy G. Salicylate pharmacokinetics in the human neonate. In: Morselli PL, Garattini S, Sereni F, eds. *Basic and therapeutic aspects of perinatal pharmacology*. New York: Raven Press, 1975:319–329.

40. Findlay JWA, DeAngelis RL, Kearney MF, et al. Analgesic drugs breast milk and plasma. *Clin Pharmacol Ther* 1981;29:625–633.

41. McNamara PJ, Burgio D, Yoo SD. Pharmacokinetics of acetaminophen, antipyrine, and salicylic acid in the lactating and nursing rabbit, with model predictions of milk to serum concentration ratios and neonatal dose. *Toxicol Appl Pharmacol* 1991;109:149–160.

42. The WHO Working Group, Bennet PN, eds. *Drugs and Human Lactation*. New York: Elsevier, 1988:325–326.

43. Adams SS. Absorption, distribution, and toxicity of ibuprofen. *Toxicol Appl Pharmacol* 1969;15:310–330.

44. Ono M. Reproductive studies of ibuprofen by rectum in rats and rabbits. *Clin Rep* 1984;18:1537–1556.

45. Aselton PA, Jick H, Milunsky A, et al. First-trimester drug use and congenital disorders. *Obstet Gynecol* 1985;65:451–455.

46. Torfs CP, Katz EA, Bateson TF, et al. Maternal medications and environmental exposures as risk factors for gastroschisis. *Teratology* 1996;54:84–92.

47. Momma K, Takeuchi H. Constriction of fetal ductus arteriosus by nonsteroidal antiinflammatory drugs. *Adv Prostaglandin Thromboxane Leukotriene* 1983;12:499–503.

48. Turner GR, Levin DL. Prostaglandin synthesis inhibition in persistent pulmonary hypertension of the newborn. *Clin Perinatol* 1984;11:581–589.

49. Levin DL. Effects of inhibition of prostaglandin synthesis on fetal development, oxygenation, and the fetal circulation. *Semin Perinatol* 1980;4:35–44.

50. Rudolph AM. The effects of nonsteroidal antiinflammatory compounds on fetal circulation and pulmonary function. *Obstet Gynecol* 1981;58:63s–67s.

51. Wilkinson AR, Mitchell M, Aynsley-Green A, et al. Persistent pulmonary hypertension and abnormal prostaglandin E levels in preterm infants after maternal treatment with naproxen. *Arch Dis Child* 1979;54:942–945.

52. Wiggins DA, Elliott JP. Oligohydramnios in each sac of a triple gestation caused by Motrin-fulfilling Kock's postulates. *Am J Obstet Gynecol* 1990;162:460–461.

53. Hendricks S, Smith J, Moore D, et al. Oligohydramnios associated with prostaglandin synthetase inhibitors in preterm labour. *Br J Obstet Gynecol* 1990;97:312–316.

54. Townsend RJ, Benedetti T, Erickson S, et al. Excretion of ibuprofen into breast milk. *Am J Obstet Gynecol* 1984;149:184–186.

55. Weibert RT, Townsend R, Kaiser D, et al. Lack of ibuprofen secretion into human milk. *Clin Pharm* 1982;1:457–459.

56. Moise KJ, Ou C, Kirshon B, et al. Placental transfer of indomethacin in the human pregnancy. *Am J Obstet Gynecol* 1990;162:549–554.

57. Katz Z. Absence of teratogenicity of indomethacin in ovarian hyperstimulation syndrome. *Int J Fertil* 1984;29:186–188.

58. Csaba IF, Sulyok E, Ertl T. Relationship of maternal treatment with indomethacin to persistence of the fetal circulation syndrome. *J Pediatr* 1978;92:484–489.

59. Besinger RE, Niebyl JR, Keyes WG, et al. Randomized comparative trial of indomethacin and ritodrine for the long-term treatment of preterm labor. *Am J Obstet Gynecol* 1991;164:981–988.

60. Norton ME, Merrill J, Cooper BAB, et al. Neonatal complications after the administration of indomethacin for preterm labor. *N Engl J Med* 1993;329:1602–1607.

61. Ajram J, Almirall Pisonero MJ, Valls I. Neonatal morbidity in newborns from mothers treated with indomethacin. *J Perinat Med* 1992;20 [Suppl 1]:176–181.

62. Rasanen J, Jouppila P. Fetal cardiac function and ductus arteriosus during indomethacin and sulindac therapy for threatened preterm labor: a randomized study. *Am J Obstet Gynecol* 1995;173:20–25.

63. Bivins HA Jr, Newman RB, Fyfe DA, et al. Randomized trial of oral indomethacin and terbutaline for the long-term suppression of preterm labor. *Am J Obstet Gynecol* 1993;169:1065–1070.

64. Murray HG, Stone PR, Strand L, et al. Fetal pleural effusion following maternal indomethacin therapy. *Br J Obstet Gynaecol* 1993;100:277–279.

65. Moise KJ Jr. Effect of advancing gestational age on the frequency of fetal ductal constriction in association with maternal indomethacin use. *Am J Obstet Gynecol* 1993;168:1350–1353.

66. Baerts W, Fetter WP, Hop WC. Cerebral lesions in preterm infants after tocolytic indomethacin. *Dev Med Child Neurol* 1990;32:910–918.

67. Herson VC, Krause PJ, Eisenfeld LI, et al. Indomethacin-associated sepsis in very-low-birth-weight infants. *Am J Dis Child* 1988;142:555–558.

68. Major CA, Lewis DF, Harding JA, et al. Tocolysis with indomethacin increases the incidence of necrotizing enterocolitis in the low-birth-weight neonate. *Am J Obstet Gynecol* 1994;170:102–106.

69. Gardner MO, Owen J, Skelly S, et al. Preterm delivery after indomethacin. A risk factor for neonatal complications? *J Reprod Med* 1996;41:903–906.

70. Van der Heijden BJ, Carlus C, Narcy F, et al. Persistent anuria, neonatal death, and renal microcystic lesions after prenatal exposure to indomethacin. *Am J Obstet Gynecol* 1994;171:617–623.

71. Walker MPR, Moore TR, Brace RA. Indomethacin and arginine vasopressin interaction in the fetal kidney. A mechanism of oliguria. *Am J Obstet Gynecol* 1994;171:1234–1241.

72. Itskovitz J, Abramovici H, Brandes J. Oligohydramnion, meconium and perinatal death concurrent with indomethacin treatment in human pregnancy. *J Reprod Med* 1980;24:137–140.

73. Schoenfeld A, Freedman S, Hod M, et al. Antagonism of antihypertensive drug therapy in pregnancy by indomethacin? *Am J Obstet Gynecol* 1989;161:1204–1205.

74. Sorensen TK, Eastering TR, Carlson KL, et al. The maternal hemodynamic effect of indomethacin in normal pregnancy. *Obstet Gynecol* 1992;79:661–663.

75. Mousavy SM. Indomethacin induces hypertensive crisis in preeclampsia irrespective of prior antihypertensive drug therapy [Letter, Comment]. *Am J Obstet Gynecol* 1991;165:1577.

76. Eeg-Olofsson O, Malmros I, Elwin CE, et al. Convulsions in a breast-fed infant after maternal indomethacin. *Lancet* 1978;2:215.

77. Suhonen R. Hydroxychloroquine administration in pregnancy. *Arch Dermatol* 1983;119:185–186.

78. Smith DW. Dysmorphology (teratology). *J Pediatr* 1966;69:1150–1169.

79. Parke AL. Antimalarial drugs, systemic lupus erythematosus and pregnancy. *J Rheumatol* 1988;15:607–610.

80. Levy M, Buskila D, Gladman DD, et al. Pregnancy outcome following first trimester exposure to chloroquine. *Am J Perinatol* 1991;8:174–178.

81. Parke A, West B. Hydroxychloroquine in pregnant patients with systemic lupus erythematosus. *J Rheumatol* 1996;23:1715–1718.

82. Buchanan NM, Toubi E, Khamashta MA, et al. Hydroxychloroquine and lupus pregnancy: review of series of 36 cases. *Ann Rheum Dis* 1996;55:486–488.

83. Wolfe MS, Cordero JF. Safety of chloroquine in chemosuppression of malaria during pregnancy. *BMJ* 1985;290:1466–1477.

84. Hart CW, Naunton RF. The ototoxicity of chloroquine phosphate. *Arch Otolaryngol* 1964;80:407.

85. Nation RL, Hackett L, Dusci E, et al. Excretion of hydroxychloroquine in human milk. *Br J Clin Pharmacol* 1984;17:368–369.

86. Rocker I, Henderson WJ. Transfer of gold from mother to fetus. *Lancet* 1976;1:1246.

87. Cohen DL, Orzel J, Taylor A. Infants of mothers receiving gold therapy [Letter]. *Arthritis Rheum* 1981;24:1045.

88. Tarp U, Graudal H. A follow-up study of children exposed to gold compounds *in utero*. *Arthritis Rheum* 1985;28:235–236.

89. Miyamoto T, Miyajl S, Horiuchi Y. Gold therapy in bronchial asthma—special emphasis upon blood levels of gold and its teratogenicity. *J Jpn Soc Intern Med* 1974;63:1190–1197.

90. Needs CJ, Brooks PM. Antirheumatic medication in pregnancy. *Br J Rheumatol* 1985;24:282–290.

91. Blau SP. Metabolism of gold during lactation. *Arthritis Rheum* 1973;16:777–778.

92. Rooney TW, Lorber A, Veng-Pedersen P, et al. Gold pharmacokinetics in breast milk and serum of a lactating woman. *J Rheumatol* 1987;14:1120–1122.

93. Ostensen M, Skavdal K, Myklebust G, et al. Excretion of gold into human breast milk. *Eur J Clin Pharmacol* 1986;31:251–252.

94. Bennett PN, Humphries SJ, Osborne JP, et al. Use of sodium aurothiomalate during lactation. *Br J Clin Pharmacol* 1990;29:777–779.

95. Beckman DA, Brent RL. Mechanisms of teratogenesis. *Annu Rev Pharmacol Toxicol* 1984;24:483–500.

96. Wilson JG, Scott W, Ritter E, et al. Comparative distribution and embryotoxicity of methotrexate in pregnant rats and rhesus monkeys. *Teratology* 1979;19:71–80.

97. Ichinoe K, Wake N, Shinkai N, et al. Nonsurgical therapy to preserve oviduct function in patients with tubal pregnancies. *Am J Obstet Gynecol* 1987;156:484–487.

98. Patsner B, Kenigsberg D. Successful treatment of persistent ectopic pregnancy with oral methotrexate therapy. *Fertil Steril* 1988;50:982–983.

99. Feldkamp M, Carey JC. Clinical teratology counseling and consultation case report: low dose methotrexate exposure in the early weeks of pregnancy. *Teratology* 1993;47:533–539.

100. Hausknecht RU. Methotrexate and misoprostol to terminate early pregnancy. *N Engl J Med* 1995;333:537–540.

101. Schardein JL. *Chemically induced birth defects,* 2nd ed. New York; Marcel Dekker, 1993:474–478.

102. Johns D, Rotherford L, Leighton P, et al. Secretion of methotrexate into human milk. *Am J Obstet Gynecol* 1972;112:978–980.

103. Greenberg LH, Tanaka KR. Congenital anomalies probably induced by cyclophosphamide. *JAMA* 1964;188:423–426.

104. Coates A. Cyclophosphamide in pregnancy. *Aust NZJ Obstet Gynaecol* 1970;10:33–34.

105. Toledo TM, Harper R, Moser R. Fetal effects during cyclophosphamide and irradiation therapy. *Ann Intern Med* 1971;74:87–91.

106. Murray CL, Reichert M, Anderson J. Multimodal cancer therapy for breast cancer in the first trimester of pregnancy. *JAMA* 1984;252:2607–2613.

107. Kirshon B, Wasserstram N, Willis R, et al. Teratogenic effects of first trimester cyclophosphamide therapy. *Obstet Gynecol* 1988;72:462–467.

108. Zemlickis D, Lishner M, Erlich R, et al. Teratogenicity and carcinogenicity in a twin exposed in utero to cyclophosphamide. *Teratog Carcinog Mutagen* 1993;13:139–143.

109. Mutchinick O, Aizpuru E, Grether P. The human teratogenic effect of cyclophosphamide. *Teratology* 1992;45:329.

110. Pizzuto J, Aviles A, Norrega L, et al. Treatment of acute leukemia during pregnancy: presentation of nine cases. *Cancer Treat Rep* 1980;64:679–683.

111. Nicholson HO. Cytotoxic drugs in pregnancy: review of reported cases. *J Obstet Gynaecol Br Commonw* 1968;75:307–312.

112. Wiernik PH, Duncan JH. Cyclophosphamide in human milk. *Lancet* 1971;1:912.

113. Durodola JI. Administration of cyclophosphamide during late pregnancy and early lactation: a case report. *J Natl Med Assoc* 1979;71:165.

114. Voogd CD. Azathioprine, a genotoxic agent to be considered non-genotoxic in man. *Mutat Res* 1989;221:133–152.

115. Golby M. Fertility after transplantation. *Transplantation* 1970;10:201–212.

116. Haagsma EB, Visser G, Klompmaker I, et al. Successful pregnancy after orthotopic transplantation. *Obstet Gynecol* 1989;74:442–443.

117. Baxi LV, Rho RB. Pregnancy after cardiac transplantation. *Am J Obstet Gynecol* 1993;169:33–34.

118. Pirson Y, VanLierde M, Ghgsen J, et al. Retardation of fetal growth in patients receiving immunosuppressive therapy [Letter]. *N Engl J Med* 1985;313–328.

119. Coulam CB, Moyer TP, Jiang NS, et al. Breast-feeding after renal transplantation. *Transplant Proc* 1982;14:605–609.

120. Grekas DM, Vasiliou SS, Lazarids AN. Immunosuppressive therapy and breast-feeding after renal transplantation. *Nephron* 1984;37:68.

The contents of this chapter were originally published as Rayburn WF. Connective tissue disorders and pregnancy; limitations with drug prescribing. *J Reprod Med* 1998;43:341–349. Written permission to reprint this information was obtained from the publisher.

18

Antibiotic Prophylaxis: Patients with Joint Prostheses and Ventricular Shunts—Prevention of Bacterial Endocarditis

Robert H. Ball

Departments of Obstetrics and Gynecology, University of Utah Health Sciences Center, Salt Lake City, Utah

INTRODUCTION AND PREVENTION OF BACTERIAL ENDOCARDITIS

Antibiotic prophylaxis in patients with either significant cardiac valvular abnormalities or with valve replacements is standard of care to prevent the development of endocarditis (1). It is thought that endocarditis can develop from seeding of the heart valves during the transient bacteremia that may result from surgical or dental procedures. In the most recent recommendations by the American Heart Association (1), the approach to prophylaxis has become less aggressive. Specifically, the range of procedures for which prophylaxis is recommended has narrowed, and the dosing has been reduced. This partly resulted from a realization that the majority of cases of endocarditis are not related to invasive procedures. The need for prophylaxis depends on the underlying cardiac condition and the procedure the patient will undergo. Table 18.1 lists high, moderate, and negligible risk categories. The most recent recommendations are that endocarditis prophylaxis is not recommended for vaginal deliveries (except perhaps for high-risk patients) and cesarean sections (1). Yet, bacteremia occurs in 1% to 5% of uncomplicated vaginal deliveries. Urethral catheterization is complicated by bacteremia in 8% of procedures, and prophylaxis is not recommended for this procedure either. Table 18.2 lists antibiotic regimens for genitourinary procedures.

This information is relevant to the subsequent discussion regarding prophylaxis in cases of indwelling ventricular shunts and joint prostheses. The reason for this is that the risk related to procedure-induced bacteremia has always been thought to be most significant with respect to endocarditis. As the concern over this has waned based on accumulating epidemiologic evidence, there will likely be a trickle-down effect with respect to other clinical areas where prophylaxis is currently considered an issue.

ANTIBIOTIC PROPHYLAXIS IN PATIENTS WITH CEREBROSPINAL FLUID SHUNTS

A recent review article (2) highlighted the increasing likelihood that an obstetrician would encounter a patient with either a ventriculoatrial or ventriculoperitoneal shunt. There are now close to 50 documented cases of pregnancies in such patients in the literature, which almost certainly represents an underestimate. The incidence can be predicted by the fact that isolated hydrocephalus occurs at a rate of approximately 0.5 per 1,000 births and 1.9 per 1,000 when one includes primary and secondary hydrocephalus. The most common cause of secondary hydrocephalus is spina bifida. With the advent of ventricular shunting nearly 40 years ago, survival and quality of life in these patients changed

TABLE 18.1. *Categorization of cardiac conditions*

Endocarditis prophylaxis recommended

High-risk category
    Prosthetic cardiac valves
    Previous bacterial endocarditis
    Complex cyanotic congenital heart disease
    Surgically constructed pulmonary shunts
Moderate-risk category
    Hypertrophic cardiomyopathy
    Mitral valve prolapse with regurgitation
    Acquired valvular dysfunction
    Most other congenital cardiac malformations

Endocarditis prophylaxis not recommended

Negligible risk category (risk similar to general
    population)
    Isolated secundum atrial septal defect
    Repaired ASD, VSD, or PDA
    Previous coronary bypass
    Mitral valve prolapse with no regurgitation
    Murmurs with no known lesion
    Previous Kawasaki disease without valve damage
    Previous rheumatic fever without valve damage
    Pacemakers and implanted defibrillators

ASD, atrial septal defect; VSD, ventricular septal defect; PDA, patent ductus arteriosis. Modified from ref. 1.

dramatically, including their ability to have families.

Vaginal delivery is not considered a procedure necessitating antibiotic prophylaxis for endocarditis prevention except in those patients with high-risk cardiac conditions (prosthetic valves, previous endocarditis, complex cyanotic congenital heart disease) (1). No prophylaxis is recommended for cesarean section regardless of the type of cardiac condition. These procedures are thus considered to have a relatively low risk of producing significant bacteremia. One would therefore extrapolate that the need for prophylaxis would be even less in the case of indwelling ventricular shunts. The likelihood that a ventriculoatrial shunt could be seeded during bacteremia seems logically greater (3) in that it is an intravascular foreign body. Ventriculoperitoneal shunts should logically be at much lower risk of seeding because they are not intravascular. Unfortunately, there are no particularly helpful scientific data to support the relative benefit of antibiotic prophylaxis for either situation (2–5). In general, authors are in favor of using antibiotic prophylaxis for cases of ventriculoatrial shunts during delivery (2,3) for the reasons noted above. They grudgingly also admit that despite the complete lack of scientific or even anecdotal evidence to support the use of prophylaxis for ventriculoperitoneal shunts, the vast majority of physicians utilize it (2–4). In fact, there has not been a single case report in the literature of an infected shunt with a causative organism related to the genital tract. Thus, despite the fact that the relative risk of a significant allergic reaction to the antibiotic is probably higher than the risk of a shunt complication, antibiotics are given. The argument that is generally given to justify this action is that the consequences of shunt infection are so great,

TABLE 18.2. *Antibiotic regimens for genitourinary procedures*

Situation	Agents	Regimen
High-risk patients	Ampicillin + gentamicin	Ampicillin 2.0 g i.m. or i.v. and gentamicin 1.5 mg/kg (not to exceed 120 mg) within 30 min of start of procedure: 6 hr later, ampicillin 1 g i.m./i.v. or amoxicillin 1 g orally
High-risk patients (allergic to ampicillin)	Vancomycin + gentamicin	Vancomycin 1 g i.v. over 1–2 hr + gentamicin 1.5 mg/kg (not to exceed 120 mg) complete injection or infusion within 30 min of start of procedure
Moderate-risk patients	Amoxicillin or ampicillin	Amoxicillin 2 g orally 1 hr before procedure or ampicillin 2 g i.m./i.v. within 30 min of start of procedure
Moderate-risk patients (allergic to ampicillin or amoxicillin)	Vancomycin	Vancomycin 1 g i.v. over 1–2 hr with infusion complete within 30 min of start of procedure

Modified from ref. 1.

necessitating surgery and prolonged antibiotics. Oral or intravenous penicillin is the drug of choice for antibiotic prophylaxis.

The degree to which antibiotic prophylaxis is unsubstantiated for vaginal deliveries and cesarean sections is put into perspective when analyzing its use for dental procedures. As already mentioned, dental procedures are considered among the highest risk for producing significant bacteremia. Nevertheless, there is no consensus on the need for prophylaxis before dental procedures either. The American Academy of Pediatric Dentistry considers this a controversial area (6,7). In their 1991–1992 reference manual (6), they consider ventriculoatrial shunts to have a high relative risk of bacteremia-induced infections, and ventriculoperitoneal shunts are classified as moderate risk. At that time, their recommendation was for antibiotic prophylaxis for all high-risk patients, but only after consultation with the neurosurgeon, in cases of moderate risk. The Academy has changed its position, and in the most recent reference manual, suggests that prophylaxis be considered only for dental surgical procedures, and then primarily in patients with poor oral hygiene and periodontal or gingival infection (7). If prophylaxis is indicated, they recommend 2 g amoxicillin orally an hour before the procedure or 600 mg clindamycin if there is a sensitivity to penicillin.

Acs and Cozzi (8) surveyed 51 pediatric dental program directors and 63 neurosurgery directors regarding their views on shunt prophylaxis for different dental procedures. They found that both groups recommended prophylaxis for extractions and scaling, but that dentists were more aggressive in recommending prophylaxis for other dental work in cases of ventriculoatrial shunts. The majority of both groups used prophylaxis for extractions and scaling with ventriculoperitoneal shunts, but neither group considered it necessary for other procedures. The general lack of hard data on prophylaxis with ventriculoperitoneal shunts was the impetus for Helpin et al. (9) to perform a pilot study to see whether omission of antibiotic prophylaxis was associated with shunt infections. Fourteen children with shunts underwent dental and fluoride treatments after which none demonstrated evidence of shunt infection. They called for larger multicenter studies to explore this issue further. Unfortunately, regardless of the scientific data that will emerge, the deep-rooted bias of most clinicians will lead to continued use of prophylaxis. Indeed, at a recent neurosurgical meeting a poll of attendees demonstrated that the great majority strongly advocated the use of prophylactic antibiotics before any dental work (J. Kestle, personal communication, 1999).

ANTIBIOTIC PROPHYLAXIS IN PATIENTS WITH JOINT PROSTHESES

There are no published data or opinions on prophylactic antibiotic use in pregnant patients with joint prostheses. This is probably related to the rarity of this situation. Joint replacements are not commonly needed in reproduction-age women. The usual indication for these procedures are degenerative joint problems caused by osteoarthritis, rheumatoid arthritis, or secondary to corticosteroid use. One is therefore limited to extrapolating from the policies relating to dental procedures. As discussed in the section on cerebrospinal fluid shunts, the relative risk of significant bacteremia with dental procedures is considered to be much higher than with vaginal deliveries or cesarean sections.

Discrepancies exist between what is justifiable based on scientific data and what the usual management is in patients with joint prostheses before dental treatment. The issue was addressed in several review articles (10–12). The consensus is the same as that on antibiotic prophylaxis with cerebrospinal fluid shunts, discussed previously. Specifically, although there is no evidence to support it, prophylaxis is widely used. Several authors performed detailed analyses of the cost-benefit ratio and relative risks of antibiotic prophylaxis. Tsevat et al. (13) determined that the use of erythromycin, but not penicillin, could be justified for prophylaxis before dental work. This was because of the anaphylactic risk with the latter. They also assumed that the probability of a joint infection was 9.3 per 100,000 based on several authors' assumptions. The validity of these assumptions, however, was challenged by others (11,12).

The American Dental Association sought consensus from experts in the field of dentistry, orthopedic surgery, and infectious diseases on the issue of prophylaxis. The result of this meeting was the publication of an advisory statement (14). The panel's conclusion was that prophylaxis was not considered to be indicated in patients with plates, screws, pins, or total joint replacements. There is a small subset of high-risk patients for whom prophylaxis was considered appropriate for procedures associated with a higher incidence of bacteremia. High-risk patients include those with rheumatoid arthritis, systemic lupus erythematosus, immunosuppresion, insulin-dependent diabetes, recent joint replacements (less than 2 years), previous prosthetic infections, malnourishment, and hemophilia. High-risk procedures are those involving a greater degree of manipulation of the teeth, such as extractions. The recommended regimen for prophylaxis is a single 2-g dose of oral amoxicillin, cephalexin, or cephradine 1 hour before the procedure. Intravenous alternatives are cefazolin or ampicillin. In those patients who are allergic to penicillin, either oral or intravenous clindamycin (600 mg) is used.

SUMMARY

In those rare cases of pregnant women with indwelling orthopedic hardware, antibiotic prophylaxis for vaginal delivery or cesarean section is probably not indicated. In many cases of cesarean section, intraoperative antibiotics for the surgery itself will already be used, negating any need for additional prophylaxis. Obstetricians managing pregnant women with joint prostheses should confer with that patient's orthopedic surgeon regarding prophylaxis. If the decision is made to use prophylaxis, although unproven in its benefit, the antibiotic regimens used for dental prophylaxis should be used.

REFERENCES

1. Dajani AS, Taubert KA, Wilson W, et al. Prevention of bacterial endocarditis, recommendations by the American Heart Association. *JAMA* 1997;277:1794–1801.
2. Stevens E. Pregnancy in women with cerebrospinal shunts: a literature review and case report. *J Perinatol* 1996;16:374–380.
3. Cusimano MD, Meffe FM, Gentili F, et al. Management of pregnant women with cerebrospinal fluid shunts. *Pediatr Neurosurg* 1991;17:10–13.
4. Landwehr JB, Isada, NB, Pryde PG, et al. Maternal neurosurgical shunts and pregnancy outcome. *Obstet Gynecol* 1994;83:134–137.
5. Frohlich, EP, Russel JM, Van Gelderen CS. Pregnancy complicated by maternal hydrocephalus. *S Afr Med J* 1986;70:358–360.
6. American Academy of Pediatric Dentistry. *Reference manual 1991–1992: antibiotic chemoprophylaxis for pediatric dental patients*. Chicago: American Academy of Pedatric Dentistry, 1991.
7. American Academy of Pediatric Dentistry. Antibiotic chemoprophylaxis for pediatric dental patients at risk; revised April 1991. *Pediatr Dent* 1996;18:67–71.
8. Acs G, Cozzi E. Antibiotic prophylaxis for patients with hydrocephalus shunts: a survey of pediatric dentistry and neurosurgery program directors. *Pediatr Dent* 1992;14:246–250.
9. Helpin ML, Rosenberg HM, Sayany Z, et al. Antibiotic prophylaxis in dental patients with ventriculo-peritoneal shunts: a pilot study. *J Dent Child* 1998;4:244–247.
10. Norden CW. Prevention of bone and joint infections. *Am J Med* 1985;78:229–232.
11. Norden CW. Antibiotic prophylaxis in orthopedic surgery. *Rev Infect Dis* 1991;13[Suppl 10]:S842–S846.
12. Field EA, Martin MV. Prophylactic antibiotics for patients with artificial joints undergoing oral and dental surgery: necessary or not? *Br J Oral Maxillofac Surg* 1991;29:341–346.
13. Tsevat J, Durand-Zaleski I, Pauker SG. Cost-effectiveness of antibiotic prophylaxis for dental procedures in patients with artificial joints. *Am J Public Health* 1989;79:739–743.
14. ADA, AAOS. Antibiotic prophylaxis for dental patients with total joint replacements. *J Am Dent Assoc* 1997;128:1004–1007.

19

Antiviral Treatment in Pregnancy

Asha Rijhsinghani

Department of Obstetrics and Gynecology, The University of Iowa Hospitals and Clinics, Iowa City, Iowa

Viral infections during pregnancy are responsible for much maternal, fetal, and neonatal morbidity and occasionally mortality. The fetus can acquire the infection through vertical transmission *in utero*, at the time of delivery, and with close contact during breast-feeding. The majority of maternal infections are subclinical. Serologic testing has been used extensively in diagnosing viral infections, especially primary maternal infections. Fetal infections are more difficult to diagnose. Some fetuses may show obvious abnormalities on ultrasound examination increasing the suspicion of intrauterine viral infection. Invasive testing is required to confirm the diagnosis. Recently, polymerase chain reaction (PCR) has been increasingly used to diagnose intrauterine infections. Maternal and fetal management of several viruses are described here.

CYTOMEGALOVIRUS

Human cytomegalovirus (CMV) is a herpesvirus composed of a double-stranded DNA core enclosed in a lipid envelope. The virus is species specific, and there are many different strains that can infect humans. Antigenic cross-activity between the strains is common. CMV is the most frequent cause of intrauterine viral infections. In developed countries, the incidence of congenital CMV infection is as high as 1.2% of all live-births (1). In a pregnant woman, primary infection is diagnosed if seroconversion can be documented during the pregnancy or if a woman who was seronegative in the first trimester gives birth to a newborn with congenital CMV infection.

The CMV-immunoglobulin M (IgM) antibody can last as long as 3 to 6 months. Diagnosis of recurrent CMV infection requires either the presence of CMV-IgG antibody before pregnancy or in the first trimester in the absence of CMV-IgM antibody (2). The risk of transmission of the CMV infection to the fetus depends on the type of infection in the mother. In a primary CMV infection, the rate of transmission ranges from 25% to 67.9% (3–5). The infection can also occur perinatally in 40% to 50% of infants born to mothers with positive cervical cultures at the time of birth and in as many as 70% of breast-fed children of seropositive mothers who are excreting the virus in the breast milk (6,7).

The risk of congenital infection is greater when infection occurs in the first half of pregnancy. Congenital CMV infection after a primary maternal infection can affect neurodevelopment leading to mental retardation, visual impairment, and sensorineural hearing loss. Fetal infection after recurrent CMV infection in the mother will more often lead to only congenital sensorineural hearing loss. Rarely does early recurrent infection affect fetal neurodevelopment (8).

To differentiate primary maternal CMV infection from secondary infection, the presence of IgM antibody is not reliable enough unless seroconversion can be documented during the pregnancy. In these cases, measurements of CMV-IgG avidity can be helpful. High CMV-IgG avidity index during the first trimester of pregnancy is a good indicator of past CMV infection (9). Prenatal diagnosis of congenital CMV infection is based on detecting the virus in the amniotic fluid by viral culture or PCR. The overall sensitivity of the viral culture is 88.6% with the best sensitivity (95.5%) obtained in pregnancies of 23 weeks or more of gestation and after a delay of 6 weeks or more and least sensitivity (35.7%) in pregnancies of 22 weeks or less of gestation with 5 weeks or less of delay (5). Amniotic fluid culture and PCR are reported to have comparable sensitivities, although some reports suggested that PCR may be more sensitive than culture and may detect viral load that is very low and not associated with congenital infection.

The risk of perinatal mortality and morbidity as well as long-term morbidity is increased in fetuses with congenital CMV infection, and therefore a few attempts have been made to treat the fetus prenatally. At the present time, there are no antiviral agents that have been approved for treatment of the fetus *in utero*. Ganciclovir (GCV), a homolog of acyclovir, is used for the prevention of CMV disease in patients who are recipients of solid organ transplant. In animals, GCV is teratogenic. GVC crosses the human placenta by simple diffusion at therapeutic levels (10). It has been used in all three trimesters of pregnancy for maternal indications without evidence of teratogenicity in the fetus (11,12). Prenatal treatment of congenital CVM infection by intravascular administration to the fetus has been attempted unsuccessfully (13). The investigators documented fetal infection at 27 weeks by CMV isolation from fetal blood and blood amniotic fluid. Cord blood studies revealed a low platelet count of 66×10^9/L and elevated γGT of 190 IU/L. Ultrasound examination was normal. GCV therapy was administered by direct intravascular injection to the fetus for 12 days. A transient reduction in fetal movements was noted after each treatment. The amniotic fluid volume decreased, although the fetal heart rate tracings remained reactive. At 32 weeks, the patient experienced preterm labor and delivered a fresh stillborn.

CMV-specific immunoglobulin has been administered to the fetus and the pregnant woman to treat CMV infection. In a case of twin gestation, 400 U were injected into the amniotic fluid of the infected fetus diagnosed with growth restriction. Additionally, the mother was given 200 U kg^{-1}/d^{-1} for 3 days intravenously because transplacental passage is not immediate (14). At 2 years of age, the infected twin was reported to have good mental and motor development without visual or auditory impairment. In the other case, 2.5 g CMV hyperimmunoglobulin was injected into the fetal abdomen of a hydropic fetus at 28 and 29 weeks of gestation (15). The patient was delivered at 34 weeks for fetal distress. The neonate had slight hepatosplenomegaly and ascites at birth. A brain computed tomography scan at 2 weeks of age revealed small calcifications adjacent to the right ventricle. At 1 year of age, the child did not have any neurologic symptoms.

Summary

There are no approved medications for treatment of maternal CMV infection or prevention of congenital infection. Ganciclovir and CMV specific immunoglobulin have been used experimentally in a very small number of cases without clear benefit. Nonpregnant women receiving GCV should be recommended to use contraceptives.

HERPES SIMPLEX VIRUS

The human herpes group of viruses has six recognized strains. Herpes simplex virus (HSV) is a double-stranded DNA enveloped virus. HSV is one of the most common sexually transmitted diseases. In the pregnant population, 76% of women were found to be seropositive for either HSV-1, HSV-2, or both (16). Seroprevalence of HSV-2 antibodies is approximately 28% to 32% among pregnant women in the United States (16,17). Women who are seronegative have a 3.5% chance of seroconversion during the pregnancy. Those who are seronegative for HSV-2 but positive for HSV-1 antibodies have an estimated chance of 1.7% of seroconversion (16). HSV in the mother has been described as primary, nonprimary first episode, or recurrent genital HSV infection. Women who have no detectable antibodies to HSV but later seroconvert to either HSV-1 or HSV-2 are described as having primary HSV infection. Patients with HSV-1 antibodies who develop antibodies to HSV-2 during pregnancy or those who are positive for HSV-2 antibodies and later seroconvert to HSV-1 antibodies as well are considered to have a nonprimary first episode of HSV infection. The third category is recurrent genital HSV infection. Two thirds of the patients who seroconvert during pregnancy have subclinical infections and one third have symptomatic infections. Patients with recurrent infections can have clinical signs and symptoms similar to those of primary genital herpes infections in the second and third trimesters of pregnancy (18). These symptoms consist of systemic symptoms such as fever, headache, malaise, myalgia, bilateral lesions with severe local pain, and tender inguinal lymphadenopathy. The only way to differentiate primary infection from recurrent infection in such cases would be by documentation of seroconversion. In rare cases, HSV infection in pregnant women can cause disseminated disease involving the lungs, liver, and brain (19). Although extremely rare, congenital infection of the fetus has been reported (20), and in the first trimester can lead to anomalies such as microcephaly, microphthalmia, intracranial calcifications, and chorioretinitis. More commonly, the neonates are infected when the mother acquires genital HSV infection near the onset of labor and has not seroconverted at the time of labor (16). The risk of neonatal infections in such patients who are diagnosed with primary or nonprimary first episode of genital HSV infection is approximately 44% (16). Both HSV-1 and HSV-2 can cause neonatal HSV infection. Although HSV-1 and HSV-2 are both equally responsible for neonatal infections, the disease secondary to HSV-1 may be less severe in the neonate compared with HSV-2.

Guidelines for clinical management of HSV infection during pregnancy were published recently by the American College of Obstetrics and Gynecology (ACOG) (21). Indications for treatment included primary infections and recurrent infections as well as daily suppressive therapy for women at risk of recurrent infections. It is also suggested that administration of acyclovir given after 36 weeks of gestation in women with recurrent genital HSV infection may decrease clinical recurrences (22,23). ACOG recommends that women with symptomatic primary HSV infection during pregnancy should be treated with

antiviral therapy. Also, women with a first episode of HSV infection at or beyond 36 weeks of gestation should be considered for treatment with antiviral medications.

An acyclovir (24) and valacyclovir pregnancy registry was maintained by GlaxoWellcome, Inc., in cooperation with the Centers for Disease Control (CDC) until July 1998. This registry was continually updated with information on women treated systemically with acyclovir or valacyclovir during pregnancy. Among women treated with systemic acyclovir in the first trimester, 4.4% to 5.4% of livebirths were found to have congenital anomalies (24,25). No recurrent pattern of anomalies was seen in these neonates. In fetuses exposed to the medication in the second and third trimesters, no apparent adverse effects were noted (23,26). Information on valacyclovir use during pregnancy is limited. A total of 56 pregnancies exposed to valacyclovir were reported to the registry of which 14 were in the first trimester. There was no evidence of increased risk of congenital defects in this small population. In a clinical study, 10 patients received the medication from 36 weeks to delivery (27). There was no evidence of increased toxicity in these patients.

There are no studies of use of famciclovir in pregnant women. Valacyclovir, acyclovir, or famciclovir can be used for treatment of HSV infection during pregnancy.

Daily suppressive therapy consists of:

- Acyclovir 400 mg twice daily or
- Famciclovir 250 mg twice daily or
- Valacyclovir 500 mg once daily

Therapy of recurrent episodes is

- Acyclovir 200 mg five times daily or 400 mg three times daily for 5 days or
- Famciclovir 125 mg twice daily for 5 days or
- Valacyclovir 500 mg twice daily for 5 days

Treatment of first clinical episode is

- Acyclovir 200 mg five times daily or 400 mg three times daily for 7 to 14 days or
- Famciclovir 250 mg three times daily for 7 to 14 days or
- Valacyclovir 1,000 mg twice daily for 7 to 14 days

Disseminated HSV infection is rare but can be fatal. Patients who develop systemic symptoms such as fever, malaise, myalgia, and signs of hepatitis should be hospitalized and treated with intravenous acyclovir.

VARICELLA

Varicella is a highly contagious disease caused by the varicella-zoster virus, which belongs to the herpesvirus family. The infection usually occurs in childhood and is self-limited. In the United Kingdom, the incidence of varicella in pregnancy is reported to be 3 per 1,000 (28). Estimates in the United States are lower. The disease is usually characterized by fever, malaise, and a generalized vesicular rash typically consisting of 250 to 500 lesions lasting 4 to 5 days. Rarely, there can be life-threatening complications such as pneumonitis and encephalitis.

The infection can be prevented by administration of varicella vaccine to individuals at risk of infection. In the adult population, the vaccine is recommended for susceptible individuals in high-risk groups, which include nonpregnant women of childbearing age (29). Among health care workers, 94.9% had detectable antibodies after the first dose of the vaccination and 100% after the second dose (30). Because it is an attenuated live virus vaccine, it should not be given to patients who are pregnant or attempting to conceive. Pregnant women can contract primary varicella infection from exposure to close contacts that have been vaccinated with the varicella vaccine (31).

Susceptible pregnant women exposed to the infection should receive postexposure prophylaxis with anti–varicella-zoster immune globulin. Such prophylaxis has been documented to attenuate the disease and prevent congenital varicella syndrome or zoster in infancy (32).

The infection in the first half of pregnancy carries an approximately 2% risk of congenital varicella syndrome. The risk is highest when the mother is infected between 8 and 21 weeks of gestation (32,33). Maternal varicella infection can lead to spontaneous abortion, intrauterine death, or the congenital varicella syndrome, which consists of hypoplasia or contractions of limbs, severe cutaneous lesions and scars, microphthalmia, and encephalitis, microcephaly, and organ involvement secondary to disseminated disease (32,33). Later in pregnancy, maternal infection can result in postnatal zoster in the infant. When maternal varicella occurs 7 days before to 7 days after delivery, the neonatal infection rate can be as high as 60% (34). Neonatal infection is more severe when the mother develops a skin rash 4 days before and up to 2 days after delivery. The majority of women who contract the infection during pregnancy do not have a history of definite exposure and therefore do not receive the postexposure prophylaxis, increasing their risks as well as those of the fetus.

One of the complications of adult varicella is pneumonia (35). The incidence of varicella pneumonia in the adult population with varicella who seek emergency care is approximately 10% (36). The risks of pregnant women developing varicella pneumonia may be increased (35), although there are conflicting reports (36). When pregnant women develop pneumonia, risks of respiratory failure and death are increased (36). Several reports recommend aggressive and timely treatment of the pregnant woman with varicella pneumonia to reduce maternal and fetal morbidity and mortality.

Summary

Prophylaxis in nonpregnant women consists of 0.5 mL varicella virus live vaccine subcutaneously, two doses given 4 to 8 weeks apart. The risk of transmission of the varicella vaccine virus from the fetus to the pregnant mother, although possible, is extremely small (31,37). Women of childbearing age should avoid pregnancy for 3 months after the vaccination. An international registry has been established by Merck Research Laboratories to follow pregnancies that have been exposed to varicella-zoster virus vaccine. There has not been evidence of teratogenic effect.

Postexposure prophylaxis is treatment with human varicella-zoster immune globulin. The dose is 125 U/10 kg and as much as 625 U given within 96 hours of the exposure. The injection is administered deep into the intramuscular (gluteal) region. Because of the large volume of the injection, it should be administered in multiple sites to minimize discomfort.

Varicella pneumonia is treated with acyclovir, given intravenously for as long as 7 days. The dose is 10 mg/kg infused at a constant rate over 1 hour, every 8 hours in patients with normal renal functions. In patients who are treated for a shorter duration with intravenous acyclovir, consideration should be given to additional oral therapy.

VIRAL HEPATITIS

Several different types of hepatitis viruses have been identified. These are the hepatitis A, B, C, D, E, and G viruses. Chronic hepatitis can occur with hepatitis B, C, and D. Chronic viral hepatitis is a major cause of chronic liver disease in the United States. The incidence of chronic hepatitis B infection in the pregnant population is 5 to 15 per 1,000. Chronic hepatitis C is more common, with a reported prevalence of 1% to 8%. Chronic hepatitis D occurs in approximately 20% to 25% of patients infected with chronic hepatitis B virus.

In the United States, hepatitis A virus is responsible for approximately one third of the cases of acute hepatitis. Hepatitis B infection occurs in 40% to 45% of all cases of hepatitis (38). Hepatitis E is rarely reported in the United States but can, occasionally, cause serious disease and maternal death. Hepatitis A and E do not have a chronic carrier state. Hepatitis G is more likely to occur in women already infected with hepatitis B or C. It does not cause chronic disease.

Hepatitis A

For postexposure prophylaxis, it is recommended that close contacts be given intramuscular immunoglobulin within 2 weeks after exposure. In the adult, 0.02 mL/kg will protect for as long as 3 months.

Prophylaxis treatment is with hepatitis A vaccine, which consists of noninfectious viral antigens. In adults, a single dose of Havrix 1440 ELISA units (EL.U) 1 mL is given by intramuscular injection. For those requiring both immediate and long-term protection, the vaccine can be administered concomitantly with the immunoglobulin. There are no reports on administration of hepatitis A vaccine during pregnancy or lactation. Patients who are at higher risks of hepatitis A infection can be vaccinated during pregnancy, if clearly indicated.

Hepatitis B

When acute hepatitis B occurs in the first trimester of pregnancy, as many as 10% of neonates will test positive for the hepatitis B surface antigen (HB_sAg). In the third trimester, the incidence of seropositive neonates is 80% to 90% (39). The risks of vertical transmission increases when the mother is seropositive for both HB_sAg and HB_eAg (hepatitis B e antigen). The vast majority of the cases of perinatal transmission of hepatitis B virus occurs during the intrapartum period. Other modes of transmission include transplacental as well as through breast-feeding and close contact in the neonatal period. Neonates born to mothers who are positive for HB_sAg at the time of delivery should receive hepatitis B immunoglobulin as well as the hepatitis B vaccine within the first 12 hours of birth followed by two additional injections of hepatitis B vaccine in the first 6 months of life.

Postexposure prophylaxis for adults previously not vaccinated against hepatitis B or those with inadequate or unknown titers consists of intramuscular administration of hepatitis immunoglobulin. The dose is 0.06 mL/kg. It should be administered as soon as possible and within 24 hours of exposure. The patient can receive concomitant hepatitis B vaccine.

Prophylaxis with hepatitis B vaccination is recommended for all individuals at increased risk of infection with hepatitis B virus. In cases of exposure, the first dose should be given within 7 days of exposure, the second dose 1 month later, and the third dose 6 months after the first dose. In the adult, each dose is 10 μg (1.0 mL) of the recombinant hepatitis B vaccine. There was no increase in abnormalities in fetuses exposed to the vaccine in the first trimester (40). Its use has also been reported in the second and third trimesters (41,42). The vaccination may not offer protection to all pregnant patients. In one study, women who smoked, were obese, or at least 25 years of age were less likely to respond to the vaccine after two vaccinations (41). After the vaccination, approximately 49% of women were reported to seroconvert (41,43). However, not all women received the three vaccinations in these studies.

Hepatitis C

Hepatitis C virus (HCV) infection is the most common blood-borne infection in the United States. Approximately 1.8% of Americans have been infected with the virus. Antibodies against the virus are not protective; most infected people have chronic infections. The prevalence of HCV RNA in mothers with HCV infection in the United States is reported to be as high as 84% (44). Vertical transmission of HCV occurs in 5% to 6% of infants when the mother is human immunodeficiency virus (HIV) negative and in as many as 17% of neonates if the mother is HIV positive (45,46). The risk is greatest in mothers who are HIV positive and HCV RNA positive (47). Although the virus can be secreted in breast milk, it is rare for neonates to become infected via breast-feeding. The average rate of infection is 4% in both breast-fed and bottle-fed infants (45). Immunoglobulins are not effective for postexposure prophylaxis of HCV.

Chronic Hepatitis

In the nonpregnant patient, antiviral agents used in the treatment of chronic viral hepatitis consist of interferon (alfa-2a, alfa-2b, and alfacon-1) and ribavirin. Therapy for chronic hepatitis B is recommended for patients with persistent elevations in the serum aminotransferase concentrations; detectable levels of HB_sAg, HB_eAg, and HBV DNA in serum; chronic hepatitis on liver biopsy; and compensated liver disease. For patients with chronic HCV infection, only those who have elevated serum aminotransferase concentrations, serum anti-HCV, and chronic hepatitis on liver biopsy are candidates for therapy. There are case reports of interferon alfa use in pregnancy for treatment of various medical conditions that include essential thrombocytopenia (48,49), chronic myelogenous leukemia (50–52), Hodgkin's disease (53), and acute progressive

and fulminant hepatitis (54). In cases in which the treatment occurred during the first trimester, only one child had congenital anomalies consisting of ambiguous genitalia and multiple hemivertebrae (55). Based on pharmacokinetic studies in two pregnant women, interferon alfa does not transfer across the placenta in significant amounts (56). Therapeutic doses of interferon alfa are unlikely to pose a substantial risk during pregnancy, but data on human pregnancies are insufficient. Spontaneous abortion was reported in four patients exposed to interferon beta at the time of conception (57). Ribavirin has been used in the second half of pregnancy in nine women for severe measles. No adverse effects were noted in the infants (58). Treatment with antiviral agents for chronic hepatitis is not recommended during pregnancy unless the maternal condition is rapidly deteriorating. Ribavirin may be teratogenic in the first trimester and patients should avoid becoming pregnant during therapy and for 6 months posttherapy because of a long half-life. Women with hepatitis B and C infections can breastfeed provided the neonate receives appropriate immunoprophylaxis (59).

HUMAN IMMUNODEFICIENCY VIRUS

Antiretroviral therapy is recommended for patients who are infected with HIV if the HIV-1 RNA level is greater than 5,000 to 10,000 copies/mL. The viral load is a strong and independent predictor of clinical outcome. The International Aids Society—USA Panel recommends treatment for patients who are committed to a complex and long-term therapy with close adherence to the regimen (60). For patients who are asymptomatic with low plasma HIV RNA levels of less than 5,000 copies/mL and high CD4+ cell count greater than 350 to 500/μL, the therapy can be deferred with close follow-up examinations. The management of pregnant women changes frequently, and the most current literature should be consulted. At the time this chapter was written, there was increasing evidence that any detectable viral load increases vertical transmission. This raises the issue of whether all pregnant women would benefit (by reduced vertical transmission)

TABLE 19.1. *Antiretroviral drugs used during pregnancy*

Antiretroviral drug	Dose	Fetal/neonatal effects
nRTI		
Zidovudine (ZDV) (62,63,65,66,68–74)	100 mg 6 times/d	No adverse immunologic, neurologic, or growth effects with average follow-up to age 4.2 y; possible anemia
Zalcitabine (ddc) (65)[a]	0.75 mg t.i.d.	1/7 infants exposed to ddc and ZDV with hepatosplenomegaly and large tongue
Didanosine (ddl) (63,65,71)[a]	≥60 kg: 200 mg b.i.d.	No reported adverse effects
Stavudine (d4T) (63,65,73,74)[a]	≥60 kg: 40 mg b.i.d.	No reported adverse effects
Lamivudine (3TC) (63,65,72–74)	150 or 300 mg b.i.d.	No reported adverse effects
NNRTI		
Nevirapine (63–65)	200 mg q.d. × 2 wk then 200 mg b.i.d.	No reported adverse effects
Delavirdine (63)[a]	400 mg t.i.d.	Manufacturer reported 7 inadvertent pregnancies: 3 ectopic, 3 normal term, 1 preterm with a VSD
PI		
Indinavir (63,74)[a]	800 mg q 8h	The protease inhibitors have been associated with SGA infants (62)
Ritonavir (RTV) (65,73,74)[a]	600 mg b.i.d.	
Saquinavir (SQV) (63,65,73,74)[a]	600 mg t.i.d.	Less severe but prolonged metabolic acidosis with RTV and SQV (72)
Nelfinavir (63,65,74)[a]	750 mg t.i.d.	

[a]Very limited data.

SGA, small for gestational age; VSD, ventricular septal defect; nRTI, nucleoside analog reverse transcriptase inhibitors; NNRTI, non-nucleoside reverse transcriptase inhibitors; PI, protease inhibitors.

Data from refs. 61, 65, and 67.

from antiviral therapy. If the CD4+ cell count decreases or the HIV RNA level increases, therapy should be recommended. The antiretroviral regimens consist of combination therapy.

Combinations in current use in the treatment-naive patients include (i) protease inhibitor (PI) and two nucleoside reverse transcriptase inhibitors (nRTIs), (ii) one nonnucleoside analog reverse transcriptase inhibitor (NNRTI) and two nRTIs, (iii) two PIs with or without one or two nRTIs, (iv) one PI and one NNRTI with or without one or two nRTIs, and (v) three nRTIs (60). Data regarding the pharmacokinetics and safety of antiretroviral drugs during pregnancy are limited (61). Zidovudine (ZDV) has been studied the most. In a prospective cohort study, children exposed to ZDV in the perinatal period through Pediatric AIDS Clinical Trials Group Protocol 076 were studied until a median age of 4.2 years. No adverse effects were observed in these children (62). Combination antiretroviral therapy when used in pregnancy has not been associated with major infant toxicity even when the therapy was initiated in the first trimester (63).

Nevirapine has been used in the peripartum period in HIV-1 infected pregnant women in Uganda with a reduction of nearly 50% of HIV transmission to the neonate. The babies were followed for 14 to 16 weeks of life and nearly all were breast-fed (64). PIs have been the least studied antiretroviral drug. A summary of the antiretroviral medications used during pregnancy is given in Table 19.1.

The International Antiretroviral Registry was established in 1993 to detect any major teratogenic effect of the antiretroviral drugs. The registration process protects patient anonymity. The information available from the registry is based on voluntary reporting of prenatal exposure to the antiretroviral drugs. Because of the nature of the exposure-registration study, rates of drug-associated adverse events may not reflect true rates. Through July 1999, 916 pregnancies were enrolled into the study. Of 916 exposures, 403 were first trimester exposures. Prenatal exposure has been reported in all three trimesters of pregnancy to almost all the antiretroviral drugs alone or in combination, with the exception of zalcitabine and delavirdine. Exposure to the latter two drugs has been reported in the first and second trimesters. The number of pregnancies exposed to the different drugs has been small, and it is not possible to draw conclusions regarding the effects of individual drugs on the fetus. Overall, birth defects complicated two per 100 live-births among women with first-trimester exposure to the antiretroviral drug. It is recommended that health care professionals report pregnancy exposure of these drugs to the registry (Antiretroviral Pregnancy Registry; the contact number in the United States is 1-800-722-9292, ext. 38465).

ZDV significantly reduces the rate of mother-to-child transmission of HIV from 25.5% in the placebo group to 8.3% in the intervention group (64). All pregnant patients should be offered the three-part ZDV chemoprophylaxis, either alone or in combination with other antiretrovirals, to reduce the risk of perinatal HIV transmission after the first trimester (64). In National Institutes of Health–sponsored clinical trials, nevirapine is currently being studied in pregnant women to decrease HIV transmission to the offspring.

Recommendation for Chemoprophylaxis to Reduce Perinatal HIV Infection

- Antepartum 100 mg ZDV orally five times daily
- Intrapartum 2 mg/kg of body weight ZDV given intravenously over 1 hour, then 1 mg/kg per hour until delivery
- ZDV for the newborn, 2 mg/kg orally every 6 hours for 6 weeks

During pregnancy, HIV-1–positive patients should be monitored similar to those who are not pregnant. The HIV-1 RNA level should be obtained every trimester. The CD4+ count should also be evaluated. Initiation of therapy for women currently not receiving antiretroviral therapy and alterations in therapy for those who are currently receiving antiretroviral therapy should be based on the same parameters as those for the non-pregnant patient. The decision regarding initiation or alteration of therapy should be made by the patient after discussion with the HIV

specialists and the health care provider regarding risks and benefits of the treatment to her and her fetus. In pregnant women who require HIV treatment with combination therapy, it is advisable to delay initiation of therapy until after 10 to 12 weeks of gestation if possible because the risks of antiretroviral therapy during the first trimester are unknown. The CDC recommends that HIV-infected women should be advised against breast-feeding to prevent transmission of the virus to the infant.

INFLUENZA

Typical influenza infection is caused by influenza A or B viruses. Influenza A viruses are categorized into subtypes based on the surface antigens hemagglutinin and neuraminidase. Influenza B virus are not categorized into subtypes. Since 1977, influenza A, H1N1 and H3N2 subtypes, and influenza B viruses have been in global circulation. The infection is characterized by sore throat, nonproductive cough, myalgia, fevers, and occasionally severe malaise. Primary influenza pneumonia or secondary bacterial pneumonia can occur leading to serious illness. During pregnancy, the relative risk of hospitalization for cardiopulmonary complications increases from 1.4 at 14 to 20 weeks of gestation to 4.7 at 37 to 42 weeks compared with postpartum patients (73). In the third trimester, the rate of hospitalization of 0.25% was comparable with that of nonpregnant women having high-risk medical conditions.

Immunoprophylaxis

The CDC recommends all pregnant women who will be in the second or third trimester during the influenza season be vaccinated. In other words, women who will be beyond the first trimester of pregnancy (more than 14 weeks of gestation) during the influenza season should be vaccinated. Those with medical conditions should be vaccinated regardless of the stage of pregnancy (74). Data on more than 2,000 pregnant women demonstrated no adverse fetal effects in association with the vaccine (75). Breast-feeding is not a contraindication for vaccination. The vaccine contains inactivated killed viruses, usually two type A and one type B. The dose is 0.5 mL given intramuscularly.

Antiviral Treatment

Four drugs are currently licensed for the control and prevention of influenza in the United States: amantadine, rimantadine, zanamivir, and oseltamivir. Amantadine and rimantadine are chemically related with activity against influenza A but not B viruses. Zanamivir and oseltamivir are neuraminidase inhibitors with activity against both influenza A and B viruses and were approved in 1999 (74). In a surveillance study of 333,000 liveborn infants based on a Medicare study, 64 pregnancies were exposed to amantadine (76). Five of the children were diagnosed with congenital anomalies. The expected number was 3.1. Three other children born to women who were treated with amantadine throughout the first trimester were reported to have anomalies. One child had tetralogy of Fallot and tibial hemimelia (77), one had pulmonary atresia and a single cardiac ventricle (78), and one had inguinal hernia (79). The drug is secreted into breast milk. There are no reports of use of rimantadine during human pregnancy.

Chemoprophylaxis is 70% to 90% effective in preventing illness from influenza A infection. However, in pregnancy, it is not recommended unless the patient has additional high-risk factors that put her at significantly high risk of complications from influenza A. Chemoprophylaxis is not a substitute for vaccination. In otherwise healthy, nonpregnant patients diagnosed with influenza A, treatment with antiviral agents does not alter the course significantly, especially if given after 48 hours of onset of illness.

The CDC states that because of the unknown effects of influenza antiviral drugs on pregnant women and their fetuses, these four drugs should be used during pregnancy only if the potential benefit justifies the potential risk to the embryo or fetus (74).

At least one group prefers use of the neuraminidase inhibitors because no teratogenicity or reproductive toxicity has been found in laboratory animals (80).

REFERENCES

1. Lazaretto T, Spezzacatena P, Pradelli P, et al. Cytomegalovirus infection in pregnancy: a still complicated diagnostic problem. *Intervirology* 1998;41:149–157.
2. Williamson DW, Demmler GJ, Percy AK, et al. Progressive hearing loss in infants with asymptomatic congenital cytomegalovirus infection. *Pediatrics* 1992;90: 862–866.
3. Lazzarotto T, Guerra B, Spezzacatena P, et al. Prenatal diagnosis of congenital cytomegalovirus infection. *J Clin Microbiol* 1998;36:3540–3544.
4. Stagno S, Pass RF, Dworsky ME, et al. Congenital cytomegalovirus infection: the relative importance of primary and recurrent maternal infection. *N Engl J Med* 1982;306:945–949.
5. Bodéus M, Hubinont C, Bernard P, et al. Prenatal diagnosis of human cytomegalovirus by culture and polymerase chain reaction: 98 pregnancies leading to congenital infection. *Prenat Diagn* 1999;19:314–317.
6. Reynolds DW, Stagno S, Hosty TS, et al. Maternal cytomegalovirus excretion and perinatal infection. *N Engl J Med* 1973;289:1–5.
7. Stagno S, Reynolds DW, Pass RF, et al. Breast milk and the risk of cytomegalovirus infection. *N Engl J Med* 1980;302:1073–1076.
8. Benshushan A, Brzezinski A, Ben-David A, et al. Early recurrent CMV infection with severe outcome to the fetus. *Acta Obstet Gynecol Scand* 1998;77:694–698.
9. Bodéus M, Goubau P. Predictive value of maternal-IgG avidity for congenital human cytomegalovirus infection. *J Clin Virol* 1999;12:3–8.
10. Gilstrap LC, Bawdon RE, Roberts SW, et al. The transfer of the nucleoside analog ganciclovir across the perfused human placenta. *Am J Obstet Gynecol* 1994;170:967–973.
11. Pescovitz MD. Absence of teratogenicity of oral ganciclovir used during early pregnancy in a liver transplant recipient. *Transplantation* 1998;67:758–759.
12. Miguelez M, Gonzalez A, Perez F. Severe cytomegalovirus hepatitis in a pregnant woman treated with ganciclovir. *Scand J Infect Dis* 1998;30:304–305.
13. Revello MG, Percivalle E, Baldanti F, et al. Prenatal treatment of congenital human cytomegalovirus infection by fetal intravascular administration of ganciclovir. *Clin Diagn Virol* 1993;1:61–67.
14. Nigro G, La Torre R, Anceschi MM, et al. Hyperimmunoglobulin therapy for a twin fetus with cytomegalovirus infection and growth restriction. *Am J Obstet Gynecol* 1999;180:1222–1226.
15. Negishi H, Yamada H, Hirayama E, et al. Intraperitoneal administration of cytomegalovirus hyperimmunoglobulin to the cytomegalovirus-infected fetus. *J Perinatol* 1998;18:466–469.
16. Brown ZA, Selke S, Zeh J, et al. The acquisition of herpes simplex virus during pregnancy. *N Engl J Med* 1997;337:509–515.
17. Kulhanjian JA, Soroush V, Au DS, et al. Identification of women at unsuspected risk of primary infection with herpes simplex virus type 2 during pregnancy. *N Engl J Med* 1992;326:916–920.
18. Hensleigh PA, Andrews WW, Brown Z, et al. Genital herpes during pregnancy: inability to distinguish primary and recurrent infections clinically. *Obstet Gynecol* 1997;89:891–895.

19. Lagrew DC, Furlow TG, Hager WD, et al. Disseminated herpes simplex virus infection in pregnancy. Successful treatment with acyclovir. *JAMA* 1984;252: 2058–2059.
20. Monif GRG, Kellner KR, Donnelly WH. Congenital herpes simples type II infection. *Am J Obstet Gynecol* 1985;152:1000–1002.
21. Management of herpes in pregnancy. *ACOG Pract Bull* 1999;No. 8.
22. Brocklhurst P, Kinghorn G, Carney O, et al. A randomised placebo controlled trial of suppressive acyclovir in late pregnancy in women with recurrent genital herpes infection. *Br J Obstet Gynecol* 1998;105:275–280.
23. Scott LL, Sanchez PJ, Jackson GL, et al. Acyclovir suppression to prevent cesarean delivery after first-episode genital herpes. *Obstet Gynecol* 1996;87:69–73.
24. Andrews EB, Yankaskas BC, Cordero JF, et al. Acyclovir in pregnancy registry: six years' experience. *Obstet Gynecol* 1992;79:7–13.
25. Eldridge R, Andrews E, Tilson H, et al. Pregnancy outcomes following systemic prenatal acyclovir exposure— June 1, 1984–June 30, 1993. *MMWR Morb Mortal Wkly Rep* 1993;42:806–809.
26. Stray-Pedersen B. Acyclovir in late pregnancy to prevent neonatal herpes simplex. *Lancet* 1990;336:756.
27. Kimberlin DF, Weller S, Whitley RJ, et al. Pharmacokinetics of oral valacyclovir and acyclovir in late pregnancy. *Am J Obstet Gynecol* 1998;179:846–851.
28. Miller E, Marshall R, Vurdien JE. Epidemiology, outcome and control of varicella zoster virus infection. *Rev Med Microbiol* 1993;4:222–230.
29. Centers for Disease Control. Prevention of varicella updated recommendations of the advisory committee on immunization practices (ACIP). *MMWR Morb Mortal Wkly Rep* 1999;48:1–5.
30. Burgess MA, Cossart YE, Wilkins TD, et al. Varicella vaccination of health-care workers. *Vaccine* 1999;17:765–769.
31. Salzman MB, Sharrar RG, Steinberg S, et al. Transmission of varicella vaccine virus from a healthy 12-month-old child to his pregnant mother. *J Pediatr* 1997;131:151–154.
32. Enders G, Miller E, Cradock-Watson J, et al. Consequences of varicella and herpes zoster in pregnancy: prospective study of 1739 cases. *Lancet* 1994;343:1548–1551.
33. Sauerbrei A. Varicella-zoster virus infections in pregnancy. *Intervirology* 1998;41:191–196.
34. Miller E, Cradock-Watson JE, Ridehalgh MKS. Outcome in newborn babies given anti-varicella-zoster immunoglobulin after perinatal maternal infection with varicella-zoster virus. *Lancet* 1989;2:371–373.
35. Haake DA, Zakowski PC, Haake DL, et al. Early treatment of acyclovir for varicella pneumonia in otherwise healthy adults: retrospective controlled study and review. *Rev Infect Dis* 1990;12:788–798.
36. Baren JM, Henneman PL, Lewis RJ. Primary varicella in adults; pneumonia, pregnancy, and hospital admission. *Ann Emerg Med* 1996;28:165–169.
37. Long SS. Toddler-to-mother transmission of varicella-vaccine virus: how bad is that? *J Pediatr* 1997;131:10–12.
38. Viral hepatitis in pregnancy. *ACOG Educ Bull* 1998;248:880–886.
39. Sweet RL. Hepatitis B infection in pregnancy. *Obstet Gynecol Rep* 1990;2:128–139.
40. Levy M, Koren G. Hepatitis B vaccine in pregnancy; maternal and fetal safety. *Am J Perinatol* 1991;8:227–232.
41. Ingardia CJ, Kelley L, Steinfeld JD, et al. Hepatitis B vaccination in pregnancy: factors influencing efficacy. *Obstet Gynecol* 1999;93:983–986.
42. Ayoola EA, Johnson AOK. Hepatitis B vaccine in pregnancy: immunogenicity, safety and transfer of antibodies to infants. *Int J Gynaecol Obstet* 1987;25:297–301.
43. Ingardia CJ, Kelley L, Lerer T, et al. Correlation of maternal and fetal hepatitis B antibody titers following maternal vaccination in pregnancy. *Am J Perinatol* 1999;16:129–132.
44. Hunt CM, Carson KL, Sharara AI. Hepatitis C in pregnancy. *Obstet Gynecol* 1997;89:883–890.
45. Centers for Disease Control. Recommendations for prevention and control of hepatitis C virus (HCV) infection and HCV-related chronic disease. *MMWR Morb Mortal Wkly Rep* 1998;47:1–39.
46. La Torre A, Biadaioli R, Capobianco T, et al. Vertical transmission of HCV. *Acta Obstet Gynecol Scand* 1998;77:889–892.
47. Ohto H, Terazawa S, Sasaki N, et al. Transmission of hepatitis C virus from mothers to infants. *N Engl J Med* 1994;330:744–750.
48. Delage R, Demers C, Cantin G, et al. Treatment of essential thrombocythemia during pregnancy with interferon-alpha. *Obstet Gynecol* 1996;87:814–817.
49. Pulik M, Lionnet F, Genet P, et al. Platelet counts during pregnancy in essential thrombocythaemia treated with recombinant alpha-interferon. *Br J Haematol* 1996;93:495.
50. Delmer A, Rio B, Bauduer F, et al. Pregnancy during myelosuppressive treatment for chronic myelogenous leukaemia. *Br J Haematol* 1992;82:783–784.
51. Haggstrom J, Adriansson M, Hybbinette T, et al. Two cases of CML treated with alpha-interferon during second and third trimester of pregnancy with analysis of the drug in the new-born immediately postpartum. *Eur J Haematol* 1996;57:101–102.
52. Kuroiwa M, Gondo H, Ashida K, et al. Interferon-alpha therapy for chronic myelogenous leukemia during pregnancy. *Am J Hematol* 1998;59:101–102.
53. Ferrari VD, Juirillo F, Lonardi G, et al. Pregnancy during alfa-interferon (INF) therapy in patient (PT) with advanced Hodgkin disease (HD). *Ann Oncol* 1994;5:194.
54. Levin S, Leibowitz E, Torten J, et al. Interferon treatment in acute progressive and fulminant hepatitis. *Isr J Med Sci* 1989;25:364–372.
55. Perez-Encinas M, Bello JL, Perez-Crespo S, et al. Familial myeloproliferative syndrome. *Am J Hematol* 1994;46:225–229.
56. Pons JC, Lebon P, Frydman R, et al. Pharmacokinetics of interferon-alpha in pregnant women and fetoplacental passage. *Fetal Diagn Ther* 1995;10:7–10.
57. Faulds D, Benfield P. Interferon beta-1b in multiple sclerosis. An initial review of its rationale for use and therapeutic potential. *Clin Immunother* 1994;1:79–87.
58. Atmar RL, Englund JA, Hamill H. Complications of measles during pregnancy. *Clin Infect Dis* 1992;14:217–226
59. Breastfeeding: Maternal and Infant Aspects. ACOG Educational Bulletin July 2000. No. 258.
60. Carpenter CCJ, Fischl MA, Hammer SM, et al. Antiretroviral therapy for HIV infection in 1998: updated recommendations of the International AIDS Society—USA Panel. *JAMA* 1998;280:78–86.

61. Centers for Disease Control. Public Health Service Task Force. Recommendations for the use of antiretroviral drugs in pregnant women infected with HIV-1 for maternal health and for reducing perinatal HIV-1 transmission in the United States. *MMWR Morb Mortal Wkly Rep* 1998;47:1–30.

62. Culnane M, Fowler MG, Lee SS, et al. Lack of long-term effects of *in utero* exposure to zidovudine among uninfected children born to HIV-infected women. *JAMA* 1999;281:151–157.

63. McGowan JP, Crane M, Wiznia AA, et al. Combination antiretroviral therapy in human immunodeficiency virus-infected pregnant women. *Obstet Gynecol* 1999;94:641–646.

64. Guay LA, Musoke P, Fleming T, et al. Intrapartum and neonatal single-dose nevirapine compared with zidovudine for prevention of mother-to-child transmission of HIV-1 in Kampala, Uganda: HIVNET 012 randomised trial. *Lancet* 1999;354:795–802.

65. Connor EM, Sperling RS, Gelber R, et al. Reduction of maternal-infant transmission of human immunodeficiency virus type 1 with zidovudine treatment. *N Engl J Med* 1994;331;1173–1180.

66. Minkoff H, Augenbraun M. Antiretroviral therapy for pregnant women. *Am J Obstet Gynecol* 1997;176:478–489

67. Fiscus SA, Adimora AA, Schoenbach VJ, et al. Trends in human immunodeficiency virus (HIV) counseling, testing, and antiretroviral treatment of HIV-infected women and perinatal transmission in North Carolina. *J Infect Dis* 1999;180:99–105.

68. Sperling RS, Stratton P, O'Sullivan MJ, et al. A survey of zidovudine use in pregnant women with human immunodeficiency virus infection. *N Engl J Med* 1992;326:857–861.

69. Frenkel LM, Wagner LE II, Demeter LM, et al. Effects of zidovudine use during pregnancy on resistance and vertical transmission of human immunodeficiency virus type 1. *Clin Infect Dis* 1995;20:1321–1326.

70. Wang Y, Livingston E, Patil S, et al. Pharmacokinetics of didanosine in antepartum and postpartum human immunodeficiency virus-infected pregnant women and their neonates: an AIDS clinical trials group study. *J Infect Dis* 1999;180:1536–1541.

71. Clarke JR, Braganza R, Mirza A, et al. Rapid development of genotypic resistance to Lamivudine when combined with Zidovudine in pregnancy. *J Med Virol* 1999;59:364–368.

72. Grubert TA, Wintergerst U, Lutz-Friedrich R, et al. Long-term antiretroviral combination therapy including Lamivudine in HIV-1 infected women during pregnancy. *AIDS* 1999;13:1430–1431.

73. Lorenzi P, Spicher VM, Laubereau B, et al. Antiretroviral therapies in pregnancy: maternal, fetal and neonatal effects. *AIDS* 1998;12:F241–F247.

74. Neuzil KM, Reed GW, Mitchel EF, et al. Impact of influenza on acute cardiopulmonary hospitalizations in pregnant women. *Am J Epidemiol* 1998;148:1094–1102.

75. Centers for Disease Control. Prevention and control of influenza—recommendations of the Advisory Committee on Immunization Practices. *MMWR Morb Mortal Wkly Rep* 2000;49:1–38.

76. Heinonen OP, Shapiro S, Monson RR, et al. Immunization during pregnancy against poliomyelitis and influenza in relation to childhood malignancy. *Int J Epidemiol* 1973;2:229–235.

77. Rosa F. Amantadine pregnancy experience. *Reprod Toxicol* 1994;8:531.

78. Pandit PB, Chitayat D, Jefferies AL. Tibial hemimelia and tetralogy of Fallot associated with first trimester exposure to amantadine. *Reprod Toxicol* 1994;8:89–92.

79. Nora JJ, Nora AH, Way GL. Cardiovascular maldevelopment associated with maternal exposure to amantadine. *Lancet* 1975;2:607.

80. Golbe KI. Parkinson's disease and pregnancy. *Neurology* 1987;37:1245–1249.

81. Gubareva LV, Kaiser L, Hayden FG. Influenza virus neuraminidase inhibitors. *Lancet* 2000;355:827–835.

20

Anticonvulsants in Pregnancy

Michele Wylen* and Jerome Yankowitz†

*Department of Obstetrics and Gynecology, Georgetown University, Washington, D.C.
†Department of Obstetrics and Gynecology, The University of Iowa Hospitals and Clinics,
Iowa City, Iowa

Seizure disorders affect approximately 0.5% to 1% of the general and pregnant population (1–6), and thus it is estimated that 800,000 to 1.1 million reproduction-age women have seizure disorders (5) in the United States alone. Epilepsy constitutes the most common neurologic disorder in pregnancy (1).

Seizures are episodic disturbances of movement, feeling, or consciousness caused by sudden synchronous, inappropriate, and excessive electrical discharges in the cerebral cortex (2). Seizures are classified as either generalized (deep bilateral onset) or partial (focal onset). In partial seizures, although focal areas of the brain are initially involved, there may be spread to the entire brain. With generalized seizures, the entire brain is affected at the outset (2,7).

Five percent of the population report having had a seizure at some point in their lives. There is a very high remission rate even among those individuals who are never treated (8). Approximately 15% of all seizures are acquired as a result of an identifiable etiology such as infection, trauma, metabolic aberration, or a space-occupying lesion. Alternatively, 85% of seizures are idiopathic or cryptogenic in nature, meaning no specific cause can be identified. Epilepsy is defined as recurrent, idiopathic seizures (7). With the administration of anticonvulsant drugs (AEDs), seizures can be controlled in approximately 60% to 70% of epileptic patients, often with one AED (2).

EFFECT OF PREGNANCY ON EPILEPSY

Most women with epilepsy will have uneventful pregnancies. The effect of pregnancy on seizure frequency can be variable. Sources cite that 15% to 50% of patients will have an increase in the frequency of seizure activity during pregnancy (3,4,6,9–12). Approximately 25% of patients will have a decrease in seizure frequency, whereas the vast majority of women with epilepsy will experience no change in seizure frequency as a result of pregnancy (9,10). In a review of 27 studies involving 2,165 pregnancies in epileptic women, 24% had an increase in seizure frequency, 23% a decrease, and 53% had no change in seizure frequency (4).

The patient's age, seizure type, AED regimen, or seizure frequency during a previous pregnancy cannot predict changes in seizure frequency for a particular pregnant woman. Knight and Rhind (13) concluded that women were not at increased risk of having increased seizure frequency during pregnancy if they had experienced less than one seizure every 9 months before conception. Conversely, women who experienced more than one seizure per month before pregnancy were likely to experience an increased seizure frequency during pregnancy. In addition, Tanganelli and Regesta (14) reported that a history of frequent seizures before conception and women with focal epilepsy were at greater risk of undergoing increased seizure frequency during pregnancy.

Other investigators have not confirmed these conclusions (9). Sabers et al. (15) recently found that 21% of 151 pregnancies in 124 women with epilepsy had increased seizure frequency during the gestation. The increased seizure frequency was not related to the seizure type.

Many different factors have been proposed as playing a role in increasing seizure frequency in some pregnant epileptics including noncompliance, hyperventilation (causing a mild compensatory alkalosis), dilutional hypocalcemia, hyponatremia, hypomagnesemia, emotional stress, sleep deprivation, altered gastric motility, nausea and vomiting, and hepatic clearance (3,6). Hormonal influences may play a role. Estrogens appear to be epileptogenic in some animal models by decreasing seizure thresholds and increasing the severity of seizures. In addition, animal studies also suggest that increased gonadotropin levels can increase the frequency of paroxysmal discharges in the brain. In a review of why epilepsy is special in women, Morrell points out that ovarian steroids effect the seizure threshold at the membrane and the genome. Estrogen affects the γ-aminobutyric acid-A receptor by increasing excitability, whereas progesterone, for example, has inhibitory effects. Thus, pregnancy as well as puberty, the menstrual cycle, and menopause may all be times of altered seizure activity (16).

Sleep deprivation and emotional stress can provoke seizures (3,11,17). Pregnancy in general can be a time of sleep deprivation because women find it difficult to get comfortable secondary to musculoskeletal pain. In addition, pregnancy often is associated with emotional stress and anxiety as new mothers prepare for a life-altering event (9).

One of the most important factors that affects seizure frequency in pregnancy is the change in AED serum levels. Total plasma concentrations of AEDs tend to decrease during pregnancy. Many women are poorly compliant with their medications when they become pregnant for fear that the AED will harm the fetus or because they fear the medication will initiate or exacerbate nausea and emesis (10). In turn, nausea and vomiting may need to be treated more aggressively to assist the otherwise compliant patient in maintaining serum levels of AEDs (18).

Impaired absorption of AEDs may occur in pregnancy, resulting in decreased serum levels. Hyperemesis impairs drug absorption. In addition, the increased calcium and antacid intake that occurs in pregnancy may decrease absorption of antiepileptic drugs (7). The increased volume of distribution and an increase in renal clearance may reduce serum drug levels. Folate supplementation, routinely administered in pregnancy, can decrease levels of antiepileptic drugs by inducing hepatic enzymes that result in increased metabolism of the AED.

It is important to keep in mind that even though total AED levels decline in almost all women during pregnancy, the majority of these women do not have increased seizure activity. This is because serum albumin levels decrease in pregnancy, resulting in an increase in the percentage of drug that is free. Because most laboratory drug assays measure total drug levels, the patient's clinical status should always be considered before initiating dosing changes. A decrease in total plasma levels of an AED should not automatically dictate an increase in the dose of the drug being administered. One must keep in mind that it is the level of free drug that correlates with seizure control and central nervous system effects (9).

If a patient has been seizure free, some obstetricians will monitor AED levels each trimester. Anytime the patient is exhibiting signs of drug toxicity, the dose should be reduced even in the case of stable total serum levels because free levels may be increased. It takes four to five half-lives for dose changes to reach a steady state, so physicians should be careful to avoid measuring drug levels too frequently. When measuring drug levels, it is better to get free levels and the blood draw should occur just before dose administration so trough levels can be obtained. Last, it is important to keep in mind that levels of AEDs may rise rapidly during the first few postpartum weeks because of decreases in both renal clearance and volume of distribution. Moreover, there is enhanced maternal compliance with drug ingestion after delivery because the pregnant woman with epilepsy no longer fears the potential adverse effects that AEDs can have on the unborn fetus. Therefore, drug dosing may need to be rapidly tapered in the postpartum period, especially if doses had been increased in the antepartum period (1).

EFFECT OF EPILEPSY ON PREGNANCY

Although the vast majority of women with epilepsy will have uneventful pregnancies, several adverse pregnancy outcomes have been reported more frequently in women with epilepsy compared with control groups in some but not all studies. These adverse outcomes include preterm delivery, low birth weight, smaller head circumference, stillbirth, depressed Apgar scores, preeclampsia, cesarean delivery, congenital malformations, developmental delay, and perinatal mortality (1,7,9).

Pregnant women with epilepsy who ingest AEDs have a fetal congenital anomaly rate of 4% to 8% instead of the 2% to 3% background incidence quoted for the general population (10,12,19). There is also a twofold increased risk of minor malformations to 6% to 20% (12).

In addition to AED use, other factors proposed as being responsible for the increased rates of congenital malformations include maternal seizures, the genetics of maternal epilepsy, physical trauma during seizures, lower socioeconomic status, and limited access to prenatal care (19). However, most investigators have concluded that maternal seizures during pregnancy have no impact on the frequency of malformation in the offspring of these women (9,19). It has been proposed that the underlying epilepsy in the mother is hereditary, and the inheritance of this genetic abnormality produces an increased frequency of birth defects in their offspring (20). Holmes et al. (21) attempted to refute this unproved theory. They studied children aged 6 to 16 years of women who had a history of seizures ($n = 57$) but took no medications during the pregnancy and matched controls ($n = 57$). There were no differences in physical features or cognitive function in the two groups. Unfortunately, this study was confounded by the seizure group being somewhat atypical and probably milder as they had no need for the AEDs. Also this was a retrospective study, and although 11 women stated

they had seizures during the index pregnancies, the seizures were described as "feeling strange," experiencing strange smells. In fact, none of the women in the study group had tonic-clonic seizures during the index pregnancy. Therefore, it remains to be shown whether adverse pregnancy outcomes of epileptic women can be attributed to some innate factor versus use of AEDs or occurrence of tonic-clinic seizures during the pregnancy. It is hoped that the establishment of a large registry (5) will answer these questions. The objective of The North American Registry for Epilepsy and Pregnancy is to identify possible associations between fetal exposure to AEDs and adverse pregnancy outcomes.

The consensus is that the AEDs used in the treatment of epilepsy, and not the epilepsy itself, are largely responsible for the adverse pregnancy outcomes in women with epilepsy, particularly the increase in fetal congenital malformations (22).

USE OF AEDs IN PREGNANCY

All AEDs cross the placenta and therefore have some potential for teratogenicity (20). Because one of every 250 fetuses is exposed to an AED, the potential impact of antiepileptic drugs is great (22).

A study by Holmes et al. (23) supports the hypothesis that AEDs are responsible for the congenital malformations found in the offspring of pregnant women with epilepsy. In this prospective study carried out from 1986 to 1988, three groups of women were followed prospectively for pregnancy outcome. One group consisted of 180 epileptic women who were exposed to AEDs. The second group was 218 epileptics who were not exposed to any AEDs. The third group of women consisted of 979 controls. In this study, there was no difference between the two epileptic groups in terms of the types of epilepsy they had. There was a significant increase in major malformations, microcephaly, or growth retardation among the drug-exposed infants compared with both the epileptic women not exposed to drugs and the control infants. In addition, there was no statistically significant difference in outcomes between the epileptic women not exposed to AEDs and the control group. One flaw of this study, however, is that seizure frequency differed among the two epileptic groups. Of the women with epilepsy who took AEDs, 50% of the subjects experienced seizures, whereas only 10% of the mothers not on any medications reported seizures during pregnancy (23).

In a recent study of 211 women with epilepsy and 355 healthy controls, pregnancy outcomes were documented prospectively. There were 174 pregnancies characterized by maternal epilepsy available for analysis. Of these, 159 pregnancies involved exposure to AEDs. No abnormal outcomes as defined by death or congenital anomalies occurred in the offspring of epileptic women not exposed to AEDs. In the 159 epileptic women exposed to AEDs, 10.7% had abnormal outcomes compared with 3.4% in the control group. This was statistically significant. In this study, there was no correlation between seizure frequency and adverse outcome (24).

In a large multiinstitutional study involving 902 epileptic women, the incidence of malformations in epileptic women on AED therapy was approximately five times that of women with epilepsy not taking any medications (25).

Additional evidence that AEDs are teratogenic is that as serum drug levels of AEDs increase, so do malformation rates, and as additional medications are added to drug regimens, malformation rates also increase (11). When two AEDs are used, the incidence of congenital malformations increases to 5.5%. The malformation rates are increased to 11% and 23%, respectively, when three and four AEDs are used (6,10). This can be compared with 2% in the general population and approximately 3% with one AED (6). Koch et al. (26) recently showed that there were long-term electroencephalographic (EEG) changes in children whose mothers were treated with AEDs during their pregnancy. IQs also decreased as the number of AEDs increased, whereas the EEG changes were not related to the number of maternal seizures during the pregnancy.

Last, the timing of AED exposure during embryogenesis is important in terms of resultant congenital malformations. Neural tube defects occur when exposure to some AEDs occurs from weeks 5 to 6 by last menstrual period (LMP).

Cleft lip and palate result when drug exposure occurs before week 7 by LMP and week 10 by LMP, respectively. Congenital heart disease occurs with drug exposure before 8 weeks by LMP (10).

Physicians should consider weaning women off their AEDs before conception if they have been seizure free for more than 2 years. The ideal that the patient should be on the fewest medications, if any, at the lowest dose needed to control the seizures was the conclusion of an international consensus guideline (27).

MECHANISMS OF AED TERATOGENICITY

Many mechanisms have been proposed to explain the teratogenicity of AEDs. One mechanism involves the formation of toxic epoxides as a metabolite of the AEDs. For example, during metabolism of phenytoin, unstable epoxides, arene oxides, are formed. These substances are known to have mutagenic effects in animal and human studies. Detoxification of the arene oxides requires epoxide hydrolase enzymes, which may be genetically absent or deficient in some fetuses, making them more susceptible to congenital malformations when exposed to AEDs (28). However, alternative mechanisms must exist because embryopathies have also been described in fetuses exposed to mephenytoin whose metabolism does not involve the formation of an arene oxide metabolite (10,19,29).

Metabolism of some AEDs results in the formation of free radicals that can bind to cell molecules including DNA and proteins and are cytotoxic because they can disrupt transcription, translation, cell division, and cell migration (29). Therefore, the formation of free radicals during AED metabolism may be an alternative mechanism by which congenital malformations are increased in epileptic women. In the metabolism of phenytoin, free radical intermediates are produced. In animal studies, pretreatment of pregnant mice with compounds that reduce phenytoin free radicals reduced the number of cleft lips and palates in the offspring. Moreover, glutathione is believed to detoxify the free radical intermediates by forming nontoxic conjugates. Studies show that substances that inhibit glutathione production increase rates of phenytoin embryopathy (19). Some fetuses may possess low levels of free radical scavenging enzymes and therefore higher levels of the free radicals themselves as a result of a genetic defect; these fetuses may be more at risk for congenital malformations. Polytherapy may have an additive effect on congenital anomaly rates because of cumulative effects of toxic metabolite formation (29).

The antifolate effects of AEDs may contribute to their teratogenicity. AEDs can decrease serum folate levels by inducing folate metabolism in the liver (10). In women without epilepsy, folate deficiency is associated with adverse pregnancy outcomes and with fetal malformations that include ventriculoseptal and neural tube defects (29). In pregnant women with epilepsy, low red blood cell levels of folate have been associated with increased malformation rates in their offspring (10,19). However, folic acid deficiency cannot be the entire explanation because phenytoin and the barbiturates induce the most marked changes in folic acid status yet pose the lowest risk for neural tube defects. Conversely, valproate and carbamazepine are associated with the highest rates of neural tube defects and have a much lesser effect on quantitative folic acid parameters (22). Folate supplementation substantially reduces the risk of adverse fetal outcome in women without epilepsy. A reduction in first occurrence of neural tube defects has been demonstrated when folic acid is supplemented at 0.4 mg per day. Folate supplementation of 4 mg per day reduces recurrent neural tube defects 3.5% to 0.7% (19). To reduce the risk of neural tube defects, folate supplementation must be present between days 1 and 28 of gestation, the time of posterior neuropore closure (29). Its safety in women receiving antiepileptic medications is unknown. Some investigators believe that women taking AEDs should not universally be treated with high doses of folic acid until there is clear evidence from controlled clinical trials that it is effective and without any adverse fetal effects (22). Folic acid ingestion can increase the activity of hepatic microsomal enzymes and lower AED concentrations. The American College of Obstetricians and Gynecologists states that it would

seem appropriate that women taking AEDs that are specifically associated with neural tube defects (i.e., valproate and carbamazepine) take a preconception dose of folic acid equivalent to 4 mg per day (1). Despite clear evidence of benefit in this particular population, others have also recommended 4 to 5 mg per day of folate supplementation for 3 months before conception and through the first trimester (3,6,18).

ANTICONVULSANT MEDICATIONS

No congenital malformations appear to be specific to one specific AED. German et al. in 1970 described the first syndrome associated with an AED, the fetal trimethadione syndrome (30). This syndrome is characterized by dysmorphic features in the exposed fetus and developmental delays in the neonate in greater than 50% of the offspring of mothers using this AED. A number of other similar syndromes have been described with the use of other AEDs. The characteristics of these syndromes are so similar that the broad term *fetal anticonvulsant syndrome* has been applied to almost any AED. The fetal anticonvulsant syndrome primarily includes orofacial, cardiovascular, and digital malformations (29).

Orofacial clefts are the most commonly reported malformation in the offspring of epileptic women who ingest AEDs. These anomalies constitute 30% of all major malformations. Midline cardiac defects and spina bifida aperta rank two and three, respectively. Valproic acid is associated with a 1% to 2% incidence of spina bifida and carbamazepine exposure is associated with a 0.5% to 1% risk of neural tube defects. In addition, various syndromes consisting of minor anomalies have been associated with fetal exposure to AEDs.

Phenytoin

Phenytoin (Dilantin) is a hydantoin anticonvulsant. Other AEDs in this class of drugs include ethotoin, mephenytoin and phenacemide. Phenytoin is used for the treatment of partial tonic-clonic seizures and status epilepticus. The usual dose is 300 to 600 mg per day administered in three divided doses. If extended release is used, a single daily dose may be appropriate. The therapeutic level is 10 to 20 μg/mL. More than 90% of the drug is protein bound. Phenytoin is eliminated by hepatic metabolism and it induces hepatic microsomal oxidative enzymes. The toxic side effects of phenytoin are dose dependent and include ataxia, nystagmus, nausea, gingival hyperplasia, depression, megaloblastic anemia, and dysrhythmias.

There is a 2% to 5% risk of major congenital anomalies that primarily include midline heart defects, orofacial clefts, and urogenital defects (1,10). The fetal hydantoin syndrome was first described and named by Hanson and Smith in 1975 (31). The risk of an exposed fetus of having the fetal hydantoin syndrome is approximately 10%. The fetal hydantoin syndrome is a constellation of minor anomalies including craniofacial abnormalities (short nose, flat nasal bridge, wide lips, hypertelorism, ptosis, epicanthal folds, low-set ears, and low hairline), and limb anomalies (distal digital hypoplasia, absent nails, and altered palmar crease). In addition, neonatal growth and performance delays have been documented.

Phenytoin may act as a competitive inhibitor of the placental transport of vitamin K. This results in a decrease of the fetal coagulation factors II, VII, IX, and X. Additionally, phenytoin may induce fetal hepatic metabolism of the coagulation factors. The resultant decrease in fetal coagulation factors is associated with an increased risk of hemorrhagic disease in the newborn. To help prevent this coagulopathy, some advocate oral vitamin K supplementation (10 mg daily) to the pregnant epileptic patient during the last month of pregnancy in addition to administering vitamin K injections to the neonate at birth (1,3,10,18).

Phenytoin is considered compatible with breast-feeding. In breast milk, it is present in levels of 15% of that in maternal serum (32).

Carbamazepine

Carbamazepine (Tegretol) is an iminostilbene; it is used to treat all types of seizure disorders with the exception of petit mal epilepsy. It is most commonly used in the treatment of psychomotor

(temporal lobe) and grand mal epilepsy. Carbamazepine is administered in doses of 200 to 1,200 mg per day with therapeutic levels from 4 to 12 μg/mL (33; product information for Tegretol, Novartis Pharmaceutical Corp., East Hanover, NJ, 1998). Dose-dependent side effects of carbamazepine include dizziness, headache, nausea, drowsiness, neutropenia, and hyponatremia (10).

In a prospective study involving 72 women with epilepsy taking carbamazepine, there was an increased incidence of congenital anomalies among the 35 fetuses exposed to the drug. There was an 11% incidence of craniofacial defects, a 26% incidence of fingernail hypoplasia, and a 20% incidence of developmental delay (34). This constellation of fetal effects has been referred to as the fetal carbamazepine syndrome and closely resembles the malformations seen in cases of fetal hydantoin syndrome.

In addition, maternal carbamazepine exposure has been specifically associated with spina bifida. An analysis of all available data involving cohorts of pregnant women ingesting carbamazepine supports the conclusion that fetal exposure to this drug carries an approximate risk of 0.5% to 1% of spina bifida (35).

Like phenytoin, carbamazepine is eliminated via hepatic metabolism and induces hepatic microsomal enzymes. In addition, carbamazepine interferes with vitamin K–dependent coagulation factors and can therefore cause hemorrhagic disease of the newborn (10).

Maternal use of carbamazepine is considered compatible with breast-feeding. It enters breast milk at levels of 25% to 70% that of maternal serum levels. According to the WHO Working Group on Human Lactation (36), its use when breast-feeding is "probably safe."

Phenobarbital

Phenobarbital is one of the most commonly used AEDs in the barbiturate class of medications. Of the barbiturates, phenobarbital, mephobarbital, and metharbital have been used in the treatment of epilepsy. Phenobarbital is used in the treatment of partial and generalized tonic-clonic seizures and status epilepticus (10,33).

Phenobarbital is administered in doses of 60 to 240 mg per day and has therapeutic plasma levels ranging from 10 to 40 μg/mL (10,37). Dose-dependent side effects of phenobarbital include drowsiness, ataxia, nystagmus, fatigue, listlessness, and depression. Phenobarbital is eliminated via hepatic metabolism and induces hepatic microsomal oxidative enzymes (10).

Fetal exposure to phenobarbital has been associated with such major malformations as congenital heart defects and orofacial clefting. A fetal phenobarbital syndrome is characterized by similar minor dysmorphic features as seen with the fetal hydantoin syndrome (10). Fetal phenobarbital exposure has also been associated with decreased intellectual and cognitive development in neonates and children. Maternal phenobarbital use during pregnancy can result in hemorrhagic disease of the newborn and neonatal withdrawal symptoms after delivery. The withdrawal symptoms consist mostly of irritability and begin at approximately 7 days of life and usually last from approximately 2 to 6 weeks (7,10,32).

Phenobarbital use in breast-feeding mothers may result in neonatal sedation and infant withdrawal symptoms when breast-feeding is discontinued (10). Occasionally, the neonate can develop sedation owing to phenobarbital in the breast milk. Breast-feeding should be discontinued in this situation (12).

Primidone

Primidone (Mysoline, Primaclone), is metabolized to phenobarbital and phenylethylmalonamide. All these compounds have anticonvulsant activity and are effective against partial and generalized tonic-clonic seizures. They may control seizures refractory to phenobarbital.

Primidone is administered in doses of 500 to 2,000 mg per day to give therapeutic levels ranging from 5 to 12 μg/mL (33,38; and product information, Mysoline, Wyeth-Ayerst Laboratories, Philadelphia, PA, 1995). Dose-dependent side effects of primidone include fatigue, depression, psychosis, nausea, ataxia, and nystagmus (10).

It has been difficult to assess the teratogenicity of primidone because many studies involving the use of primidone alone are lacking. There are cases in the literature in which fetal exposure to primidone has been associated with similar dysmorphic features as those characterizing the fetal hydantoin syndrome. Congenital heart defects, orofacial clefting, and microcephaly have been associated with primidone exposure in utero (10,39–44).

As in the case of phenobarbital, fetal primidone exposure has been associated with neonatal withdrawal syndrome and hemorrhagic disease of the newborn (10).

Primidone should be used with caution by lactating women. In fact, the WHO Working Group on Human Lactation (36) classifies the use of this AED as unsafe in lactating women. Neonatal sedation, hypotonia, and feeding problems have been reported in breast-feeding infants exposed to primidone (32,45,46).

Valproic Acid

Valproic acid (Depakene, Depakote) is used to treat absence and generalized tonic-clonic seizures. It is administered in three to four divided doses daily for a total of 10 to 15 mg/kg per day. Therapeutic levels range from 50 to 100 μg/mL. Dose-dependent side effects include dyspepsia, nausea, tremor, weight gain, alopecia, and peripheral edema.

Infants exposed to valproic acid have a 1% to 2% risk of spina bifida. The neural tube defect tends to be lumbosacral in location. Fetal valproic acid exposure has also been associated with cardiac defects, orofacial clefting, and genitourinary anomalies. A fetal valproate syndrome has been described that is characterized by the following dysmorphic features: epicanthal folds, shallow orbits, hypertelorism, low-set ears, flat nasal bridge, up-turned nasal tip, microcephaly, thin vermillion borders, down-turned mouth, thin overlapping fingers and toes, and hyperconvex fingernails (7,9,10).

Valproic acid is metabolized in the liver and is an inhibitor of hepatic microsomal enzymes. It is associated with neonatal hemorrhage and liver damage.

Maternal use of valproic acid is compatible with breast-feeding and is present in breast milk in amounts of 15% of maternal plasma levels (10,32).

Ethosuximide

Ethosuximide (Zarontin) and its related compounds phensuximide and methsuximide are from the class of compounds known as succinimides. Ethosuximide primarily is used to treat uncomplicated petit mal, absence seizures. It is administered in amounts of 500 to 2,000 mg per day in divided doses to achieve therapeutic levels of 40 to 100 μg/mL. Dose-dependent side effects include nausea, emesis, anorexia, irritability, headache, drowsiness, and abdominal pain. Maternal use of ethosuximide in pregnancy may be associated with congenital heart disease, orofacial clefting, and hydrocephalus. Fetal exposure to this AED has also been associated with hemorrhagic disease of the newborn. Finally, maternal ingestion of ethosuximide when breast-feeding may be associated with poor suckling and hyperexcitability in the newborn (10). The American Academy of Pediatrics deems this medication compatible with breast-feeding (32).

Clonazepam

Clonazepam (Klonopin) is from the benzodiazepine class of medications and is used in the setting of refractory myoclonic seizures. The usual dose administered is a starting dose of 1.5 mg per day with daily doses not to exceed 20 mg. There are no guidelines in the literature regarding therapeutic levels. Its use is limited because of its tendency to cause sedation, fatigue, and dizziness and because of its potential for the development af drug tolerance. The maternal use of clonazepam has been noted to potentially increase the risk of congenital cardiac defects, but there is no conclusive evidence of human teratogenicity. Clonazepam must be used with caution in lactating women because of the potential risk of apnea in the neonate (10). The American Academy of Pediatrics only advises caution with use of the benzodiazepines because of possible concern, although no adverse effects have been reported (32).

Diazepam (Valium) is also a benzodiazepine anticonvulsant. Diazepam is primarily used in the treatment of acute seizures and status epilepticus. Status epilepticus occurs when there are prolonged or repetitive seizures in a patient. Specifically, it is defined by seizure activity lasting longer than 30 minutes or the occurrence of three or more seizures in 30 minutes without intervening recovery of consciousness. Status epilepticus can occur in epileptic as well as nonepileptic women and can result in irreversible brain damage or death in the mother and/or fetus. Diazepam is the drug of choice in the treatment of status epilepticus (20).

New Antiepileptic Drugs

The ideal AED should control seizures adequately when used as monotherapy, have little or no protein binding, not utilize the hepatic cytochrome P-450 system, have no arene oxide metabolites, and not alter folate-mediated biological processes (29).

Among the new antiepileptics are felbamate, gabapentin, lamotrigine, oxcarbazepine, topiramate, tiagabine, and vigabatrin (47).

Felbamate (Felbatol) was approved by the US Food and Drug Administration for monotherapy use but was later severely restricted secondary to its association with aplastic anemia and hepatic failure. It is an inhibitor of the cytochrome P-450 system, has little to no protein binding, and does not result in any significant arene oxide metabolite formation (29).

Gabapentin (Neurontin) was initially released in the United States as an adjunctive treatment for partial seizures and secondarily generated tonic-clonic seizures. Gabapentin inhibits dopamine release in the central nervous system. Studies in mice, rats, and rabbits have not linked this AED to developmental toxicity. Gabapentin has little to no protein binding activity and no effect on the cytochrome P-450 system. Last, its metabolism does not result in any significant formation of arene oxide metabolites (29,48).

Lamotrigine (Lamictal) is a phenyltriazine AED. It appears to have efficacy comparable with that of carbamazepine in the monotherapy of partial epilepsy. Teratology testing has been done in mice, rats, and rabbits. No increase in congenital malformations has been noted with fetal exposure to this antiepileptic in any of the species tested. Maternal and fetal toxicity as characterized by delayed ossification and decreased weight was seen at the top doses used in the rodent studies. At three times the estimated human maintenance dose, fetal intrauterine death was increased in rats. Lamotrigine is an inhibitor of dihydrofolate reductase and decreases embryonic folate levels in experimental animals. This raises the concern that human use of lamotrigine may result in developmental toxicity. At present, there is a registry set up by the manufacturer (GlaxoWellcome, Research Triangle Park, NC) to evaluate this possibility. A preliminary report from this registry indicates a 6% congenital malformation rate in fetuses exposed to this drug, which is not a clear increase in malformations. However, there have not been sufficient numbers of fetal exposures to draw any definite conclusions from the data (6). Last, lamotrigine is not protein bound, has no effect on the cytochrome P-450 system, and does not appear to result in significant accumulations of arene oxide metabolites (27,49; Eldridge, unpublished).

Many patients are presenting to prenatal clinics already using the newer AEDs. We routinely counsel patients that, at present, there is no evidence of teratogenicity but little information is available. Several authors have suggested avoiding the newer AEDs until evidence of safety has accumulated (6,47).

PRECONCEPTION AND POSTNATAL ISSUES

It would be prudent to attempt to provide preconception counseling to all epileptic women. They should be informed of the association between AEDs in general and their specific AED regimen with malformations. The patient should be aware of the controversy surrounding whether the disease itself contributes to malformations or other adverse outcomes. The patient should be offered ultrasonography to detect evidence of fetal malformations or growth restriction and serum screening to assist in detecting neural tube defects. Individual practitioners must decide on the appropriateness of offering amniocentesis to ascertain amniotic fluid α-fetoprotein. The patient

should understand the potential deleterious effects of tonic-clonic seizures during gestation. Folate supplementation can be considered. If no seizures have occurred in 2 years, stopping the AED or attempting to convert from polytherapy to monotherapy can be considered (3).

Postnatally, the issues include breast-feeding and neonatal bleeding. It is usually safe to breast-feed and take AEDs. Generally, AEDs cross into breast milk in an inverse proportion to protein binding (12). Although breast-feeding is certainly not contraindicated, epileptic women tend to breast-feed less than the general population (11). Given interference with vitamin K, diligence should be used in confirming neonatal administration of supplemental vitamin K (3,18). Although sometimes considered, maternal vitamin K supplementation has not been proven to be effective in reducing neonatal hemorrhagic complications (1).

REFERENCES

1. *ACOG Educ Bull* 1996;231:1–7.
2. Brodie MJ, French JA. Management of epilepsy in adolescents and adults. *Lancet* 2000;356:323–329.
3. Rochester JA, Kirchner JT. Epilepsy in pregnancy. *Am Fam Physician* 1997;56:1631–1636, 1638.
4. Swartjes JM, van Geijn HP. Pregnancy and epilepsy. *Eur J Obstet Gynecol Reprod Biol* 1998;79:3–11.
5. The North American Pregnancy and Epilepsy Registry. A North American Registry for Epilepsy and Pregnancy, a unique public/private partnership of health surveillance. *Epilepsia* 1998;39:793–798.
6. Nulman I, Laslo D, Koren G. Treatment of epilepsy in pregnancy. *Drugs* 1999;57:535–544.
7. Eller PE, Patterson CA, Webb GW. Maternal and fetal implications of anticonvulsant therapy during pregnancy. *Obstet Gynecol Clin North Am* 1997;24:523–532.
8. Brodie MJ, Dichter MA. Antiepileptic drugs. *N Engl J Med* 1996;334:168–174.
9. Yerby MS, Devinsky O. Epilepsy and pregnancy. In: Devinsky O, Feldman E, Hainline B, eds. *Neurologic complications of pregnancy*. New York: Raven Press, 1994.
10. Malone FD, D'Alton ME. Drugs in pregnancy: anticonvulsants. *Semin Perinatol* 1997;21:114–123.
11. Zahn C. Neurologic care of pregnant women with epilepsy. *Epilepsia* 1998;39[Suppl 8]:526–531.
12. Morrell MJ. Guidelines for the care of women with epilepsy. *Neurology* 1998;51[Suppl 4]:S21–S27.
13. Knight AH, Rhind EG. Epilepsy and pregnancy: a study of 153 pregnancies in 59 patients. *Epilepsia* 1975;16:99–110.
14. Tanganelli P, Regesta G. Epilepsy, pregnancy, and major birth anomalies: an Italian prospective, controlled study. *Neurology* 1992;42:89–93.

15. Sabers A, a'Rogvi-Hansen B, Dam M, et al. Pregnancy and epilepsy: a retrospective study of 151 pregnancies. *Acta Neurol Scand* 1998;97:164–170.

16. Morrell MJ. Epilepsy in women: the science of why it is special. *Neurology* 1999;53[Suppl 1]:S42–S48.

17. Pedley TA. The epilepsies. In: Bennett JC, Plum F, eds. *Cecil textbook of medicine.* Philadelphia: WB Saunders, 1996.

18. El-Sayed YY. Obstetric and gynecologic care of women with epilepsy. *Epilepsia* 1998;39[suppl 8]:517–525.

19. Yerby SY. Pregnancy, teratogenesis, and epilepsy. *Pediatr Neurogenet* 1994;12:749–765.

20. Shuster EA. Seizures in pregnancy. *Emerg Clin North Am* 1994;12:1013–1025.

21. Holmes LB, Rosenberger PB, Harvey EA, et al. Intelligence and physical features of children of women with epilepsy. *Teratology* 2000;61:196–202.

22. Lindhout D, Omizigt JGC. Teratogenic effects of antiepileptic drugs: implications for the management of epilepsy in women of childbearing age. *Epilepsia* 1994;35[Suppl 4]:S19–S28.

23. Holmes LB, Harvey EA, Brown KS, et al. Anticonvulsant teratogenesis: I. A study design for newborn infants. *Teratology* 1994;49:202–207.

24. Waters CH, Belai Y, Gott PS, et al. Outcomes of pregnancy associated with antiepileptic drugs. *Arch Neurol* 1994;51:250–253.

25. Nakane Y, Okuma T, Takahashi R, et al. Multi-institutional study on the teratogenicity and fetal toxicity of antiepileptic drugs: a report of a collaborative study group in Japan. *Epilepsia* 1980;21:663–680.

26. Koch S, Titze K, Zimmermann RB, et al. Long-term neuropsychological consequences of maternal epilepsy and anticonvulsant treatment during pregnancy for school-age children and adolescents. *Epilepsia* 1999:40:1237–1243.

27. Delgado-Escueta AV, Janz D. Consensus guidelines: preconceptional counseling, management, and care of the pregnant woman with epilepsy. *Neurology* 1992;42 [Suppl 5]:149–160.

28. Buehler BA, Delimont D, van Waes M, et al. Prenatal prediction of risk of the fetal hydantoin syndrome. *N Engl J Med* 1990;322:1567–1572.

29. Morrell MJ. The new antiepileptic drugs and women: efficacy, reproductive health, pregnancy and fetal outcome. *Epilepsia* 1996;37[Suppl 6]:S34–S44.

30. German J, Kowal A, Ehlers KH. Trimethadione in human teratogenesis. *Teratol* 1970;3:349–362.

31. Hanson JW, Smith DW. The fetal hydantoin syndrome. *J Pediatr* 1975;87:285–290.

32. Committee on Drugs. American Academy of Pediatrics. The transfer of drugs and other chemicals into human milk. *Pediatrics* 1994;93:137–150.

33. Levy RH, Yerby MS. Effects of pregnancy on antiepileptic drug utilization. *Epilepsia* 1985;26[Suppl 1]:S52–S57.

34. Jones KL, Lacro RV, Johnson KA, et al. Patterns of malformations in the children of women treated with carbamazepine during pregnancy. *N Engl J Med* 1989; 320:1661–1666.

35. Rosa FW. Spina bifida in infants of women treated with carbamazepine during pregnancy. *N Engl J Med* 1991;324:674–677.

36. The WHO Working Group on Human Lactation. In: Bennet PN, ed. *Drugs and human lactation.* Amsterdam: Elsevier, 1988:335–340.

37. Dalessio DJ. Current concepts: seizure disorders and pregnancy. *N Engl J Med* 1988;312:559–563.

38. Battino D, Binelli S, Bossi L, et al. Changes in primidone/phenobarbital ratio during pregnancy and the puerperium. *Clin Pharmacokinet* 1984;9:252–260.

39. Schardein JL. *Chemically induced birth defects.* New York: Marcel Dekker, 1985.

40. Krauss CM, Holmes LB, Van Lang Q, et al. Four siblings with similar malformations after exposure to phenytoin and primidone. *J Pediatr* 1984;105:750–755.

41. Myhree SA, William R. Teratogenic effects associated with maternal primidone therapy. *J Pediatr* 1981;99:160–162.

42. Rudd NL, Freedom RM. A possible primidone embryopathy. *J Pediatr* 1979;94:835–837.

43. Kristjansson K, Flannery DB, et al. Possible dose response in primidone teratogenicity. *Clin Res* 1988;36:59A.

44. Hoyme HE, et al. Fetal primidone effects. *Teratology* 1986;33:76C.

45. Nau H, Rating D, Hauser I, et al. Placental transfer and pharmacokinetics of primidone and its metabolites phenobarbital, PEMA, and hydroxyphenobarbital in neonates and infants of epileptic mothers. *Eur J Clin Pharmacol* 1980;18:31–42.

46. Kuhnz W, Koch S, Ehelge H, et al. Primidone and phenobarbital during the lactation period in epileptic women: total and free drug serum levels in the nursed infants and their effects on neonatal behavior. *Dev Pharmacol Ther* 1988;11:147–154.

47. Morrell MJ. The new antiepileptic drugs and women: efficacy, reproductive health, pregnancy, and fetal outcome. *Epilepsia* 1996;37[Suppl 6]:S34–S44.

48. Petrere JA, Anderson JA. Developmental toxicity studies in mice, rats and rabbits with the anticonvulsant gabapentin. *Fundam Appl Toxicol* 1994;23:588–589.

49. Eldridge RR. Three prospective registries to monitor prenatal maternal exposures: the acyclovir in pregnancy, the antiretroviral in pregnancy and the lamotrigine in pregnancy registries. *Reprod Toxicol* 1993;7:637.

21

Headaches, Pregnancy, and Lactation

Stephen D. Silberstein

Department of Medicine, Thomas Jefferson University, Philadelphia, Pennsylvania

The International Headache Society (IHS) divides headaches into two broad categories: primary and secondary headache disorders. Secondary headaches are symptoms of another disease and can be caused by intracranial or extracranial structural abnormalities or by systemic or metabolic conditions. In primary headache disorders, the headache itself is the illness (Table 21.1). The primary headache disorders include migraine, tension-type headache (TTH), and cluster headache. Chronic daily headache (CDH), a term in common use but not recognized by the IHS, may be due to chronic TTH, prolonged or transformed migraine, or hemicrania continua and is often associated with abortive medication overuse (1).

Headache prevalence is age dependent. Migraine prevalence peaks near age 40 and declines thereafter. With aging, not only is there a change in prevalence of the primary headache disorder, but a shift to new or organic causes of headache may occur (2).

The first step in establishing a diagnosis is a complete history that should include the patient's age at headache onset; the location, severity, and type of pain; the attack frequency (including any change in frequency); associated symptoms; precipitating and relieving factors; the patient's sleep habits; and the family history. A complete medication history should be taken to evaluate the doses, duration of use, and effectiveness of previous headache medications, as well as to determine whether any medications that could exacerbate headaches are being used or overused (3). This will not only serve as a baseline but will help with preconception counseling.

Migraine and TTH are primary headache disorders whose diagnosis is primarily clinical, with normal physical and neurologic examinations and a history that satisfies the IHS criteria (1). However, conditions that mimic migraine may also occur during pregnancy (4). New-onset migraine with aura can be due to a symptomatic disorder such as vasculitis, brain tumor, or occipital arteriovenous malformation (AVM) (5). Some disorders that produce headache, such as stroke, cerebral venous thrombosis, eclampsia, and subarachnoid hemorrhage (SAH), occur more frequently during pregnancy. Sinusitis, meningitis, and idiopathic intracranial hypertension can present as intractable headache (5). SAH can present as a severe bout of acute-onset headache. These symptomatic conditions require neuroimaging and/or a lumbar puncture to diagnose them. Some disorders are more common or occur exclusively during pregnancy and produce headache. These include stroke, cerebral venous thrombosis, eclampsia, SAH, pituitary tumor, and choriocarcinoma (6,7). Idiopathic intracranial hypertension does not occur more commonly during pregnancy.

Investigation of headache, and migraine in particular, is controversial and few guidelines exist. In fact, in a typical healthy migraineur, laboratory tests may not be necessary for diagnosis; some, however, are usually recommended before treatment. Even less is known about the need to investigate other types of headache. Systemic secondary causes of headache often cannot be diagnosed by physical examination; therefore, laboratory studies are performed to rule them out (5).

TABLE 21.1. *IHS classification*

Primary disorders
  Migraine
  Tension-type headache
  Cluster headache and chronic paroxysmal
    hemicrania
  Miscellaneous headaches unassociated with
    structural lesion
Secondary disorders
  Headache associated with head trauma
  Headache associated with vascular disorders
  Headache associated with nonvascular intracranial
    disorder
  Headache associated with substances
    or their withdrawal
  Headache associated with noncephalic infection
  Headache associated with metabolic disorder
  Headache or facial pain associated with disorder
    of cranium, neck, eyes, ears, nose, sinuses, teeth,
    mouth, or other facial or cranial structures
  Cranial neuralgias, nerve trunk pain,
    and deafferentation pain

TABLE 21.2. *Guidelines for neuroimaging the patient who is or may be pregnant*

Determine the necessity and the potential risks
  of the procedure.
Pick the procedure with the highest accuracy
  balanced by the lowest radiation.
Use magnetic resonance imaging, if possible.
Avoid direct exposure to the abdomen and pelvis.
Do not avoid radiologic testing purely for the sake
  of the pregnancy.
If significant exposure is incurred by a pregnant
  patient, consult a radiation biologist.
Consent forms are neither required nor recommended.

Adapted from Schwartz RB. Neurodiagnostic Imaging of the Pregnant Patient. In: Devinsky O, Feldmann E, Hainline B, eds. *Neurological Complications of Pregnancy*. New York: Rowen Press, 1994.

Diagnostic testing functions to (i) confirm the diagnosis, (ii) exclude other causes of headache, (iii) rule out comorbid and coexistent diseases that could complicate headache and its treatment, (iv) establish a baseline for and exclude contraindications to drug treatment, and (v) measure drug levels to determine absorption, patient compliance, or medication overuse (8).

LUMBAR PUNCTURE

Lumbar puncture is crucial in four distinct clinical situations: (i) a "first or worst" headache, with the suspicion of an intracranial infection or SAH; (ii) a severe, rapid-onset, recurrent headache; (iii) a progressive headache; and (iv) a chronic intractable or atypical headache disorder (9). If increased intracranial pressure is suspected, lumbar puncture should be performed after neuroimaging, except when meningitis is suspected, in which case it should not be delayed.

NEUROIMAGING

Head computed tomography is relatively safe during pregnancy and is the study of choice for head trauma and possible nontraumatic subarachnoid, subdural, or intraparenchymal hemorrhage. For all other nontraumatic or nonhemorrhagic

craniospinal pathology, magnetic resonance imaging is preferred. Use magnetic resonance angiography first to evaluate any suspected vascular pathology, but, when necessary, angiography is reasonably safe in the pregnant patient (Table 21.2).

Indications for computed tomography or magnetic resonance imaging in headache investigation during pregnancy include the first or worst headache of the patient's life, particularly if it is of abrupt onset (thunderclap headache); a change in the frequency, severity, or clinical features of the headache attack; an abnormal neurologic examination; a progressive or new daily persistent headache; neurologic symptoms that do not meet the criteria of migraine with typical aura; persistent neurologic defects; definite electroencephalographic evidence of a focal cerebral lesion; an orbital or skull bruit suggestive of AVM; and new comorbid partial (focal) seizures (5).

MIGRAINE

Migraine is an episodic headache disorder that may be preceded by a prodrome and initiated by an aura. In the past, migraine headaches were known as either classic migraine or common migraine, based on the presence or absence of an aura (4). Common migraine is now called migraine without aura. Classic migraine is now called migraine with aura. Migraine with or without aura may be associated with premonitory phenomena that develop hours to days before the headache attack. Examples include hyper- or hypoactivity, depression, irritability, difficulty concentrating, or food cravings, especially for chocolate (4).

Prevalence

Migraine occurs in 4% of children, 6% of men, and 18% of women. Sixty-two percent of migraineurs also have TTH (10). Migraine usually begins in the first three decades of life, and prevalence peaks in the fifth decade (10). The prognosis for migraine sufferers is good because migraine prevalence decreases with increasing age (11). Migraine in women is influenced by hormonal changes throughout the life cycle: menarche, menstruation, oral contraceptive use, pregnancy, menopause, and hormonal replacement therapy. Migraine can occur for the first time during pregnancy; preexisting migraine may worsen, particularly during the first trimester; or the patient may become headache free in later pregnancy. Some women have no change in their headache during pregnancy (12). The true incidence of migraine in pregnancy is uncertain, and most reported cases have been of migraine with aura or prolonged aura. Migraine prevalence decreases with menopause, although the prevalence does not fall to premenarche levels.

Clinical Features

Migraine diagnosis depends on the characteristics of the pain and associated features. A diagnosis of migraine without aura, according to the IHS criteria (Table 21.3), requires the patient to have at least five headache attacks (1). A diagnosis of migraine with aura (classic migraine) requires the patient to have at least two attacks with at least three characteristics listed in Table 21.4. If the aura lasts longer than 1 hour but less than a week, the condition is called migraine with prolonged aura (1). The migraine aura may occur without the headache, and migraine may remit or become transformed into CDH (with or without medication overuse).

Migraine aura occurs in approximately 20% of migraineurs. It usually develops over 5 to

TABLE 21.3. *Migraine without aura*

Diagnostic criteria
A. At least 5 attacks fulfilling B–D
B. Headache lasting 4–72 hr (untreated or unsuccessfully treated)
C. Headache has at least two of the following characteristics:
  1. Unilateral location
  2. Pulsating quality
  3. Moderate or severe intensity (inhibits or prohibits daily activities)
  4. Aggravation by walking stairs or similar routine physical activity
D. During headache at least one of the following:
  1. Nausea and/or vomiting
  2. Photophobia and phonophobia
E. No evidence of organic disease

Criteria from ref. 1.

20 minutes, lasts 20 to 30 minutes, and consists of focal neurologic symptoms (visual, sensory, motor, or speech) that accompany the headache or occur up to an hour before it begins (13). Visual symptoms are the most common and include scintillations (fluorescent flashes of light in the visual field), fortification spectra or teichopsia (alternating light and dark lines in the visual field), photopsia (flashing lights), positive scotomata (bright geometric lights in the visual field), and negative scotomata (blind spots that may move across the visual field). Sensory symptoms are less common and include numbness, tingling, or paresthesias of the face or hand. Motor symptoms are usually hemiparetic, whereas

TABLE 21.4. *Migraine with aura*

Diagnostic criteria
A. At lest 2 attacks fulfilling B
B. At least 3 of the following 4 characteristics:
  1. One or more fully reversible aura symptoms indicating focal cerebral cortical, brain stem dysfunction, or both
  2. At least one aura symptom develops gradually over more than 4 min or 2 or more symptoms occur in succession
  3. No aura symptom lasts more than 60 min. If more than one aura symptom is present, accepted duration is proportionally increased
  4. Headache follows aura with a free interval of less than 60 min (it may also begin before or simultaneously with the aura)
C. No evidence of organic disease

Criteria from ref. 1.

language disturbances consist of difficulty speaking (aphasia) or understanding (14,15).

The headache of migraine can begin at any time during the day, usually developing gradually and subsiding after 4 to 72 hours (16). A headache lasting longer than 72 hours defines status migrainosus. The pain is moderate to severe in intensity and usually described as throbbing or pulsating. It is usually unilateral, but may begin as, or become, bilateral (16). Unilateral headaches are not of concern because they occur in 20% of migraineurs. Accompanying symptoms are common: most patients are anorectic and have nausea; some vomit or have diarrhea. Photophobia and phonophobia cause patients to seek relief in a dark, quiet room to decrease sensory stimulation. Most patients have one to four attacks a month (15).

After the headache phase, some patients experience a postdrome, or recovery, phase that may last up to 24 hours. Some patients feel tired, others feel alert, some feel depressed, others feel euphoric, some feel worn out, whereas some feel refreshed. Some may complain of poor concentration, food intolerance, or scalp tenderness (13).

TENSION-TYPE HEADACHE

TTH is the most common headache type, with a lifetime prevalence of 69% in men and 88% in women. TTH can begin at any age, but onset during adolescence or young adulthood is most common. The IHS criteria for TTH are listed in Table 21.5. The headache may be shorter or longer in duration than migraine. TTH is mild or moderate in intensity and has no accompanying autonomic symptoms. The cause of this common disorder is unknown, but it is not related to muscular tension (in fact, patients with migraine have more muscle tension than patients with TTH).

Acute TTH often responds to nonpharmacologic treatment. If the headache does not respond to this approach and medication is needed, many patients self-medicate with over-the-counter analgesics (aspirin, acetaminophen, ibuprofen, naproxen), with or without caffeine. Combination analgesics contain sedatives or caf-

TABLE 21.5. *Tension-type headache (IHS)*

Episodic tension-type headache
  Diagnostic criteria
  A. At least 10 previous headache episodes
    fulfilling criteria B–D listed below. Number
    of days with such headache <180/yr (<15/mo)
  B. Headache lasting from 30 min to 7 d
  C. At least 2 of the following pain characteristics:
    1. Pressing/tightening (nonpulsating) quality
    2. Mild or moderate intensity (may inhibit, but
      does not prohibit activities)
    3. Bilateral location
    4. No aggravation by walking stairs or similar
      routine physical activity
  D. Both of the following:
    1. No nausea or vomiting (anorexia may occur)
    2. Photophobia and phonophobia are absent,
      or one but not the other is present
Chronic tension-type headache
  Diagnostic criteria
  A. Average headache frequency >15 days/mo
    (180 d/yr) for >6 mo fulfilling criteria B–D
  B. At least 2 of the following pain characteristics:
    1. Pressing/tightening quality
    2. Mild or moderate severity (may inhibit but
      does not prohibit activities)
    3. Bilateral location
    4. No aggravation by walking stairs or similar
      routine physical activity
  C. Both of the following:
    1. No vomiting
    2. No more than one of the following: nausea,
      photophobia, or phonophobia

Criteria from ref. 1.

feine, and their use should be limited, as overuse may cause dependence. Narcotic analgesics and benzodiazepines should be avoided because of their abuse potential. Overusing symptomatic medications, including tranquilizers and analgesics, can cause episodic TTH to convert to chronic TTH (17). In women who are attempting to become or who are pregnant, the drugs should be used with the precautions outlined in the treatment section later in the chapter.

CHRONIC DAILY HEADACHE

CDH (Table 21.6) may be due to chronic TTH (Table 21.5) or transformed migraine and is often associated with abortive medication overuse. It is important to determine the cause of the CDH so that the appropriate treatment can be chosen. When concurrent depression and medication dependence accompany CDH, treatment is difficult

TABLE 21.6. *Chronic daily headache*

Primary
  Headache duration >4 hr
    Transformed migraine
    Chronic tension-type headache
    New daily persistent headache
    Hemicrania continua
  Headache duration <4 hr
    Cluster headache
    Chronic paroxysmal hemicrania
    Hypnic headache
    Idiopathic stabbing headache
Secondary
  Posttraumatic headache
    Cervical spine disorders
    Headache associated with vascular disorders
    [arteriovenous malformation, arteritis (including
    giant cell arteritis), dissection, subdural
    hematoma]
    Headache associated with nonvascular
    intracranial disorders [intracranial hypertension,
    infection (EBV, HIV), neoplasm]
    Other (temporomandibular joint disorder, sinus
    infection)

EBV, Epstein–Barr virus; HIV, human immunovirus.
Criteria from ref. 17.

TABLE 21.7. *Cluster headache*

A. At least 5 attacks fulfilling B–D
B. Severe unilateral orbital, supraorbital,
   and/or temporal pain lasting 15–180 min untreated
C. Headache is associated with at least 1 of the
   following signs that have to be present on the pain
   side:
   1. Conjunctival injection
   2. Lacrimation
   3. Nasal congestion
   4. Rhinorrhea
   5. Forehead and facial sweating
   6. Miosis
   7. Ptosis
   8. Eyelid edema
D. Frequency of attacks: from 1 every other day to 8/d
E. No evidence of organic disease

Criteria from ref. 1.

Episodic cluster features bouts lasting 1 week to a year with remission periods lasting at least 14 days, whereas chronic cluster has either no remission periods or remissions that last less than 14 days. Cluster attacks may begin with slight discomfort that rapidly increases (within 15 minutes) to excruciating pain. The attacks often occur at the same time each day and frequently awaken patients from sleep. Attacks generally last for 30 to 90 minutes but may last as long as 180 minutes and often occur once or twice a day. Patients may say "It's like driving a hot poker in my eye." Tearing occurs in most patients. Patients with cluster headaches should avoid alcohol and nitroglycerin.

and detoxification may be required. This is particularly important in women who want to become pregnant. Under these circumstances, both the amounts and the types of medicine used must be limited. Refractory rebound headaches may occur when aspirin, acetaminophen, or opiate-containing analgesics are overused or when analgesics or triptans are taken more frequently than 3 days per week or ergotamine tartrate more often than 2 days per week. To avoid this situation, headache medication must be used within defined limits (17).

PREGNANCY AND MIGRAINE

Mechanisms

The relationship between migraine and sex hormones is well-known. Menarche, menstruation, oral contraceptive use, pregnancy, menopause, and hormonal replacement therapy affect migraine, in part by changing a woman's estrogen levels. Estrogen levels do not differ in nonpregnant women with or without menstrual migraine. Rising or sustained high estrogen levels have been proposed as the mechanism of migraine relief that often occurs during pregnancy; this mechanism, however, cannot explain the worsening or new appearance of migraine that sometimes occurs (19). The rapid fall of estrogen

CLUSTER HEADACHE

Cluster headache prevalence is lower than that of migraine or TTH, with a rate of 0.01% to 0.24% in various populations. In contrast to migraine, prevalence is higher in men (70% to 90%) than in women (Table 21.7). Cluster headache can begin at any age: it most commonly begins in the late 20s, rarely in childhood, and occasionally (10%) in patients in their 60s (2,18). The prognosis of cluster headaches is guarded; it is a chronic headache disorder that may last for the patient's entire life.

levels may be responsible for menstrual and postpartum migraine. Women with a history of migraine are more likely to develop postpartum migraine (20).

Migraine relief during pregnancy is not dependent on adequate "protective" levels of progesterone. No statistical differences in progesterone levels, measured near term, are found between women who did not have migraine relief during pregnancy and those who did, suggesting that migraine relief does not depend on the absolute blood level of progesterone (21).

The key to the genesis of migraine may be the intrinsic estrogen receptor sensitivity of the hypothalamic neurons. In most women, rising or sustained estrogen levels decrease headache. In some women, these same changes could induce headache (22).

Course of Migraine During Pregnancy

Approximately 60% to 70% of migraineurs will improve during pregnancy, whereas some women who have not had migraine will experience their first migraine headache (Table 21.8). Case reports of migraine that occur for the first time during pregnancy emphasize the presence of focal neurologic symptoms (migraine with aura), probably because patients with these dramatic presentations are more likely to be referred to a neurologist. Wright and Patel (23) presented a series of 10 women with headache and focal neurologic symptoms (visual or sensory aura,

dysphasia, weakness, or a combination of these symptoms): two presented in the first trimester, six in the third trimester, and two postpartum. Seven had a history of migraine before pregnancy and four had migraine with aura. Massey (24) reported a 19-year-old woman who, in her 27th week of pregnancy, developed two episodes (24 hours apart) of anomia; blurred vision; and right arm, face, and mouth numbness, followed by a pounding bifrontal headache with photophobia. The patient had no history of headache but did have a positive family history of migraine.

Chancellor and Wroe (19) presented a series of nine women who developed migraine for the first time while pregnant. One woman had migraine without aura and eight had migraine with aura. Two women developed migraine in the first trimester of pregnancy, two in the second trimester, and five in the third. These women were referred for neurologic consultation because of focal neurologic symptoms.

Uknis and Silberstein (12) reported a 27-year-old woman with no family or personal history of migraine who presented with a headache associated with unilateral paresthesias and blurred vision. This was her first attack of migraine with aura and led to the diagnosis of her pregnancy.

Most women with migraine improve during pregnancy. Some women have their first attack during pregnancy. Migraine often recurs postpartum and can begin for the first time in general. Despite drug use, migraineurs do not differ from

TABLE 21.8. *Migraine and pregnancy*

	Lance & Anthony (25)	Callaghan (26)	Somerville (21)	Ratinahirana et al. (28)	Granella et al. (29)	Rasmussen (30)	Chen & Leviton (31)	Maggioni et al. (33)
Women studied		200	200	703	1300	975	55,000	428
History of migraine and pregnancies	120	41	38	116	943	80	484	80
No. of pregnancies	252	200	200	147	943	—	484	?
New migraine during pregnancy	0	33/41 (80%)	7/38 (18%)	16/147 (11%)	12 (1.3%)	?	0	1/428
New migraine postpartum	—	—	—	?	42 (4.5%)	?	0	?
Prior migraine	252	8	31	131	571	80	484	91
Prior migraine improved	145/252 (58%)	4 (50%)	24/31 (77%)	102/131 (78%)	384/571 (67.3%)	48%	382/484 (79%)	80%
Prior migraine unchanged or worsened	107/252 (42%)	3 (38%)	7/31 (23%)	29/131 (22%)	187/571 (32.7%)	52%	102/484 (21%)	20%
Type series	R, H	R, H	R, H	R, O	R, H	R, POP	P, O	R, H

H, headache or neurologic; P, prospective; R, retrospective; POP, population base; ?, not available.

TABLE 21.9. *Menstrual migraine and migraine improvement with pregnancy*

	Lance (25)	Ratinahirana et al. (28)
Menstrual		
Disappeared or improved	64%	86%
Worsened	36%	7%
Nonmenstrual		
Disappeared or improved	48%	60%
Worsened	52%	15%

nonmigraineurs in miscarriages, toxemia, congenital anomalies, or stillbirths.

Several series are available (Table 21.8) that evaluate the behavior of migraine in pregnancy (25–33). Two of the studies (25,28) specifically evaluate whether there are differences in how those with menstrual migraine behave during pregnancy versus those with nonmenstrual migraine (Table 21.9).

In addition to the above studies, Scharff et al. (32) recruited 30 women who were more than 10 weeks pregnant. They reported a nonsignificant decrease in all headache types including migraine and TTH, more so for the primiparous women. Marcus et al. (34) recruited 49 women who were no more than 16 weeks pregnant. Headache that was reported at the end of the first trimester was likely to continue during pregnancy and not worsen postpartum. There was a nonsignificant trend toward improvement in women with migraine.

Outcome of Pregnancy in Migraineurs

Wainscott and Volans (35) found that the incidence of miscarriage, toxemia, congenital anomalies, and stillbirth was not increased in a sample of 777 migraine sufferers compared with the national averages or controls. In Chancellor's small series (19), four of nine patients developed complications, including preeclampsia in two. Again, this may be due to selection artifact.

Postpartum Migraine

Stein (20) prospectively followed 71 randomly selected women during their first postpartum week. Postnatal headache (PNH) occurred in 39%. It was most frequent on days 3 to 6 postpartum and was associated with a history or a family history of migraine. PNH, although less severe than the patients' typical migraine, was bifrontal, prolonged, and associated with photophobia, nausea, and anorexia.

MacArthur et al. (36) investigated 11,701 women who gave birth in one hospital in Birmingham between 1978 and 1985. Follow-up information was obtained using a mailed questionnaire. By 3 months postpartum, newly occurring frequent headache occurred in 3.6% of the women and migraine in 1.4%. The definition of migraine was not stated. Two of the cases of focal neurologic migraine of Wright and Patel (23) presented postpartum. Both had a history of migraine with aura. Migraine frequently restarts in the postpartum period and can begin *de novo*.

HEADACHE TREATMENT

The major concerns in the management of the pregnant patient are the effects of both the medication and the disease on the fetus. Medication use is appropriate during pregnancy (8,37,38). Because migraine usually improves after the first trimester, many women can manage their headaches with this reassurance and nonpharmacologic means of coping, such as ice, massage, and biofeedback (8,37,39,40). Some women, however, will continue to have severe, intractable headaches, sometimes associated with nausea, vomiting, and possible dehydration. Not only are these conditions disruptive to the patient, but they may pose a risk to the fetus that is greater than the potential risk of the medications used to treat the pregnant patient (8,39).

Symptomatic treatment, designed to reduce the severity and duration of symptoms, is used to treat an acute headache attack (Tables 21.10–21.15). Individual attacks should be treated with rest, reassurance, and ice packs. For headaches that do not respond to nonpharmacologic treatment, symptomatic drugs are indicated. The nonsteroidal antiinflammatory drugs (NSAIDs) (in limited doses), acetaminophen (alone or with codeine), codeine alone, or other opioids can be used during pregnancy (41). Aspirin in low

TABLE 21.10. *Ergots and serotonin agonists*

	Fetal risk (from TERIS)	Breast-feeding
Ergots		
Ergotamine	Min	Contraindicated
Dihydroergotamine	U	Contraindicated
Methylergonovine	U	Caution
Methysergide	U	Caution
Triptans		
Sumatriptan	U	Caution
Naratriptan	U	Caution
Rizatriptan	U	Caution
Zolmitriptan	U	Caution

See ref. 63.

TABLE 21.11. *Analgesics*

	Fetal risk (from TERIS)	Breast-feeding
Simple analgesics		
Aspirin	N–Min	Caution
Acetaminophen	N	Compatible
Caffeine	N–Min	Compatible
NSAIDs		
Fenoprofen	U	Compatible
Ibuprofen	N–Min	Compatible
Indomethacin	N	Compatible
Ketorolac	U	Caution
Meclofenamate	U	Compatible
Naproxen	U	Compatible
Sulindac	U	Compatible
Tolmetin	U	Caution

NSAIDs, nonsteroidal antiinflammatory drugs; N–Min, none to minimal; N, none; U, unknown.

TABLE 21.12. *Opioids*

	Fetal risk (from TERIS)	Breast-feeding
Butorphanol	N–Min	Compatible
Codeine	N–Min	Compatible
Hydromorphone	N–Min	Compatible
Meperidine	N–Min	Compatible
Methadone	N–Min	Compatible
Morphine	N–Min	Compatible
Propoxyphene	N–Min	Compatible

N–Min, none to minimal.

TABLE 21.13. *Corticosteroids*

	Fetal risk (from TERIS)	Breast-feeding
Cortisone	N–Min	Compatible
Dexamethasone	N–Min	Compatible
Prednisone	N–Min	Compatible
Triamcinolone	N–Min	Compatible

N–Min, none to minimal.

TABLE 21.14. *Neuroleptics/antiemetics*

	Fetal risk (from TERIS)	Breast-feeding
Other		
Emetrol	U	Compatible
Doxylamine and vitamin B_6	N	NA
Trimethobenzamide	N–Min	NA
Neuroleptics		
Phenothiazines		
Chlorpromazine	N–Min	Concern
Prochlorperazine	N	Compatible
Promethazine	N	NA
Promazine	U	NA
Butyrophenones		
Droperidol	U	Unknown
Haloperidol	N–Min	Concern
Thioxanthenes		
Thiothixene	U	NA
Other		
Metoclopramide	N–Min	Concern

U, unknown; N, none; N–Min, none to minimal; NA, not available.

intermittent doses is not a significant teratogenic risk, although large doses, especially if given near term, may be associated with maternal and fetal bleeding. Aspirin use should probably be reserved unless there is a definite therapeutic need for it (other than headache). In general, NSAIDs may be safely taken for pain during the first trimester of pregnancy. However, their use should be limited during later pregnancy, as some NSAIDs may constrict or close the fetal ductus arteriosus (41). Byron (42) believes

TABLE 21.15. *Sedatives/hypnotics/ antihistamines*

	Fetal risk (from TERIS)	Breast-feeding
Antihistamines		
Cyclizine	U	NA
Cyproheptadine	U	Contraindicated
Dimenhydrinate	U	NA
Meclizine	N–Min	NA
Barbiturates		
Butalbital	N–Min	Caution
Phenobarbital	N–Min	Caution
Benzodiazepines		
Chlordiazepoxide	N–Min	Concern
Clonazepam	U	Concern
Diazepam	N–Min	Concern
Lorazepam	U	Concern
Other		
Zolpidem	U	Not recommended

U, unknown; N–Min, none to minimal; NA, not available.

that the most potent inhibitors of prostaglandin synthesis, such as salicylates and indomethacin, should be avoided throughout pregnancy if possible and certainly during the last trimester. Barbiturate and benzodiazepine use should be limited. Ergotamine, dihydroergotamine, and the triptans (sumatriptan, naratriptan, rizatriptan, and zolmitriptan) should be avoided (8,37,40).

Acute Specific Antimigraine Drugs (Table 21.10)

Ergotamine

Ergotamine (Table 21.10) is an older nonspecific serotonin agonist used for migraine treatment. The use of ergot alkaloids during pregnancy is contraindicated (43,44). The abortifacient action of uterotonic ergots in humans has been known for years, but the teratogenic effects of ergotamine and dihydroergotamine are less certain. Attempted (but failed) abortion has rarely been associated with some congenital defects. The Collaborative Perinatal Project (45) reported on 25 exposures to ergotamine and 32 exposures to other ergot derivatives, with the relative risk of malformation being one per 24 and one per 45, respectively. Six case reports have described adverse fetal outcomes attributable to ergotamine (45–52) including multiple congenital anomalies. In the Hungarian Case-Control Surveillance of Congenital Anomalies, 1980 to 1986 (53), among controls (normal infants, but including those with Down's syndrome), 0.11% (18 of 16,477) had used ergotamine during pregnancy, whereas 0.14% (13 of 9,460) of pregnancies with a birth defect had been exposed to the drug (difference not significant). Four of the index cases, however, involved neural tube defects compared with none of the controls ($p < 0.01$), a finding that prompted the author to state that further study was required (46).

The accidental use at 38 weeks of gestation of a rectal suppository containing ergotamine (2 mg) and caffeine (100 mg) in a woman with nonproteinuric hypertension produced sudden fetal distress that led to an emergency cesarean section (54). Because many of the reports of adverse outcomes after the use of the drug during pregnancy are consistent with vascular injury

and because ergotamine toxicity is known to cause vasospasm, the author recommended that the drug should be avoided during pregnancy (55).

In summary, small, infrequent doses of ergotamine do not appear to be fetotoxic or teratogenic, but idiosyncratic responses may occur that endanger the fetus. Larger doses or frequent use, however, may cause fetal toxicity or teratogenicity that is probably caused by maternal or fetal vascular disruption (46).

Breast-feeding

A 1934 study reported that 90% of nursing infants of mothers using an ergot preparation for migraine therapy had symptoms of ergotism (56). Ergotamine is a member of the same chemical family as bromocriptine, an agent that is used to suppress lactation. Although no specific information has been located relating to the effects of ergotamine on lactation, ergot alkaloids may hinder lactation by inhibiting maternal pituitary prolactin secretion (57). Ergot alkaloids can enter breast milk and have been reported to cause vomiting, diarrhea, and convulsions in nursing infants.

Specific Serotonin Receptor Agonists

Sumatriptan

Sumatriptan (Table 21.10) is a selective serotonin subtype receptor agonist that is safe and effective in the treatment of the nonpregnant migraineur. It is available in injection, nasal spray, and tablet formulations. There is no evidence that sumatriptan is a human teratogen, but no adequate, well-controlled studies have been done in pregnant women.

An interim report of the Sumatriptan Pregnancy Registry by GlaxoWellcome, covering the period of January 1, 1996, through April 30, 1998, reported 245 prospective reports of prenatal exposure to sumatriptan. The outcomes of 27 pregnancies were still pending and 11 were lost to follow-up. Among the remaining 208 outcomes (207 pregnancies, one set of twins), 193 had their earliest exposure to sumatriptan during the first trimester, 11 had their earliest exposure during the second trimester, and one occurred during the third trimester. The number of congenital malformations reported prospectively with first-trimester exposure to sumatriptan (3.0%; 95% confidence interval, 1.1%, 7.1%) did not appear to be different from those in a nonexposed population. Moreover, there was no consistent pattern among the reported defects to suggest a common cause.

Shuhaiber et al. (58) conducted a controlled prospective cohort study to determine the fetal safety of sumatriptan exposure. The study cohort consisted of pregnant women who used sumatriptan during pregnancy and who voluntarily contacted a teratogen information service. Two control groups were used: disease-matched controls (pregnant women contacting Motherisk who had migraine headache and used other drugs such as acetaminophen, NSAIDs, and narcotic analgesics) and nonteratogen controls (pregnant women who contacted Motherisk requesting counseling about medications known to be safe in the human fetus).

A total of 96 women who were exposed to sumatriptan during pregnancy were prospectively followed up. Ninety-five pregnant women were exposed during the first trimester, of whom 12 were also exposed during the second trimester, and six were also exposed during the third trimester. The incidence of major birth defects did not differ among the groups (relative risk, 1.05 in the study versus disease-matched groups; relative risk, 1.06 in the study versus the nonexposed groups).

Although these data are reassuring, the number of exposed pregnancies is still too limited to assess with confidence the safety of the agent (46).

Sumatriptan is excreted in breast milk. The mean weight-adjusted dose (i.e., μg sumatriptan/kg of infant body weight as a percentage of mother's dose in μg/kg) for infants is approximately 3.5%. The risk to a nursing infant from this exposure is not significant. In adults, the mean oral bioavailability of sumatriptan is 14% to 15%, indicating that absorption from the gastrointestinal tract is inhibited. Although the oral absorption in infants may be markedly different from adults, the amount of sumatriptan reaching the systemic circulation of a breast-feeding infant is probably negligible. Discarding the milk

for 8 hours after a dose, an interval during which approximately 88% of the amount excreted into milk can be recovered, would reduce even more the small amounts present in milk. Sumatriptan can be used with this precaution in nursing women.

Naratriptan

Naratriptan is a new selective serotonin receptor agonist that is safe and effective in the acute treatment of migraine.

Through April 30, 1998, 10 women exposed to naratriptan during pregnancy were registered prospectively in the GlaxoWellcome pregnancy registry. Of these 10, three are pending delivery. All the remaining seven pregnancies reported the livebirth of an infant without birth defects (GlaxoWellcome Sumatriptan and Naratriptan Pregnancy Registry, January 1, 1996 to April 30, 1998). This sample is of insufficient size for reaching definitive conclusions regarding the possible teratogenic risk of naratriptan.

Naratriptan-related material is excreted in the milk of rats. Therefore, caution should be exercised when considering giving naratriptan tablets to a nursing woman.

Zolmitriptan

Zolmitriptan is another of the new serotonin receptor agonists that is safe and effective in the treatment of migraine.

There are no adequate and well-controlled studies in pregnant women; therefore, zolmitriptan should be used during pregnancy only if the potential benefit justifies the potential risk to the fetus.

It is not known whether zolmitriptan is excreted in human milk. Because many drugs are excreted in human milk, caution should be exercised when zolmitriptan is administered to a nursing woman.

Rizatriptan

Rizatriptan is another new serotonin agonist that is safe and effective in the treatment of migraine.

There are no adequate and well-controlled studies in pregnant women.

It is not known whether this drug is excreted in human milk. Because many drugs are excreted in human milk, caution should be exercised when rizatriptan is administered to women who are breast-feeding.

ASSOCIATED SYMPTOMS

The associated symptoms of migraine, such as nausea and vomiting, can be as disabling as the headache pain itself. In addition, some medications that are used to treat migraine can produce nausea. Metoclopramide, which decreases the gastric atony seen with migraine and enhances the absorption of coadministered medications, is extremely useful in migraine treatment (8). Mild nausea can be treated with phosphorylated carbohydrate solution (Emetrol) or doxylamine succinate and vitamin B$_6$ (pyridoxine) (8,41). More severe nausea may require the use of injections or suppositories. Trimethobenzamide, chlorpromazine, prochlorperazine, and promethazine are available orally, parenterally, and as a suppository and can all be used safely. We frequently use promethazine and prochlorperazine suppositories. Corticosteroids can be utilized occasionally. Some use prednisone in preference to dexamethasone (which crosses the placenta more readily). Domperidone is an antiemetic used outside the United States. In the United Kingdom (59), its use is not advised during pregnancy because of variable embryotoxic effects in animal tests. In France, on the contrary, the product summary indicates no teratogenicity in animals or humans. Minimal amounts are transferred in breast milk.

Severe acute attacks of migraine should be treated aggressively (37,60). We start intravenous fluids for hydration and then use 10 mg intravenous prochlorperazine to control both nausea and head pain. Intravenous opioids or intravenous corticosteroids can supplement this. This is an extremely effective way of handling status migrainosus during pregnancy.

PREVENTIVE TREATMENT

Increased frequency and severity of migraine associated with nausea and vomiting may justify the use of daily prophylactic (preventive) medication. This treatment option should be a last resort and used only with the consent of the patient and her partner after the risks have been completely explained. Preventive therapy is designed to reduce the frequency and severity of headache attacks. Consider prophylaxis when patients experience at least three or four prolonged, severe attacks per month that are particularly incapacitating or unresponsive to symptomatic therapy and may result in dehydration and fetal distress (40). β-Adrenergic blockers such as propranolol have been used under these circumstances, although adverse effects, including intrauterine growth retardation, have been reported (8,41). If the migraine is so severe that drug treatment is essential, the patient should be told of the risks posed by all the drugs that are used (Tables 21.16–21.20) (8,40). If the patient has

TABLE 21.16. *Anticonvulsants*

	Fetal risk (from TERIS)	Breast-feeding
Carbamazepine	S	Compatible
Gabapentin	U	Uncertain
Lamotrigine	U	Not recommended
Phenobarbital	M–S	Compatible
Phenytoin	S–Mod	Compatible
Primidone	S–Mod	Caution
Topiramate	U	Uncertain
Valproic Acid	S–Mod	Compatible
Vigabatrin	U	Uncertain

S, slight; U, unknown; M–S, minimum to small; S–Mod, slight to moderate.

TABLE 21.17. *Antidepressants*

	Fetal risk (from TERIS)	Breast-feeding
Tricyclics		
Amitriptyline	N–Min	Concern
Amoxapine	U	Concern
Desipramine	U	Concern
Doxepin	U	Concern
Imipramine	N–Min	Concern
Nortriptyline	U	Concern
Protriptyline	U	Concern
SSRIs		
Fluoxetine	N	Caution
Paroxetine	U	Concern?
Sertraline	U	Concern?
MAOIs		
Phenelzine	U	Concern
Others		
Bupropion	U	Concern

N–Min, none to minimal; U, unknown; N, none; SSRIs, specific serotonin reuptake inhibitors.

TABLE 21.18. *Antihypertensives*

	Fetal risk (from TERIS)	Breast-feeding
Beta blockers		
Atenolol	U	Caution
Metoprolol	U	Compatible
Nadolol	U	Compatible
Propranolol	U	Compatible
Timolol	U	Compatible
Adrenergic blockers		
Clonidine	U	Compatible
Calcium channel blockers		
Diltiazem	U	Compatible
Nifedipine	U	Compatible
Nimodipine	U	Uncertain
Verapamil	U	Compatible

U, unknown.

a coexistent illness that requires treatment, one drug should be chosen that will treat both disorders. For example, propranolol (41) can be used to treat hypertension and migraine, and fluoxetine can be used to treat comorbid depression.

DRUG EXPOSURE

If a woman inadvertently takes a drug while she is pregnant or becomes pregnant while taking a drug, determine the dose, timing, and duration of the exposure(s). Ascertain the patient's past and present state of health and the presence of mental retardation or chromosomal abnormalities in the family. Using a reliable source of information (such as TERIS), determine whether the drug is a known teratogen (although for many drugs this is not possible) (46,61–63).

If the drug is teratogenic or the risk is unknown, confirm the gestational age by ultrasonography. If the exposure occurred during

TABLE 21.19. *Other drugs*

	Fetal risk (from TERIS)	Breast-feeding
Diphenoxylate	U	Compatible
Lidocaine	None[a]	NA
Lithium	Small	Contraindicated
Paregoric	U	Compatible

[a]As local anesthetic.
U, unknown; NA, not available.

TABLE 21.20. *Drugs and breast-feeding*

Contraindicated
Require temporary cessation of breast-feeding
Effects unknown but may be of concern
Use with caution
Usually compatible

embryogenesis, then high-resolution ultrasonography can be performed to determine whether damage to specific organ systems or structures has occurred. If the high-resolution ultrasonography is normal, it is reasonable to reassure the patient that the gross fetal structure is normal (within the 90% sensitivity of the study) (46). However, fetal ultrasonography cannot exclude minor anomalies or guarantee the birth of a normal child. Delays in achieving developmental milestones, including cognitive development, are potential risks that cannot be predicted or diagnosed prenatally. Discuss the results of these studies with the mother and the significant other; formal prenatal counseling may be helpful in uncertain cases (46).

BREAST-FEEDING

Milk is a suspension of fat and protein in a carbohydrate–mineral solution. A nursing mother secretes 600 mL of milk per day that contains sufficient protein, fat, and carbohydrate to meet the nutritional demands of the growing and developing infant (46). The transport of a drug into breast milk depends on its lipid solubility, molecular weight, degree of ionization, protein binding, and the presence or absence of active secretion (64). Species differences in the composition of milk can result in differences in drug transfer. Because human milk (pH usually more than 7.0) has a much higher pH than cow's milk (pH usually <6.8), bovine drug transfer data may not be accurate in humans (46).

Many drugs can be detected in breast milk at levels that are not clinically significant to the infant. The concentration of drug in breast milk is a variable fraction of the maternal blood level. The infant dose is usually 1% to 2% of the maternal dose, which is usually trivial. However, any exposure to a toxic drug or potential allergen may be inappropriate (64).

Drug concentration in breast milk depends on drug characteristics (pKa, lipid solubility, molecular weight, protein binding) and breast milk characteristics (composition and volume). Breast milk is given its unique physicochemical properties by the active transport of electrolytes and the formation and excretion of lactose and proteins by glandular epithelial cells in the breast with passive diffusion of water. The volume produced depends on nutritional factors, the amount of milk removed by the suckling infant, and the increase in mammary blood flow that occurs with breast-feeding. Volume production slowly increases from an average of 600 mL to 800 mL per day by the time the infant is 6 months old and undergoes a diurnal variation, with the greatest quantity occurring in the morning. For the first 10 days of production, milk composition is characterized by a gradual increase in fat and lactose from a milk that is higher in protein content (colostrum).

Because most drugs are either weak acids or bases, the transfer across a biological membrane will be greatly influenced by the ionization characteristics (pKa) and pH differences across the membrane. Because the pH of breast milk (7.0) is slightly lower than that of plasma (7.4), there is a tendency toward ion-trapping of basic compounds.

CLASSIFICATION OF DRUGS USED DURING LACTATION

The American Academy of Pediatrics Committee on Drugs reviewed drugs in lactation and categorized the drugs (Table 21.20) (65). When prescribing drugs to lactating women, consider the following: Is the drug necessary? If so, use the safest drug (e.g., acetaminophen instead of aspirin). If there is a possibility that a drug may present a risk to the infant (e.g., phenytoin, phenobarbital), consider measuring the blood level in the nursing infant. The nursing infant's exposure may be minimized by having the mother take the medication just after completing a breast-feeding (66).

The migraineur who is breast-feeding should avoid bromocriptine, ergotamine, and lithium and use the triptans, benzodiazepines, antidepressants, and neuroleptics only when clearly indicated. Acetaminophen is compatible with breast-feeding and is preferred to aspirin. Moderate caffeine use is compatible with breast-feeding, although accumulation may occur in infants whose mothers use excessive amounts. Narcotic use is compatible with breast-feeding. Phenobarbital has caused sedation in some nursing infants.

SUMMARY

Migraine and TTH are primary headache disorders that are common during pregnancy. Migraine sometimes occurs for the first time with pregnancy. The majority of migraineurs improve while pregnant; however, migraine often recurs postpartum. Some disorders that produce headache, such as stroke, cerebral venous thrombosis, eclampsia, and SAH, occur more frequently during pregnancy. Diagnostic testing serves to exclude organic causes of headache, to confirm the diagnosis, and to establish a baseline before treatment. If neurodiagnostic testing is indicated, the study that will provide the most information with the least fetal risk is the study of choice (8).

Drugs are commonly used during pregnancy despite insufficient knowledge about their effects on the growing fetus. Most drugs are not teratogenic. Adverse effects, such as spontaneous abortion, developmental defects, and various postnatal effects, depend on the dose and route of administration and the timing of the exposure relative to the period of fetal development.

Although medication use should be limited, it is not absolutely contraindicated in pregnancy. In migraine, the risk of status migrainosus may be greater than the potential risk of the medication used to treat the pregnant patient. Nonpharmacologic treatment is the ideal solution; however, analgesics such as acetaminophen and narcotics can be used on a limited basis. Preventive therapy is a last resort.

Many drugs are present in breast milk at nonclinically significant levels. However, exposure to any toxic drug is inappropriate. Most drugs used to treat headache can be used in lactating women.

REFERENCES

1. Headache Classification Committee of the International Headache Society. Classification and diagnostic criteria for headache disorders, cranial neuralgia, and facial pain. *Cephalalgia* 1988;8:1–96.

2. Silberstein SD, Young WB. Headache. In: Pathy MSJ, ed. *Principles and practice of geriatric medicine.* New York: John Wiley & Sons, 1998:733–746.

3. Dalessio DJ, Silberstein SD. Diagnosis and classification of headache. In: Dalessio DJ, Silberstein SD, eds. *Wolff's headache and other head pain,* 6th ed. New York: Oxford University Press, 1993:3–18.

4. Silberstein SD, Saper JR. Migraine: diagnosis and treatment. In: Dalessio DJ, Silberstein SD, eds. *Wolff's headache and other head pain,* 6th ed. New York: Oxford University Press, 1993:96–170.

5. Silberstein SD, Lipton RB, Goadsby PJ. *Headache in clinical practice.* Oxford: Isis Medical Media, 1998.

6. Fox MV, Harms RW, Davis DH. Selected neurologic complications of pregnancy. *Mayo Clin Proc* 1990;65:1595–1618.

7. Hainline B. Headache. *Headache* 1994;12:443–460.

8. Silberstein SD. Migraine and pregnancy. *Neurol Clin* 1997;15:209–231.

9. Silberstein SD, Corbett JJ. The forgotten lumbar puncture. *Cephalalgia* 1993;13:212–213.

10. Stewart WF, Lipton RB, Celentano DD, et al. Prevalence of migraine in the United States. *JAMA* 1992;267:64–69.

11. Lipton RB, Silberstein SD, Stewart WF. An update on the epidemiology of migraine. *Headache* 1994;34:319–328.

12. Uknis A, Silberstein SD. Review article: migraine and pregnancy. *Headache* 1991;31:372–374.

13. Silberstein SD, Lipton RB. Overview of diagnosis and treatment of migraine. *Neurology* 1994;44:6–16.

14. Silberstein SD, Young WB. Migraine aura and prodrome. *Semin Neurol* 1995;45:175–182.

15. Silberstein SD. Migraine symptoms: results of a survey of self-reported migraineurs. *Headache* 1995;35:387–396.

16. Selby G, Lance JW. Observation on 500 cases of migraine and allied vascular headaches. *J Neurol Neurosurg Psychiatry* 1960;23:23–32.

17. Silberstein SD, Lipton RB. Chronic daily headache. In: Goadsby PJ, Silberstein SD, eds. *Headache.* Newton: Butterworth-Heinemann, 1997:201–225.

18. Silberstein SD. Pharmacological management of cluster headache. *CNS Drugs* 1994;2:199–207.

19. Chancellor MD, Wroe SJ. Migraine occurring for the first time in pregnancy. *Headache* 1990;30:224–227

20. Stein GS. Headaches in the first postpartum week and their relationship to migraine. *Headache* 1986;21:201–205.

21. Somerville BW. A study of migraine in pregnancy. *Neurology* 1972;22:824–828.

22. Silberstein SD, Merriam GR. Sex hormones and headache. In: Goadsby PJ, Silberstein SD, eds. *Headache.* Newton: Butterworth-Heinemann, 1997:143–173.

23. Wright DS, Patel MK. Focal migraine and pregnancy. *BMJ* 1986;293:1557–1558.

24. Massey EW. Migraine during pregnancy. *Obstet Gynecol Surv* 1977;32:693–696.

25. Lance JW, Anthony M. Some clinical aspects of migraine. *Arch Neurol* 1966;15:356–361.

26. Callaghan N. The migraine syndrome in pregnancy. *Neurology* 1968;18:197–201.

27. Somerville BW. The role of estradiol withdrawal in the etiology of menstrual migraine. *Neurology* 1972;22:355–365.

28. Ratinahirana H, Darbois Y, Bousser MG. Migraine and pregnancy: a prospective study in 703 women after delivery. *Neurology* 1990;40:437.

29. Granella F, Sances G, Zanferrari C, et al. Migraine without aura and reproductive life events: a clinical epidemiologic study in 1300 women. *Headache* 1993;33:385–389.

30. Rasmussen BK. Migraine and tension-type headache in a general population: precipitating factors, female hormones, sleep pattern, and relation to lifestyle. *Pain* 1993;53:65–72.

31. Chen TC, Leviton A. Headache recurrence in pregnant women with migraine. *Headache* 1994;34:107–110.

32. Scharff L, Marcus DA, Turk DA. Headache during pregnancy and in the postpartum: a prospective study. *Headache* 1997;37:203–210.

33. Maggioni F, Alessi C, Maggino T, et al. Headaches during pregnancy. *Cephalalgia* 1997;17:765–769.

34. Marcus DA, Scharff L, Turk D. Longitudinal prospective study of headache during pregnancy and postpartum. *Headache* 1999;39:625–632.

35. Wainscott G, Volans GN. The outcome of pregnancy in women suffering from migraine. *Postgrad Med J* 1978;54:98–102.

36. MacArthur C, Lewis M, Knox EG. Health after childbirth. *Br J Obstet Gynaecol* 1991;98:1193–1204.

37. Pitkin RM. Drug treatment of the pregnant woman: the state of the art. Proceedings from the Food and Drug Administration conference on regulated products and pregnant women, Virginia, 1994.

38. Raskin NH. Migraine treatment. In: Raskin NH, ed. *Headache,* 2nd ed. New York: Churchill-Livingstone, 1988.

39. Silberstein SD. Appropriate use of abortive medication in headache treatment. *Pain Manage* 1991;4:22–28.

40. Silberstein SD. Headaches and women: treatment of the pregnant and lactating migraineur. *Headache* 1993; 33:533–540.

41. Koren G, Pastuszak A, Ito S. Drugs in pregnancy. *N Engl J Med* 1998;338:1128–1137.

42. Byron MA. Prescribing in pregnancy: treatment of rheumatic disease. *BMJ* 1987;294:236–238.

43. Dalessio DJ. Classification and treatment of headache during pregnancy. *Clin Neuropharmacol* 1986;9:121–131.

44. Saameli K. Effects on the uterus. In: Berde B, Schild HO, eds. *Ergot alkaloids and related compounds.* Berlin: Springer-Verlag, 1978:231–319.

45. Heinonen OP, Sloan S, Shapiro S. Birth defects and drugs in pregnancy. Littleton, MA: Publishing Sciences Group, 1977.

46. Briggs GG, Freeman RK, Yaffe SJ. *Drugs in pregnancy and lactation,* 6th ed. Baltimore: Williams & Wilkins, 1998.

47. Hughes HE, Goldstein DA. Birth defects following maternal exposure to ergotamine, beta-blockers, and caffeine. *J Med Genet* 1988;25:396–399.

48. Peeden JN, Wilroy RS, Soper RG. Prune perineum. *Teratology* 1979;20:233–236.

49. Spranger JW, Schinzel A, Myers T, et al. Cerebroarthrodigital syndrome: a newly recognized formal genesis

syndrome in three patients with apparent arthromyodysplasia and sacral agenesis, brain malformation and digital hypoplasia. *Am J Med Genet* 1980;5:13–24.

50. Graham JM, Marin-Padilla M, Hoefnagel D. Jejunal atresia associated with cafergot ingestion during pregnancy. *Clin Pediatr* 1983;22:226–228.

51. Au KL, Woo JS, Wong VC. Intrauterine death from ergotamine overdosage. *Eur J Obstet Gynecol Reprod Biol* 1985;19:313–315.

52. Verloes A, Emonts P, Dubois M, et al. Paraplegia and arthrogryposis multiplex of the lower extremities after intrauterine exposure to ergotamine. *J Med Genet* 1990;27:213–214.

53. Czeizel A. Teratogenicity of ergotamine. *Teratology* 1989;51:344–347.

54. DeGroot AN, VanDongen PW, VanRoosmalen J, et al. Ergotamine-induced fetal stress: review of side effects of ergot alkaloids during pregnancy. *Eur J Obstet Gynecol Reprod Biol* 1993;51:73–77.

55. Raymond GV. Teratogen update: ergot and ergotamine. *Teratology* 1995;51:344–347.

56. Fomina PI. Untersuchungen uber den ubergang des aktiven agens des mutterkorns in die milch stillender mutter. *J Pediatr* 1965;66:1068–1082.

57. Briggs GG, Freeman RK, Yaffe SJ. A reference guide to fetal and neonatal risk. In: Drugs in pregnancy and lactation, 5/e. Philadelphia: Williams and Wilkins, 1998.

58. Shuhaiber S, Pastuszak A, Schick B, et al. Pregnancy outcome following first trimester exposure to sumatriptan. *Neurology* 1998;51:581-583.

59. MacGregor A. Treatment of migraine during pregnancy. *IHS News Headache* 1994;4:3–9.

60. Rayburn WF, Lavin JP. Drug prescribing for chronic medical disorders during pregnancy: an overview. *Am J Obstet Gynecol* 1986;155:565–569.

61. Little BB, Gilstrap LC. Counseling and evaluation of the drug-exposed patient. In: Little BB, Gilstrap LC, eds. *Drugs and pregnancy,* 2nd ed. New York: Elsevier, 1998:25–32.

62. Blake DA, Niebyl JR. Requirements and limitations in reproductive and teratogenic risk assessment. In: Niebyl JR, ed. *Drug use in pregnancy,* 2nd ed. Philadelphia: Lea & Febiger, 1988:1–9.

63. Friedman JM, Polifka JE. Teratogenic effects of drugs: a resource for clinicians (TERIS). Baltimore: Johns Hopkins University Press, 1994.

64. Niebyl JR. Teratology and drugs in pregnancy and lactation. In: Winters R, ed. *Danforth's obstetrics and gynecology,* 6th ed. Philadelphia: Lippincott, 1990.

65. American Academy of Pediatrics Committee on Drugs. The transfer of drugs and other chemicals into human milk. *Pediatrics* 1994;93:137–150.

66. Murray L, Seger D. Drug therapy during pregnancy and lactation. *Emerg Med Clin N Am* 1994;12:129–149.

22

The Use of Antineoplastic Agents in Pregnancy

Mark S. Shahin and Joel I. Sorosky

Division of Gynecologic Oncology, Department of Obstetrics and Gynecology,
The University of Iowa Hospitals and Clinics, Iowa City, Iowa

Cancer is the second leading cause of mortality for women of reproductive age (1). However, it accounts rarely for maternal death. One in 1,000 to 1,500 pregnancies are complicated by cancer (2). The American College of Obstetricians and Gynecologists estimates that 3,500 cases of cancer occur in pregnant women annually in the United States. The most common malignancies associated with pregnancy include carcinoma of the cervix and breast, lymphoma, melanoma, leukemia, and carcinoma of the ovary and colon (3,4). Pregnancy per se does not appear to increase the risk of developing a malignancy; however, it presents an opportunity for screening examinations, which may result in a cancer diagnosis. In fact, the incidence of specific malignancies during pregnancy mirrors that of nongravid women of comparable age. It is estimated that the incidence of cancer diagnosed during pregnancy will increase as childbearing is delayed to later reproductive years.

The decision to proceed with or to postpone treatment of the malignancy becomes increasingly difficult when the pregnancy is desired and the fetus has not reached maturity. Parents and their health care professionals need to participate in the decision-making process and make informed judgments. Counseling should include a thorough discussion of maternal and fetal effects of therapy including surgery, chemotherapy, radiation, and other biological agents. For patients with breast cancer, ovarian cancer, leukemia, and lymphomas, chemotherapy plays a major role in treatment (5). Examples of antineoplastic agents used in specific malignancies complicating pregnancy are provided in Table 22.1. Administration of chemotherapy agents in pregnancy requires knowledge of the mechanism of action, effects on the cell cycle phase, and toxicity. There are, however, no large randomized trials to address the issues encountered when chemotherapy is used in pregnancy. Hence, most physicians have been forced to formulate treatment plans based on case reports, series, or at best small retrospective studies.

The main concern of a pregnant mother afflicted with cancer is the well-being of her developing child. A conflict may arise as the simultaneous needs of the mother and her fetus are considered. Potential benefits of chemotherapy must be weighed carefully against the possible harm to the fetus. Maternal physiologic alterations and the developmental stage of the fetus will simultaneously dictate the final effects of antineoplastic agents on the developing fetus. This chapter provides information regarding the use of chemotherapy in pregnancy as well as fetal and maternal effects based on current literature and recommendations.

MATERNAL PHYSIOLOGIC CONSIDERATIONS

The physiologic alterations associated with pregnancy have an enormous impact on the dosing and toxicity of chemotherapeutic agents. These are outlined in Chapter 2 (Pharmacokinetics of Drugs During Pregnancy and Lactation). In general, the resultant changes in the drug concentration are likely to be greatest for drugs of low lipid

TABLE 22.1. *Classification of common cancers in pregnancy and chemotherapeutic agents utilized*

Cancer	Drugs currently preferred
Breast	Cyclophosphamide, methotrexate, 5-fluorouracil
Leukemia	Vincristine, doxorubicin, cytarabine, asparaginase, thioguanine
Lymphoma	Doxorubicin, bleomycin, vinblastine, dacarbazine, cyclophosphamide, methotrexate
Melanoma	Interleukin-2, dacarbazine, dactinomycin
Ovary	Paclitaxel, cisplatin, etoposide, topotecan, bleomycin
Colorectal	5-Fluorouracil, mitomycin, topotecan

solubility that are tightly bound to proteins. Obesity may cause maternal sequestration of lipid-soluble drugs. Amniotic fluid may act as a potential third space. This is relevant to agents such as methotrexate, in which distribution into a third space such as pleural or ascitic fluid delays excretion and may increase toxicity. Decreased gastrointestinal motility may interfere with the absorption of oral agents (6).

In pregnancy, altered pharmacokinetics of antineoplastic agents is inevitable. Doses used during the nonpregnant state must therefore be used with a high degree of caution, given the various maternal physiologic alterations.

TRANSPLACENTAL AND FETAL CONSIDERATIONS

Virtually all chemotherapy agents cross the placenta. The features shared by these agents facilitating transplacental transfer include a preferential uptake of nonionized, slightly lipophilic molecules, molecular weights less than 1,000 d, and a low degree of protein binding (7). The exceptions are high molecular weight proteins such as *L*-asparaginase or interferon alpha. Transplacental passage of doxorubicin and cisplatin has been reported (8–10). Once the chemotherapeutic agent crosses the placenta, the same pharmacokinetic principles as in the mother apply, but on a much smaller scale. Recently, the multidrug resistance (MDR) glycoprotein was described on the gravid endometrium, and thus it may serve as a natural fetal barrier for some antineoplastic agents (11). The chemotherapy agents in the fetal system may be metabolized through oxidation by the fetal liver and excreted via the fetal kidneys. Once the agents or their metabolites

are returned to the amniotic fluid, they may be ingested by the fetus or may return to the maternal circulation (12). In the event these substances are active, further toxicity to the mother and fetus is possible. All chemotherapy agents are theoretically teratogenic and mutagenic. Almost all controlled experiments in this field have been performed on gravid animals. Caution must be exercised when extrapolating animal data to human subjects.

PRINCIPLES OF CHEMOTHERAPY ADMINISTRATION DURING PREGNANCY

Chemotherapeutic agents act on rapidly dividing cells and are potentially dangerous to the fetal tissue. The effects on the fetus are dependent on the timing of exposure, duration and frequency of the exposure, and the ability of the drug to cross the placenta. Chemotherapeutic toxicity may be enhanced when combination therapy is used or concurrent radiation is administered. As reviewed earlier, maternal factors that affect fetal drug exposure include hypoalbuminemia, obesity, expanded plasma volume, and increased creatinine clearance (7).

The trimester of exposure is the most critical determinant for teratogenesis in the developing fetus. The first trimester is most critical with respect to exposure to chemotherapy. Chemotherapy may prove deleterious during the period of organogenesis. The stem cell population is limited early in development, and destruction of small numbers of cells may result in significant anatomic defects. The early blastocyst is resistant to teratogens in the first 2 weeks of life. If it is not destroyed by a teratogen, the surviving blastocyst may not manifest any aberrations caused by the chemotherapeutic agent. If severe damage is sustained by the blastocyst up to 2 weeks, spontaneous abortion will ensue. The weeks 3 to 8 after conception represent a time of maximal susceptibility to teratogenic insult. Sublethal damage occurring during this time period results in teratogenesis (13,14). Doll et al. (7) reported rates of 16% and 17% of congenital malformations with the use of single agent and combination chemotherapy, respectively, during the first trimester. However, this rate fell to 6% when folate antagonists were excluded. The background rate of malformations for all births in the general population is 2% to 3%. It is during this period when the most difficult decisions occur as to whether to proceed with therapeutic termination or risk teratogenicity from chemotherapy. In general, chemotherapy must be delayed until after 10 weeks after the last menstrual period.

The second trimester of pregnancy and beyond is heralded by completion of organogenesis, with the exception of brain and gonadal tissue. During the second and third trimesters, the risk of developing a malformation from exposure to chemotherapy agents is greatly diminished and intrauterine growth restriction becomes the dominant effect. Low birth weight, premature birth, and spontaneous abortion have also been reported (15). The incidence of such events is not clear because data in this field are lacking. Nevertheless, because the central nervous system continues to grow during this time, chemotherapy agents potentially affect cortical brain function. In a review of 110 cases of chemotherapy in pregnancy, Nicholson (16) reported no abnormalities in the offspring of the 73 mothers who received chemotherapy during the second trimester. Fifteen of 57 infants exposed to chemotherapeutic agents during the first trimester had congenital malformations.

CHEMOTHERAPY, DELIVERY, AND POSTNATAL CARE

Careful planning and coordination are required for administration of chemotherapy near term or time of delivery. The maternal status including her blood counts must be optimal at the time of delivery whenever possible. Ideally, chemotherapy should be avoided for 3 weeks before birth to allow recovery from neutropenia or thrombocytopenia. Timing of the delivery is of importance also to the fetus because the placenta acts as a vehicle for drug delivery to the fetus and a route of fetal drug excretion. Cases of neonatal cytopenias have been reported in association with cancer chemotherapy (17,18). Delivery of the fetus soon after administration of an antineoplastic agent may impede the excretion of the drug in the infant and result in toxicity owing to prolonged exposure. This is especially true in the preterm infant whose liver and kidneys may have limited capacity to metabolize chemotherapeutic agents (12).

Many chemotherapy agents including hydroxyurea, cyclophosphamide, cisplatin, doxorubicin, and methotrexate can be found in human breast milk. Therefore, breast-feeding is contraindicated in women receiving chemotherapy (19,20). Little is known regarding the delayed effects of *in utero* exposure to antineoplastic agents. Areas of concern include physical and mental development, gonadal function, carcinogenesis, and second-generation teratogenesis. Impaired growth has been documented with exposure to folic acid antagonists during the first trimester (21). Avilez and Nil (22) reported a 92% normal follow-up in 50 children born to women receiving treatment for leukemias and lymphomas in pregnancy. Of 50 children, 21 were exposed to chemotherapy in the first trimester and only one reportedly has multiple congenital abnormalities and has later developed neuroblastoma and thyroid carcinoma. Antineoplastic agents can induce gonadal dysfunction and failure through cytotoxic effects in the germinal cell (23). In a large cohort of survivors of childhood cancers, prior exposure to alkylating agents reduced fertility by 33%, compared with no apparent increase associated with exposure to nonalkylating agents (24). Secondary malignancy is also a well-recognized feature of antineoplastic agents; increases in mutations in lymphocytes and chromosomal aberrations are documented in humans (25,26). The long-term effects of such alterations may not be demonstrable until later life and subsequent generations (27).

NATIONAL REGISTRY

In 1985, the National Cancer Institute established a national registry for *in utero* exposure to chemotherapeutic agents (28). Of the first 210 cases studied, 29 outcomes were abnormal with a total of 52 birth defects. Although extensive generalization is not possible because of the small number of birth defects, the data are reassuring in that only two abnormal outcomes were associated with exposure after the first trimester. Such data are voluntarily reported and potential for bias exists. The precise number of drug exposures is not known, and the registry may include excess abnormal or normal outcomes. Information from this database may be obtained by calling (412) 641-4168. Cases of cancer in pregnancy should be reported to this number.

CHEMOTHERAPY AGENTS

The common antineoplastic agents used during the pregnancy complicated by cancer and their mechanism of action and side effects are shown in Table 22.2.

ALKYLATING AGENTS

Alkylating agents crosslink DNA strands, causing an interruption of RNA and protein synthesis in a cell-cycle, nonspecific manner. They provide a significant role in curative or palliative therapeutic regimens. Such agents including busulfan, chlorambucil, cyclophosphamide, and nitrogen mustard are associated with an increased risk of congenital anomalies if administered during the first trimester. The risk of fetal malformations is reported to be 14% with exposure during organogenesis. Later administration has been reported to cause only a 4% malformation rate (29). The "chlorambucil syndrome" is characterized by renal aplasia, cleft palate, and skeletal anomalies after first-trimester exposure and has been reported by Nicholson (16) in one of six infants.

ANTIBIOTICS

The antibiotic class is composed of naturally occurring compounds that act by DNA intercalation. In humans, there are no reports of fetal adverse outcomes associated with administration

TABLE 22.2. *Classification of chemotherapeutic agents and common side effects*

Agent	Side effects
Alkylating agents	
Busulfan	Myelosuppression, pulmonary fibrosis
Chlorambucil	Myelosuppression
Cyclophosphamide	Alopecia, myelosuppression, hemorrhagic cystitis
Antibiotics	
Doxorubicin	Alopecia, myelosuppression, cardiomyopathy, radiation recall
Dactinomycin	Alopecia, myelosuppression, stomatitis
Mitomycin	Myelosuppression
Bleomycin	Pneumonitis, pulmonary fibrosis
Antimetabolites	
Methotrexate	Myelosuppression, stomatitis
5-Fluorouracil	Myelosuppression, diarrhea
Cytarabine	Myelosuppression, stomatitis
Taxanes	
Paclitaxel	Alopecia, myelosuppression, major hypersensitivity reaction
Docetaxel	Myelosuppression, fluid retention syndrome
Topoisomerase interactive agents	
Etoposide	Alopecia, myelosuppression
Topotecan	Myelosuppression
Vinca alkaloids	
Vincristine	Neurotoxicity, constipation
Vinblastine	Myelosuppression, stomatitis, neurotoxicity
Miscellaneous	
Cisplatin	Nephrotoxicity, neurotoxicity, ototoxicity
Hexalen	Myelosuppression, neurotoxicity

of chemotherapeutic antibiotics. Bleomycin may cause maternal pulmonary toxicity. In women exposed to bleomycin who require general anesthesia, oxygen must be administered at room air concentrations. Furthermore, the common practice of increasing maternal oxygen concentration during labor may result in significant maternal pulmonary toxicity. Bleomycin is used with curative intent for ovarian germ-cell tumors. We have successfully used the combination of bleomycin, etoposide, and cisplatin in a woman diagnosed with an immature teratoma during the second trimester of pregnancy. The mother and the baby are well 2 years after delivery.

Anthracycline antibiotics including doxorubicin and daunorubicin have been administered during pregnancy without any associated fetal malformations. In a review of 28 patients, including four cases of combination therapy during the first-trimester exposure, Turchi and Villasis (30) reported two maternal and fetal deaths and two spontaneous abortions. Actinomycin D has been administered during the second and third trimesters without congenital malformations (31).

ANTIMETABOLITES

The folic acid antagonists aminopterin and methotrexate are the agents most commonly associated with fetal malformations when given during the first trimester of pregnancy (21). Indeed, a syndrome of congenital anomalies has been recognized (the "aminopterin syndrome"). This syndrome is characterized by cranial dysostosis, hypertelorism, a wide nasal bridge, anomalies of the external ear, and micrognathia. Other features including limb deformities, below-average intelligence, and poor speech development have also been described. Methotrexate, another folate antagonist, has long been recognized as a human teratogen and an abortifacient (7). Multiple birth defects including cranial defects and malformed extremities have been described in association with first-trimester exposure to methotrexate. Kozlowski et al. (32), however, recently reported the experience of eight pregnant women undergoing therapy with low-dose methotrexate for rheumatoid arthritis during the first trimester. Five normal term neonates were delivered; three spontaneous abortions and two elective terminations were also reported. These findings illustrate that methotrexate does not always behave as a teratogen.

Birth defects associated with other antimetabolites have rarely been described in the literature. 5-Fluorouracil, a pyrimidine antagonist, has been reported to result in congenital malformation; however, concurrent radiation was administered (33). Topical and intravaginal 5-fluorouracil has been used in pregnancy without adverse effects (34,35). No cases of neonatal birth defects have been documented in association with the use of 6-mercaptopurine in 20 patients (7). Cytarabine, an analog of the nucleoside deoxycytidine, has been used alone or in combination during pregnancy. Caliguiri and Mayer (36) reported two cases of congenital malformations in six infants.

TAXANES

Paclitaxel is an antineoplastic agent of extreme importance in treatment of epithelial ovarian cancer and metastatic breast cancer. It prevents cellular replication by preventing depolymerization of tubulin. Paclitaxel has been shown to cause increased fetal deaths in the rat model (37). Severe embryotoxicity was also demonstrated in chicks. To date, there are no published reports of taxane administration during pregnancy. We recently treated a woman in early third trimester with paclitaxel and cisplatin for primary therapy of advance-stage epithelial ovarian cancer after optimal cytoreductive surgery. At 6 months postnatal follow-up, the infant appears to be normal without any developmental deficiencies (unpublished data). A recent report suggested liposomal encapsulation diminishes the toxic side effects of this agent (38). Docetaxel, a semisynthetic analog of paclitaxel, has not been administered to date in pregnancy.

TOPOISOMERASE INTERACTIVE AGENTS

Topotecan, an inhibitor of DNA topoisomerase I, is an active agent in treatment of colorectal and ovarian carcinomas. Myelosuppression is the most notable side effect of this agent. No published reports of topotecan administration in pregnancy exist in the literature.

Etoposide, an inhibitor of DNA topoisomerase II, is another important anticancer drug. An association with neonatal pancytopenia has been reported for second-trimester chemotherapy regimens that include etoposide (39). No report of first-trimester exposure is available at this time.

VINCA ALKALOIDS

Vinca alkaloids bind tubulin and cause dissociation of the microtubule apparatus. They are specific to the M phase of the cell cycle. Vinblastine and vincristine are often used in combination curative chemotherapeutic regimens. These agents have shown to be teratogenic in the animal model; however, reports of usage in pregnancy do not support the animal model. Schpira and Chudley (40) reported no abnormalities in 10 neonates with first-trimester exposure. In a review, Gilliland and Weinstein (31) reported no congenital anomalies in three neonates who had first-trimester exposure to these agents. There has only been one report of abnormality observed in the offspring of 14 women treated with vinblastine during first trimester (12). It is therefore concluded that these agents may be used safely during pregnancy.

CISPLATIN

Cisplatin exerts its antitumor activity by binding to DNA and creating intrastructural crosslinks that affect DNA replication. No outcome data are available regarding first-trimester cisplatin exposure (37). Cisplatin administration has been reported during the second and third trimesters without adverse neonatal outcomes. Tomlinson et al. (41) reported on 10 pregnant women treated with cisplatin during second and third trimesters. One half of the infants demonstrated evidence of growth restriction at birth. Moderate hearing loss was evident at birth in one infant. Transient leukopenia and alopecia were observed in two separate cases.

COMBINATION CHEMOTHERAPY

A combination of chemotherapeutic agents that have been effectively used as single agents individually may be utilized for the therapy of many cancers, e.g., breast cancer, leukemias, and lymphomas. The apparent rate of fetal malformations associated with combination chemotherapy is similar to that observed with single agents (12,42,43). Definitive conclusions regarding the use of combination chemotherapy in the first trimester is hampered by the paucity of data and variability of the individualized regimen. In a review of combination therapy during the second and third trimesters, Doll and Yarbo (12) reported two cases of malformation among 166 patients treated.

RECOMMENDATIONS

When chemotherapy is given with the curative intent, therapy modification should not be made to compromise the goal. If palliation, however, is the intended goal, the primary concern would be to decrease harm to the fetus. The therapy of the pregnant patient with cancer must be individualized. A team including her primary care provider, perinatologist, oncologist, and neonatologist should facilitate her care.

The most toxic chemotherapeutic agents administered during the pregnancy are methotrexate and aminopterin, and both agents should be avoided during the pregnancy, particularly during the first trimester. Delivery of the fetus should occur optimally when the mother is neither neutropenic nor thrombocytopenic. Breast-feeding should be avoided if postpartum chemotherapy is planned.

REFERENCES

1. Landis SH, Murray T, Bolden S, et al. Cancer statistics, 1998. *CA Cancer J Clin* 1998;48:6–29.
2. Waalen J. Pregnancy poses tough questions for cancer treatment. *J Natl Cancer Inst* 1991;83:900–902.
3. Betson JR, Golden ML. Cancer and pregnancy. *Am J Obstet Gynecol* 1961;81:718–728.
4. Haas JF. Pregnancy in association with a newly diagnosed cancer: a population-based epidemiologic assessment. *Int J Cancer* 1984;34:229–235.
5. Doll DC, Ringenberg QS, Yarbo JW. Management of cancer during pregnancy. *Arch Intern Med* 1988;148:2058–2064.

6. Redmond GP. Physiological changes during pregnancy and their implications for pharmacological treatment. *Clin Invest Med* 1985;8:317–322.

7. Doll DC, Ringenberg QS, Yarbo JW. Antineoplastic agents and pregnancy. *Semin Oncol* 1989;16:337–346.

8. Karp GI, von Oeyen P, Valone F, et al. Doxorubicin in pregnancy: possible transplacental passage. *Cancer Treat Rep* 1983;67:773–777.

9. Henderson CE, Elia G, Garfinkel D, et al. Platinum chemotherapy during pregnancy for serous cystadenocarcinoma of ovary. *Gynecol Oncol* 1993;49:92–97.

10. Shamkhani H, Anderson LM, Henderson CE, et al. DNA adducts in women and patas monkey: maternal and fetal tissues induced by platinum drug chemotherapy. *Reprod Toxicol* 1994;8:207–216.

11. Anceci RJ, Croop JM, Horitz SB, et al. The gene encoding multidrug resistance is induced and expressed at high levels during pregnancy in the secretory epithelium of the uterus. *Proc Natl Acad Sci USA* 1988;85:4350–4354.

12. Doll DC, Yarbo JW. Chemotherapy in pregnancy. In: Perry MC, ed. *The Chemotherapy source book,* 2nd ed. Baltimore: Williams & Wilkins, 1997:803–811.

13. DeVita VT. Principles of cancer management: chemotherapy. In: DeVita VT, Hellman S, Rosenberg SA, eds. *Cancer: principles and practice of oncology,* 5th ed. Philadelphia, Lippincott–Raven, 1997:333–348.

14. Buekers TE, Lallas TA. Chemotherapy in pregnancy. *Obstet Gynecol Clin* 1998;25:323–329.

15. Landon MB. Malignant diseases. In: Gabbe SG, Niebyl JR, Simpson JL, eds. *Obstetrics: normal and problem pregnancies,* 2nd ed. New York: Churchill-Livingstone, 1992:1199–1214.

16. Nicholson HO. Cytotoxic drugs in pregnancy. *J Obstet Gynaecol Br Commonw* 1968;75:307–312.

17. Reynosa E, Shepard F, Messner H, et al. Acute leukemia in pregnancy: the Toronto Leukemia Study Group experience with long-term follow-up of children exposed in utero to chemotherapeutic agents. *J Clin Oncol* 1987;5:1098–1106.

18. Okun DB, Groncy PK, Sieger L, et al. Acute leukemia in pregnancy: transient neonatal myelosuppression after combination chemotherapy in the mother. *Med Pediatr Oncol* 1979;7:315–319.

19. Ben-Baruch G, Menczer J, Goshen R, et al. Cisplatin excretion in human milk. *J Natl Cancer Inst* 1992;84:451–452.

20. Egan PC, Costanza M, Dadion P, et al. Doxorubicin and cisplatin excretion into human breast milk. *Cancer Treat Rep* 1985;69:1387–1389.

21. Warkany J. Aminopterin and methotrexate: folic acid deficiency. *Teratology* 1978;17:353–358.

22. Avilez A, Nil J. Long Term follow-up of children born to mothers with acute leukemia during pregnancy. *Med Pediatr Oncol* 1988;16:3–6.

23. Shahin MS, Puscheck E. Reproductive sequelae of cancer treatment. *Obstet Gynecol Clin* 1998;25:423–433.

24. Byrne J, Mulvihill JJ, Myers MH, et al. Effects of treatment on fertility in long-term survivors of childhood or adolescent cancer. *N Engl J Med* 1987;317:1315–1321.

25. Kyle PA. Second malignancies associated with chemotherapy. In: Perry MC, Yarbo JW, eds. *Toxicity of chemotherapy.* Orlando, FL: Grune & Stratton, 1984:479–506.

26. Dempsey JL, Seshadri RS, Morley AA. Increased mutation frequency following treatment with cancer chemotherapy. *Cancer Res* 1985;45:2873–2877.

27. Bender RA, Young RL. Effects of cancer treatment on individual and generational genetics. *Semin Oncol* 1978;5:47–56.

28. Randall T. National registry seeks scarce data on pregnancy outcomes during chemotherapy. *JAMA* 1993;269:323.

29. Glantz JC. Reproductive toxicology of alkylating agents. *Obstet Gynecol Surv* 1994;49:709–715.

30. Turchi JJ, Villasis C. Anthracyclins in the treatment of malignancy in pregnancy. *Cancer* 1988;61:435–440.

31. Gilliland J, Weinstein L. The effects of cancer chemotherapeutic agents on developing fetus. *Obstet Gynecol Surv* 1983;3:6–11.

32. Kozlowski RD, Steinbrunner JV, MacKenzie AH, et al. Outcome of first trimester exposure to low dose methotrexate in eight patients with rheumatoid arthritis. *Am J Med* 1990;8:589–592.

33. Stephens JD, Golbus MS, Miller TR, et al. Multiple congenital anomalies in a fetus exposed to 5-fluorouracil during the first trimester. *Am J Obstet Gynecol* 1980;137:747–749.

34. Le L, Pizzutic DJ, Greenberg M, et al. Accidental use of low-dose 5-fluorouracil in pregnancy. *J Reprod Med* 1991;36:872–874.

35. Kopelman JN, Miyazawa K. Inadvertent 5-fluorouracil treatment in early pregnancy: a report of three cases. *Reprod Toxicol* 1990;4:233–235.

36. Caliguiri MA, Mayer RJ. Pregnancy and leukemia. *Semin Oncol* 1989;16:388–396.

37. Weibe VJ, Sipila PEH. Pharmacology of antineoplastic agents in pregnancy. *Crit Rev Oncol Hematol* 1994;16:75–112.

38. Scialli AR, Waterhouse TB, Desesso JM, et al. Protective effect of liposome encapsulation on paclitaxel developmental toxicity in the rat. *Teratology* 1997,56:305–310.

39. Hsu KF, Chang CH, Chou CY. Sinusoidal fetal heart pattern during chemotherapy in a pregnant woman with acute myelogenous leukemia. *J Formos Med Assoc* 1995;94:562–565.

40. Schpira DV, Chudley AE. Successful pregnancy following continuous treatment with combination chemotherapy before conception and throughout pregnancy. *Cancer* 1984;54:800–803.

41. Tomlinson MW, Tredwell MC, Deppe G. Platinum based chemotherapy to treat recurrent Sertoli-Leydig cell ovarian carcinoma during pregnancy. *Eur J Gynecol Oncol* 1997;18:44–46.

42. Sorosky JI, Scott-Conner CEH. Breast disease complicating pregnancy. *Obstet Gynecol Clin* 1998;25:353–363.

43. Sorosky JI, Sood AK, Buekers TE. The use of chemotherapeutic agents during pregnancy. *Obstet Gynecol Clin* 1997;27:591–599.

23

Radiologic Examinations During Pregnancy

Martin Fielder* and John M. Thorp, Jr.†

*University of North Carolina at Chapel Hill, Chapel Hill, North Carolina
†Department of Obstetrics and Gynecology, University of North Carolina School of Medicine,
Chapel Hill, North Carolina

Many diagnostic imaging modalities can be used by physicians caring for pregnant women. Radiographic and nuclear medicine studies in particular can cause anxiety for patients, their families, and even their physicians. This anxiety can be needless, lead to litigation, refusal of necessary procedures, and termination of pregnancies. Nearly all diagnostic imaging studies pose little risk to the developing fetus. The American College of Radiology states that no single diagnostic radiographic procedure results in radiation exposure that would threaten the well-being of an embryo, preembryo, or fetus. Thus, diagnostic radiographic exposure is not an indication for therapeutic abortion (1).

Pregnant women may inadvertently have an abdominal radiograph during the first trimester of pregnancy (2). It is therefore vital for the obstetric care provider to understand the risks of ionizing radiation to counsel properly the patient. This chapter provides the physician with basic knowledge about the risks of imaging studies on a developing fetus and provides adequate resources of further information. For specific cases, the reader is encouraged to seek advice from an experienced radiologist and/or medical physicist.

IONIZING RADIATION

Ionizing radiation includes radiographs, radioisotope examinations, radiation therapy, and environmental exposures, such as to an atomic bomb or nuclear reactor. The latter three are important because many of our available data come from exposure to these sources. However, our discussion focuses on diagnostic studies, such as plain film radiographs, computed tomography scans, fluoroscopy, and nuclear medicine studies.

Radiation effects can be divided into two categories: stochastic and deterministic. Stochastic effects are caused by a mutation in a cell or small group of cells. The dose given is not important for the severity of the effect, but it is important for the probability that a given effect will occur (3). Examples of effects include malignancies (such as leukemia) and heritable effects. There is no safe threshold below which no effects are seen. As the dose increases, the probability of the effect increases, until a dose when cell killing may take place, resulting in an apparent decrease in the probability of an effect (3).

For deterministic effects to occur, many cells must be killed or adversely affected, and there is a threshold dose. The magnitude of the threshold depends on the dose rate, the organ, and the clinical effect (4). Both the probability and severity increase with increasing doses above the threshold dose. Examples of deterministic effects are malformations, growth restriction, mental retardation, and fetal death. Protracted radiation exposures may affect many tissues throughout pregnancy, but, in general, such exposures probably have less overall teratogenic effect than a brief radiation exposure of high intensity (5).

The classic deterministic effects of radiation on the developing mammal are gross congenital malformations, mental retardation, intrauterine growth retardation, and embryonic death.

Central nervous system (CNS) effects are the hallmark of malformations seen; in fact, no other malformations secondary to radiation are seen in humans without having a CNS malformation or growth restriction (6). The most common radiation effects reported are growth restriction, microcephaly, mental retardation, microphthalmia, retinal pigment changes, genital and skeletal malformations, and cataracts (6). It is believed that the CNS is more susceptible to radiation because of its complex nature and interactions and that it maintains a sensitivity throughout the gestation. Because it maintains susceptibility for an extended period of time versus other organ systems, it is more likely to be randomly affected. An excellent review of CNS effects can be found in Schull et al. (7).

It is well established that the effects of radiation are dependent on the age of the developing fetus. At earlier gestational ages, the fetus is much more sensitive to radiation than later, when large doses cause fewer effects. Lethality is the most worrisome in the very early stages, whereas malformations are the concern during organogenesis. Later, mental retardation, microcephaly, and growth restriction occur. These risks are further evaluated by stage of the developing fetus in Table 23.1.

PREIMPLANTATION STAGE

There are relatively few human data on the preimplantation stage [0 to 8 days postconception or 14 to 22 days from last menstrual period (LMP)]. From animal data, it appears that there is an "all-or-none" phenomenon of embryonic mortality. It appears that the threshold is approximately 5 to 10 rad (8). After this threshold is reached, a maximum excess mortality is approximately 1% per rad (3). No malformations or growth restriction have been observed with exposure at this gestational stage. This may be because the tissues at this age are extraembryonic and the primitive streak has yet to be formed (9).

EMBRYONIC STAGE

There is a continued but reduced risk of embryonic death in this period (9 to 60 days postconception or 23 to 74 days after LMP). Many would extend the all-or-none period to 35 days after the LMP. The threshold for death is higher, probably approximately 25 to 50 rad. The excess fetal mortality is 6.9% with a 50-rad exposure in the preimplantation period; it is 4.8% during the embryonic stage (10). The principal risks are malformations of the CNS system, mostly microcephaly, and growth retardation. The threshold of malformation is considered to be approximately 10 rad, with an increased risk of 0.5% per rad above the threshold (4,11,12). Growth retardation has a threshold of approximately 5 to 25 rad (13). Data from Hiroshima survivors place a risk of microcephaly without mental retardation at approximately 1% per rad, above a threshold of 10 to 20 rad (14,15).

TABLE 23.1. *Risks of irradiation per gestational age*

Defect and gestational age (d)	Occurence	Threshold (rad)	Risk per rad
Lethality			
0–8 (p.c.)	+++	5–10	1% max
9–60	+	25–50	ND
61–104	+	50	ND
105–175	–	–	–
>175	–	–	–
Malformation			
0–8	–	–	–
9–60	+++	10–20	0.50%
61–104	–	–	–
105–175	–	–	–
>175	–	–	–
Mental retardation			
0–8	–	–	–
9–60	–	–	–
61–104	+++	12	0.40%
105–175	+	65	0.10%
>175	–	–	–
Microcephaly			
0–8	–	–	–
9–60	++	10–20	1%
61–104	++	10–20	1.00%
105–175	–	–	–
>175	–	–	–
Growth retardation			
0–8	–	–	–
9–60	+++	5–25	ND
61–104	++	5–25	ND
105–175	–	–	–
>175	–	–	–

Adapted from refs. 3, 6, and 13.
p.c., postconception; –, no observed effect; +, demonstrated effect; ++, readily apparent effect; +++, occurs in high incidence; ND, no data.

EARLY FETAL STAGE

Lethality is much less common in the early fetal stage (61 to 104 days postconception or 75 to 118 days from LMP) with a threshold of 50 rad and large increases do not increase the risk substantially (3). Microcephaly and mental retardation are the principal risks at this stage (13). Using data from the Hiroshima survivors, the threshold for mental retardation is 12 rad with a risk of 0.4% per rad above this threshold (16,17). The risk of growth restriction is less than during the embryogenesis phase (13), although the risk of microcephaly is approximately the same, especially early in this phase (18).

MIDFETAL STAGE

The risks are much less in the midfetal stage (105 to 175 days postconception or 119 to 189 from LMP), with the threshold of mental retardation being 65 rad, the threshold of microcephaly and growth retardation being 50 rad, and a much higher threshold for fetal death (13). Hobbs (19) reported a pregnancy in which the fetus was exposed to 12.8 Gy without abnormalities noted after birth. The risk of mental retardation per rad in this period has been reported as 0.1% per rad above threshold (17).

LATE FETAL STAGE

The risks of death, malformation, and mental retardation are negligible at this stage (>175 days). Growth restriction remains the only deterministic effect seen, with a threshold of 50 rad (13).

The primary stochastic effect of concern is carcinogenesis. Because there is no threshold below which a stochastic effect cannot be found, this is the concern of radiation at diagnostic levels. The other stochastic effect discussed in the literature is the risk of heritable diseases. This effect carries a very low risk from ionizing radiation, with the risk estimated to be between 0.012% and 0.099% per rad. This is well below the baseline risk of 1.6% (3).

The natural prevalence of fatal childhood cancer up to the age of 15 years of age is one per 1,300 (0.08%) (10). The risk of excess fatal cancer has been estimated from 0.03% to 0.07% per rad (4,10,13,20–22). Therefore, a 1- to 2-rad exposure increases the risk by 1.5 to twofold. This is very different from that for the adult, in whom this amount of exposure does not make a perceptible change in risk (6). Leukemias are the cancers most reported, but other solid tumors have been reported as well (3,6). This increased risk has been challenged by many authors, including Brent (6), Miller (23), Totter and MacPherson (24), and the UNSCEAR report (11). They point out flaws in the studies, challenge the biological plausibility, and propose that there is merely an association but not a causal relationship between radiation and childhood malignancy (5). There is also debate about whether this risk is higher or lower early in gestation. Some state that this risk is higher in the first trimester (25), whereas others (10) argue that it is less. Clearly there is still debate about this relationship.

There are several approaches to limit the radiation exposure to the fetus. First, if there is another modality that does not use ionizing radiation, it should be considered. Shielding of the fetus should be done whenever possible. The study should be limited to the views that are necessary. Limiting the number of radiographs taken for a particular study is helpful as well. It must also be said that the study's usefulness should not be limited or compromised using the techniques above. Stovall et al. (13) and Wagner et al. (26) provide excellent reviews of ways to limit radiation exposure.

The estimated doses of radiation to the fetus from selected diagnostic studies are listed in Table 23.2. The actual amount of radiation received can be quite variable, depending on shielding, equipment, operator, and body habitus. Again, for an accurate estimate for a specific study, consultation should be requested from the radiologist or medical physicist. Their calculations will include the type of study, their knowledge of the equipment used, and distance of the fetus from the focus of the study. Please note that virtually all the studies listed give an exposure well below any threshold listed previously. Thus, threshold levels are rarely reached by diagnostic studies but can take place during an extensive evaluation for abdominal pain and/or gastrointestinal bleeding or when fluoroscopy is necessary.

TABLE 23.2. *Typical radiation exposure to the fetus for selected diagnostic studies*

Study	Radiation exposure (mrad)
Chest radiograph	2–8
Dental x-rays	<1
Mammography	7–10
Abdominal radiograph	200–700
Lumbar spine radiograph	300–600
Hip radiograph	200–500
Upper gastrointestinal series	100–550
Barium enema	800–1,300
Intravenous pyelogram	600–1,000
Cholecystography	100
Head computed tomography	50
Chest computed tomography	1,000
Abdomen computed tomography	3,000–4,000
Pelvimetry computed tomography	250
Cardiac catheterization	<500

1 rad = 1,000 mrad.
Adapted from refs. 1, 2, and 26.

NUCLEAR MEDICINE STUDIES

Nuclear medicine studies are frequently used in reproduction-age women resulting in use during pregnancy. The exposure of the fetus is determined by the physical and biological properties of the isotope employed (27) and the gestational age (28). It is difficult to determine specific radiation exposure from a particular type of nuclear medicine study because of a lack of information on human subjects regarding placental uptake and fetal distribution to various organs. Most data are therefore extrapolated from animal studies and the few human studies available. In general, the fetus-absorbed dose tends to decrease throughout gestation unless the fetal and/or placental uptake increases during gestation, such as with sodium iodide I 131 or sodium I or ^{131}I/Na I (28).

The majority of nuclear medicine studies will likely have fetal doses of less than 1 rad. With typical use, only studies with gallium citrate Ga 67, ^{131}I/Na I, ^{131}I red blood cells, and thallous chloride Tl 201 could result in fetal doses higher than 1 rad (28). One of the most common exposures occurs with diagnostic tests related to thyroid problems. Iodide 131 is commonly used, but ^{123}I or technetium-99m (^{99m}Tc) may be a better choice if a thyroid study is essential during pregnancy (29). The half-life of ^{131}I is approxi-

mately 8 days versus 13 hours for [123]I. Although neither has known teratogenic effects in doses used for diagnostic tests, both, but particularly ^{131}I, can cause fetal thyroid damage, goiter, and local effects when concentrated by the fetal thyroid after 70 days post-LMP. Therapeutic levels of ^{131}I for treatment of hyperthyroidism or thyroid cancer should be avoided in pregnancy and while breast-feeding if possible. Doses can reach 1,000 to 10,000 times that used for diagnostic tests. When treating hyperthyroidism and/or ablating the thyroid, fetal exposure can vary from 14 rad in early gestation to 50 rad at term, compared with levels secondary to diagnostic uses such as a thyroid uptake scan (100 mrad) (28).

The most widely used radioisotope in pregnancy is [99m]Tc. This isotope can be "tagged" to various chemical agents to perform brain, renal, lung, bone, and cardiovascular scans (1). [99m]Tc can cross the placenta depending on the agent to which it is tagged, but the amount of radiation from any routine study is small (1). A typical ventilation/perfusion scan uses ^{99m}Tc and xenon gas and gives an exposure of approximately 50 mrad.

Breast-feeding decisions will depend on the particular isotope. Suggestions about thallium vary from no delay in breast-feeding to a delay of several days. Although neonatal exposure may be relatively low, at least one report describes the isotope concentrating in the testes. Breast-feeding should probably be avoided with gallium use, but one could test the level of radioactivity in the breast milk to safely resume or initiate breast-feeding. A delay of 7 to 14 days or testing for radioactivity in breast milk is also prudent for maternal ^{131}I exposure. Breast-feeding can probably safely resume after 24 to 48 hours after ^{99m}Tc exposure.

MAGNETIC RESONANCE IMAGING

The use of magnetic resonance imaging (MRI) in obstetrics has become more common. Evaluation of the fetus, placenta, maternal abdominal/pelvic masses, and pelvimetry are some of the typical uses. No radiation is generated by a MRI scan, as its images are generated from four magnetic fields (26). There are very few studies that adequately evaluate the effects of MRI on fetuses. There have been no documented adverse fetal effects noted in humans in the available literature. Two small animal studies (30,31) suggested that *in utero* exposure may result in intrauterine growth restriction, but this was refuted by Myers et al. (32). The only published study of the safety of MRI in human pregnancy was a 3-year follow-up, uncontrolled study of 20 children imaged *in utero*. No disease or disability attributed to MRI was found (33). However, because data are limited, the National Radiological Protection Board arbitrarily advises against its use in the first trimester (1). Levine and Edelman (34) describe using a fast MRI technique to enhance fetal studies and to limit the length of the procedure.

Gadolinium is the nonionic contrast agent typically used for MRI evaluations. There are few data about its use in pregnancy. The manufacturer's package insert reports fetal growth retardation in rabbits and rats after high-dose exposure, but no malformations were seen (Magnevist package insert, Berlex Laboratories, Wayne, NJ). There have been no reports of adverse fetal effects in humans (Reprotox review). Gadolinium is excreted into breast milk in small amounts (35), and one group estimated the amount to be less than 0.5% of the total injected dose (36). This led the authors to recommend the suspension of breast-feeding for 36 to 48 hours after administration; however, this is not based on any available data regarding infant morbidity.

ULTRASONOGRAPHY

Ultrasonography remains the diagnostic imaging study of choice in pregnancy. There is no radiation exposure with ultrasonography. No documented teratogenic effects have been found for diagnostic ultrasound procedures (6). A randomized, controlled trial involving intensive use of ultrasonography (five scheduled procedures) versus less intensive use (one procedure) showed a significant increase in growth restriction based on birth weight less than either the tenth or third centile. The authors suggested that ultrasonography be used only when it offers a clinical benefit (37,38). A follow-up showed no difference at 1 year of age.

SUMMARY

Many women will require the use of diagnostic imaging during their pregnancy. Nearly every study provides little to no risk to the developing fetus, regardless of gestational age. The risk of childhood malignancy justifies the judicious use of ionizing radiation but should not restrict a necessary study. MRI and ultrasonography appear to have no effect on a developing fetus and should be preferentially used when possible.

Imaging studies are safe when breast-feeding, and use of individual radioisotopes should be considered on a case-by-case basis.

REFERENCES

1. Guidelines for diagnostic imaging in pregnancy. ACOG Committee Opinion, 158.
2. Mossman KL, Hill LT. Radiation risks in pregnancy. *Obstet Gynecol* 1982;60:237–242.
3. Steenvoorde P, Pauwels E, Harding L, et al. Diagnostic nuclear medicine and risk for the fetus. *Eur J Nucl Med* 1998;25:193–199.
4. ICRP Publication 73. Radiological protection and safety in medicine. *Ann ICRP* 1996;26.
5. Mettler FA, Upton AC. Radiation exposure in utero. In: *Medical effects of ionizing radiation*. Philadelphia: WB Saunders, 1995:319–341.
6. Brent RL. The effects of embryonic and fetal exposure to x-ray, microwaves, and ultrasound. *Clin Perinatol* 1986;13:615–648.
7. Schull WJ, Norton S, Jensh RP. Ionizing radiation and the developing brain. *Neurotoxicol Teratol* 1990;12:249–260.
8. ICRP Publication 62. Radiological protection in biomedical research. *Ann ICRP* 1991;22.
9. ICRP Publication 52. Protection of the patient in nuclear medicine. *Ann ICRP* 1987;17.
10. NRPB. *Board statement on diagnostic medical exposures to ionising radiation during pregnancy and estimates of late radiation risks to the UK population.* Chilton, Didcot, Oxon: National Radiological Protection Board, 1993.
11. UNSCEAR. *Sources and effects of ionizing radiation. United Nations Scientific Committee on the Effects of Atomic Radiation.* New York: United Nations, 1993.
12. Streffer C. Biological effects of prenatal irradiation. In: Lake JV, Bock GR, Cardew G, eds. *Health impacts of large releases of radioisotopes.* New York: John Wiley & Sons, 1997:155–166.
13. Stovall M, Blackwell CR, Cundiff J, et al. Fetal dose from radiotherapy with photon beams: report of AAPM radiation therapy committee task group no. 36. *Med Phys* 1995;22:63–82.
14. Otake M, Schull WJ. Radiation-related small head sizes among prenatally exposed A-bomb survivors. *Int J Radiat Biol* 1993;63:255–270.
15. Miller RW. Effects of prenatal exposure to ionizing radiation. *Health Phys* 1990;59:57–61.

16. ICRP Publication 49. Developmental effects of irradiation on the brain of the embryo and the fetus. *Ann ICRP* 1986;16.

17. Otake M, Schull WJ. *In utero* exposure to A-bomb radiation and mental retardation: a reassessment. *Br J Radiol* 1984;57:409–414.

18. Schull WJ. Report of risk task group of committee 1: Ionizing radiation and the developing human brain. *Ann ICRP* 1991.

19. Hobbs AA. Fetal tolerance to roentgen rays: a case report. *Radiology* 1950;54:242–246.

20. Mole R. The biology and radiobiology of *in utero* development in relation to radiological protection. *Br J Radiol* 1993;66:1095–1102.

21. Doll R, Wakeford R. Risk of childhood cancer from fetal irradiation. *Br J Radiol* 1997;70:130–139.

22. ICRU Report 33. *Radiation quantities and units.* Washington: International Commission of Radiation Units and Measurements, 1980.

23. Miller RW. Epidemiological conclusions from radiation toxicity studies. In: Fry RJM, Grahn D, Griem ML, et al. eds. *Late effects of radiation.* London: Taylor and Francis, 1970.

24. Totter JR, MacPherson HG. Do childhood cancers result from prenatal x-rays? *Health Phys* 1981;40:511–524.

25. Bithell JF, Stewart AM. Prenatal irradiation and childhood malignancy, a review of British data from the Oxford survey. *Br J Cancer* 1975;31:271–287.

26. Wagner LK, Lester RG, Saldana LR. *Exposure of the pregnant patient to diagnostic radiations,* 2nd ed. Madison, WI: Medical Physics Publishing, 1997.

27. Twickler DM, Clarke G, Cunningham FG. *Diagnostic imaging in pregnancy. Supplement to Williams obstetrics,* 18th ed. Norwalk, CT: Appleton and Lange, 1992.

28. Russell JR, Stabin MG, Sparks RB, et al. Radiation absorbed dose to the embryo/fetus from radiopharmaceuticals. *Health Phys* 1997;73:756–69.

29. Ginsberg JS, Hirsh J, Rainbow AJ. Risks to the fetus of radiologic procedures used in the diagnosis of maternal venous thromboembolic disease. *Thromb Haemost* 1989;61:189–196.

30. Carnes KI, Magin RL. Effects of *in utero* exposure to 4.7 T MR imaging conditions on fetal growth and testicular development in the mouse. *Magn Reson Imaging* 1996;14:263–274.

31. Tyndall DA. MRI effects on crania facial size and crown/rump length in C57bl/6J mice in 1.5 T fields. *Oral Surg Oral Med Oral Perfo* 1993;76:655–660.

32. Myers C, Duncan KR, Gowland PA, et al. Failure to detect intrauterine growth restriction following in utero exposure to MRI. *Br J Radiol* 1998;71:549–551.

33. Baker PN, Johnson IR, Gowland PA, et al. Measurement of fetal brain, liver, and placental volumes with echo planar magnetic resonance imaging. *Br J Obstet Gynaecol* 1995;102:35–39.

34. Levine D, Edelman RR. Fast MRI and its application in obstetrics. *Abdom Imag* 1997;22:589–596.

35. Schmiedl U, Maravilla KR, Gerlach R, et al. Excretion of gadopentetate dimeglumine in human breast milk. *AJR Am J Roentgenol* 1990;154:1305–1306.

36. Padhani AR, Lopez AJ, Revell PB, et al. Eye and testicular pain after administration of gadopentetate dimeglumine. *AJR Am J Roentgenol* 1995;165:484–485.

37. Newnham JP, Evans SF, Michael CA, et al. Effects of frequent ultrasound during pregnancy: a randomised controlled trial. *Lancet* 1993;342:887–891.

38. Berlin L. Malpractice issues in radiology. *Am J Radiol* 1996;167:1377–1379.

24

Anticoagulation in Pregnancy

Jerome Yankowitz

Department of Obstetrics and Gynecology,
University of Iowa Hospitals and Clinics, Iowa City, Iowa

Thromboembolism is a leading cause of morbidity and mortality in pregnancy and during the postpartum period. It is the second most common cause of pregnancy-related maternal mortality in the United States (1). Pregnant women have a fivefold increased risk of venous thrombosis (2). Data from the United Kingdom from 1973 to 1993 show that although deaths from hemorrhage, eclampsia, and sepsis have gradually decreased, the maternal death rate from pulmonary embolism has shown little or no change (3). The report agreed with previously reported data and found that the death rates during the antepartum and postpartum periods were the same. Antepartum deaths occurred with the same frequency in each trimester. Because the antepartum period is longer than the usual risk period postpartum, there is a 2.5-fold increased risk of thrombotic events during pregnancy and a 20-fold increase in the puerperium relative to the risk for nonpregnant women of the same age. Cesarean delivery increases the risk 10 times that of vaginal delivery and the risk also increases with maternal age.

For the clinician faced with the need to use anticoagulation, there are three concerns: the indications, the level of anticoagulation desired, and the agents to achieve anticoagulation. The anticoagulants available are the coumarin derivatives, unfractionated heparin, and low molecular weight heparin (LMWH).

INDICATIONS FOR ANTICOAGULATION AND LEVEL OF ANTICOAGULATION

Thromboembolism

Thromboembolism is one of the leading causes of maternal mortality, occurring in 0.5 to 3 per 1,000 pregnancies. In a study of 35,000 deliveries, there were 20 deep vein thromboses (DVT) and 10 pulmonary emboli (PE) for a 0.09% incidence between 1970 and 1980 (4). The incidence of PE after DVT is dependent on whether there has been adequate treatment. When patients are treated, PE occurs in only 4.5%, with mortality of less than 1%. In the United Kingdom, PE is the leading cause of maternal death (5). In the United States, PE is the second leading cause of death during pregnancy and accounts for 12% of deaths postpartum (6).

Consideration of risk factors goes back at least to Virchow's triad, described in 1856 and consisting of injury to the vessel wall, stasis, and changes in local clotting factors. The triad represents the characteristics predisposing an individual to intravascular coagulation. In pregnancy, veins distend starting in the first trimester, and by the third trimester venous flow velocity is reduced by half in the lower extremities. Levels of several clotting factors increase in pregnancy, whereas there may be decreased fibrinolytic activity. In addition to these risk factors, cesarean section carries a ninefold increased risk over vaginal delivery. Thus, normal pregnancy is a time when at least two elements of Virchow's triad exist. Endothelial damage to pelvic vessels can occur during vaginal or abdominal delivery, setting the stage for the development of thrombosis (5). DVT can be diagnosed by a variety of modalities including clinical presentation, venography, Doppler ultrasonography. Diagnosis is not reviewed in this chapter.

Early data showed that postpartum events were much more frequent than antepartum, but at the time these older studies were published, there was increased use of postpartum bed rest and hospitalization. Currently, antepartum events are at least as common as postpartum events (2). Recently, McColl et al. (7) evaluated risk factors for pregnancy-associated venous thromboembolism. They retrospectively evaluated 72,000 patients in the United Kingdom. There were 62 confirmed venous thrombotic events (51 DVTs, 11 PEs). The incidence of DVT was 0.72 per 1,000 deliveries and PE 0.15 per 1,000 deliveries. Antepartum, the incidence of DVT was 0.50 per 1,000 and PE 0.07 per 1,000. Postpartum incidence of DVT was 0.21 per 1,000 and PE 0.08 per 1,000. Of those affected 28% had no risk factor for the episode, 12% had antithrombin III (ATIII) deficiency; factor V Leiden mutation was found in 8%, and 1% each had a protein C deficiency and antiphospholipid syndrome. The authors derived thrombotic risk based on the population prevalence of each disorder. The risk for an event was one per 437 for those with factor V Leiden mutation, one per 113 for protein C deficiency, one per 2.8 for type I ATIII deficiency, and one per 42 for type II ATIII deficiency.

Treatment of acute DVT includes bed rest with elevation of the involved extremity to promote venous return and decrease edema. Heparin is the acute treatment of choice and reduces the risk of recurrence by 11 to 15 times. Optimal treatment targets an activated partial thromboplastin time (aPTT) of 1.5 to 2.5 times control or a heparin level of 0.3 U/mL. A loading dose of 100 or 150 U/kg for uncomplicated DVT or PE, respectively, can be used with a minimum of 5,000 U. An infusion rate of 15 to 25 U/kg per hour can then be given. aPTTs can be obtained 4 hours

after the loading dose or any changes. When a steady state is achieved, aPTTs can be done daily. After 3 to 5 days, therapy can be switched to subcutaneous heparin in pregnant patients. For nonpregnant patients, warfarin would be the drug of choice. Because of good absorption after subcutaneous delivery, the patient's intravenous daily dose can be divided into two or three boluses to be given every 8 or 12 hours. After DVT, therapy is maintained until 6 to 12 weeks postpartum, and as long as 6 months postpartum after a PE.

For patients with a more remote history of DVT, the risk of recurrence has not been unequivocally established but is estimated at 4% to 15% (8–10). For these women, a prophylactic minidose may be used. The rationale is that it takes less heparin to inhibit factor Xa than to prevent clotting once thrombin has been formed. One standard regime is to administer 5,000 U subcutaneously every 12 hours, with some advocating an increase to 7,500 to 10,000 U twice daily in the second to third trimesters. The higher doses have been shown to provide the same factor Xa suppression in the latter part of pregnancy, but whether more appropriate prophylaxis is provided is not known.

Few or no data exist to guide the clinician on the precise starting time of prophylaxis based on specific histories (Table 24.1).

Valvular Heart Disease

The optimal management of valvular heart disease and specifically pregnant patients with prosthetic valves is controversial. The rate of embryopathy using warfarin is uncertain, with a range of 4% to 67% cited in the literature (11). There have been reports of catastrophic heparin failure leading to maternal and fetal morbidity and mortality. There has been a 4.5-fold increase in valve thrombosis when using heparin versus warfarin, but in eight of 12 cases, there was suboptimal treatment (11). Heparin administered to maintain the aPTT at 1.5 to 2.5 times the control level has failed, resulting in thromboembolic complications in pregnant women with mechanical heart valves (12). The concerns about the adverse effects of warfarin were previously

TABLE 24.1. *Anticoagulation in pregnancy*

Feature	Care in pregnancy
APS with recurrent pregnancy loss or prior fetal death	Heparin prophylactically 15,000–20,000 U/d, administered s.c. in divided doses, and low-dose aspirin
APS with prior thrombotic event	Heparin full anticoagulation or prophylactically 15,000–20,000 U/d
APS without pregnancy loss or thrombosis	Uncertain; options include no treatment, or low-dose aspirin, or prophylactic heparin at 5,000–20,000 U divided q12h and low-dose aspirin with all of the above
Antiphospholipid antibodies without APS	Uncertain; no treatment reasonable, or low-dose aspirin or prophylactic heparin and low-dose aspirin
Other antibodies	Uncertain; no treatment or low-dose aspirin
Previous DVT or PE before current pregnancy	Surveillance with warfarin postpartum for 4–6 wk or heparin 5,000 U q12h with warfarin postpartum or low molecular weight heparin or 5,000 U q12h in 1st and 2nd trimesters and increase in the third to prolong aPTT to 1.5× or 10,000 q12h throughout pregnancy or prophylaxis intrapartum and 6 wk postpartum or 7,500–10,000 U q12h throughout pregnancy with postpartum prophylaxis
DVT or PE during this pregnancy	i.v. heparin then q12h heparin to elevate PTT to therapeutic range
Mechanical heart valves	Heparin to prolong aPTT in therapeutic range or heparin in first trimester and end of third trimester with warfarin (INR 2.5–3.5) other times

APS, antiphospholipid syndrome; DVT, deep vein thromboses; PE, pulmonary embolism; PTT, partial thromboplastin time; aPTT, activated partial thromboplastin time; INR, international normalized ratio. Modified from refs. 10, 16, 30, and 33.

described. There are also concerns that bioprosthetic heart valves may deteriorate at an accelerated rate during pregnancy.

Iturbe-Alessio et al. (13) studied 72 pregnant women with artificial heart valves. Among those who received warfarin, 25% to 30% had embryopathy, but there were fatal valve prosthesis thromboses using low-dose heparin. The authors concluded that low-dose heparin is not appropriate for prophylaxis in patients with heart valves and that warfarin is a teratogen. Similar results were found in a study of 92 pregnancies in 59 women. In 31 women, oral anticoagulants were discontinued when pregnancy was diagnosed and subcutaneous heparin was started with a goal of adjusting the aPTT to two times control. In 61 pregnancies, the oral anticoagulant was continued throughout the first trimester. There was one case of hydrocephalus from a pregnancy maintained on oral anticoagulation. There were more embolic events in the group who received heparin (14).

Ginsberg and Hirsh (15) recommended using a heparin dose to maintain the aPTT at 1.5 times control. However, Salazar et al. (12) had two fatal thromboses using such a protocol, and more recent recommendations suggest the need for more intensive anticoagulation (16).

The controversy over the use of warfarin was stirred up after a report describing 151 pregnan-cies in 133 women with mechanical valves. All thromboses occurred during heparin use. No warfarin embryopathy was seen in 56 women treated with warfarin, and the authors stated that they thought its use in pregnancy was safer than previously thought (17). This recommendation is feared to cause a reemergence of warfarin embryopathy because two cases of embryopathy were described after the increased use of warfarin in pregnant patients with cardiac lesions (18).

Chan et al. (19) reviewed the literature to evaluate reports of oral anticoagulation versus heparin in first-trimester and second/third-trimester oral anticoagulation versus heparin use. Spontaneous abortion occurred in 196 of 792 (24.7%) women using oral anticoagulation alone. Congenital abnormalities were found in 6.4% of the remaining 549 fetuses. The spontaneous loss rate was similar across the groups, but only 3.4% (6/174) using heparin in the first trimester and warfarin later had malformations, and none of the 17 patients who received only heparin had malformations. Conversely, the risk of thromboembolic complications and death was much higher with decreased use of warfarin, and low-dose heparin was associated with a particularly high complication rate and therefore absolutely should not be used as prophylaxis for patients with prosthetic valves.

Lecuru et al. (20) compared women who used heparin during the critical teratogenic period and warfarin in the remainder of the pregnancy versus women who used warfarin more extensively during the pregnancy. In the heparin group, despite attempting to maintain the PTT at two times control, there was one valve thrombosis in 43 patients. The group with more extensive warfarin use had no thromboses, but one of 11 had coumadin embryopathy.

The American College of Chest Physicians offer guidelines about prophylaxis of patients with mechanical prosthetic valves. They recommend heparin every 12 hours to prolong the 6-hour postinjection aPTT into the therapeutic range or heparin up to the 12th week and after the middle of the third trimester until delivery with use of warfarin [target international normalized ratio (INR), 2.5 to 3.5] between these time periods. The higher INR goal is in contrast to most indications for which an INR of 2.0 to 3.0 is appropriate (16,21). Elkayam (22) suggests the use of a higher INR (3 to 4.5) in patients with older, higher risk mechanical valves like Starr-Edwards or Bjork-Shiley in the mitral position.

Although use of warfarin during pregnancy is generally discouraged in publications of the American College of Obstetricians and Gynecologists (23), it is noted that some investigators recommend it after the first trimester in some situations involving artificial heart valves. It is appropriate to fully counsel such a patient concerning the risk to the fetus versus the significant risks to the mother (and therefore fetus) of the different treatment protocols (11). As others have said, a large, prospective, randomized trial to evaluate the efficacy and safety of various anticoagulation regimens to treat pregnant women with heart valves is needed (24).

Inherited Thrombophilias

In a general outpatient population presenting with an objectively documented DVT, the prevalence of deficiencies of ATIII, protein C, or protein S is relatively low. These conditions tend to be identified among younger patients and those with recurrent thrombotic events. Resistance to activated protein C, usually owing to the factor

V Leiden mutation, can be present in as many as 20% to 50% of patients in some populations presenting with venous thrombosis. These conditions are usually inherited in autosomal dominant fashion. The risk of thrombosis is approximately 2% to 4% per year after age 15 years, so that by 50 years of age, 50% to 70% of patients will develop a thrombosis (25). After diagnosis, a family evaluation should be encouraged as other affected individuals may be found. Long-term warfarin therapy is usually not recommended until at least one event has occurred. With a history of two or more thrombotic events, life-time oral anticoagulation is suggested.

In pregnancy, ATIII deficiency has the highest risk of thrombotic complications of the inherited thrombophilias. Without prophylaxis, 18% of those with ATIII deficiency had thrombotic events versus 7% for protein C deficiency and none in 17 cases of protein S deficiency. Postpartum thrombosis developed in 33%, 19%, and 17%, respectively. ATIII deficiency has a prevalence between one per 600 and one per 5,000 and is caused by one of more than 80 mutations. Protein S and C deficiencies have a prevalence of approximately 1 per 500 (26,27).

The concentration of these factors can change in pregnancy, making diagnosis of a thrombophilia problematic. Although protein C changes little, both free and total protein S fall appreciably (28).

The Leiden mutation of blood coagulation factor V is the most common genetic abnormality associated with venous thromboembolism and is found in approximately 5% of Caucasian people. There is still much to learn about this genetic alteration because, although it increases the risk of DVT, it appears to be protective against pulmonary embolism (29).

The congenital thrombophilias have also been associated with increased risk of fetal loss and other adverse outcomes such as growth restriction and preeclampsia (5).

Although treatment with heparin during pregnancy is suggested, an optimal dose is not known. Depending on level of risk, full anticoagulation (to a aPTT of 1.5 times control), low-dose heparin, and even observation without anticoagulation have been suggested.

Antiphospholipid Syndrome

Antiphospholipid syndrome (APS) is an autoimmune condition. Diagnosis of APS is made in a patient with one or more specific clinical signs (recurrent pregnancy loss, venous or arterial thrombosis, or autoimmune thrombocytopenia) combined with the appropriate laboratory abnormality (presence of the lupus anticoagulant using one of several clotting assays such as aPTT and/or presence of anticardiolipin antibodies, generally of the IgG type) (30).

Although there is clear evidence supporting anticoagulation for the patient with a previous thrombotic event and use of low-dose or therapeutic heparin for the patient with previous pregnancy loss, whether to treat the patient with laboratory findings but one loss or none is not straightforward. It is also common to see patients with antibodies but no definitive evidence of the clinical criteria for APS. These patients can either be left untreated or given low-dose aspirin. There is clear evidence that use of heparin and aspirin provides the most protection against pregnancy loss when APS is present. Low-dose heparin (10,000 U every 12 hours) and aspirin versus high-dose heparin (approximately 20,000 U every 12 hours) were compared. The low dose was meant to keep the PTT in the upper normal range, whereas the high dose was adjusted to a PTT of 1.2 to 1.5 times control. The rate of livebirths was similar in both groups and between 76% and 80% (31). The heparin component, however, may be the sole source of this improvement. We reserve use of both heparin and aspirin only for the most clear-cut and high-risk cases. A pregnancy-related death was reported for a woman treated with heparin and aspirin after *in vitro* fertilization. She had no prolongation of her clotting parameters but had a lethal intracranial hemorrhage (32).

ANTICOAGULANTS

Coumarin Derivatives

Warfarin sodium (Coumadin) is a coumarin anticoagulant that is administered orally and works by depressing vitamin K–dependent clotting factors (II, VII, IX, and X). It interferes with the cyclic interconversion of vitamin K and its 2,3-epoxide, thus inhibiting the carboxylation of the glutamic acid residues of the vitamin K–dependent factors. This interferes with the ability of these factors to bind calcium or phospholipids, resulting in defective hemostasis. Warfarin also limits activation of the anticoagulant proteins C and S (33). It has a low molecular weight and therefore readily crosses the placenta, potentially resulting in teratogenic and other fetal effects (34).

The effectiveness of warfarin anticoagulation is measured by use of the prothrombin time (PT), which is expressed as an INR, making comparison between laboratories possible and accurate. Factor VII and protein C have short half-lives (6 to 8 hours) and their levels fall first after initiation of warfarin. Thus, there may be an initial hypercoagulable state. Also the anticoagulant effect precedes the antithrombotic effect by approximately 24 hours. For these reasons, loading with warfarin has been abandoned as ineffective and potentially unsafe.

DiSaia (35) reported the first case of teratogenicity due to warfarin in 1966. The patient had a Starr-Edwards mitral valve prosthesis and was treated with warfarin throughout most of the pregnancy. The term infant weighed 2,275 g and had nasal obstruction secondary to hypoplasia of the nasal structures as well as bilateral optic atrophy, blindness, and mental retardation. Three reports simultaneously recognized this association as fetal warfarin syndrome in 1975 (36–38). In 1980, Hall et al. (39) reviewed all published and communicated cases. They found 418 pregnancies complicated by coumarin use. One sixth of the livebirths had abnormalities, one in six of the pregnancies ended in stillbirth or spontaneous abortion, and approximately two thirds had a normal outcome. For the 45 pregnancies with only first-trimester exposure, 31 had some type of problem including 22 (49%) abortions and nine (20%) with a malformation. For those with isolated second- and/or third-trimester exposure, the overall problem rate was 20% to 30%, but this was not further defined as to losses versus malformations. At least one source (40) states that based on three prospective studies of women exposed only in the second and third trimesters, the incidence of malformations in this group must be exceedingly low as there was no evidence of fetal/neonatal CNS or eye abnormalities. Warfarin embryopathy, similar to the X-linked chondrodysplasia punctata (CDPX), has been reported in as many as 67% of fetuses exposed between the sixth and twelfth weeks of gestation. This may be owing to inhibition of arylsulfatase E by warfarin. Deficiency of arylsulfatase E is responsible for CDPX. The period between the sixth and ninth weeks is particularly critical. This fetal warfarin syndrome consists of nasal hypoplasia, depressed nasal bridge, often with a deep groove between the alae and nasal tip, stippled epiphyses, nail hypoplasia, mental retardation, and growth restriction. Second- and third-trimester exposure can also lead to fetal effects secondary to bleeding and includes CNS and eye abnormalities such as microcephaly, blindness, deafness, and growth restriction.

Although the American College of Obstetricians and Gynecologists (41) suggests women taking warfarin consider switching to heparin before conception, we suggest counseling the patient to either use effective contraception or report for prenatal care with a missed or late menses to allow time to switch from warfarin to heparin before the 6- to 12-week window. Conception can take a lengthy period of time, and for some patients, the use of heparin without a confirmed pregnancy can be both inconvenient and dangerous (as in the case of mechanical heart valves). The Australasian Society of Thrombosis and Haemostasis mentions pregnancy in its consensus guidelines for warfarin therapy but does not offer specific suggestions for anticoagulation of pregnant women with mechanical heart valves (42).

The precise effect of warfarin has been difficult to determine because patients have been treated with different doses and a clinical geneticist may not have examined the child for mild abnormalities. The embryopathy may affect as few as 5% to 10% of fetuses exposed in the first trimester, although others cite that as many as one third to two thirds of all exposed fetuses can be affected. Twenty-two women with prosthetic heart valves delivered 29 liveborn infants between 1978 and 1989. When warfarin was ad-

ministered throughout the pregnancy ($n = 18$), the rate of nasal hypoplasia was 66% and hypertelorism 61% (43). In a review of 1,325 pregnancies in 186 studies, a 16.9% incidence of adverse outcomes was reported with use of warfarin. The discrepant results in terms of the number of exposed fetuses exhibiting the embryopathy may be owing to treatment at different times in pregnancy with different doses. There is some evidence that a lower dose may have less teratogenic potential (44). Further, the studies differ in how thoroughly evidence of teratogenic features is sought and whether a dysmorphologist is involved in the study. Finally, studies that do not include close evaluation of abortus material may underestimate the teratogenic effects. In the United States and elsewhere, warfarin is reserved for pregnant women with mechanical heart valves at high risk of failure if other agents are used.

Some drugs can influence the pharmacokinetics of warfarin. Carbamazepine, barbiturates, phenytoin, nafcillin, dicloxacillin, and smoking generally cause a need for an increase in dose of warfarin (21).

Warfarin activity has not been found in breast milk or infant circulation and is thus approved as compatible with breast-feeding by the American Academy of Pediatricians (http://www.aap.org/policy/00026t6.htm).

Unfractionated Heparin

Unfractionated heparin has a molecular weight of 20,000 to as high as 40,000 and is highly charged. These characteristics prevent heparin from crossing the placenta. It is not associated with adverse fetal effects. Heparin is a glycosaminoglycan and it has high-affinity binding to AT. It is composed of chains of alternating residues of D-glucosamine and a uronic acid (21). This causes a conformational change in AT that increases its ability to inactivate the coagulation factors IIa (thrombin), Xa, and IXa.

Unfractionated heparin must be administered parenterally and is associated with a few complications. Heparin-induced thrombocytopenia can occur in as many as 3% at 2 weeks. Heparin-induced osteoporosis resulting in symptomatic fractures can occur in 2.2%. As many as 17% of pregnant women treated with prophylactic heparin may develop osteopenia.

Pregnant women require a greater amount of heparin than nonpregnant women to achieve the same level of anticoagulation. Further, an increasing dose is needed as pregnancy advances. There is less bioavailability when given subcutaneously versus intravenously (45).

Bleeding complications have been reported in as many as 5% to 10% of patients receiving standard unfractionated heparin but is most likely closer to the 2% reported in the nonpregnant population and similar to the rate reported with use of warfarin (10). If rapid reversal of the anticoagulation is needed to treat serious bleeding, protamine sulfate can be administered as a slow intravenous injection over 10 minutes. Each milligram neutralizes approximately 100 U heparin and more than 50 mg protamine should not be administered as a single dose or 100 mg over a short period of time (9).

A review of anticoagulation in pregnancy identified 1,325 pregnancies. It found that the reported high rates of adverse fetal/infant outcomes associated with heparin use during pregnancy were largely owing to comorbid conditions of the mother and not the heparin itself (15).

Although heparin is compatible with breastfeeding, most patients who require continued anticoagulation will be switched to oral anticoagulants postpartum.

Low Molecular Weight Heparin

LMWH is fragments of unfractionated heparin produced by controlled enzymatic or chemical depolymerization that yields chains with a mean molecular weight of 5,000. LMWH also functions by activating AT but is thought to produce a more predictable anticoagulant response because of better bioavailability, longer half-life, and a dose-dependent clearance. LMWH has been shown to have a comparable or better effect than that of unfractionated or standard heparin as thromboprophylaxis for general surgical procedures, orthopedic procedures of the lower limb including total hip and knee replacements, and hip fractures. The benefits that have been

ascribed to LMWH include an easier dosing regime and less thrombocytopenia, and one paper stated it to be the anticoagulant of choice in pregnancy (46), although no data were provided or are, in fact, available to support that statement.

The American College of Obstetricians and Gynecologists (47) stated that experience with LMWH use during pregnancy supports the conclusions that patients with history of thromboembolic events or thrombophilic disorders can be treated as effectively with LMWH as with traditional heparin and that ease of administration and less need for laboratory monitoring may provide advantages. Further, there is no greater risk of bone demineralization. LMWH is four to six times more costly, but the ease of use and less need for laboratory monitoring may compensate for this cost difference. There are inadequate data to suggest use with mechanical heart valves. Use of regional anesthesia may be limited because of the possibility of epidural hematomas. LMWH has less binding to platelets, which may theoretically decrease the risk of thrombocytopenia and less binding to osteoblasts may reduce the risk of osteopenia (45).

Although LMWH is very much an acceptable alternative to unfractionated heparin, many questions require additional study. Lev-Ran et al. (48) reported failure of enoxaparin at 40 mg per day to prevent valve thrombosis in a pregnant patient. This report was severely criticized in the accompanying editorial for failure to use the appropriate dose of 1 mg/kg every 12 hours. As recently as 1999, review of the published data on LMWH in pregnancy concluded that there were insufficient data on the efficacy of LMWH versus unfractionated heparin in terms of the impact on thrombocytopenia and bone loss, other adverse reactions, whether monitoring of anti-Xa activity is needed, and, given the greater expense of LMWH, which is more cost-effective (49).

Although initially touted for once per day dosing, there is evidence that a sustained 24-hour elevation of the anti-Xa level may require injections every 12 hours, particularly in late pregnancy (26). Others have shown that the anti-Xa level falls with increasing weight of the patient (50).

Overall LMWH has appeared safe in the management of more than 480 pregnancies (51). In one study, both LMWH heparin ($n = 50$) and LMWH ($n = 55$) completely prevented thrombotic events in women with previous or current thromboembolisms. LMWH does not appear to cross the placenta and should therefore not pose a teratogenic risk (52).

SUMMARY

Use of anticoagulants is common in pregnancy and fraught with controversy. Generally heparin, unfractionated or LMWH, is used. In the case of maternal mechanical heart valves, the patient should be counseled about the risks and benefits of the various treatment options as no clear consensus is available to guide treatment.

Other conditions warranting treatment include a history of DVT, PE, thrombophilia, or APS. The suggestions that make the most sense involve stratifying patients based on underlying risk of a thrombotic event and treating accordingly. Using a variety of sources, general guidelines can be provided to cover most situations (Table 24.1).

Both heparin and coumadin are compatible with breast-feeding.

REFERENCES

1. Berg CJ, Atrash HK, Koonin LM, et al. Pregnancy-related mortality in the United States, 1987–1990. *Obstet Gynecol* 1996;88:161–167.
2. Warkany J. Warfarin embryopathy. *Teratology* 1976; 14:205–209.
3. Bonnar J. Can more be done in obstetric and gynecologic practice to reduce morbidity and mortality associated with venous thromboembolism? *Am J Obstet Gynecol* 1999;180:784–791.
4. Letsky E, de Swiet M. Thromboembolism in pregnancy and its management. *Br J Haematol* 1984;57:543–552.
5. Greer IA. Thrombosis in pregnancy: maternal and fetal issues. *Lancet* 1999;353:1258–1265.
6. Pettila V, Kaaja R, Leinonen P, et al. Thromboprophylaxis with low molecular weight heparin (dalteparin) in pregnancy. *Thromb Res* 1999;96:275–282.
7. McColl MD, Ramsay JE, Tait RC, et al. Risk factors for pregnancy associated venous thromboembolism. *Thromb Haemost* 1997;78:1183–1188.
8. Dizon-Townson D, Branch DW. Anticoagulant treatment during pregnancy: an update. *Semin Thromb Hemost* 1998;24:55–62.
9. Brown HL, Bobrowski RA. Anticoagulation. *Clin Obstet Gynecol* 1998;41:545–554.
10. Ginsberg JS. Thromboembolism and pregnancy. *Thromb Haemost* 1999;82:620–625.
11. Frewin R, Chisholm M. Anticoagulation of women with prosthetic heart valves during pregnancy. *Br J Obstet Gynaecol* 1998;105:683–686.
12. Salazar E, Izaguirre R, Verdejo J, et al. Failure of adjusted doses of subcutaneous heparin to prevent thromboembolic phenomena in pregnant patients with mechanical cardiac valve prostheses. *J Am Coll Cardiol* 1966;27:1698–1703.
13. Iturbe-Alessio I, del Carmen Fonseca M, Mutchinik O, et al. Risks of anticoagulant therapy in pregnant women with artificial heart valves. *N Engl J Med* 1986;315:1390–1393.
14. Meschengieser SS, Fondevila CG, Santarelli MT, et al. Anticoagulation in pregnant women with mechanical heart valve prostheses. *Heart* 1999;82:23–26.
15. Ginsberg JS, Hirsh J, Turner DC, et al. Risks to the fetus of anticoagulant therapy during pregnancy. *Thromb Haemost* 1989;61:197–203.
16. Ginsberg JS, Hirsh J. Use of antithrombotic agents during pregnancy. *Chest* 1998;114:524S–530S.
17. Sbarouni E, Oakley CM. Outcome of pregnancy in women with valve prostheses. *Br Heart J* 1994;71:196–201.
18. Wellesley D, Joore I, Heard M, et al. Two cases of warfarin embryopathy: a re-emergence of this condition. *Br J Obstet Gynaecol* 1998;105:805–806.
19. Chan WS, Anand S, Ginsberg JS. Anticoagulation of pregnant women with mechanical heart valves. *Arch Intern Med* 2000;160:191–196.
20. Lecuru F, Desnos M, Taurell R. Anticoagulant therapy in pregnancy. Report of 54 cases. *Acta Obstet Gynecol Scand* 1996;75:217–221.
21. Hirsch J, Dalen JE, Anderson DR, et al. Oral anticoagulants: mechanism of action, clinical effectiveness, and optimal therapeutic range. *Chest* 1998;114:445S–469S.
22. Elkayam U. Pregnancy through a prosthetic heart valve. *J Am Coll Cardiol* 1999;33:1642–1645.
23. American College of Obstetricians and Gynecologists. Thromboembolism in pregnancy. *ACOG Pract Bull* 2000;19:1–10.
24. Elkayam U. Anticoagulation in pregnant women with prosthetic heart valves: a double jeopardy. *J Am Coll Cardiol* 1996;27:1705–1706.
25. Bauer KA. Management of patients with hereditary defects predisposing to thrombosis including pregnant women. *Thromb Haemost* 1995;74:94–100.
26. Bonnar J, Green R, Norris L. Inherited thrombophilia and pregnancy: the obstetric perspective. *Semin Thromb Hemost* 1998;24:49–53.
27. Bonnar J, Green R, Norris L. Perinatal aspects of inherited thrombophilia. *Semin Thromb Hemost* 1999;25:481–485.
28. Clark P, Brennand J, Conkle JA, et al. Activated protein C sensitivity, protein C, protein S and coagulation in normal pregnancy. *Thromb Haemost* 1998;79:1166–1170.
29. Bounameaux H. Factor V Leiden paradox: risk of deep-vein thrombosis but not of pulmonary embolism. *Lancet* 2000;356:182–183.
30. American College of Obstetricians and Gynecologists. Antiphospholipid syndrome. *ACOG Educ Bull* 1998; 244:1–10.
31. Kutteh WH, Ermel LD. A clinical trial for the treatment of antiphospholipid antibody-associated recurrent pregnancy loss with lower dose heparin and aspirin. *Am J Reprod Immunol* 1996;35:402–407.

32. Anonymous. From the Centers for Disease Control and Prevention. Pregnancy-related death associated with heparin and aspirin treatment for infertility. *JAMA* 1996;279:1860–1861.

33. Barbour LA. Current concepts of anticoagulant therapy in pregnancy. *Obstet Gynecol Clin N Am* 1997;24: 499–521.

34. Ramin SM, Ramin KD, Gilstrap LC. Anticoagulants and thrombolytics during pregnancy. *Semin Perinatol* 1997;21:149–153.

35. DiSaia PJ. Pregnancy and delivery of a patient with Starr-Edwards mitral valve prosthesis. *Obstet Gynecol* 1966;28:469–472.

36. Becker MH, Genieser NB, Finegold M, et al. Chondrodysplasia punctata. Is warfarin therapy a factor? *Am J Dis Child* 1975;129:356–359.

37. Shaul WL, Emery H, Hall JG. Chondrodysplasia punctata and maternal warfarin use during pregnancy. *Am J Dis Child* 1975;129:360–362.

38. Pettifor JM, Benson R. Congenital malformation associated with the administration of oral anticoagulants during pregnancy. *J Pediatr* 1975;86:459–462.

39. Hall JG, Pauli RM, Wilson KM. Maternal and fetal sequelae of anticoagulation during pregnancy. *Am J Med* 1980;68:122–140.

40. Jones KL. *Smith's recognizable patterns of human malformation,* 5th ed. Philadelphia: WB Saunders, 1997.

41. American College of Obstetricians and Gynecologists. Preconceptional care. *ACOG Tech Bull* 1995;205:1–6.

42. Gallus AS, Baker RI, Chong BH, et al. Consensus guidelines for warfarin therapy. Recommendations from the Australasian Society of Thrombosis and Haemostasis. *Med J Aust* 2000;172:600–605.

43. Wong V, Cheng CH, Chan KC. Fetal and neonatal outcome of exposure to anticoagulants during pregnancy. *Am J Med Genet* 1993;45:17–21.

44. Vitale N, De Feo M, De Santo LS, et al. Dose-dependent fetal complications of warfarin in pregnant women with mechanical heart valves. *J Am Coll Cardiol* 1999;33:1637–1641.

45. Hirsch J, Warkentin TE, Raschke R, et al. Heparin and low-molecular-weight heparin: mechanisms of action, pharmacodynamics, dosing considerations, monitoring, efficacy, and safety. *Chest* 1998;114:489S–510S.

46. Weitz JI. Low-molecular-weight heparins. *N Engl J Med* 1997;337:688–698.

47. American College of Obstetricians and Gynecologists. Anticoagulation with low-molecular-weight heparin during pregnancy. ACOG Committee Opinion 1998;211:1–2.

48. Lev-Ran O, Kramer A, Gurevitch J, et al. Low-molecular-weight heparin for prosthetic heart valves. treatment failure. *Ann Thorac Surg* 2000;69:264–266.

49. Ensom MHH, Stephenson MD. Low-molecular-weight heparins in pregnancy. *Pharmacotherapy* 1999;19:1013–1025.

50. Crowther MA, Spitzer K, Julian J, et al. Pharmacokinetic profile of a low-molecular-weight heparin (reviparin) in pregnant patients. A prospective cohort study. *Thromb Res* 2000;98:133–138.

51. Sanson BJ, Lensing AW, Prins MH, et al. Safety of low-molecular-weight heparin in pregnancy: a systematic review. *Thromb Haemost* 1999;81:668–672.

52. Melissari E, Parker CJ, Wilson NV, et al. Use of low molecular weight heparin in pregnancy. *Thromb Haemost* 1992;68:652–656.

25

Poisoning During Pregnancy and Lactation

Alfredo F. Gei and George R. Saade

Department of Obstetrics and Gynecology, The University of Texas Medical Branch at Galveston, Galveston, Texas

INTRODUCTION

Scope of the Problem

It is estimated that 4.6 million poisonings occur per year in the United States, for a rate of nine per 1,000 population (1). A little more than 50% of the toxic exposures in 1998 occurred in women, and more than 300,000 took place in women of reproductive age. Although overall toxic exposures are more frequent in children, the age distribution of the fatal exposures peaks in the late reproductive years (1).

In 1998, 8,120 poisonings during pregnancy were reported to the 65 Poison Control Centers in the United States, with about an equal distribution among the trimesters (1). The number of toxic exposures accounted for by pregnant patients has increased since 1993 in parallel with the total number of exposures reported (Table 25.1).

Emergency department studies have shown that as many as 6.3% of the female patients may have an unrecognized pregnancy (2). For this reason, it has been recommended that a pregnancy test should be part of the evaluation of any woman of childbearing age presenting with an overdose or poisoning (3).

Pregnancy and Medications

Despite the reluctance that most pregnant women have toward the use of medications, pregnancy, independently of comorbid conditions, increases the average intake of medications (4). Pregnancy is therefore a time of predisposition for adverse effects of medications, including overdosing.

Over a 12-year period, poisoning was the leading cause of hospitalization for injury among pregnant women (5).

Fortunately, the incidence of poisoning during pregnancy is low (Table 25.1). Women are most likely aware of the potential adverse effects of medications on the fetus and wish to maximize fetal well-being (6,7). The incidence of intentional toxic exposures is higher among women carrying unwanted pregnancies, after voluntary terminations, or after delivering a stillbirth (6,8,9).

Toxicologic Considerations in Pregnancy

The poisoned pregnant woman poses particular challenges to obstetricians, emergency department physicians, and toxicology experts. These challenges are related to the variability of physiologic changes of pregnancy on absorption, distribution, and metabolism of different potentially toxic agents (10–12). Table 25.2 summarizes the most important gestational changes affecting the diagnosis or treatment of poisoning in pregnant patients.

In addition to the physiologic changes, immediate, latent, and delayed fetal effects must be considered. Once the acute maternal condition is addressed and resolved, a specific discussion regarding these fetal effects and short- or long-term follow-up is warranted. Often the maternal effects are limited to the immediate period after poisoning, but fetal effects can progress as a result of continued exposure to circulating metabolites or toxic compounds

TABLE 25.1. *Toxic exposures reported to Poison Control Centers in the United States: 1993–1998*

Year	Total	N (%) Pregnant	1st trim. (%)	2nd trim. (%)	3rd trim. (%)
1993	1,751,476	6,443 (0.36)	32	38	30
1994	1,926,438	6,147 (0.32)	31	38	31
1995	2,023,089	6,484 (0.32)	30	39	31
1996	2,155,952	7,103 (0.33)	30	39	31
1997	2,192,088	7,250 (0.33)	31	38	31
1998	2,241,082	8,120 (0.36)	32	38	30

Trim., trimester.

Between 1993 and 1998, the number of toxic exposures reported by pregnant women represents only a fraction of all the exposures. During this period, both the total of exposures and the ones reported by pregnant women increased steadily by a factor of 1.6% to 10% per year. The distribution of toxic exposures per trimester of pregnancy has been stable over the past 6 years, with a slightly higher predominance of the second over the other two trimesters.

Data from 1998, 1997, 1996, 1995, 1994, and 1993 Annual Reports of the American Association of Poison Control Centers Toxic Exposure Surveillance System.

released from body stores. Although the maternal condition stabilizes, the continued risk to the fetus requires long-term follow-up (13–15).

There is little information on the appropriate treatment of poisoning in pregnancy, and the use of antidotes raises ethical and medicolegal questions (16). Several instances have been reported in which treatment was withheld from women because of pregnancy, with catastrophic results for both mother and fetus (17–19).

TABLE 25.2. *Physiologic changes of pregnancy and their toxicologic impact*

System	Gestational change	Toxicologic implication
Digestive	Pica, decreased intraesophageal pressure, delayed gastric emptying, delayed transit time, hepatic flow unchanged, reduced hepatic enzymatic activity	Pros: window of opportunity for gastric lavage potentially longer Cons: increased risk of exposure, increased gastric absorption, increased risk of aspiration, increased enteral absorption, increased risk of hepatotoxicity
Respiratory	Hyperemia of upper respiratory tract, increased minute ventilation, decreased residual lung volume, increased diffusing capacity	Pros: higher sensitivity to hypoxemia and hypercarbia (protective against respiratory depression) Cons: increased absorption of inhaled agents
Circulatory	30–50% increase in cardiac output, 50% increase in plasma volume, 25% decrease in serum albumin, increased oxygen consumption	Pros: dilutional effect Cons: higher concentrations in organs with rich perfusion (uterus, placental bed, kidneys, skin), higher free fraction of toxins and greater placental passage
Renal	Increase in glomerular filtration rate, increased tubular reabsorption	Pros: increased renal clearance of protein bound and unbound substances Cons: increased nephrotoxicity potential
Skin	Increased surface, increased blood flow	Cons: increased absorption of contact agents
Uterus/placenta	Volume increased by 2,000% at term, increased blood perfusion, pronounced liposolubility	Pros: maternal protection for certain exposures Cons: fetal exposure to toxic agents
Others Body mass Oxygen consumption Fat	 Increased by 25% at term Increased by 20% Increased storage, third-trimester mobilization	Pros: larger distribution volumes Cons: potential for reexposure during third trimester

Data from refs. 10–12.

There are approximately 250,000 substances that are potentially toxic to humans (20). We provide an overview of the agents most commonly responsible for lethal exposure in the United States (1) as applies to the pregnant or lactating woman, fetus, and newborn. For more detailed information about these agents, as well as others not covered here, a list of suggested readings and resources is provided at the end of the chapter.

A FEW DEFINITIONS

Although the terms, *poisoning* and *overdose* are frequently used interchangeably, poisoning denotes the morbid state produced by a toxic agent (poison) causing a functional disturbance (e.g., renal failure or hepatitis) and/or structural damage (e.g., chemical burn). Overdose or overdosage refers to a state produced by excess or abuse of a drug or substance (21). Consequently, overdoses can be considered as a particular type of poisoning.

EVALUATION OF THE POISONED PREGNANT PATIENT

Although both the poisoning and the pregnancy may not be apparent at initial presentation, the most common scenario is that of a second-trimester pregnant woman with a history of an acute exposure to a known toxic agent. The ideal setting for the evaluation of these patients is the emergency department, as the situation can range from very straightforward and of no consequence to life-threatening and complex requiring a multidisciplinary team and elaborate forms of treatment. The algorithms presented here (Figs. 25.1 and 25.2) summarize our guidelines for evaluation and management of pregnant patients with a known or suspected toxic exposure, regardless of the agent(s) in question. The most relevant aspects of the algorithms, noted by numbers, are discussed.

Initial Evaluation

The initial assessment (Fig. 25.1) consists of rapidly determining whether the patient is conscious or unconscious. If unconscious, is she in cardiac or respiratory arrest? The management (Fig. 25.2) of the unconscious pregnant patient differs little from nonpregnant patients with the exception of two considerations:

1. Special positioning with a pelvic tilt to the left and/or manual displacement of the uterus off the midline to the left is recommended to relieve the aortocaval compression by the gravid uterus and improve venous blood return.
2. Prompt consultation with the obstetric service as these patients need an expert assessment of gestational age with the capability to proceed with a bedside cesarean section if the resuscitative efforts are not successful within 5 minutes of the cardiac arrest (Fig. 25.2) (22).

The rapid removal of all clothes (including footwear) is critical. The personnel involved in the patient care should handle the clothes with gloves and set them aside in a labeled plastic bag. Absorption of toxins, organic chemicals, and industrial compounds through the skin is generally the rule rather than the exception. The garments can potentially be used for sampling later and should not be disposed of (21).

In the unconscious patient with history of or suspected toxic exposure, trauma should be strongly considered and the cervical spine should be stabilized until evaluated and cleared (23).

Altered Mental Status

If the patient is unconscious but hemodynamically stable or conscious but disoriented, the diagnosis of altered mental status is made.

Hypoxemia and hypoglycemia should immediately be considered as possible etiologies and oxygen and a parenteral glucose infusion (50 g of 50% intravenous glucose) started without delay, even before the diagnosis is confirmed through an arterial blood gas (ABG) and a glucose determination (23,24). Forcing oral intake in a patient with altered mental status is actively discouraged.

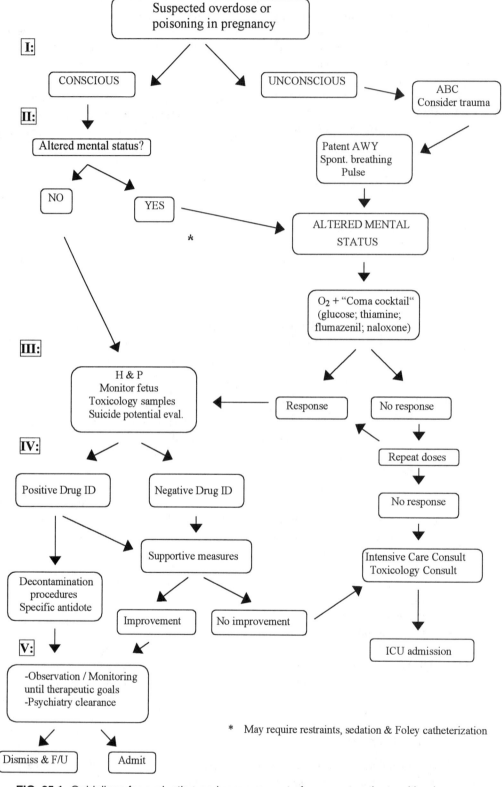

FIG. 25.1. Guidelines for evaluation and management of pregnant patients with a known or suspected toxic exposure.

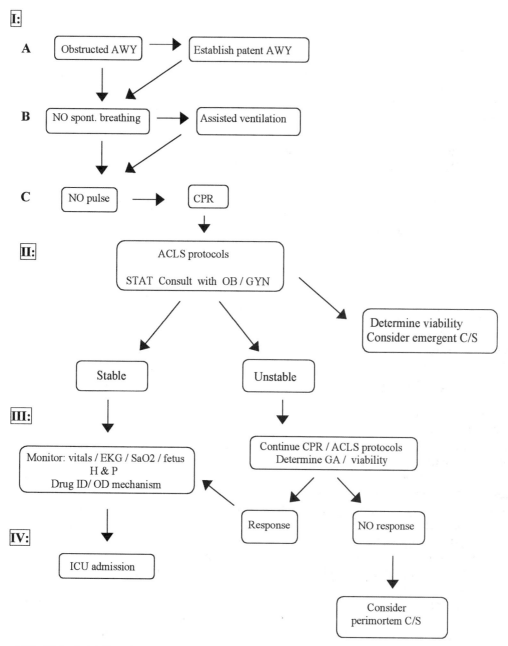

FIG. 25.2. Guidelines for the evaluation of the unconscious pregnant patient with a known or suspected toxic exposure.

The use of padded restraints, the insertion of an indwelling bladder catheter, and intravenous sedation may be required for the management of uncooperative and belligerent patients. The use of sedatives should ideally be delayed until the toxic agent(s) of exposure is identified to avoid unforeseeable interactions and possibly compound central nervous system (CNS) depression.

Other components of the so-called "coma cocktail" (thiamine, naloxone, and flumazenil) should not be given routinely but as considered appropriate by the treating physicians. Specific recommendations for their use are (25–27):

Naloxone (Narcan): Altered mental status and miosis, respiratory rate of 12 or less or circumstantial evidence of opioid use.

Thiamine: Altered mental status and suspected thiamine deficiency (ethanol abuse, malnutrition, hyperemesis gravidarum, eating disorders, TPN, acquired immunodeficiency syndrome, cancer, dialysis patients).

Flumazenil (Romazicon): Altered mental status, suspected or known benzodiazepine exposure, and no contraindications such as use of benzodiazepines for seizure control, coexposure to tricyclics, or head injury.

No epidemiologic studies of the relationship of use of naloxone, thiamine, or flumazenil during pregnancy with resultant congenital malformations are available. Therefore, these agents would be appropriate for the acutely ill parturient.

Secondary Evaluation

Every effort should be made to obtain as much information from as many sources as possible (the patient, her relatives or friends, any witnesses, and the paramedic personnel if she was brought by ambulance). Besides the obstetric and general history, specific information that needs to be obtained regarding the toxic exposure include time of exposure, substances exposed to, amount of exposure (including strength of prescription, if pills or medications), route of exposure, treatment before arrival (including emetics, diluents, and adsorbents), vomitus (number of times and content), diarrhea (number of times and content), and symptoms.

A high degree of caution needs to be exercised with the interpretation of the histories, as the information obtained can be contradictory and, in the case of suicide attempts/gestures, deceitful. As a rule of thumb, the worse scenario (most severe history of exposure) obtained should be used as a clinical parameter.

The collection of samples for toxicologic analysis is of paramount importance in the identification of the toxic agent(s). As a general rule,

at least one sample of all biologic fluids obtained should be saved for toxicologic analysis. Depending on the clinical circumstances, this will include blood, urine, saliva, vomit, gastric lavage material, feces, cerebrospinal fluid, amniotic fluid if collected, breast milk, and meconium if the patient delivers soon after admission (28–30).

Toxic Identification

The mainstay of treatment for all poisonings is supportive measures. For some toxic agents, three additional actions can be implemented to (a) decrease the exposure (decontamination procedures), (b) enhance elimination (diuresis, hemofiltration, hemoperfusion, hemodialysis, plasmapheresis), and (c) counteract the toxicity of the agent (antidotes) (21,31). All these types of measures have their specific indications.

Decontamination Procedures

Skin (21,32)

Substances that can cause significant systemic toxicity through transdermal absorption include organophosphate insecticides, organochlorines, nitrates, and industrial aromatic hydrocarbons. Organophosphates in particular can pass through intact skin at a remarkable speed and without causing any specific skin sensation of burning or itching. Given the physiologic increase in skin perfusion throughout gestation (Table 25.2), pregnancy would theoretically contribute to increased toxicity by this route.

The skin should be flushed thoroughly with warm soapy water. It may be worthwhile to use an industrial shower (as is used for corrosive exposure) to thoroughly rinse the entire body. Be generous both with volume and velocity of irrigation.

A rare exception to immediate decontamination with water would be exposure to agents that react violently with water (e.g., the chemical may ignite, explode, or produce toxic fumes if contact with water occurs). Examples of such chemicals include chlorosulfonic acid, titanium tetrachloride, and calcium oxide.

Gastrointestinal (21,32–34)

Several strategies exist for decontamination of the gastrointestinal (GI) tract.

Dilution. Lacking other alternatives (see below), 200 to 300 mL of milk may be given orally (but not through gastric tubes) when ingestion of caustic chemicals (acids or alkalis) is suspected.

Emesis. After lavage, emesis is considered the second choice for gastric emptying. The dose in adults is 30 mL ipecac with water and repeated in 15 to 30 minutes if vomiting is not induced. It is indicated in ingestion of drugs that can form gastric concretions (e.g., salicylates, meprobamate, barbiturates, glutethimide) or delay gastric emptying (e.g., tricyclics, narcotics, salicylates) or in conditions producing adynamic ileus. Its use is controversial for the following reasons:

1. Not immediately effective.
2. The effect may persist for 2 hours, delaying the administration of adsorbents.
3. With exceptions, it is unlikely to be effective after 1 to 2 hours after ingestion.
4. It has not been proven to be better than lavage.
5. Several contraindications are caustic ingestion, altered mental status, inability to protect airway, seizures or seizure potential, hemorrhagic diathesis, hematemesis, ingestion of drugs that can lead to rapid change in the patient's condition (tricyclics, beta-blockers, phencyclidine, isoniazid).
6. It has no value in ethanol intoxication and the ingestion of some hydrocarbons.
7. In case of failure to induce emesis (approximately 5% of cases), the stomach should be evacuated by other means because ipecac can be cardiotoxic (theoretical risk).

The frequency of congenital anomalies was no greater than expected among the infants of 68 women who took ipecac during the first 4 lunar months or among the infants of 379 women who used the drug anytime during pregnancy in the Collaborative Perinatal Project (35).

Gastric Lavage. Use of gastric lavage is indicated when emesis is inappropriate or contraindicated, the patient is comatose or mentally altered, or the substance ingested can cause seizures or is lethal and rapidly absorbed (i.e., delay while waiting for emesis can result in death). It is also contraindicated in cases of ingestion of caustics and in hemorrhagic diathesis. It has the advantages that it can be performed immediately on arrival of the patient, takes only 15 to 20 minutes to complete, and facilitates the administration of charcoal.

A large gastric tube (Ewald, Lavaculator, or others) size 36 to 40 F should be passed orally with lubricant. Consideration for intubation needs to be made in patients with depressed mental status, altered gag reflex, or seizures or seizure potential. The patient needs to be placed in the Trendelenburg or sitting position and aspiration before lavage needs to be made to confirm placement of the tube and collect a sample for analysis. Lavage is done with normal saline or water in runs of 1.5 mL/kg (up to 200 mL) until clear and then with at least 1 L more. Some recommend slight movement changes of the patient or position changes to dislodge potential residues of medications or undissolved pills.

Adsorption with Activated Charcoal. Activated charcoal is a finely divided powder made by pyrolysis of carbonaceous material. It consists of small particles with an internal network of pores that adsorb substances. It is indicated after gastric emptying procedures, whether successful or not. It should be repeated every 2 to 4 hours for drugs with enterohepatic circulation (e.g., theophylline, digoxin, nortriptyline, amitriptyline, salicylates, benzodiazepines, phenytoin, and phenobarbital). This effect has been called GI dialysis.

It may be used immediately after ipecac (does not interfere with its action; some believe that this is the best way to give it) and N-acetylcysteine. It is contraindicated in caustic ingestion and ineffective in ingestion of elemental metals (e.g., iron), some pesticides (malathion, DDT), cyanide, ethanol, or methanol.

The typical dose is 30 to 100 g in adults (or 1 g/kg) and is usually given with a cathartic (50 mL of 70% sorbitol or 30 g of magnesium sulfate) to accelerate the transit time of the toxin–charcoal complex. A superactivated charcoal formulation capable of adsorbing two to three times the conventional capacity of the charcoal is available.

Neutralizing Agents. In some types of poisoning, the use of a neutralizing agent instead of charcoal is preferable. Examples of such chemicals and the neutralizing agent(s) used are

1. Mercury: Sodium formaldehyde sulfoxylate (20 g) neutralizes $HgCl$ to metallic mercury, which is less soluble.
2. Iron: Sodium bicarbonate (200 to 300 mL given after lavage) converts the ferrous ion to ferrous carbonate, which is less soluble.
3. Iodine: Starch solution (75 g of starch in 1 L of water) given repeatedly until the aspirate is no longer blue.
4. Strychnine, nicotine, quinine, physostigmine: Potassium permanganate (1:10,000).

Cathartics. These are used as adjunctive treatment with charcoal and should be used only when needed. They are contraindicated in diarrhea, dehydration, electrolyte imbalances, abdominal trauma, intestinal obstruction, and adynamic ileus. The agent most frequently used in poisoning treatment is sorbitol because of the onset of action (less than an hour), duration of effect (8 to 12 hours), and no interaction with charcoal. Oil cathartics are contraindicated because they can be extremely harmful if aspirated and can increase the absorption of hydrocarbons. Complications such as fluid and electrolyte imbalance may result from overaggressive use of cathartics.

Whole Bowel Irrigation. This procedure refers to the administration of polyethyleneglycol at a rate of 500 to 2,000 mL per hour orally or through a nasogastric tube with the purpose of cleaning the bowel of whole or undissolved pills. It may be helpful in clearing the GI tract of iron or delayed-release formulations not adsorbed by charcoal as well as when onset of treatment is delayed. The procedure takes 3 to 5 hours and may be complicated by bowel perforation, bowel obstruction, ileus or GI hemorrhage.

SPECIFIC AGENTS

The following agents, discussed in alphabetical order, are responsible for the majority of fatal exposures reported in the United States (1).

Acetaminophen (10,21,23,36–41)

Common trade-name medications containing acetaminophen are Alka-Seltzer (some formulations), Anacin, Benadryl (some formulations), Comtrex, Contac, Coricidin, Darvocet, Dimetapp, Drixoral, Esgic, Excedrin (some formulations), Fioricet, Goody's Body Pain Relief, Lortab, Midol, Midrin, Nyquil, Pamprin, Panadol, Parafon, Percocet, Phenaphen, Robitussin, Sudafed, Tavist, Thera-Flu, Triaminic, Tylenol, Tempra, Unisom, Vicodin, Wygesic.

As a cause of morbidity: 1 (other analgesics included) (1).
As a cause of mortality: 1 (other analgesics included) (1).
Most frequent route of exposure: ingestion.
Most frequent reason for exposure: unintentional overdose.

Maternal Considerations

Symptoms: Nausea, vomiting, anorexia, right upper quadrant pain.
Signs: Icterus, right upper abdominal tenderness, lethargy, evidence of bleeding.
Diagnostic tests: Blood: acetaminophen plasma or serum level (at 4 or more hours of ingestion), transaminases (elevated), lactic dehydrogenase (elevated), prothrombin time (PT) (prolonged), amylase (elevated), lipase (elevated), creatinine (elevated). Plot acetaminophen values in the Rumack-Matthew nomogram to assess risk of hepatotoxicity. Urinalysis. Electrocardiography (ECG): nonspecific ST/T changes.
Short-term problems: Oliguria, pancreatitis, hypotension, myocardial ischemia, necrosis, premature contractions, potential for premature delivery.
Long-term problems: Diffuse hepatic necrosis (potential for 1% to 2% late mortality).

Fetal Considerations

Acetominaphen crosses the placenta; fetus is at risk of poisoning, particularly late in pregnancy.

Signs: Decreased fetal movements, decreased beat-to-beat variability, absence of fetal heart rate accelerations, falling baseline heart rate.

Teratogenic potential: No support for association, potential for fetal liver damage (hepatocellular necrosis), increased risks of spontaneous abortion and stillbirth.

Fetal distress potential: This has been reported.

Indications for delivery: Non-reassuring fetal condition.

Neonatal period: Hyperbilirubinemia.

Management Considerations

Supportive: Induced emesis may be indicated for home treatment of a large dose (more than 100 mg/kg or 6 g). Gastric lavage + activated charcoal (1 g/kg in water or sorbitol).

Specific measures/antidotes: Indications for antidotal use: **a.** If the ingestion is known to be greater than 6 g (or 100 mg/kg); **b.** If plasma acetaminophen levels (at 4 or more hours after exposure) are 150 μg/mL or greater (993 μmol/L); **c.** When exposure to other hepatotoxic agents or history of liver disease is present along with the acetaminophen exposure (including ethanol, carbamazepine, and isoniazid); **d.** If the results of the acetaminophen levels are not available by 7 to 8 hours after the exposure.

Route of administration: Oral: methionine (2.5 g every 4 hours for four doses) or *N*-acetylcysteine (140 mg/kg loading dose followed by 70 mg/kg every 4 hours for 17 doses); parenteral (preferred in pregnancy): *N*-acetylcysteine (150 mg/kg in 200 mL of 5% dextrose over 15 minutes or 100 mg/kg in 1,000 mL of 5% dextrose over 16 hours).

Monitoring: Vital signs, mental status, intake, and output; blood: transaminases, PT, and acetaminophen level every 4 hours (first 24 hours), then daily or as indicated; EFM: indicated.

Therapeutic goals: Asymptomatic patient, normal liver function tests (transaminases and PT).

Disposition considerations: Intensive care unit (ICU) admission if hepatic failure or encephalopathy. Consider psychiatric evaluation for all exposures. Contemplate induction of labor in third trimester in severe exposures. May discharge after 72 to 96 hours after exposure if therapeutic goals met.

Follow-up: Caution the patient about the possibility of spontaneous abortion, premature delivery, and risk of stillbirth. Counsel against the use of potentially hepatotoxic agents. Consider serial biophysical profiles in viable pregnancies and severe exposure (value not established).

Aspirin (10,23,36,42–47)

Common trade-name medications containing aspirin are Alka-Seltzer, Ascriptin, BC Powder, Bufferin, Darvon, Ecotrin, Excedrin, Fiorinal, Goody's Body Pain Relief, Norgesic, Pepto-Bismol, Percodan, Soma, Talwin.

As a cause of morbidity: 1 (other analgesics included) (1).

As a cause of mortality: 1 (other analgesics included) (1).

Main route of exposure: oral (transdermal is possible).

Main mechanism of exposure: intentional.

Maternal Considerations

Symptoms: None, nausea and vomiting, abdominal pain, tinnitus, decreased hearing, dyspnea.

Signs: Hyperventilation, altered mental status, flushing, diaphoresis, hyperpyrexia, GI bleeding, petechiae, bruising, hypovolemia, pulmonary edema, seizures, acute respiratory distress syndrome, coma.

Diagnostic tests: ABG, respiratory alkalosis, compensated metabolic acidosis or metabolic acidosis, increased anion gap (greater than 14 mEq/L); blood: salicylate levels, creatinine, blood urea nitrogen (BUN), electrolytes, glucose, complete blood count (CBC), PT and PTT; urinalysis: specific gravity, volume, and ferric chloride test (bedside calorimetric test: add 10% $FECL_3$ in equal amounts to a 1 mL of urine at least 2 hours after ingestion; purple to purple brown indicates salicylate presence); chest radiograph, edema.

Short-term problems: Volume depletion, shock, hemorrhage, seizures.

Long-term problems: Higher risk of peripartum hemorrhage soon after exposure.

Fetal Considerations

Salicylate crosses the placenta freely and concentrates in the fetus, particularly the CNS.

Signs: Constriction of the ductus arteriosus, growth restriction.

Teratogenic potential: No.

Fetal distress potential: Yes.

Indications for delivery: Non-reassuring fetal condition. Avoidance of instrumental delivery soon after poisoning is recommended (fetal risk of cephalohematomata and intracranial bleeding).

Neonatal period: Hyperbilirubinemia, clinical evidence of thrombocytopenia.

Management Considerations

Supportive: Generous intravenous fluid (glucose-containing solutions) replacement; if hypotension is refractory, may use plasma or blood. May need invasive cardiovascular monitoring (pulmonary artery catheter) to manage fluid administration. If assisted ventilation is required, hyperventilation (16 to 20 breaths/minute) as needed to keep P_2 near 35 mm Hg. Keep serum glucose above 90 mg/dL.

Specific measures/antidotes: **a.** Induced emesis is not recommended; **b.** Gastric lavage (even if more than 4 hours have elapsed since ingestion); **c.** Forced alkaline diuresis (0.45% saline solution + 5% glucose + 44 mEq of bicarbonate and 20 mEq of KCl added per liter); goal: 5 to 10 mL/min of urine with pH of 7.5. Administer intravenous or intramuscular vitamin K 10 mg (aspirin inhibits prothrombin formation and production of factors II, V, VII, and X); **d.** Hemodialysis may be indicated (severe CNS deterioration, pulmonary edema, renal failure, salicylate level greater than 90 mg/dL (6.6 mmol/L), inability to alkalinize urine and/or no improvement with decontamination and urine alkalinization).

Monitoring: Vital signs, mental status, intake, and output, ECG, oxymetry; blood: ABG + potassium every 2 to 4 hours (monitor alkalinization), serial determination of salicylate levels (every 2 hours) until declining trend noted and levels fall below 30 mg/dL (2.2 mmol/L), serial blood glucose; urine: pH every hour. If fetus is viable, inform the neonatology or pediatrics service of the potential delivery of a salicylate-exposed infant.

Therapeutic goals: Asymptomatic patient, salicylate level less than 30 mg/dL (2.2 mmol/L) more than 2 hours after exposure.

Disposition considerations: Contemplate induction of labor in severe exposures in the third trimester. May discharge if asymptomatic, appropriate treatment administered, decreasing serum salicylate levels, and absence of electrolyte or acid-base imbalances.

Follow-up: Establish. Consider evaluation of fetal growth. Consider psychiatric evaluation.

Barbiturates (21,23,24,36,48–50)

Common generic or trade-name medications containing barbiturates are amobarbital, barbital, butabarbital, pentobarbital, phenobarbital, secobarbital, thiamylal, thiopental, veronal, Amytal, Arco-Lase, Butisol, Donnatal, Esgic, Fioricet, Fiorinal, Luminal, Membaral, Nembutal, Phrenilin, Sedapap, Tuinal.

As a cause of morbidity: 4 (sedatives, hypnotics, and antipsychotics) (1).

As a cause of mortality: 5 (sedatives, hypnotics, and antipsychotics) (1).

Most frequent route of exposure: ingestion.

Most frequent reason for exposure: unintentional overdose; acute or chronic.

Maternal Considerations

Symptoms: Weakness, fatigue, sleepiness.

Signs: Sedation, altered mental status, miosis, bradypnea, respiratory depression, ataxia, nystagmus, extraocular muscle palsy, dysarthria, hyporeflexia, decreased bowel sounds, hypothermia, hypotension, cardiovascular collapse.

Diagnostic tests: Blood: CBC; electrolytes, glucose, creatinine, BUN, PT, PTT, phenobarbital level (levels may not correlate with symptoms); urinalysis: drug screen, pH.

Short-term problems: Respiratory failure, coma, anoxic encephalopathy [interpretation of electroencephalogram (EEG) is unreliable with elevated serum barbiturate levels].

Long-term problems: Withdrawal syndrome in chronic user/abuser (insomnia, excitement, delirium, psychosis, seizures, hypotension).

Fetal Considerations

Signs: Potential for decreased beat-to-beat variability, bradycardia, abnormal biophysical profile in severe maternal poisoning.

Teratogenic potential: Controversial, usually risk is multifactorial and may be related to the combined effects of the seizure disorder and medication.

Fetal distress potential: Only in severely symptomatic exposures (if respiratory depression, hypoxemia, or cardiovascular collapse).

Indications for delivery: Obstetric indications. Caution is suggested when interpreting electronic fetal heart rate monitoring and biophysical profile.

Postnatal: Risk of hemorrhagic disease of the newborn, risk of withdrawal syndrome in chronic users (occurs on average 6 days and up to 2 weeks later), neonatal sedation of some breast-fed infants (caution patient about it).

Management Considerations

Supportive: Respiratory support is the priority; measures needed may range from supplemental O_2 to endotracheal intubation and mechanical ventilation. Maintaining an adequate volume expansion and diuresis is critical. Forced alkaline diuresis recommended for symptomatic patients (add potassium to the bicarbonate infusion).

Specific measures/antidotes: Induced emesis may be indicated if no significant depression; gastric lavage (even after 8 hours after the exposure) followed by activated charcoal and cathartics recommended. Multiple doses of activated charcoal (every 4 hours) are recommended. Alkaline diuresis through the combination of sodium bicarbonate, intravenous fluids, and diuretics enhances elimination (goal: 5 to 10 mL/min of urine with pH 8.0). In chronic overdose, a gradual withdrawal (200 mg of phenobarbital is indicated to prevent withdrawal complications). Hemoperfusion (resin over charcoal) or hemodialysis may be indicated in cases of toxic/lethal exposures (phenobarbital level of 100 μg/mL or 430 μmol/L) and/or if uremia develops. No specific antidote.

Monitoring: Vital signs, mental status, airway, blood pressure, oxygen saturation, electrolytes, and serum calcium levels need to be followed.

Therapeutic goals: Asymptomatic patient, no need for supplemental oxygen or volume expansion, therapeutic or subtherapeutic level.

Discharge considerations: Dose adjustment if patient is epileptic. Psychiatric consult recommended if mechanism of exposure is deemed intentional.

Follow-up: Follow phenobarbital levels. Notify primary physician (obstetrician and neurologist) before discharge. Consider folate supplementation in chronic users.

Benzodiazepines (10,21,23,25–27,36,51–56)

Common generic and trade-name medications containing benzodiazepines are lorazepam, oxazepam, clonazepam, diazepam, temazepam, chlordiazepoxide, Ativan, Centrax, Dalmane, Diastat, Halcion, Klonopin, Librium, Limbitrol, ProSom, Restoril, Serax, Tranxene, Valium, Versed, Xanax.

As a cause of morbidity: 4 (sedatives, hypnotics, and antipsychotics) (1).

As a cause of mortality: 5 (sedatives, hypnotics, and antipsychotics) (1).

Most frequent route of exposure: ingestion.

Most frequent reason for exposure: unintentional overdose.

Maternal Considerations

Symptoms: Drowsiness, ataxia, nystagmus, dysarthria, paradoxical irritability, excitation, delirium, hallucinations.

Signs: Lethargy, altered mental status, slurred speech, ataxia, bradycardia or tachycardia, decreased bowel sounds, respiratory depression, hypotension, dyskinesia, acute dystonic reactions, coma (rare in the absence of co-ingestants).

Diagnostic tests: Blood: CBC, electrolytes and glucose, toxicology screen (detects most barbiturates except clonazepam). Serum levels of no value in the emergency treatment. Calculation of osmolal and anion gaps recommended if suspicion of co-ingestion or in severe clinical manifestations. Urinalysis: drug screen, specific gravity.

Short-term problems: Respiratory depression, hypotension, anoxic encephalopathy (interpretation of EEG is unreliable with elevated levels of benzodiazepines).

Long-term problems: Withdrawal syndrome (anxiety, insomnia, dysphoria, nausea, palpitations, fatigue, confusion, delirium, muscle twitching, seizures, psychosis) may appear 1 to 7 days after abrupt cessation of benzodiazepines.

Fetal Considerations

Signs: Potential for decreased beat-to-beat variability, bradycardia, abnormal biophysical profile in severe maternal poisoning.

Teratogenic potential: Majority of the evidence does not support it.

Fetal distress potential: Only in the presence of severe maternal toxicity and secondary to maternal hypovolemia or hypoxemia.

Indications for delivery: Obstetric indications. Caution is suggested when interpreting electronic fetal heart rate monitoring and biophysical profile.

Postnatal: Potential for neonatal hypotonia, lethargy, and apnea needing resuscitation; risk of neonatal withdrawal may produce seizures 2 to 6 days after delivery. Inform pediatrician of perinatal exposure.

Management Considerations

Wide therapeutic index; low lethal potential if isolated poison. Suspect co-ingestion (particularly alcohol and tricyclics).

Supportive: Respiratory assistance may be required; crystalloid infusion to maintain adequate volume; dopamine and norepinephrine infusions may be required in refractory hypotension.

Specific measures/antidotes: Induced emesis not recommended; gastric lavage recommended in pregnancy followed by activated charcoal (50 to 60 g) in sorbitol (1 g/kg) and repeated (25 to 30 g) every 4 hours (the sorbitol added only every 12 hours). Flumazenil (Romazicon, category C): give if vital signs are not stable, tricyclic co-ingestion excluded, and if no history of chronic use or abuse of benzodiazepines (possibility of inducing seizures).

Monitoring: Vital signs, mental status, oxymetry, intermittent fetal heart rate monitoring. Repeat drug levels not indicated.

Therapeutic goals: Asymptomatic patient, normal mental status without benzodiazepine antagonism (at least more than 4 hours since last dose of flumazenil), normal bowel sounds, completed decontamination procedures, no evidence of co-ingestion, reassuring fetal condition, consults completed.

Discharge considerations: Investigate chronic use/abuse of benzodiazepines. Consider drug counselor and psychiatric and social worker evaluations.

Follow-up: Notify primary care physician (obstetrician, psychiatry).

Carbon Monoxide (10,21,23,57–64)

Examples of situations leading to carbon monoxide exposure are fires, motor vehicle fumes, and heat stoves.

As a cause of morbidity: 11 (1).
As a cause of mortality: 8 (1).
Main route of exposure: inhalation.
Reasons for exposure: unintentional; intentional (suicide attempt).

Maternal Considerations

Symptoms: Depends on concentration (% CO-Hb), headache, shortness of breath, nausea, dizziness, dim vision, weakness.

Signs: Vasodilation, disturbed judgment, collapse, coma, convulsions, Cheyne-Stokes respiration.

Diagnostic tests: ECG: sinus tachycardia, ST depression, atrial fibrillation, prolonged PR and QT intervals, AV or bundle branch block; ABG: % CO-Hb (correlates with symptoms and signs); others: CBC, transaminases, electrolytes, creatinine, and urinalysis. If patient rescued from a fire, consider a serum cyanide level.

Short-term problems: Myocardial ischemia/infarction, rhabdomyolysis, renal failure, pulmonary edema, blindness, hearing loss.

Long-term problems: Delayed CNS toxicity (perivascular infarction, demyelination of basal ganglia) in comatose or acidotic patients on arrival.

Fetal Considerations

Carbon monoxide crosses the placenta; higher affinity for fetal than adult hemoglobin results in 10% to 15% higher fetal compared with maternal levels and higher risk of mortality for the fetus.

Teratogenic potential: Potential for fetal brain damage, subsequent developmental delay.

Fetal distress potential: Yes, high.

Indications for delivery: Obstetric indications, fetal distress.

Management Considerations

Supportive: Remove the patient from contaminated environment; absolute rest to decrease oxygen consumption.

Specific measures/antidotes: Oxygen at 100% via tight-fitted nonrebreather mask; some authorities recommend the administration of oxygen for five times as long as it is expected for the maternal levels to normalize (58). Hyperbaric oxygen if CO-Hb is greater than 20% (versus greater than 40% in the nonpregnant state), signs of non-reassuring fetal condition or any unfavorable neurologic signs in the mother (10).

Monitoring: Admit if CO-Hb greater than 25%; cardiovascular disease with CO-Hb more than 15%; pregnant (CO-Hb more than 10%); impaired mentation or metabolic acidosis.

Therapeutic goals: CO-Hb less than 5% and no symptoms. Discharge considerations: Identification (and avoidance) of source of exposure if not obvious (social services consult may be helpful). Suicidal evaluation (psychiatric consult) if circumstances suggest such possibility. Counsel regarding long-term fetal effects.

Follow-up: Establish. Consider follow-up of intrauterine growth.

Cocaine (10,21,23,36,65–73)

Other names for cocaine are crack, rock, blow, snow, liquid lady (alcohol + cocaine), speedball (heroine + cocaine).

As a cause of morbidity: N/A.
As a cause of mortality: 3 (1).
Most frequent route of exposure: inhalation.
Most frequent reason for exposure: unintentional overdose.

Maternal Considerations

Symptoms: Anxiety, chest pain, respiratory difficulty, palpitations, dizziness, headache, nausea.

Signs: Agitation, altered mental status (up to frank psychosis), tachycardia, hypertension, hyperthermia, mydriasis, tachypnea, diaphoresis, hyperactive bowel sounds, pulmonary edema, uterine contractions (up to tetany), vaginal bleeding.

Diagnostic tests: Blood: CBC, electrolytes and glucose, creatinine and BUN, creatine phosphokinase and isofractions, myoglobin, troponine I, amylase, lipase; urine: microhematuria, myoglobinuria; ECG: tachycardia, ischemia, ST segment elevation, acute myocardial infarction; chest radiograph: pulmonary edema, pulmonary infarction. Consider other radiologic surveys if history of recent traveling (possibility of body packing). Computed tomography and lumbar puncture if seizures.

Short-term problems: Arrhythmias, myocardial infarction, seizures, pulmonary infarction, intracranial hemorrhage or infarcts, visceral infarcts, preterm delivery, abruptio placentae.

Long-term problems: Malnutrition, sexually transmitted diseases, growth restriction, stillbirth, preeclampsia.

Fetal Considerations

Cocaine crosses the placenta with ease.

Signs: Fetal tachycardia, decreased beat-to-beat variability, bradycardia, late decelerations.
Teratogenic potential: Controversial data, potential for growth restriction.
Fetal distress potential: Yes, secondary to uterine hyperstimulation, uterine vasoconstriction, and maternal seizures.
Indications for delivery: Non-reassuring fetal condition and severe growth restriction.
Postnatal: Risk of withdrawal syndrome (seizures, cardiovascular collapse), antenatal notification of the neonatology service recommended, risk for fetal neurodevelopmental delay (when cocaine is a component of polydrug abuse).

Management Considerations

Rectal and vaginal examinations indicated to rule out occult drug packing.

Supportive: Hydration (forced alkaline diuresis if myoglobinuria detected or if creatinine elevated on arrival).
Specific measures/antidotes: Activated charcoal and whole bowel irrigation may decrease absorption if history of ingestion ("stuffing"). Avoid use of beta-blockers for arrhythmia treatment (may worsen coronary vasoconstriction and induce seizures). Benzodiazepines (5 to 10 mg intravenous diazepam or 2 to 4 mg intravenous lorazepam) are the first line of treatment for supraventricular arrhythmia, hypertension, ischemic chest pain, anxiety, and seizures. Lidocaine (1.5 mg/kg intravenous bolus followed by infusion of 2 mg/min) and serum alkalinization are the treatments of choice for ventricular arrhythmia. Phenobarbital is the second choice for seizures. In ischemic chest pain, may also use nitroglycerin (0.4 mg sublingually every 5 minutes and continuous intravenous drip thereafter). In refractory cases: 1 mg intravenous phentolamine (repeat in 5 minutes). Heparinize if ischemic chest pain (5,000 IU intravenous bolus + 1,000 IU/hr infusion). External cooling is needed to control hyperthermia (neuromuscular blockade may be needed in severe cases). Hemodialysis may be indicated for renal failure secondary to myoglobinuria. No specific antidote available.
Monitoring: Vital signs, mental status, oxymetry, cardiac for at least 24 hours after the exposure. Consider repeat ECGs and cardiac enzymes every 6 hours if significant exposure, risk factors for coronary artery disease, or chest pain on arrival.
Therapeutic goals: Asymptomatic patient, normal laboratory values, no contractions or bleeding, reassuring fetal condition, more than 24 hours of observation. Consults obtained (see below)
Disposition considerations: Admit to an ICU if seizures, ventricular arrhythmia, or hyperthermia. Drug counselor, psychiatric, and social work consults recommended. Evaluate for sexually transmitted diseases.
Follow-up: Establish because most of these patients do not have prenatal care. Consider follow-up of fetal growth.

Ethanol (14,21,23,32,74–79)

As a cause of morbidity: 9 (1).
As a cause of mortality: 6 (1).
Most frequent route of exposure: ingestion.
Most frequent reason for exposure: unintentional overdose.

Maternal Considerations

Clinical presentation may vary with acute and/or chronic ethanol abuse or withdrawal. Acute overdose is considered here.

Symptoms: Euphoria, incoordination, impaired judgment and reflexes. Social inhibitions are loosened. Aggressive or boisterous behavior is common. Hypoglycemia may occur.

Signs: As above plus ataxia, nystagmus, altered mental status, small pupils, characteristic breath smell. In severe overdoses: decreased temperature, pulse, and blood pressure; respiratory depression; respiratory distress; coma.

Diagnostic tests: Glucose, electrolytes, BUN, creatinine, transaminases, PT, magnesium, ABG, or pulse oxymetry, chest radiograph if aspiration is suspected.

Short-term problems: Respiratory depression, pulmonary aspiration, hypoglycemia, coma, less frequently GI bleeding or rhabdomyolysis.

Long-term problems: organic and social. Organic: pancreatitis, hepatitis, cirrhosis, hepatic encephalopathy, portal hypertension, GI bleedings, anemia, thiamine deficiency, alcoholic ketoacidosis, decreased resistance to infections, hypomagnesemia, hypokalemia, hypophosphatemia; social: malnutrition, isolation, depression, suicidal attempts.

Fetal Considerations

Signs: Decrease in fetal heart rate accelerations and variability, suppression of fetal breathing movements.

Teratogenic potential: Fetal alcohol syndrome: **a.** Craniofacial dysmorphology; **b.** Fetal growth restriction (body length affected more than weight); **c.** CNS dysfunction; **d.** Other abnormalities (mainly cardiac, urogenital, and hemangiomas) in 30% to 40% or more of the infants exposed. Other features: short palpebral fissures, ptosis, strabismus, epicanthal folds, myopia, microphthalmia, hypoplastic philtrum and maxilla, short upturned nose, posterior rotation of ears, poorly formed concha, mild to moderate mental retardation, hypotonia, poor coordination, microcephaly. Diagnosis may be delayed until 9 to 12 months of age.

Fetal distress potential: Not likely unless the acute intoxication is complicated by trauma. Transient lack of reactivity to fetal movements or to external stimuli has been described in acute intoxication.

Indications for delivery: Obstetric indications. Allow metabolism of alcoholic load before

acting on non-reassuring fetal heart rate monitoring.

Postnatal: Potential for withdrawal syndrome. Ethanol passes freely into breast milk; potential for sedation and dose-related psychomotor development delay in breast-fed infants.

Management Considerations

Decontamination: Emesis is not indicated unless a substantial ingestion has occurred within minutes of presentation or other drug ingestion is suspected. Gastric lavage indicated if intake of large amounts within 30 to 45 minutes of presentation. Charcoal does not efficiently adsorb ethanol; useful if other drugs were (or suspected to be) ingested.

Supportive: Airway protection. Treatment of coma and seizures if they occur. Elimination of ethanol occurs at a fixed rate.

Specific measures/antidotes: No specific antidote; flumazenil and naloxone may alleviate respiratory depression (anecdotal arousal after use of naloxone). Give glucose and thiamine.

Monitoring: Pulse oxymetry if the patient is asleep or initial reading is abnormal.

Therapeutic goals: Sobriety; no acute complications in 6 to 8 hours of observation.

Disposition considerations: Consider admission for social reasons. Social work, drug counseling, and psychiatric evaluations may be helpful. Consider folate supplementation.

Follow-up: Establish. Fetal growth follow-up recommended. Social work and psychiatric follow-up recommended.

Iron (10,23,36,46,80–82)

Common generic or trade-name drugs containing iron are ferrous gluconate, ferrous fumarate, ferrous sulfate, Chromagen, Feosol, Fergon, Ferlecit, Ferro-Folic, Ferro-Grad, Iberet, Irospan, Megadose, Nephro-Fer, Nephro-Vite, Prenate, Slow Fe, Trinsicon.

As a cause of morbidity: 2 (80), 6 (1).
As a cause of mortality: rare.
Most frequent route of exposure: ingestion.

Most frequent reason for exposure: intentional overdose; suicidal gesture.

Maternal Considerations

Symptoms: Abdominal pain, indigestion, nausea, vomiting, hematemesis, diarrhea.

Signs: As above + bloody stools, fever, shock, and acidosis in severe cases.

Diagnostic tests: CBC: leukocytosis, serum iron levels (<18 μmol/L = nontoxic, 18–59 μmol/L = minimal toxicity, 60–89 μmol/L = moderate toxicity, more than 90 μmol/L = severe toxicity); other tests: glucose (mild hyperglycemia), liver function tests, ABG if patient's mental status is altered or patient is in shock.

Short-term problems: Shock, hemorrhage, hepatic failure, pulmonary edema/hemorrhage, disseminated intravascular coagulopathy.

Long-term problems: GI scarring, small intestine infarction, hepatic necrosis, achlorhydria.

Fetal Considerations

Signs: Contractions.

Teratogenic potential: None specific.

Fetal distress potential: None unless associated maternal acidosis or bleeding.

Indications for delivery: Obstetric indications.

Management considerations

Supportive: Vigorous intravenous hydration and gastric lavage. Ipecac emesis recommended within the first hour in the conscious patient if lavage and bicarbonate (see below) not available.

Specific measures/antidotes: 1% sodium bicarbonate (200–300 mL) after lavage or induced emesis (converts the ferrous ion to ferrous carbonate, which is less soluble). Deferoxamine at an intramuscular dose of 1 g followed by 500 mg intramuscularly every 4 hours for two doses is recommended for patients with serum iron levels of 300 μg/dL or greater or a calculated ingestion of 30 mg/kg of elemental iron. Intravenous infusion at the same doses is preferred in patients in shock (infusion not to exceed 15 mg/kg per hour).

Monitoring: Check serum iron levels every 4 to 6 hours until they are within normal range.

Therapeutic goals: Normal serum iron levels.

Disposition considerations: Evaluate suicidal potential (psychiatric consult).

Follow-up: Establish.

Organophosphates (10,23,46,83–87)

The insecticides belonging to the family of the carbamates (e.g., Carboryl and Bendiocarb) have the same mechanisms of poisoning, manifestations, and therapy. Examples of compounds containing organophosphates: diazinon, dichlorvos, dimethoate, malathion, parathion, Quinalphos, sarin (nerve gas).

As a cause of morbidity: 12 (1).

As a cause of mortality: 16 (1).

Most frequent route of exposure: ingestion (followed by contact).

Most frequent reason for exposure: intentional overdose.

Maternal Considerations

Symptoms: Nausea, vomiting, blurred vision, headache, dizziness, respiratory difficulty, abdominal pain (cramping usually), diarrhea, urinary incontinence, coma.

Signs: Agitation, altered mental status, fever, miosis, fasciculations or tremors, sialorrhea, bronchorrhea, bronchospasm, pulmonary edema, tachycardia or bradycardia, hypotension or hypertension, respiratory arrest.

Diagnostic tests: Blood: decrease by 80% to 90% of erythrocyte cholinesterase (serum pseudocholinesterase is less specific); CBC: leukocytosis with bandemia baseline transaminases, lactic dehydrogenase, and bilirubin; urine: hematuria, glycosuria, proteinuria, drug screen (intentional use can coexist with cocaine, used to potentiate cocaine effects); ECG: initial tachycardia, subsequent bradycardia, variable degrees of atrioventricular block, prolonged QT interval.

Short-term problems: Respiratory failure, aspiration pneumonia, ventricular arrhythmia, acute respiratory distress syndrome.

Long-term problems: Hepatic failure. Relapse after apparent recovery is a well-described phenomenon in organophosphate poisoning. The "intermediate syndrome" has been described 24 to 96 hours after exposure and manifests itself as muscular paralysis developing after recovery from the cholinergic phase. Another form of delayed toxicity is explained by the hepatic metabolism to more toxic compounds within 72 hours of the exposure. CNS dysfunction characterized by impaired memory, confusion, and depression and a form of peripheral neuropathy with paresthesias, anesthesia, and weakness have been described.

Fetal Considerations

Signs: Hypotonia, bradycardia, loss of beat-to-beat variability, death.

Teratogenic potential: Not enough evidence (one case reported of multiple anomalies after exposure to oxydemeton-methyl at 4 weeks).

Fetal distress potential: Yes, from maternal hypoxia.

Indications for delivery: Obstetric indications. Non-reassuring fetal condition. Notify pediatrician of third-trimester exposure (neonatal respiratory depression requiring mechanical ventilation has been reported after resolution of maternal symptoms).

Management Considerations

Supportive: Maintenance of airway, respiratory support may be necessary, ICU setting suggested.

Specific measures/antidotes: Induced emesis may be indicated in prehospital setting; gastric lavage followed by activated charcoal and sorbitol (for catharsis) are indicated. Remove clothing and shoes and have the patient washed thoroughly with soap and water. Pralidoxime chloride 1 g intravenously over several minutes is effective in reversing the action of the poison on the cholinesterases if given within 24 to 36 hours of the exposure (can be repeated

within 30 to 40 minutes if no response is observed). Repeat boluses every 12 hours. Atropine 2 mg intravenously in repeated doses for control of the muscarinic effects (salivation, lacrimation, urination, defecation, GI distress and emesis); an atropine drip may be necessary if multiple doses required. Intravenous diazepam can be used for seizures.

Monitoring: Vital signs, pulse oxymetry, ECG, mental status, symptoms. Daily cholinesterase levels. EFM: indicated during therapy.

Therapeutic goals: Asymptomatic patient with normal levels of erythrocyte cholinesterase. Normal antenatal fetal testing.

Disposition considerations: Discharge can be considered more than 72 hours after significant exposure; easy accessibility to the hospital and therapeutic goals met. Evaluate suicide potential (psychiatric consult).

Follow-up: Establish. Social work and psychiatric follow-ups recommended.

Tricyclics (10,23,32,36,49,78,88–90)

Generic or trade-name medications containing tricyclics are imipramine, amitriptyline, doxepin, trimipramine, trazadone, fluoxetine, Anafranil, Asendin, Elavil, Etafron, Limbitrol, Norpramin, Pamelor, Sinequan, Surmontil, Tofranil, Triavil, Vivactil.

As a cause of morbidity: 5 (1).
As a cause of mortality 2 (1).
Most frequent route of exposure: ingestion.
Most frequent reason for exposure: unintentional overdose.

Maternal Considerations

Symptoms: Dry mouth, urinary retention, delirium.

Signs: No evident toxicity, agitation, mydriasis, hyperthermia, tachycardia, hypotension, dry axilla, absent bowel sounds, urinary retention, myoclonus, slurred speech, lethargy, rapid loss of consciousness, seizures, cardiac dysrhythmias.

Diagnostic tests: ECG (best predictor of toxicity): R wave in aVR, wide QRS, right axis deviation in the frontal plane, prolonged QT, ventricular tachycardia; blood: serum levels not indicated (correlate poorly with toxicity); ABG: acidosis, CBC, electrolytes, glucose, baseline creatinine, and BUN.

Short-term problems: Cardiac dysrhythmias, hypotension, respiratory depression, seizures, urinary retention, GI hypomotility.

Long-term problems: Rhabdomyolysis, permanent neurologic sequelae.

Fetal Considerations

Signs: Fetal tachycardia, exaggerated accelerations.

Teratogenic potential: Multiple congenital effects have been reported after overdose including microcephaly, cleft palate, micrognathia, ambiguous genitalia, foot deformities, and undetectable dermal ridges. Limb reduction defects also reported.

Fetal distress potential: Yes, secondary to maternal hypoxia or acidosis.

Indications for delivery: Obstetric indications and non-reassuring fetal condition. Notify pediatrician of perinatal exposure.

Management Considerations

Supportive: ICU admission is indicated. Intubation may be necessary to control airway; if so, hyperventilation recommended (avoid hyperalkalinization when combined with bicarbonate infusions).

Specific measures/antidotes: Induced emesis is contraindicated. Orogastric lavage followed by activated charcoal (1 g/kg initially) in multiple doses (at 0.5 g/kg every 2 to 4 hours with intact gut motility). Continuous suction (30% excreted into stomach) recommended in the interim: **a**. Alkalinization with sodium bicarbonate (1 to 3 mEq/kg intravenous bolus, followed by an infusion) in the presence of ventricular arrhythmias, hypotension, or a QRS more than 100 milliseconds (goal: keep arterial pH 7.5); **b**. Lidocaine is the drug of choice for management of ventricular arrhythmias and diazepam for seizures (preferred over phenytoin for both indications). Quinidine, disopy-

ramide, and procainamide are contraindicated (exacerbation of cardiotoxicity); **c**. Phenobarbital (and intubation) are recommended for persistent seizures; **d**. Norepinephrine (2 to 20 μg/min titrated to blood pressure) is the drug of choice for refractory hypotension (over dopamine); **e**. Physostigmine not recommended (may exacerbate cardiac toxicity and induce seizures); **f**. Hemodialysis not effective; little support for use of hemoperfusion (large distribution volume); **g**. In severe and refractory hypotension, anecdotal survival achieved with extracorporeal circulation.

Monitoring: Vital signs (including temperature), oxymetry, mental status; EKG: at least 6 hours of cardiac monitoring recommended even after minimal exposure and no signs of toxicity. In the presence of toxic signs, cardiac monitoring is recommended for 24 hours after remission.

Therapeutic goals: Asymptomatic patient, normal mental status, no evidence of QRS prolongation on initial and follow-up ECG (6 hours later).

Disposition considerations: May consider discharge after GI decontamination, more than 6 hours have elapsed after exposure and therapeutic goals met, normal antenatal testing results. Continue observation if ECG shows sinus tachycardia. Evaluate suicide potential (psychiatric consult recommended).

Follow-up: Establish. Psychiatric follow-up recommended.

SUMMARY

- Poisoning during pregnancy represents one third of a percent of all toxic exposures in the United States.
- The number of reported toxic exposures has increased by approximately 25% over the past 6 years both in the pregnant and nonpregnant population.
- Although slightly more frequent during the second trimester, toxic exposures during pregnancy are reported with similar frequency in all trimesters.
- Even in the absence of a history suggestive of pregnancy, every female of reproductive age treated for a known or suspected toxic

exposure should have a pregnancy test as part of her evaluation.

- The emergency treatment and stabilization of the mother should take priority over the monitoring and treatment of the fetus.

- A prompt consultation with the obstetric service is recommended in the emergency management of the compromised poisoned pregnant patient. The goals of this consult are the assessment of fetal viability and the decision/skill to proceed with an emergent or perimortem cesarean section, if the patient's condition worsens and/or the resuscitative efforts are not successful.

- The mechanism of exposure needs to be sought and established because intentional toxic exposure usually indicates severe social, emotional, and/or psychiatric pathology. When identified, the need for additional and aggressive intervention (e.g., hospital admission, social work, and psychiatric consults) may prevent a potentially fatal recurrence.

- Regardless of their severity, all toxic exposures need to be reported to the respective Poison Control Center.

REFERENCES

1. Litovitz TL, Klein-Schwartz W, Martin E, et al. 1998 American Annual Report of the American Association of Poison Control Centers Toxic Exposure Surveillance System. *Am J Emerg Med* 1999;17:435–487.
2. Stengel CL, Seaburg DC, MacLeod BA. Pregnancy in the emergency department: risk factors and prevalence among all women. *Ann Emerg Med* 1994;24:697–700.
3. Jones JS, Dickson K, Carlson S. Unrecognized pregnancy in the overdosed or poisoned patient. *Am J Emerg Med* 1997;15:538–541.
4. UNICEF. Drug use in pregnancy. *The Prescriber* 1992;1.
5. Greenblatt JF, Dannenberg AL, Johnson CJ. Incidence of hospitalized injuries among pregnant women in Maryland, 1979–1990. *Am J Prev Med* 1997;13:374–379.
6. Appleby L. Suicide during pregnancy and in the first postnatal year. *BMJ* 1991;302:137–140.
7. Kendell RE. Suicide in pregnancy and the puerperium. *BMJ* 1991;302:126–127.
8. Perrone J, Hoffman RS. Toxic ingestions in pregnancy: abortifacient use in a case series of pregnant overdose patients. *Acad Emerg Med* 1997;4:206–209.
9. Houston H, Jacobson L. Overdose and termination of pregnancy: an important association? *Br J Gen Pract* 1996;46:737–738.
10. Erickson TB, Neylan VD. Management principles of overdose in pregnancy. In: Haddad LM, Shannon MW, Winchester JF, eds. *Clinical management of poisoning and drug overdose,* 3rd ed. Philadelphia: WB Saunders, 1998.
11. Cruikshank DP, Wigton TR, Hays PM. Maternal physiology in pregnancy. In: Gabbe SG, Nyebyl JR, Simpson JL, eds. *Obstetrics. normal and problem pregnancies,* 3rd ed. New York: Churchill-Livingstone, 1996.
12. Doan-Wiggins L. Medical illness in the pregnant patient. In: Howell JM, Altieri M, Jagoda AS, et al, eds. *Emergency medicine.* Philadelphia: WB Saunders, 1998.
13. Tenenbein M. Methanol poisoning during pregnancy-prediction of risk and suggestions for management. *Clin Toxicol* 1997;35:193–194.
14. Koren G, ed. *Maternal-fetal toxicology,* 2nd ed. New York: Marcel Dekker, 1994.
15. Timar L, Czeizel AE. Birth weight and congenital anomalies following poisonous mushroom intoxication during pregnancy. *Reprod Toxicol* 1997;11:861–866.
16. McElhatton PR, Roberts JC, Sullivan FM. The consequences of iron overdose and its treatment with desferrioxamine in pregnancy. *Hum Exp Toxicol* 1991;10:251–259.
17. Strom RL, Schiller P, Seeds AE, et al. Fatal iron poisoning in a pregnant female: case report. *Minn Med* 1976;59:483–489.
18. Olenmark M, Biber B, Dottori O, et al. Fatal iron intoxication in late pregnancy. *Clin Toxicol* 1987;25:347–359.
19. Richards S, Brooks SHE. Ferrous sulphate poisoning in pregnancy (with apofibrinogenaemia as a complication). *West Ind Med J* 1966;15:134–140.
20. Olson K. *Poisoning and drug overdose,* 2nd ed. Norwalk, CT: Appleton & Lange, 1994.
21. Gei AF, Wen T, Belfort MA. Overdose and poisoning. In: Clark SL, Cotton DB, Hankins GDV, et al., eds. *Critical care obstetrics,* 3rd ed. Malden: Blackwell Science, 1997:636–669.
22. Kloeck A, Cummins RO, Chamberlain D, et al. Special Resuscitation Situations. An advisory statement from the International Liaison Committee on Resuscitation. *Circulation* 1997;95:2196–2210.
23. Goldfrank LR, Flomenbaum NE, Lewin NA, et al, eds. *Goldfrank's toxicologic emergencies,* 6th ed. Norwalk, CT: Appleton & Lange, 1998.
24. Nicholson DP. The immediate management of overdose. *Med Clin North Am* 1983;67:1279–1293.
25. Doyon S, Roberts JR. Reappraisal of the "coma cocktail." Dextrose, flumazenil, naloxone and thiamine. *Emerg Clin North Am* 1994;12:301–316.
26. Hoffman RS, Goldfrank LR. The poisoned patient with altered consciousness. Controversies in the use of a "coma cocktail." *JAMA* 1995;274:562–569.
27. Weinbroum AA, Flaishon R, Sorkine P, et al. A risk-benefit assessment of flumazenil in the management of benzodiazepine overdose. *Drug Saf* 1997;17:181–196.
28. Dickson PH, Lind A, Studts P, et al. The routine analysis of breast milk for drugs of abuse in a clinical toxicology laboratory. *J Forensic Sci* 1994;39:207–214.
29. Sim MR, McNeil JJ. Monitoring chemical exposure using breast milk: a methodological review. *Am J Epidemiol* 1992;136:1–11.
30. Kim E, Brion LP, Meenan G, et al. Perinatal toxicology screening: comparison of various maternal and neonatal samples. *J Perinatol* 1998;18:116–121.
31. Bolgiano EB, Barish RA. Use of new and established antidotes. *Emerg Clin North Am* 1994:12:317–334.

32. Gossel TA, Bricker JD, eds. *Principles of clinical toxicology,* 3rd ed. New York: Raven Press, 1994.

33. Shannon MW, Haddad LM. The emergency management of poisoning. In: Haddad LM, Shannon MW, Winchester JF, eds. *Clinical management of poisoning and drug overdose,* 3rd ed. Philadelphia: WB Saunders, 1998.

34. Smilkstein MJ. Techniques used to prevent gastrointestinal absorption of toxic compounds. In: Goldfrank LR, Flomenbaum NE, Lewin NA, et al., eds. *Goldfrank's Toxicologic Emergencies,* 6th ed. Norwalk, CT: Appleton & Lange, 1998.

35. Heinonen OP, Slone D, Shapiro S. *Birth defects and drugs in pregnancy.* Littleton, MA: John Wright-PSG, 1977:378,442.

36. PDRR Electronic Library. Version 5.1.0a. Montvale: Medical Economics, 1999.

37. McElhatton PR, Sullivan FM, Volans GN. Paracetamol overdose in pregnancy. Analysis of the outcomes of 300 cases referred to the Teratology Information Service. *Reprod Toxicol* 1997;11:85–94.

38. Wang PH, Yang MJ, Lee WL, et al. Acetaminophen poisoning in late pregnancy. A case report. *J Reprod Med* 1997;42:367–371.

39. Jones AL, Prescott LF. Unusual complications of paracetamol poisoning. *Q J Med* 1997;90:161–168.

40. Rutherfoord-Rose S. Acetaminophen. In: Howell JM, Altieri M, Jagoda AS, et al., eds. *Emergency medicine.* Philadelphia: WB Saunders, 1998.

41. Horowitz RS, Dart RC, Jarvie DR, et al. Placental transfer of *N*-Acetylcysteine following human maternal acetaminophen toxicity. *Clin Toxicol* 1997;35:447–451.

42. Chan TYK. Potential dangers from topical preparations containing methyl salicylate. *Hum Exp Toxicol* 1996; 15:747–750.

43. Palatnick W, Tenenbein M. Aspirin poisoning during pregnancy: increased fetal sensitivity. *Am J Perinatol* 1998;15:39–41.

44. Rejent TA, Baik S. Fatal *in utero* salicylism. *J Forensic Sci* 1985;30:942–944.

45. White S, Wong SHY. Standards of laboratory practice: analgesic drug monitoring. *Clin Chem* 1998;44:1110–1123.

46. Balaskas TN. Common poisons. In: Gleicher N, Elkayam U, Galgraith RM, et al., eds. *Principles and practice of medical therapy in pregnancy,* 2nd ed. Norwalk, CT: Appleton & Lange, 1992.

47. Kerns W II. Salicylate and nonsteroidal anti-inflammatory drug poisoning. In: Howell JM, Altieri M, Jagoda AS, et al., eds. *Emergency medicine,* Philadelphia: WB Saunders, 1998.

48. McFarland AK III. Anticonvulsants. In: Howell JM, Altieri M, Jagoda AS, et al., eds. *Emergency medicine.* Philadelphia: WB Saunders, 1998.

49. Martin CL, Babib JL, Demarquez B, et al. Intoxication néo-natale par certaines thérapeutiques psychotropes maternelles. Aspects cliniques et physiopathologiques. *Pediatrie* 1974;29:147–157.

50. Mazurek A, Mazurek J. Acute barbiturate poisoning in the 39th week of pregnancy. Case report. *Anaesth Resusc Intens Ther* 1975;3:193–196.

51. Schauben JL. Benzodiazepines. In: Howell JM, Altieri M, Jagoda AS, et al., eds. *Emergency medicine,* Philadelphia: WB Saunders, 1998.

52. Gaudreault P, Guay J, Thivierge RL, et al. Benzodiazepine poisoning. Clinical and pharmacological considerations and treatment. *Drug Saf* 1991;6:247–265.

53. Cerqueira MJ, Olle C, Bellart J, et al. Intoxication by benzodiazepines during pregnancy. *Lancet* 1988;1:1341.

54. Sakai T, Matsuda H, Watanabe N. Triazolam (Halcion) intoxication in a neonate—a first report. *Eur J Pediatr* 1996;155:1065–1068.

55. Stahl MM, Saldeen P, Vinge E. Reversal of fetal benzodiazepine intoxication using flumazenil. *Br J Obstet Gynaecol* 1993;100:185–188.

56. Dixon JC, Speidel BD, Dixon JJ. Neonatal flumazenil therapy reverses maternal diazepam. *Acta Paediatr* 1998;87:225–226.

57. Silvers SM, Hampson NB. Carbon monoxide poisoning among recreational boaters. *JAMA* 1995;274:1614–1616.

58. Longo LD. The biological effects of carbon monoxide on the pregnant woman, fetus, and newborn infant. *Am J Obstet Gynecol* 1977;129:69–103.

59. Tomaszewski C. Carbon monoxide poisoning. Early awareness and intervention can save lives. *Postgrad Med* 1999;105:39–50.

60. Rubio S, García ML, Intoxicación por monóxido de carbono. *Med Clin* 1997;108:776–778.

61. Koren G. Carbon monoxide poisoning in pregnancy. *Can Fam Physician* 1996;42:854–855.

62. Kopelman AE, Plaut TA. Fetal compromise caused by maternal carbon monoxide poisoning. *J Perinatol* 1998;18:74–77.

63. Silverman RK, Montano J. Hyperbaric oxygen treatment during pregnancy in acute carbon monoxide poisoning. A case report. *J Reprod Med* 1997;42:309–311.

64. Abramovich A, Shupak A, Ramon Y, et al. Hyperbaric oxygen for carbon monoxide poisoning. *Harefuah* 1997;132:21–24.

65. Jackson LD. Different presentations of cocaine intoxication: four cases studies. *J Emerg Nurs* 1997;23:232–234.

66. Lovejoy FH, Shannon M, Woolf AD. Recent advances in clinical toxicology. *Curr Probl Pediatr* 1992;March:119–128.

67. Miller JM, Boudreaux MC, Regan FA. A case-control study of cocaine use in pregnancy. *Am J Obstet Gynecol* 1995;172:180–185.

68. Wehbeh H, Matthews RP, McCalla S, et al. The effect of recent cocaine use on the progress of labor. *Am J Obstet Gynecol* 1995;172:1014–1018.

69. Martinez A, Larrabee K, Monga M. Cocaine is associated with intrauterine fetal death in women with suspected preterm labor. *Am J Perinatol* 1996;13:163–166.

70. Delaney DB, Larrabee KD, Monga M. Preterm premature rupture of the membranes associated with recent cocaine use. *Am J Perinatol* 1997;14:285–288.

71. Emery CL, Morway LF, Chung-Park M, et al. The Kleihauer-Betke test. Clinical utility, indication, and correlation in patients with placental abruption and cocaine use. *Arch Pathol Lab Med* 1995;119:1032–1037.

72. Nair P, Rothblim S, Hebel R. Neonatal outcome in infants with evidence of fetal exposure to opiates, cocaine, and cannabinoids. *Clin Pediatr* 1994;May:280–285.

73. Cohen HR, Green JR, Crombleholme WR. Peripartum cocaine use: estimating risk of adverse pregnancy outcome. *Int J Gynecol Obstet* 1991;35:51–54.

74. Stewart DE, Streiner D. Alcohol drinking in pregnancy. *Gen Hosp Psychiatry* 1994;16:406–412.

75. Morgan BW, Ford MD. Ethanol. In: Howell JM, Altieri M, Jagoda AS, et al., eds. *Emergency medicine,* Philadelphia: WB Saunders, 1998.
76. Brien JF, Smith GN. Effect of alcohol (ethanol) on the fetus. *J Dev Physiol* 1991;15:21–32.
77. Streissguth AP, Sampson PD, Barr HM. Neurobehavioral dose-response effects of prenatal alcohol exposure in humans from infancy to adulthood. *Ann N Y Acad Sci* 1989;562:145–158.
78. Levine B, ed. *Principles of forensic toxicology.* Washington: American Association of Clinical Chemistry, 1999.
79. Barinov EK, Burago II, Bulanakova AB. The death of a newborn infant from ethanol poisoning. *Sud Med Ekspert* 1997;40:45.
80. Rayburn W, Anonow R, Delay B, et al. Drug overdose during pregnancy: an overview from a metropolitan poison control center. *Obstet Gynecol* 1984;64:611–614.
81. Lacoste H, Goyert GL, Goldman LS, et al. Acute iron intoxication in pregnancy: case report and review of the literature. *Obstet Gynecol* 1992;80:500–501.
82. Tran T, Wax JR, Steinfield JD, et al. Acute intentional iron overdose in pregnancy. *Obstet Gynecol* 1998;92:678–680.
83. Bailey B. Organophosphate poisoning in pregnancy [Letter]. *Ann Emerg Med* 1997;29:299.
84. Okumura T. Organophosphate poisoning in pregnancy [Reply]. *Ann Emerg Med* 1997;29:299.
85. Sancewicz K, Groszek B, Pach D, et al. Acute pesticides poisonings in pregnant women. *Przegl Lek* 1997;54:741–744.
86. Saadeh AM, Al-Ali MK, Farsakh NA, et al. Clinical and sociodemographic features of acute carbamate and organophosphate poisoning: a study of 70 adult patients in North Jordan. *Clin Toxicol* 1996;34:45–51.
87. Dmochowska-Mroczek H, Lebensztejn W, Tolwinski K. Severe intoxication with Dipterex in a pregnant woman. *Pol Tygod Lek* 1972;27:1406–1407.
88. Perrone JM, Hoffman RS. Antidepressants. In: Howell JM, Altieri M, Jagoda AS, et al., eds. *Emergency medicine,* Philadelphia: WB Saunders, 1998.
89. Vree PH, Zwart P. A newborn infant with amitriptyline poisoning. *Ned Tijdschr Geneesk* 1985;129:910–912.
90. Gimovsky ML. Fetal heart rate monitoring casebook. *J Perinatol* 1995;15:246–249.

SUGGESTED READINGS

Balaskas TN. Common poisons. In: Gleicher N, Elkayam U, Galgraith RM, et al., eds. *Principles and practice of medical therapy in Pregnancy,* 2nd ed. Norwalk, CT: Appleton & Lange, 1992.
Erickson TB, Neylan VD. Management principles of overdose in pregnancy. In: Haddad LM, Shannon MW, Winchester JF, eds. *Clinical management of poisoning and drug overdose,* 3rd ed. Philadelphia: WB Saunders, 1998.
Gei AF, Wen T, Belfort MA. Overdose and poisoning. In: Clark SL, Cotton DB, Hankins GDV, et al., eds. *Critical care obstetrics,* 3rd ed. Malden: Blackwell Science, 1997:636–669.

26

Complementary and Alternative Therapy During Pregnancy

Gayle L. Olson

Department of Obstetrics and Gynecology, The University of Texas Medical Branch at Galveston, Galveston, Texas

Complementary and alternative medicine (CAM) encompasses a broad array of healing resources. CAM includes all practices and ideas that may prevent or treat illness or promote health and well-being. CAM encompasses the theories and beliefs that are other than those of the politically dominant health system of a particular society or culture in a given historical period. In practice, CAM often overlaps with the politically dominant system (1).

CAM is now a forefront issue as more and more of our patients choose to participate in CAM theories and methods. Women will use CAM more than men, and the group most likely to use CAM is affluent middle-aged women (2). Overall, 80% of patients who use CAM also use conventional medicine and 70% of these patients do not discuss CAM use with their physician (2). Estimated expenditures for CAM professional services have increased 45% between 1990 and 1997 and expenditures for CAM exceeded all out-of-pocket expenditures for U.S. hospitalization (3). CAM therapies that appear to be on the rise include herbal, massage, megavitamins, self-help groups, folk remedies, energy healing, and homeopathy (3). Many modalities have been used during pregnancy and include acupressure, acupuncture, massage, phytomedicine, homeopathy, yoga, Tai Chi Chuan, meditation, sound therapy, color therapy, light therapy, visualization, and naturopathy (4). Many of these modalities have not undergone scientific study

and only acupuncture, acupressure, massage, and phytomedicine are discussed here.

ACUPUNCTURE

Acupuncture theory and practice are grounded in the framework of traditional Chinese medicine. Simply stated, in traditional Chinese medicine yin, yang, Qi, blood, fluids, and the five elements (wood, fire, earth, metal, and water) interact and thus influence one's environment and health (5,6). An individual's energy balance can be influenced by these forces in both positive and negative directions. This energy flows along the body in meridians or rivers of energy. There are 14 main meridians that run in a paired vertical manner along the body (7). Acupuncture points are specific locations or gates along the body where the meridians come to the surface of the skin (5,6). Physiologic or emotional ailments may indicate an unbalanced positive/negative charge or blocked energy. The energy can be manipulated by the insertion of very fine needles at these specific acupoints or gates, and the imbalance is thereafter corrected. Acupuncture needles vary in size but, most important, are now disposable. Insertion techniques also vary in terms of depth and angle and depend on the ailment. A small sensation is usually noted upon insertion of the needle and may coincide with activation of nerve receptors.

Acupressure is similar to acupuncture but uses the application of pressure rather than needles at various acupuncture points (4). Indications for the use of acupuncture and acupressure during pregnancy have included hyperemesis, version, cervical ripening, stimulation of labor, stimulation of lactation, edema, preeclampsia, depression, and analgesia for delivery (6,8,9). Specific indications and the associated acupoints include:

Stimulation of labor: spleen 9 (SP 9), spleen 6 (SP 6), large intestine 4 (LI 4), stomach 36 (ST 36), and bladder 67 (BL 67) (6,10,11). However, caution is suggested, for these same points used early in pregnancy may also facilitate termination (10).
Spontaneous version: bladder 67 (BL 67) (12).
Hyperemesis: Pericardium 6 (P 6) (13,14).
Insufficient lactation postpartum: Cardiovascular (CV 17), stomach 18 (ST 18), large intestine (LI 4), and small intestine (SI 1) (13,15).

Because of the possible effect of labor stimulation, acupoints to avoid in the antenatal period include any abdominal point, the bottom of the foot, kidney (K I1), the inner lower leg, spleen 6 (SP 6), the outer thumb base, (LI 4), and the back of the shoulder, (GB 21) (8,13; personal communication, S. Rosenblatt, Board of National Accreditation for Acupuncture, 1999) (Fig. 26.1).

Although acupuncture has been practiced for more than 5,000 years, scientific investigation evaluating its effectiveness is relatively new. In the area of obstetrics, studies evaluating the effectiveness of acupuncture for spontaneous version, hyperemesis gravidarum, and anesthesia/analgesia during delivery have been conducted as follows:

Spontaneous Version

Moxibustion has been used for several thousand years in Chinese medicine to promote a breech fetus turning to a cephalic presentation in the third trimester (8,12). Moxibustion itself is the use of moxa, otherwise known as mugwort (*Artemisia vulgaris*), that is dried and finely ground. The moxa is formed into a cone, stick, or small button that is placed directly on the skin or indirectly through interfacing agents. The moxa stick is used like a cigar; it is lighted and held near the skin to cause mild warmth but not blistering. Moxibustion was scientifically evaluated by Cardini et al. (12) who recruited 260 primigravidas at gestational ages 33 to 35 weeks and randomized to either intervention (moxibustion) or no intervention. Intervention consisted of moxibustion therapy 30 minutes once daily for the first week, then twice daily during the second week. The participants were instructed to tolerate an intensity of moxibustion that would result in hyperemia from local vasodilation but not blisters. Upon completion of 35 weeks of gestation, 75% of fetuses were cephalic in the intervention group compared with 47% in the nonintervention group. Moxibustion's mechanism of action is believed to be associated with increased fetal movement. Fetal movement was in fact recorded during this trial and supports this theory, as the women in the intervention group noted significantly more fetal movements compared with the nonintervention group (12).

Hyperemesis

Acupuncture and acupressure therapy for nausea and vomiting have been investigated in multiple trials (14,16–23). In traditional Chinese medicine, hyperemesis is differentiated into three different categories. Acupoints specific for each category are then stimulated for treatment (6,8,9). Refinement, to this degree, has not been attempted in Western medicine where the single acupoint, P 6, is primarily used. Vickers (14) reviewed 33 trials involving acupuncture during chemotherapy, pregnancy, or surgery. In four of the studies, acupuncture was administered simultaneously with anesthesia and did not appear to be effective; however, in 27 of the remaining 29 trials, acupuncture stimulation was superior to placebo. In 11 of the 33 trials, the study designs were randomized and placebo-controlled and involved approximately 2,000 patients (14). These 11 trials noted a significant effect in nausea reduction by acupuncture (14). DeAloysio and Penacehioni (18) evaluated unilateral versus bilateral use of wrist bands in addition to overall effectiveness and, although acupressure was found to be superior to placebo, no difference was noted between unilateral and bilateral application for nausea reduction.

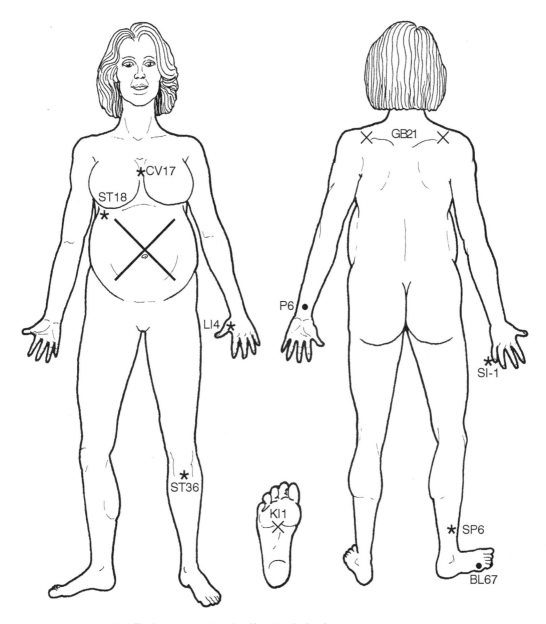

X Points contra-indicated during pregnancy
• Points beneficial for treatment during pregnancy
★ Points which are used for induction or lactation

FIG. 26.1. Approximate acupoints using anatomic landmarks.

One of the largest clinical trials by Dundee et al. (23) involved 350 participants and compared P6 acupoint versus sham or no intervention and did not find a significant benefit from acupressure. A variation of acupuncture, electro-acupuncture, uses an electric current to stimulate the acupoint, thus balancing positive and negative forces along meridians. The Relief Band is a device patented to stimulate P6 using electro-acupuncture techniques for treatment of nausea and vomiting owing to chemotherapy, motion sickness, and pregnancy. Although this device is used clinically, no randomized trials have been conducted. Clinical trials investigating acupressure for nausea and vomiting during pregnancy in most cases showed reductions in symptoms (17–20). However, all the clinical trials are hampered by the ability of researchers to conduct true blinded and placebo-controlled investigations. Evidence available in the literature appears to be equivocal concerning benefits of acupressure for nausea and vomiting of pregnancy. However, although methodologies may be debated and statistical significance disputed, acupressure of P6 appears to benefit many women and as yet has not been associated with adverse events.

Labor and Delivery

In the time frame surrounding delivery, acupuncture has been used for preparation of labor, induction, analgesia, and anesthesia.

Acupuncture in preparation for labor has been evaluated in three trials (24–26). The trials reveal conflicting results. Zeisler et al. (24) stimulated three acupoints for the study group on a weekly basis beginning at 36 weeks of gestation. The control group was established by choosing women who had delivered a pregnancy at the same time as a study participant. The first stage of labor was significantly shorter and the use of oxytocin significantly less for the study group compared with the control group. Conversely, the incidence of premature rupture of membranes (PROM) was significantly greater for the study versus control group. Lyrenas et al. (25) found no difference in an acupuncture-treated group compared with a control group for length of the first stage of labor, but noted the second stage of labor to be significantly prolonged. The acupoints utilized by Lyrenas et al. differed from those used by other investigators, otherwise study designs were similar. Finally, Kubista and Kucera (26) revealed a reduction in delivery time for primiparous women treated with acupuncture compared with a group without acupuncture. Study designs differ slightly in all three trials; nonetheless, there does not appear to be solid evidence

that acupuncture in the last weeks of pregnancy reduces labor or decreases obstetric intervention. Rather, the finding of increased PROM in one acupuncture group should raise concern regarding the application of this alternative method before term.

Electroacupuncture for induction of labor has been reported (27–29) primarily as observational studies. Uterine contractility was successfully stimulated in approximately 78% of the gravidas. These successes were attained in postterm and intrauterine demise cases (28) and did not appear to be associated with fetal or maternal complications in the postterm group (28,29). One case required electroacupuncture stimulation for 36 hours, whereas others required treatment for 5 to 18 hours (28). A different group receiving midterm terminations all failed to respond to similar electroacupuncture stimulation (28).

Abouleish and Depp (30) applied electroacupuncture in a small group of women for analgesia during labor. Each participant acted as her own control receiving regional anesthesia when electroacupuncture was no longer tolerated. Electroacupuncture primarily provided hypoalgesia when compared with regional techniques. No adverse effects were noted on fetal heart rate or uterine contractility; however, some electrical interference with the fetal heart rate tracing was appreciated (30). Finally, these authors concluded the electroacupuncture analgesia was incomplete, inconsistent, and cumbersome.

Acupuncture anesthesia at the time of cesarean section has been documented in more than 24,000 cases in the Chinese literature with success rates of 70% to 80% (31,32). However, supplemental medication and special surgical technique were required. Acupuncture anesthesia was compared with epidural anesthesia (32) and appeared associated with less blood loss, less alteration in pulse and blood pressure, and a more rapid recovery time. An additional investigation involving 14 patients had a failure rate of 43% for acupuncture anesthesia during cesarean section (33).

There are no randomized trials evaluating the efficacy of acupuncture for labor preparation, analgesia during labor, or anesthesia during cesarean section. The increased incidence of PROM during labor preparation should be considered in discussing this alternative modality. Adverse events were otherwise not noted. Women interested in acupuncture would need to be highly motivated to receive this therapy. Although efficacy cannot be confirmed, acupuncture use after 37 weeks of gestation appears not to do harm, and when used for cesarean section would most likely need to be supplemented with other modalities.

MASSAGE

Massage therapy has been advocated as a way to improve health because it has the potential to reduce tension, improve circulation and digestion, and relax muscles (4). Massage during pregnancy may prove beneficial in relieving backache, insomnia, lower extremity edema, and hyperemesis. Swedish massage techniques are among the most commonly employed and would appear the most appropriate during pregnancy.

The position of the woman during the massage in the first trimester is not of major concern; however, in the second and third trimesters, the completely supine or prone positions are not desirable. The supine position utilizing left lateral tilt may be tolerated for a short amount of time. The side-lying position (complete left lateral) is preferred for the majority of the massage (34). Special tables may be also used that accommodate the gravid abdomen. Deep abdominal massage is to be avoided during the entire pregnancy and for 3 months postpartum (35). Overstretching of muscles and overmobilizing of joints are also to be avoided because permanent laxity may result (35). As previously discussed, acupressure at specific points should be avoided during pregnancy, likewise these same points should not receive acupressure stimulation during massage.

In a prospective, randomized trial by Field et al. (36), 26 gravidas were assigned to massage or relaxation therapy for 5 weeks. Compared with the relaxation therapy group, the women in the massage group reported reduced anxiety, improved mood and sleep, and less back pain.

Norepinephrine levels were also decreased in the group receiving massage.

In a separate study, Field et al. (37) randomized women in labor to breathing alone versus breathing and massage. The massage group had significantly shorter labor and less postpartum depression.

Both of these randomized trials suggest benefit from massage therapy during pregnancy. Given proper positioning and technique, massage during pregnancy does not appear to be associated with adverse events.

PHYTOMEDICINE

Phytomedicinals have been used for health and well-being since the time of Hippocrates. In fact, many of our conventional medications are derived from herbs. In recent times, therapeutic use of herbs has been more widely practiced in Europe than the United States, and government standards have been set forth in Germany to ensure the safety and efficacy of herbal preparations (38). Herbal remedies have now become a major factor in American Health Care. Herbal products in the United States are classified as dietary supplements and as such have avoided scientific scrutiny by the US Food and Drug Administration (FDA) (39). They are not required to have proof of safety or any testing for efficacy. There are no required quality control standards.

Historic indications for the use of herbs during pregnancy are listed in Table 26.1. Herbs containing the chemicals anthraquinone and berberine may stimulate uterine activity and should not be used during pregnancy (40). Herbs containing pyrrolidine alkaloids, for example, comfrey, are associated with severe liver damage and are not to be used internally at any time (Table 26.2) (40). As a result of the limited scientific evaluation for most herbs, safety and efficacy cannot be clearly addressed. The suggestion by even one source of an unfavorable outcome or reaction associated with an herb should currently prevent its use during pregnancy (Table 26.3).

The following section discusses aromatherapy, herbal preparations, and uses of herbs during pregnancy.

TABLE 26.1. *Herbs historically used during pregnancy by CAM practitioners*

Prevention or termination of pregnancy
  Black hellebore (*Helleborus niger*)
  Burning bush (*Dictamnus albus*)
  Castor oil plant (*Ricinus communis*)
  Chinese cinnamon (*Cinnamomum aromaticum, Arsarum europaem*)
  Jequirity (*Abrus precatorius*)
  Pomegranate (*Punica granatum*)
  Rue (*Ruta graveolens*)
  Safflower (*Carthamus tinctorius*)
  Sumaruba (*Simaruba amora*)
  Wild carrot (Queen Anne's lace) (*Daucus carota*)
  Yew (*Taxus baccata*)
Postpartum hemorrhage
  Broom (*Cytisus scoparius*)
  Ergot (*Claviceps purpurea*)
Cervical ripening
  Evening primrose oil (*Oenothera biennis*)
Stimulation of lactation
  Black elder (*Sambuscus nigra*)
  Caraway (*Carum carvi*)
  Cotton (*Gossypium herbaceum*)
  Vervain (*Verbena officinalis*)
Stimulation of labor
  Black haw (*Vibernum prunifolium*)
  Black cohosh (*Cimicifuga racemosa*)
  Blue cohosh (*Caulophyllum thalictroides*)
  Broom (*Cytisus scoparius*)
  Fever bark (*Alstonia constricta*)
  Life root (*Senecio nemorensis*)
  Lily of the valley (*Convallaria majalis*)
  Motherwort (*Leonurius cardiaca*)
  Partridgeberry (*Mitchella repens*)
  Peony (*Paeonia officinalis*)
  Red raspberry (*Rubis ideius*)

Note: The editors include this section for educational purposes. Many of these herbs are at least relatively, if not absolutely, contraindicated for use in pregnancy.
  Adapted from refs. 39–41, 57, and 77.

TABLE 26.2. *Chemical agents to avoid*

Agent	Herb-containing agent
Anthranoids	Aloe (*Aloe vera/barbadensis*)
	Buckthorn berry (*Rhamnus catharticus*)
	Buckthorn bark (*Rhamnus frangula*)
	Cascara sagrada bark (*Rhamnus purshiana*)
	Rhubarb root (*Rheum officinale*)
	Senna (*Senna alexandrina, Cassia acutifolia*)
	Yellow dock (*Rumex crispus*)
Pyrrolizidine alkaloids	Borage (*Borago officinalis*)
	Coltsfoot (*Tussilago farfara*)
	Comfrey (*Symphytum officinale*)
	Gravel root (*Eupatorium purpureum*)
	Hound's-tongue (*Cynoglossum officinale*)
	Petasites (*Petasites spp*)
Berberine	Barberry (*Berberis vulgaris*)
	Celandine (*Chelidonium majus*)
	Goldenseal (*Hydrastis canadensis*)
	Oregon graperoot (*Mahonia repens*)

Adapted from refs. 39–41, 57, and 77.

Aromatherapy

Aromatherapy is a science and art using essential oils of the plant derived through a distillation process that leaves volatile, water-insoluble isolates (41). Therefore, the essential oils are the most concentrated form of an herb, and for this reason a little may be beneficial but more is definitely not better. In fact, the distillation process may remove a portion of the whole herb, thus changing the benefit profile listed in an evaluation of the whole plant. Some oils are toxic, trigger seizures, hypertension, and hypotension, stimulate the heart, promote diuresis, or simply cause skin irritation when used in excess (42).

Essential oils are often used in conjunction with massage. For this application, the essential oil is diluted and seldom dangerous. However, the safety of use has not been demonstrated during pregnancy (43). Many herbs from which essential oils are derived are used during everyday cooking, and in the form of the whole herb, they are safe to use when added to foods in this manner (41).

Essential oils can be administered through the skin, using a bath or compress, mucous membranes, using a douche or pessary, or inhaled by using candles and burners (44). Essential oils have been used during pregnancy for insomnia, nausea, vomiting, labor induction, stress, constipation, edema, relief of labor pain, and healing of the perineum after delivery (1,41). In a survey conducted in North Carolina (45), 32.9% of certified nurse-midwives reported using this form of alternative therapy during pregnancy. Essential oils that have not as yet been associated with adverse effects have been suggested as safe for use during pregnancy and include lavender, mandarin, orange, rosewood, sandalwood, ylang-ylang, geranium, and neroli (Table 26.4) (1,42). These same authors suggested that some essential oils be avoided during pregnancy (Table 26.5). No randomized trials have been

TABLE 26.3. *Herbs with at least one report indicating use is contraindicated during pregnancy*

Angelica (*Angelica archangelica*)
Autumn crocus (*Colchicum autumnale*)
Basil oil (*Ocimum basilicum*)
Bearberry (uva ursi leaf) (*Arctostaphylos uva-ursi*)
Borage (*Borago officinalis*)
California poppy (*Eschscholzia californica*)
Catnip (*Nepeta cataria*)
Cinnamon (*Cinnamomum verum*)
Coltsfoot (*Tussilago farfara*)
Fennel (*Foeniculum vulgare*)
Feverfew (*Chrysanthemum parthenium*)
Horehound (*Ballota nigra*)
Hyssop (*Hyssopus officinalis*)
Indian snakeroot (*Rauvolfia serpentina*)
Juniper berry (*Juniperus communis*)
Kava kava (*Piper methysticum*)
Licorice (*Glycyrrhiza glabra*)
Liverwort (*Anemone hepatica*)
Marjoram (*Origamun marjorana*)
Marsh tea (*Ledum latifolium*)
Mayapple (*Podophyllum peltatum*)
Mistletoe (*Phoradendron flavescens*)
Motherwort (*Leonorus cardiaca*)
Mugwort (*Artemisia vulgaris*)
Myrrh (*Commiphora molmol*)
Nutmeg (*Myristica fragrans*)
Parsley (*Petroselinum crispum*)
Pasqueflower (*Pulsatilla pratensis*)
Pennyroyal (*Hedeoma pulegiodes and Menthapulegium*)
Peppermint (*Mentha piperita*)
Roman chamomile (*Chamaemelum nobile*)
Rose (*Rose* spp)
Rosemary (*Rosmarinus officinalis*)
Safflower (*Carthamus tinctorius*)
Saffron (*Crocus sativus*)
Sage leaf (*Salvia officinalis*)
Sheperd's purse (*Capsella bursa-pastoris*)
Tansy (*Chrysanthemum vulgare*)
Thuja (*Thuja occidentalis*)
Trillium (*Trillium pendulum*)
Turmeric root (*Curcuma domestica*)
Wild bergamot (*Monarda punctata*)
Wild ginger (*Asarum canadensis*)
Wintergreen (*Gaultheria procumbens*)
Wormwood (*Artemisia absinthium*)
Yarrow (*Achillea millefolium*)

Adapted from refs. 39–41, 57, and 77.

TABLE 26.4. *Methods of administration of essential oils*

Oil	Massage	Bath	Burner
Lavender	X	X	X
Mandarin	X	X	X
Neroli			X
Orange		X	X
Rosewood		X	
Sandalwood			X
Ylang-ylang			X

Adapted from refs. 44 and 45.

jasmine, rose, lemon, and mandarin. Lavender was the oil most commonly used, and it was chosen to reduce anxiety and lighten the mood. Participants completed questionnaires and commented on lavender's relaxing effect. Only two women described increased nausea when exposed to lavender aroma. Unfortunately, evaluation of the effect on labor or birth outcome was not included in the report.

Safety and efficacy of aromatherapy during pregnancy have not been evaluated and, although some essential oils appear to have been used without untoward effects, recommendations for use during pregnancy can not be given at this time.

Herbs

Herbal preparations come in various forms, are listed as dietary supplements by the FDA, and particularly lend themselves to self-administration by patients. Herbal preparations include tea, infusion, deconcoction, poultice, compress, fomentation, tincture, and capsule

conducted to support these claims. A study by Burns and Blamey (46) did attempt to evaluate the effect of aromatherapy during childbirth. Five hundred pregnant women presenting in labor received aromatherapy treatments. The essential oils studied included lavender, clary sage, peppermint, eucalyptus, chamomile, frankincense,

TABLE 26.5. *Essential oils to avoid*

Angelica	Fennel	Oregano
Aniseed	Ginger	Parsley
Basil	Hyssop	Pennyroyal
Blue chamomile	Jasmine	Peppermint
Camphor	Juniper	Rose
Cedarwood	Marjoram	Rosemary
Cinnamon Bark	Mugwort	Sage
Clary Sage	Myrrh	Savory
Clove	Nutmeg	Thyme
Cypress	Origanum	Wintergreen

Adapted from refs. 4 and 45.

TABLE 26.6. *Emmenagogues*

Vervain	Myrrh
Corydalis (Turkey corn)	Wild ginger
Turmeric	Pennyroyal
Motherwort	Tansy
Bugleweed	Blue cohosh
Peach seed	St. John's wort
Safflower	Rose flowers
Saffron	Chaste berries
Calendula	Rue
Frankincense	Collinsonia

Adapted from refs. 40, 41, and 57.

(40). Herbs with actions specific to pregnancy can be classified as abortifacients, emmenagogues, and galactogogues (40). Emmenagogues promote uterine contraction and have been used to induce labor; conversely, if used in the early stages of pregnancy, they could also result in premature delivery. A list of herbs cited as having emmenagogue properties are included in Table 26.6. In addition to the indications for treatment of specific ailments, herbs are also used as tonics. A tonic is a term reserved for an herb that nourishes well-being. In western alternative medicine, this word generally means a safe and gentle herb that is taken daily in small amounts. Over time, this aids in restoring balance and tone to systems that are under stress (40). It is recommended that herbs used as tonics during pregnancy, if used alone, are used in very small amounts or are alternated in small amounts with other tonic herbs (40). This reduces the overall amount of any single herb. Herbs considered safe tonics for use during pregnancy include lemon balm, lavender, oats, alfalfa, spearmint, stevia, dandelion root, raspberry leaf, stinging nettle, Siberian ginseng, and green tea (40)

Antepartum Herbal Use

Hyperemesis Gravidarum

Ginger (*Zingiberis officinale*) has a long history of use in Chinese medicine for treating nausea and vomiting during pregnancy (38,39). In a recent study, Fischer-Rasmussen et al. (47) were also able to reduce symptoms of hyperemesis by administering ginger capsules (47). However,

the German Commission E Monographs caution the use of ginger because of two studies suggesting mutagenic activity (38). Admittedly, the authors of these monographs cite multiple references in which ginger has been used without adverse effects, and they acknowledge this controversy. Nevertheless, the initial stance in the Commission E Monographs was not reversed (38). Ginger can be taken as capsules and as tea (48). Tea would involve the smallest amount of the herb and would appear to be the safest. Ginger has been noted to interfere with clotting in test tubes; however, studies involving oral ginger administration did not note similar effects (48). Four of six studies evaluating ginger for the prevention of motion sickness found it beneficial (49).

Vitamin B_6 in doses of 10 to 25 mg three times daily was found to be beneficial in treating hyperemesis in some trials (21,48). A randomized, double-blind, placebo-controlled study (50) investigating B_6 treatment for nausea and vomiting during pregnancy found a significant reduction in symptoms with B_6 compared with placebo. No differences were noted between B_6 and placebo for women with mild to moderate nausea and larger doses are not recommended (51).

Additional herbal remedies found successful in the treatment of nausea include chamomile, meadowsweet, spearmint, and slippery elm, most often as infusions or frozen (52,53). In cases in which heartburn is predominant, herbs that may reduce symptoms include meadowsweet, slippery elm bark, chamomile, and Iceland moss (52,54).

Again, the smallest dose of herb is probably the safest and is obtained when consuming preparations in the form of a tea. Herbs used in treating hyperemesis may seem ineffective after prolonged use; therefore, alternating herbs can avoid both tolerance and overuse (40,52).

The supplement with the strongest evidence for use in the treatment of hyperemesis gravidarum is vitamin B_6. The safety and efficacy of herbal preparations have yet to be established. Even considering the controversy surrounding ginger, its widespread use without adverse effects supports use, especially in the form of teas and soft drinks.

Insomnia

Common therapies for insomnia include acupressure, acupuncture, and herbal and homeopathic remedies (4). An infusion consisting of hops, lime blossom, or skullcap has been noted to resolve insomnia during pregnancy (52). Essential oils of lavender, marjoram, and neroli all have sedative properties and can be used alone or in combination in a bath before bedtime. A small drop of lavender oil can also be placed on the edge of the pillow or placed in an aromatherapy dispenser (42). No alternative therapy or herbal preparation has been studied for treatment of insomnia during pregnancy. Valerian has received attention as an herb beneficial in reducing anxiety and promoting sleep in nonpregnant populations (38,39,48,55) and is discussed in detail.

Valerian (Valeriana Officinalis)

Valerian is indigenous to Europe. The underground portion of the plant and roots contains the medicinally relevant compounds, which include valepotriates, volatile oil, sesquiterpenes, pyridine alkaloids, and chlorogenic acid (39,56). Valerian is suggested as treatment for both insomnia and nervousness in the nonpregnant population (38,39,48). No contraindications for use of valerian have been suggested (38,39), and no side effects have been documented (38,39). Valerian can be taken internally or used in the bath (39). The only cautions would apply to the operation of a motor vehicle after ingesting valerian (48). Outside the context of pregnancy, valerian's effectiveness has been studied in comparison with placebo and other sleeping medications. In studies that were conducted, valerian appeared more effective than placebo and as effective as other sleeping pills (48). Animal studies as well confirm that valerian had a calming and sedative action on the animal after it was ingested (48). Although the safety of valerian has not been established during pregnancy, the herb has been mentioned for its sedative and calming effects during pregnancy in midwifery practices (54). We would hesitate to recommend an agent whose safety has not been confirmed.

Dysphoria

Herbs that treat anxiety during pregnancy primarily work through the nervous system and are broadly categorized as having either stimulating or sedating properties (54). Stapleton (54) described herbal preparations in the form of infusions for alleviating dysphoria that consist of various combinations of raspberry leaf, peppermint, spearmint, and lemon balm. Bitter tonics such as burdock, blessed thistle, vervain, and orange peel are suggested as beneficial in maintaining emotional stability (52,54). These recommendations are essentially anecdotal and, although they have been administered during pregnancy, their safety and efficacy have not been established.

Valerian, as previously mentioned, may also be beneficial in reducing nervousness (38,39,48). German chamomile (*Matricaria recutitia*) and St. John's wort (*Hypericum perforatum*) have both been used to reduce anxiety (38,48,56,57). Chamomile is often taken as a tea for insomnia and anxiety (48). St. John's wort has received much attention as a therapeutic agent for treatment of mild depression (38,58,59) as well as simply calming nervous tension (56) and promoting sleep (57). Neither German chamomile nor St. John's wort has been approved for use during pregnancy. Both herbs, at least in some sources, have been listed as possessing "emmenagogic" properties (56,57), although no studies confirming these properties have been performed. The safety for use during pregnancy is unknown.

Stretch Marks

A multitude of creams are available on the market with claims of preventing stretch marks. Stretch marks or striae may be the result of changes in collagen, elastin, and fibrillin. Watson et al. (60) noted a reorganization and diminution of the elastic fiber network in biopsies of skin with striae, whereas other investigators believe striae to be scar tissue rather than stretched connective tissue (61). A few studies have been conducted evaluating topical tretinoin and pulsed dye laser for treatment of stretch marks (62). Topical tretinoin at a concentration of 0.1% has been shown to improve significantly the clinical appearance of early active stretch marks; however, measurements of connective tissue quality were unchanged (63). Tretinoin, like other retinoids, can be a potent teratogen; however, when used topically the risk is minimal (64).

Essential oils and herbal preparations have been suggested in the prevention of stretch marks; however, no clear evidence exists to verify these claims. In any event, any cream or oil applied to the abdomen will keep it soft and moisturized. Suggestions for moistening the abdomen and attempting to ward off stretch marks include essential oils, neroli, mandarin, bergamot, lavender, and rosewood (41,42,44). Tiran (41) recommends applying the oils to the abdomen in an alternating fashion after 16 weeks of gestation. Given the previous information on essential oils, it could be suggested that use of any essential oil should be monitored by a person trained in aromatherapy. Furthermore, there are no trials evaluating the efficacy of essential oils for treatment of stretch marks. Finally, vitamin E, cocoa butter, olive oil, and sweet almond oil have all been used to combat stretch marks during pregnancy (34,65), and although these have not been subjected to scientific studies, they appear safe for use during pregnancy with unknown efficacy.

Lower Extremities

Varicose veins and pedal edema are both common during pregnancy and often increase as gestation progresses (66). In terms of traditional Chinese medicine, varicose veins are considered a result of stagnation and congestion in the body (52). With this in mind, herbal remedies to relieve varicosities are aimed at relieving congestion and include infusions of lime blossom and fresh ginger root to strengthen venous tone and garlic and onions to improve circulation. Fresh parsley and nettles added to the diet or as infusions also improve venous elasticity, and aching legs can be soothed with lotions or compresses that contain comfrey, marshmallow, marigold, plantain, yarrow, hawthorne, cypress, lemongrass, and lavender (52,67). A decoction of oak and

witch hazel barks can be added to any herbal lotion or compress to ease the pain of varicosities; however, the bark may stain the skin (54). A lukewarm footbath containing a few drops each of benzoin, rose, and orange or geranium and a cool footbath with peppermint may be beneficial (42,67).

In a review by Fugh-Berman (68), an herbal component rutoside was evaluated in one study for effects on gestational edema. Rutosides are a flavonoid and can be found in buckwheat and eucalyptus. Rutoside capsule versus placebo was administered to 69 pregnant women (68). Subjects receiving rutoside experienced significantly greater reduction in edema and associated symptoms compared to placebo. Unfortunately, this small study cannot suggest safety of use during pregnancy.

Although these remedies have been used primarily in Chinese medicine and midwifery practices, no trials have been conducted concerning safety and efficacy during pregnancy. The traditional treatment for gestational edema is leg elevation and compression by support hose.

Headache

Headaches do occur during pregnancy, and the majority of them would fall under the category of tension headache. The tension headache is often acute and short in duration, resolves spontaneously or with simple measures, and is not a sign of a serious medical condition (69). Electromyographic biofeedback has been successfully used to treat this type of headache (70,71). A migraine headache is usually more severe than a tension headache and may be accompanied by an aura. The majority of women with migraines may experience a decrease in frequency and severity of the attacks during pregnancy (72). However, for those who do not or for the women who have new-onset migraines, traditional treatment approaches may not be desirable during pregnancy. Marcus et al. (73) investigated nonpharmacologic approaches to migraine treatment during pregnancy. Thirty gravid headache sufferers were evaluated and treated with physical therapy, relaxation techniques, and biofeedback, and 80% of the participants experienced relief with the alternative method. Furthermore, when reevaluated 1 year later, 67% of the original study group maintained relief with the given alternative method they were taught.

Alternative herbal remedies have been used in the treatment and prophylaxis of migraine headache, with the most common being feverfew.

Feverfew (Tanacetum/Chrysanthemum Parthenium)

Feverfew has been used in folk and modern medicine for treatment or prophylaxis of migraine headaches (39,56,74). Parthenolide, a main constituent of the sesquiterpene lactone component of the plant, is considered the active component (75); however, the mechanism of action has yet to be definitely determined (48). There was renewed interest in its use for treatment of migraines in the 1970s. Early case reports and observations during this time supported the efficacy of feverfew for both treatment and prophylaxis of migraine (48). Subsequent placebo-controlled, blinded trials revealed a reduction in frequency and severity of migraines, whereas one study showed no difference between a feverfew preparation and placebo (48,49). The trials that showed benefit used whole-leaf preparations, whereas the one that did not used a dried ethanolic extract standardized to a parthenolide content (48,49). The *Physicians' Desk Reference for Herbal Medicines* reports that *in vitro* studies suggest but do not confirm an interaction between antithrombotic medications such as aspirin and warfarin (39) which may be mediated through inhibition of arachidonic acid. Feverfew has been widely used for years in England, and no reports of serious toxicity have been published (48). Unfortunately, another indication for feverfew in older folk medicine was to promote abortion (48). Because of this report and the absence of any clinical trials during pregnancy, the safety and efficacy of feverfew during gestation have not been evaluated and its use cannot be recommended. Furthermore, feverfew has not been recommended for use during pregnancy or lacta-

tion or for children younger than 2 years of age (39,75).

Peripartum

A national survey conducted by McFarlin et al. (76), in which 500 members of the American College of Nurse-Midwives were polled, revealed the most common herbs used for labor preparation and labor induction were blue cohosh, black cohosh, red raspberry leaf, castor oil, and evening primrose oil. Additional herbs either singly or in combination with these have been used to stimulate labor or resolve hemorrhage and include black haw, crampbark, mugwort, feverfew, pennyroyal, and goldenseal (4,40,52,76).

Although these herbs, both in the past and the present, have been used in midwifery practices, few, if any, have been studied in clinical trials. Even so, some adverse events have been documented and are discussed.

Red Raspberry (Rubus Idaeus)

Red raspberry is indigenous to Europe and Asia (39). The active components of red raspberry are tannin, flavonoid, vitamin C, vitamin E, calcium, and iron (39,53). The tannin components act as an astringent and are believed to have a tightening and toning effect on the uterus (52,54,56). For this reason, red raspberry leaf has been suggested as a tonic after 25 weeks of gestation. A scan of available literature reveals that red raspberry leaf has been used to treat hyperemesis, prevent miscarriage, and shorten labor (4,76,77). These last two indications appear contradictory and emphasize the unknown mechanisms by which herbs work (48,76). As a result of these conflicting indications for red raspberry and the lack of medical studies to evaluate its safety and efficacy, therapeutic use cannot be recommended (38). Furthermore, no data are available on teratogenesis (55). Even some proponents of red raspberry do suggest it be avoided in the first half of pregnancy (52). Finally, Ehudin-Pagano et al. (53) discuss in their article a uterine toning combination herbal (PN-6). In addition to red raspberry, PN-6 contains blue cohosh, black cohosh, squaw vine, blessed thistle pennyroyal, and lobelia. There are currently no scientific studies available for evaluation of this combination. Furthermore, several of the herbs are considered emmenagogues (56) and lobelia can be toxic (53).

Blue Cohosh (Caulophyllum Thalictroides)

Blue cohosh is an emmenagogue and has oxytocic properties (56,78). Throughout the history of its use by Native Americans until the present time, blue cohosh has been used to prevent miscarriage and induce labor (40). In fact, some authors consider it an abortifacient (56,78). Animal studies reveal that isolated components have been shown to cause coronary artery vasoconstriction and decreased blood flow, stimulate uterine muscle, and elevate blood pressure (40). In a survey of 172 providers, 64% who used labor-stimulating herbs used blue cohosh (76); however, none did so in the context of randomized trials. Adverse events have been documented from these observations and include maternal nausea, meconium staining, transient fetal tachycardia, fetal distress, and a high-pitched neonatal cry (40,76,78). Two cases of neonatal myocardial toxicity were reported after the use of blue cohosh (79,80). The FDA adverse events database also cites two additional adverse events, the first involving a stroke and the second involving aplastic anemia, both in infants (81). These cases are rare and no causal association is as yet established. However, the potential toxicity, especially in the light of excess herb ingestion by one gravida (79), must be seriously considered (80,82). Three isolated compounds in blue cohosh may possess teratogenic potential. These three compounds are the alkaloid constituents anagyrine, *N*-methylcytosine, and taspine (78). In grazing animals, anagyrine has been linked with spine and limb malformations (76,83), *N*-methylcytosine with spine malformations in rat embryos (84), and taspine as cytotoxic in rat embryo cultures (84).

Black Cohosh (Cimicifuga Racemosa)

The root of black cohosh contains the medicinally useful components triterpene glycoside and phenylpropane (39). Recent western publications site indications for the use of black cohosh for premenstrual discomfort, dysmenorrhea, and menopausal complaints (38,39,48). Black cohosh is also an emmenagogue (56) and as such was used by Native Americans to induce labor (4,76). In addition, black cohosh was used as a major ingredient of Lydia E. Pinkham's vegetable compound for menstrual cramps, a popular compound in the nineteenth century (48). A survey by McFarlin et al. (76) evaluated the use of black cohosh by midwives for stimulating labor. Forty-five percent of the respondents to the survey used black cohosh in the form of tinctures or teas (76). Again, none did so in the context of a clinical trial. Nonetheless, some interesting adverse events were noted and include increased meconium staining and transient fetal tachycardia. Furthermore, overdoses of black cohosh have been associated with the following adverse reactions: hypotension, headache, vomiting, and dizziness (39,48,76). Although black cohosh appears to have been used with some benefit in labor, no therapeutic trials have been conducted. As an emmenagogue, it should be excluded in the first half of pregnancy.

Castor Oil (Ricinus Communis)

The plant is a native to India and now can be found throughout central and southern Europe (39,76). The compounds in the plant include triglycerides, 90% of which is ricinoleic acid (39,76), fatty oil, proteins, lectins, tocopherol, and pyridine alkaloids (39). Castor oil is considered a demulcent, laxative, and purgative (56). The beans themselves are poisonous, owing to the lectin component (39,76), and as few as 12 beans may be fatal for an adult (39). Ricinoleic acid is the component responsible for stimulating bowel motor activity (76). Ricinoleic acid is absorbed systemically after ingestion and may stimulate the uterus directly or as a reflex to increased bowel activity (76). Long-term use of castor oil has the potential to alter electrolyte balance (39). One study is available that investigated the effectiveness of castor oil for labor induction and other information has been obtained by surveys (76). Wang et al. (85) compared castor oil with misoprostol for labor induction. The length of time from induction to delivery was reduced in the misoprostol compared with the castor oil group. However, significantly more cases of uterine tetany were noted in the misoprostol group. Interestingly, in this study by Wang et al., castor oil was associated with few adverse events (85). In contrast, reports in surveys of midwives who use castor oil cite tumultuous or precipitous labor, diarrhea, thrombosed hemorrhoids, and increased meconium staining (76). Two additional cases that may be associated with castor oil ingestion are also worth mentioning. The first is an infant with a constellation of features similar to fetal hydantoin syndrome whose mother ingested castor oil for 8 weeks in the first trimester (86), and the second is an amniotic fluid embolism in a women who ingested castor oil for labor induction (87). A causal association between these adverse events and castor oil is not possible. Given these concerns and the lack of scientific trials testing safety and efficacy, the use of castor oil is not recommended.

Evening Primrose Oil (Oenothera Biennis)

Evening primrose oil is indigenous to North America, and the medicinal component is contained in the oil from its seed (39). This oil can be purchased as a standardized product, and the active components include tryptophan, linoleic acid, gamma-linoleic acid, oleic acid, and palmitic acid (39,76). The components linoleic acid and gamma-linoleic acid are prostaglandin precursors and, as such, may explain the success of evening primrose oil for cervical ripening (76). In addition, evening primrose oil is also a natural source of essential fatty acids and has been suggested as a dietary supplement during pregnancy and for improving the fat content of breast milk during lactation (76). No prospective randomized trials have been conducted evaluating evening primrose oil. McFarlin et al. (76) conducted a survey and found that 60% midwives who used herbal preparations during pregnancy used evening primrose oil and remarked on superior results for cervical ripening with evening primrose oil compared with blue cohosh, black cohosh, red raspberry, and castor oil. In contrast,

a retrospective trial by Dove and Johnson (88) comparing oral evening primrose with no supplement from 37 weeks of gestation until delivery and noted no difference between the groups for length of gestation or labor. However, the evening primrose oil group appeared to have an increased incidence of PROM, oxytocin augmentation, arrest of descent, and vacuum extraction.

Clearly prospective randomized trials are in order, and until such time safety and efficacy cannot be evaluated.

Postpartum

Breast-Feeding

Breast-feeding has multiple benefits for both mother and infant. Breast-feeding is associated with less childhood illness in the first year of life including acute as well as chronic disease and possibly sudden infant death syndrome (89,90). Factors that hinder a woman's ability to successfully breast-feed her infant include anxiety over the success of breast-feeding as well as the discomforts that occur while breast-feeding including engorgement, nipple soreness, and infection. Lactation consultants are widely available and can be consulted to aid with most of these concerns, but there are simple alternative methods that have been suggested to help the mother increase milk production and decrease discomfort.

Milk production can first be promoted by ensuring adequate hydration. Garlic has been shown to improve suckling, increase letdown, and decrease engorgement (91). Herbal teas believed to further encourage an adequate supply of milk include blessed thistle, hops, red raspberry, nettles, red clover, fennel, barley, and leafy greens (4,77).

Breast engorgement has been successfully treated by placing raw cabbage leaves or a poultice of grated raw potato or carrot around the breast (77,89,91). Fresh rhubarb leaf can be substituted for cabbage with similar results (4). Essential oils of lavender and fennel have been reported as useful by adding a few drops of oil to a bowl of water, soaking a cloth in the mixture, wringing out the excess, and applying to the breast (4).

Sore nipples are a common complaint and are often associated with cracking, bruising, and bleeding at the nipple (92). Changing the position of the infant during breast-feeding and ensuring that the infant's mouth is in the proper position during suckling can be the first steps to resolving the problem (77,92,93). Soap and alcohol products can promote soreness and are best avoided (77,92). Placing a fresh geranium leaf, furry side against the nipple, aids in healing (91). In addition, sweet almond oil, olive oil, lanolin cream, and comfrey, or yarrow ointments may be of benefit in healing the cracked nipple (67,77,91). Pure essential oils must be used with caution when applied to an area that could come in contact with the infant. The breast and nipple should be washed clean, removing all traces of the oil to avoid possible transfer to the infant.

None of these suggestions have been evaluated in clinical trials. However, some measures, whether by placebo or actual effect, may be beneficial with little or no risk to mother and infant and include hydration, teas, and cabbage. Given the possibility of transfer of an essential oil to the infant, especially in unknown amounts, these remedies cannot be recommended.

Mastitis and breast abscess are not contraindications to continuing breast-feeding; however, antibiotics may be required. Therefore, contacting a health care provider rather than initially choosing an alternative method would be advisable.

POPULAR HERBAL REMEDIES

The top five conditions that prompt the use of an herbal product include common cold, flu, digestive complaints, headache, and insomnia (38). Pregnancy offers no immunity from these common ailments, some of which have already been addressed. Many of the herbal products listed as the most popular will gain the attention of pregnant women. The herbal products receiving the most attention, as evidenced by sales, include echinacea, garlic, ginkgo, goldenseal, saw palmetto, aloe, Asian ginseng, cat's claw, milk thistle, bilberry, valerian, ginger, and St. John's wort (38,94). Most of these have been addressed as they relate to complaints during pregnancy; a few others are briefly reviewed.

Echinacea (Echinacea Purpurea)

There are three species of echinacea that have made their way into commercial products, *Echinacea pallida, E. purpurea,* and *E. angustifolia* (38), and have clinically been used as supportive therapy for influenza-like infections and chronic infections of the respiratory tract and lower urinary tract (38). External applications have been used for poorly healing wounds and chronic ulcerations. The mechanism of action appears to be an increase in immune system function evidenced by an increase in immune cell mass and activity, and increase in body temperature (38). Only *E. pallida* root and *E. purpurea* herb have received approval in the Commission E Monographs (38). Although no side effects have been noted from oral consumption, echinacea is not recommended for individuals with autoimmune disorders or human immunodeficiency virus (38,48,94). The German Commission E also recommends limiting its use to 8 weeks and has not confirmed the safety during pregnancy or lactation (38), nor has efficacy been established.

Garlic (Allium Sativum)

Indications for garlic include prevention for atherosclerosis and cancer. In addition, garlic has been shown to lower cholesterol and blood pressure (38,48). Garlic is on the FDA's "generally regarded as safe" list. Side effects listed include nausea, dizziness, headache, diarrhea, flatulence, and insomnia (48). It is further suggested that the concomitant use of garlic and coumadin, heparin, aspirin, ginkgo, and vitamin E be avoided because of a risk of increased bleeding (48). Likewise, ingestion of high doses of garlic before any surgical procedure, which would include delivery, is contraindicated (48).

Saw Palmetto (Serenoa Repens)

This herb is indicated in treatment of benign prostatic hyperplasia (38,39,48). In addition, saw palmetto possesses mild diuretic properties. There appear to be no indications for considering use in pregnancy.

Bilberry (Vaccinium Myrtillus)

Indications for use of bilberry include acute diarrhea, inflammation of the mouth, diabetes, poor night vision, and varicose veins (38,39,48). Bilberry does not appear to interfere with clotting mechanisms, and there does not appear to be any adverse effects with proper administration; however, signs of poisoning have been noted in animal experiments (38,39). Bilberry has been used for treatment of varicose veins and appears to provide relief from pain and swelling in nonpregnant persons; however, safety during pregnancy has not been proven (48).

Ginkgo (Ginkgo Biloba)

Ginkgo is used in the treatment of organic brain disturbance and memory improvement (38,48). Ginkgo may interact with coumadin, heparin, and aspirin and potentiate bleeding (39,48). The simultaneous use of garlic, vitamin E, and ginkgo may have a similar effect (48). The use of ginkgo during pregnancy has not been contraindicated; however, neither has its safety clearly been established (38,48).

Asian Ginseng (Panax Ginseng)

Ginseng has been used as a tonic during convalescence and for improving invigoration and resistance to stress (38,48). No contraindications have been listed in the German Commission E Monographs (38), but other reviews suggest that ginseng can interfere with the metabolism of other drugs, specifically Digitalis and monoamine oxidase inhibitors (48). The safety of any form of ginseng has not been established for use during pregnancy, and the herb was in fact not recommended for use during pregnancy and lactation in traditional Chinese medicine (48).

Goldenseal (Hydrastis Canadensis)

Goldenseal was used by Native Americans as a dye and for skin, eye, and gastrointestinal disorders. Today, goldenseal is used externally to speed wound healing as well as being combined with other herbs that boost the immunity or control weight (48). One component of goldenseal, berberine, does possess antibacterial and antifungal activity; unfortunately for gravid women, it can also stimulate uterine activity. For this reason, it is best avoided during pregnancy (48).

Milk Thistle (Silybum Marianum)

Milk thistle is indigenous to Europe, and the ripe seeds contain its medicinal component (39). Indications for milk thistle include viral hepatitis, toxic liver damage, antidote for Death-Cap poisoning, and insufficient lactation (38,39,48). Milk thistle is considered an emmenagogue (39). In England, various parts of the milk thistle plant were used as a food source without reports of adverse effects. Because of this extensive use, it is believed to be safe during pregnancy and lactation; however, its safety has not been scientifically validated (48).

CONCLUSION

The renewed interest in complementary and alternative therapies will be accompanied by research addressing the efficacy and safety of the individual modalities. Until such time as clear evidence regarding the safety of alternative practices for the pregnant or lactating woman are available, some guidelines should be established for the use of alternative methods. Evaluate the training and experience of the herbalist, acupuncturist, or healer from which a service or advice is obtained. Validate all modalities and methods through reliable sources. Evaluate herbal safety by confirming which portion of the plant is used for treatment. Determine whether an evaluation of an herbal product was based on any scientific evidence. Examine the consistency and purity of an herbal product that you will purchase. If other medication is to be taken, determine whether there are any drug reactions. Examine the label of combination products and research any components unknown to you. Finally, determine the customary dose of the herb. Do not assume that because an herb is listed as a dietary supplement that it is always safe to take or that taking a higher dose than recommended will resolve an ailment faster.

The majority of alternative therapies as they apply to pregnancy have not been subjected to clinical trials. This lack of proof of safety and efficacy prevents recommendations for use during pregnancy for all but the most benign modality.

Particular caution is needed for the pregnant (or nonpregnant) patient who may use oral herbal supplements in addition to other pharmacologic agents. Concurrent use of herbs can mimic, magnify, or oppose the effect of drugs particularly anticoagulants, antidepressants, steroids, and a variety of cardiovascular medications (95).

GLOSSARY

Capsule: Powdered herb placed in a capsule form. Grinding the herb to a powder can promote oxidation and potency loss of plant constituents.

Carrier oil: Vegetable oil in which to place an essential oil. Jojoba or sweet almond oil act as good massage mediums during pregnancy.

Compress: Plant material placed in a cloth and then applied to the skin.

Decoctions: Preparation of roots and bark by steeping in boiling water.

Emmenagogue: Vitalizes the blood. Western medicine directs used of this type of agent for women primarily at menses and pregnancy. In Chinese medicine, however, "moving the blood" also includes treatment for heart disease, tumor, and thrombosis for both men and women. Emmenagogues are contraindicated during early pregnancy, menstruation, and menorrhagia and for individuals who bleed easily.

Essential oil: Extremely concentrated portion of the plant.

Fomentation: A cloth dipped in an infusion or decoction and then applied to the skin.

Galactogogue: An agent that increases lactation.

Infused oil: The immersion of the fresh plant in oil for 2 weeks.

Infusions: Preparation of leafy portions.

    Cold: Soak in cold water. Suggest use within 12 hours of preparation.

    Hot: Prolonged steeping in boiling water.

One-to-one extract (1:1): Alcohol extraction method using equal concentrations of plant to alcohol. This extraction method and concentration have the potential to result in different

profiles and proportions of herb other than what is known in historic, traditional herbal medicine.

Poultice: Plant material applied directly to skin.

Standardized extract: The isolation, measurements, and concentration of specific plant constituents. The method dissociates the whole plant and only removes synergistic or beneficial components.

Teas: Preparation of flower and seeds by steeping in boiling water.

Tincture: Alcohol extraction method using fresh or dried plant material. In concentrations, plant to alcohol 1 : 5 for dried material and 1 : 2 for fresh material.

REFERENCES

1. The Burton Goldberg Group. *Alternative medicine: the definitive guide.* Tiburon, CA: Future Medicine Publishing, 1997.
2. Aikins Murphy P, Kronenburg F, Wade C. Complementary and alternative medicine in women's health. *J Nurse-Midwifery* 1999;44:192–204.
3. Eisenberg DM, Davis RB, Ettner SL, et al. Trends in alternative medicine use in the United States, 1990–1997: results of a follow-up national survey. *JAMA* 1998; 280:1569–1575.
4. Charlish A. *Your natural pregnancy: a guide to complementary therapies.* Berkeley: Ulysses Press, 1996.
5. Beijing College of Traditional Chinese Medicine, Shanghai College of Traditional Chinese Medicine, Nanjing College of Traditional Chinese Medicine, The Acupuncture Institute of the Academy of Traditional Chinese Medicine. *Essentials of Chinese acupuncture.* Beijing: Foreign Languages Press, 1980.
6. Whitlocke B. *Chinese medicine for women.* Toronto: Publishers Group West, 1999.
7. Singer JA. Acupuncture, a brief introduction. *Acupuncture* 1999;1–6.
8. Flaws B. *The path of pregnancy.* Brookline, MA: Paradigm Publications, 1983.
9. Beal MW. Acupuncture and related treatment modalities. Part II: applications to antepartal and intrapartal care. *J Nurse-Midwifery* 1992;37:260–268.
10. Wensel LO. *Acupuncture in medical practice.* Reston, VA: Reston Publishing, 1980.
11. Yip SK, Pang JCK, Sung ML. Induction of labor by acupuncture electro-stimulation. *Am J Chinese Med* 1976;4:257–265.
12. Cardini F, Weixin H. Moxibustion for correction of breech presentation: a randomized controlled trial. *JAMA* 1998;280:1580–1584.
13. Tiran D. Complementary therapies for nausea in pregnancy. *Mod Midwife* 1996;6:19–21.
14. Vickers AJ. Can acupuncture have specific effects on health? A systematic review of acupuncture antiemesis trials. *J R Soc Med* 1996;89:303–311.
15. Chen E. *Cross-sectional anatomy of acupoints.* New York: Churchill-Livingstone, 1995.

16. Belluomini J, Litt RC, Lee KA, et al. Acupressure for nausea and vomiting of pregnancy: a randomized, blinded study. *Obstet Gynecol* 1994;84:245–248.

17. O'Brien B, Relyea MJ, Taerum T. Efficacy of P6 acupressure in the treatment of nausea and vomiting during pregnancy. *Am J Obstet Gynecol* 1996;174:708–715.

18. DeAloysio S, Penacehioni P. Morning sickness control in early pregnancy by Neiguan point acupressure. *Obstet Gynecol* 1992;80:852–854.

19. Bayreuther J, Lewith GT, Pickering R. A double-blind cross-over study to evaluate the effectiveness of acupressure at pericardium 6 (P6) in the treatment of early morning sickness (EMS). *Complement Ther Med* 1994;2:70–76.

20. Hyde E. Acupressure therapy for morning sickness: a controlled clinical trial. *J Nurse-Midwifery* 1989;34:171–178.

21. Aikins Murphy P. Alternative therapies for nausea and vomiting of pregnancy. *Obstet Gynecol* 1998;91:149–155.

22. Evans AT, Samuels SN, Marshall C, et al. Suppression of pregnancy-induced nausea and vomiting with sensory afferent stimulation. *J Reprod Med* 1993;38:603.

23. Dundee JW, Sourial FB, Bell PF. P6 acupressure reduces morning sickness. *J R Soc Med* 1988;81:456–457.

24. Zeisler H, Tempfer C, Mayerhofer K, et al. Influence of acupuncture on duration of labor. *Gynecol Obstet Invest* 1998;46:22–25.

25. Lyrenas S, Lutsch H, Hetta J, et al. Acupuncture before delivery: effect of labor. *Gynecol Obstet Invest* 1987;24:217–224.

26. Kubista E, Kucera H. On the use of acupuncture in the preparation for delivery. *Z Geburtshilfe Perinatol* 1974;178:224–229.

27. Tsuei JJ, Lai Y. Induction of labor by acupuncture and electrical stimulation. *Obstet Gynecol* 1974;43:337–342.

28. Tsuei JJ, Lai Y, Sharma SD. The influence of acupuncture stimulation during pregnancy: the induction and inhibition of labor. *Obstet Gynecol* 1977;50:479–480.

29. Yip S-K, Pang JCK, Sung ML. Induction of labor by acupuncture electro-stimulation. *Am J Chin Med* 1976;4:257–265.

30. Abouleish E, Depp R. Acupuncture in obstetrics. *Anesth Analg* 1975;54:82–88.

31. Wang DW, Jin YH, Present status of cesarean section under acupuncture anesthesia in China. *Fukushima J Med Sci* 1989;35:45–52.

32. Cesarean Section Acupuncture Unit, Beijing Obstetric and Gynecology Hospital. Clinical analysis of 1,000 cases of cesarean section under acupuncture anesthesia. *Chinese Med J* 1980;93:231–8.

33. Vallette C, Niboyet JEH, Imbert-Martelet M, et al. Acupuncture analgesia and cesarean section. *J Reprod Med* 1980;25:108–112.

34. Aesoph L. Pregnancy and childbirth. In: Chopra D, ed. *Alternative medicine: the definitive guide.* Tiburon, California: Future Medicine Publishers, 1999.

35. Salvo SG. *Massage therapy: principles & practice.* Philadelphia: WB Saunders, 1999:483–484.

36. Field T, Hernandez-Reif M, Hart S, et al. Pregnant women benefit from massage therapy. *J Psychosom Obstet Gynecol* 1999;20:31–38.

37. Field T, Hernandez-Reif M, Taylor S, et al. Labor pain is reduced by massage therapy. *J Psychosom Obstet Gynecol* 1997;18:286–291.

38. The American Botanical Council. *The complete German Commission E monographs: therapeutic guide to herbal medicines.* Boston: Integrative Medicine Communications, 1998.

39. *PDR for Herbal Medicines.* Montvale: Medical Economics, 1998.

40. Belew C, Herbs and the childbearing woman: guidelines for midwives. *J Nurse-Midwifery* 1999;44:231–252.

41. Tiran D. *Aromatherapy in midwifery practice.* Philadelphia: Baillière Tindall, 1996.

42. Tisserand M. *Aromatherapy for women: a practical guide to essential oils for health and beauty.* Rochester, VT: Healing Arts Press, 1996.

43. Lis-Balchin M. Possible health and safety problems in the use of novel plant essential oils and extracts in aromatherapy. *J R Soc Health* 1999;119:240–243.

44. Decoder Concept International. *Gentle aromatherapy for women decoder.* Melbourne: Dynamo House, 1999.

45. Allaire AD, Moos MK, Wells SR. Complementary and alternative medicine in pregnancy: a survey of North Carolina certified nurse-midwives. *Obstet Gynecol* 2000;95:19–23.

46. Burns E, Blamey C. Complementary medicine. Using aromatherapy in childbirth. *Nurs Times* 1994;90:54–60.

47. Fischer-Rasmussen W, Kjaer SK, Dahl C, et al. Ginger treatment of hyperemesis gravidarum. *Eur J Obstet Gynecol Reprod Biol* 1990;38:19–24.

48. Bratman S, Kron D, eds. Natural Health Bible. Roseville, California: Prima Publishing, 1999.

49. Foster S, Tyler VE. *Tyler's honest herbal: a sensible guide to the use of herbs and related remedies.* New York: The Haworth Herbal Press, 1999.

50. Sahakian V, Rouse D, Sipes S, et al. Vitamin B6 is effective therapy for nausea and vomiting of pregnancy: a randomized, double-blind placebo-controlled study. *Obstet Gynecol* 1991;78:33–36.

51. Zeidenstein L. Journal reviews: alternative therapies for nausea and vomiting of pregnancy. *J Nurse-Midwifery* 1998;43:392–393.

52. Stapleton H. Herbal medicines for disorders of pregnancy. *Mod Midwife* 1995;5:18–22.

53. Ehudin-Pagano E, Paluzzi PA, Ivory LC, et al. The use of herbs in nurse-midwifery practice. *J Nurse-Midwifery* 1987;32:260–262.

54. Stapleton H. The use of herbal medicine in pregnancy and labour. Part I: an overview of current practice. *Complement Ther Nurs Midwifery* 1995;1:148–153.

55. Youngkin EQ, Israel DS. A review and critique of common herbal alternative therapies. *Nurse Pract* 1996;21:39–60.

56. Tierra M. *Planetary herbology.* Twin Lakes: Lotus Press, 1988.

57. Shealy CN, ed. *The illustrated encyclopedia of healing remedies.* Boston: Shaftesbury, Dorset, 1998.

58. Volz HP. Controlled clinical trials of hypericum extracts in depressed patients–an overview. *Pharmacopsychiatry* 1997;30:72–76.

59. Myers J. Can an herb really help depression? *Adv Nurse Pract* 1998;6:33–34.

60. Watson RE, Parry EJ, Humphries JD, et al. Fibrillin microfibrils are reduced in skin exhibiting striae distensae. *Br J Dermatol* 1998;138:931–937.

61. Zheng P, Lavker RM, Kligman AM. Anatomy of striae. *Br J Dermatol* 1985;112:185–193.

62. Bergfeld WF. A lifetime of healthy skin: implications for women. *Int J Fertil Womens Med* 1999;44:83–95.

63. Kang S, Kim KJ, Griffiths CE, et al. Topical tretinoin (retinoic acid) improves early stretch marks. *Arch Dermatol* 1996;132:519–526.

64. Briggs GG, Freeman RK, Yaffe SJ. Captopril. In: Mitchell CW, ed. *Drugs in pregnancy and lactation.* Baltimore: Williams & Wilkins, 1994:120–126.

65. Davey CMH. Factors associated with the occurrence of striae gravidarum. *J Obstet Gynaecol Br Commonw* 1972;79:1113–1114.

66. Mittelmark RA, Posner MD. Fetal responses to maternal exercise. In: Mittelmark RA, Wiswell RA, Drinkwater BL, eds. *Exercise in pregnancy.* Baltimore: Williams & Wilkins, 1991:213–224.

67. Rippin J. *Aromatherapy for health relaxation, and wellbeing.* New York: Lorenz Books, 1997.

68. Fugh-Berman A. Treatments for leg edema in pregnancy. *Altern Ther Womens Health* 1999;1:73–75.

69. ACOG Patient Education. *Headache.* Washington: American College of Obstetricians and Gynecologists, 1998.

70. Fugh-Berman A. *Alternative medicine: what works.* Baltimore: Williams & Wilkins, 1997.

71. Andrasik F. Psychologic and behavioral aspects of chronic headache. *Neurol Clin* 1990;8:961–976.

72. Marcus DA, Scharff L, Turk DC. Nonpharmacological management of headaches during pregnancy. *Psychosom Med* 1995;57:527–535.

73. Scharff L, Marcus DA, Turk DC. Maintenance of effects in the nonmedical treatment of headaches during pregnancy. *Headache* 1996;36:285–290.

74. Lust JB. *The herb book.* New York: Bantam Books, 1974.

75. Sinclair S. Migraine headaches: nutritional, botanical and other alternative approaches. *Altern Med Rev* 1999;4:86–95.

76. McFarlin BL, Gibson MH, O'Rear J, et al. A national survey of herbal preparation use by nurse-midwives for labor stimulation: review of the literature and recommendations for practice. *J Nurse-Midwifery* 1999;44:205–216.

77. Weed SS. *Wise woman herbal for the childbearing year.* Woodstock: Ash Tree Publishing, 1986.

78. Irikura B, Kennelly EJ. Blue cohosh: a word of caution. *Altern Ther Womens Health* 1999;1:81–83.

79. Jones TK, Lawson BM. Profound neonatal congestive heart failure caused by maternal consumption of blue cohosh herbal medication. *J Pediatrics* 1998;132:550–552.

80. Gunn TR, Wright IMR. The use of black and blue cohosh in labour. *N Z Med J* 1996;109:410–411.

81. http://www.fda.gov/

82. Jones TK. Reply to the editor: neonatal effects of maternal consumption of blue cohosh. *J Pediatr* 1999;134:384–385.

83. Keeler RF. Livestock models of human birth defects, reviewed in relation to poisonous plants. *J Anim Sci* 1988;66:2414–2427.

84. Kennelly EJ, Flynn TJ, Mazzola EP, et al. Detecting potential teratogenic alkaloids from blue cohosh rhizomes using an in vitro rat embryo culture. *J Nat Prod* 1999;62:1385–1389.

85. Wang L, Shi C, Yang G. Comparison of misoprostol and ricinus oil meal for cervical ripening and labor induction. *Chung Hua Fu Chan Ko Tsa Chih* 1997;32:666–668.

86. El Mauboub M, Khallfa MM, Jaswal OB, et al. "Ricin syndrome." A possible new teratogenic syndrome associated with ingestion of castor oil seed in early pregnancy: a case report. *Ann Trop Paediatr* 1983;3:57–61.

87. Steingrub JS, Lopez T, Teres D, et al. Amniotic fluid embolism associated with castor oil ingestion. *Crit Care Med* 1988;16:642–643.

88. Dove D, Johnson P. Oral evening primrose oil: its effect on length of pregnancy and selected intrapartum outcomes in low-risk nulliparous women. *J Nurse-Midwifery* 1999;44:320–324.

89. Psychologic impact of breastfeeding. In: Lawrence RA, ed. *Breastfeeding: a guide for the medical profession.* St. Louis: Mosby, 1994:181–201.

90. American Academy of Pediatrics Work Group on Breastfeeding. Breastfeeding and the use of human milk. *Pediatrics* 1997;100:1035–1039.

91. Stapleton H. The use of herbal medicine in pregnancy and labour. Part II: events after birth, including those affecting the health of babies. *Complement Ther Nurs Midwifery* 1995;1:160–162.

92. Melnikow J, Bedinghaus JM. Management of common breast-feeding problems. *J Fam Pract* 1994;39:56–64.

93. Bell KK, Rawlings NL. Promoting breast-feeding by managing common lactation problems. *Nurse Pract* 1998;23:102–123.

94. Klausner A. EN's herbal medicine cabinet: top 10 herbs you can trust. *Environ Nutr* 1998;21:1–5.

95. Fugh-Berman A. Herb-drug interactions. *Lancet* 2000; 355:134–138.

ADDITIONAL RESOURCES

Internet

NIH Office of Dietary Supplements (www.dietary-supplements.info.nih.gov)

A Modern Herbal Home Page (www.botanical.com)
American Botanical Council (www.herbalgram.org)
Acupuncture (www.acupuncture.com)
www.fda.gov
www.altmed.od.nih.gov

Evidence-Based Books

Complementary/alternative medicine: an evidence-based approach. St. Louis: Mosby, 1999.

Journals

Focus on Alternative and Complementary Therapies
Alternative Therapies in Health and Medicine

Subject Index

Note: Page numbers followed by *f* indicate figures; page numbers followed by *t* indicate tables.